TEXT BOOK OF HUMAN OSTEOLOGY

VOLUME 2

BIOMECHANICS, PALEOPATHOLOGY, AND FORENSIC APPLICATIONS

Dr. Kavita Ramanathan

ALLIED HEALTH PRESS

Text book of Human Osteology Volume 2

Biomechanics, Paleopathology, and Forensic Applications

Author: **Dr. Kavita Ramanathan**

Allied Health Press
4164 Lakeshore Road
Burlington ON L7L 1A4
Canada
www.alliedhealthpress.com
Email: orders@arclereducation.com

ISBN: 978-1-77956-769-7

ABOUT THE AUTHOR

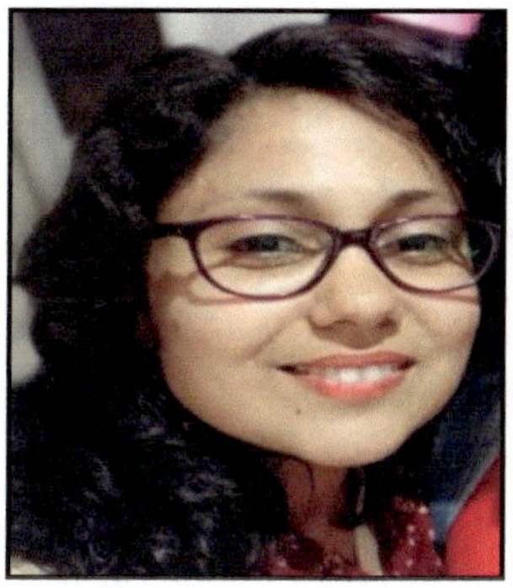

Dr Kavita Ramanathan is an accomplished medical professional with experience working through the length and breadth of India. With 16+ years in clinical and anatomic pathology, she understands the normal and abnormal functioning of the human body in depth. Also, she held positions in the senior management for 8+ years and designed business strategies. She successfully helped organisations attain profitability while maintaining quality and service standards. Additionally, during the COVID-19 pandemic, she contributed significantly by aligning operations to support government initiatives. She earned her undergraduate and graduate medical degrees from reputed institutions under the University of Mumbai, India, and she also holds an MBA in Finance. Dr Kavita volunteers with a non-profit organisation where she tutors students from low-income schools for over two decades. Post-pandemic, she quit her corporate job to pursue her passion of teaching and writing. Currently, she tutors high school and university students in biology, psychology, and medical sciences. Additionally, she authors books, articles, and blogs on topics related to health and well-being. Her strong academic background, enriched with a vast and varied experience, shapes her into a mature and sensible professional.

Brief Table of Contents

Getting Started with This Book

Chapter Openers

A list of Chapter Outline is presented providing a brief Introduction to what will be covered in the chapter.

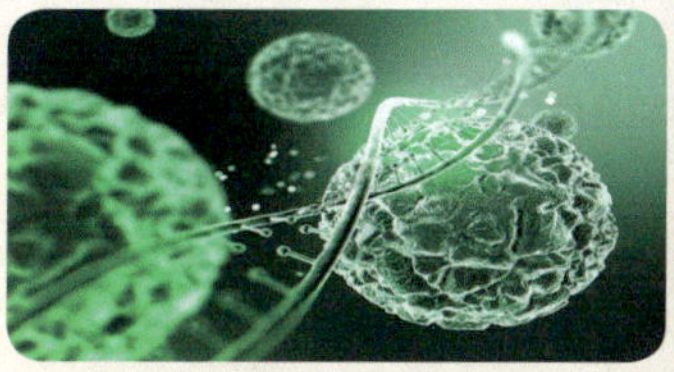

LEARNING OBJECTIVES

After studying this chapter, you will be able to:

1. Discuss the scientific method in biology;
2. Explain the cell theory;
3. Discuss the genetics and heredity;
4. Evolution and natural selection;
5. Focus on ecology and ecosystems;
6. Learn about human biology;
7. Evaluate the plant biology;
8. Explain the microbiology;
9. Focus on current trends in biology.

Introduction

Often referred to as the science of life, biology is a broad field of study aimed at comprehending the several kinds of life on Earth, from tiny creatures to sophisticated multicellular entities. Comprising several subfields, including molecular biology, ecology, and evolutionary biology, each of which advances our knowledge of living systems, this field clarifies the mechanisms controlling life events, including development, reproduction, and interaction with the surroundings, which is the central goal of biology. Moreover, biology fills in the void between the natural sciences and medicine by offering a necessary understanding of health, illness, and the interactions between organisms and their environments. Dealing with urgent global issues such as climate change, biodiversity loss, and new diseases depends on an awareness of these complex biological interactions, therefore highlighting the critical part biology plays in modern civilization. Fundamentally, biology explores and tests ideas about the living world using the scientific method. Through methodical observation and experimentation,

1.1. The Scientific Method in Biology

Learning Outcome

1. Describe the steps of the scientific method;
2. Focus on hypothesis formation;
3. Learn about experimental design.

Learning Outcomes

The beginning of each section of every chapter contains a set of Learning Outcomes that inform students of concepts they should understand. These outcomes help students understand what they should be able to do if they have mastered the material in that section.

Test Your Knowledge

Throughout each chapter, Test Your Knowledge cues you to note which topics have been covered and to self-test your understanding of the material presented.

Test Your Knowledge

1. Explain why correlation does not imply causation in scientific experiments.
2. How does the scientific method help reduce the influence of personal opinions in research?

Chapter Summary

The Summary Section appear at the end of each chapter and summarize main concepts covered throughout the chapter. These points provide key concepts in an engaging and meaningful way.

Summary

The investigation of biological principles highlights the importance of a comprehensive view of life by reflecting the intricate interactions that occur within living systems. The complexity of biology goes beyond individual species or systems, as this essay highlights; it also includes the interactions that mold ecosystems and affect biodiversity. Researchers can conduct in-depth analyses of metabolomic data using sophisticated technologies like MetaboAnalyst, which offer insights into the molecular mechanisms underlying these interactions. As demonstrated by the developments in MetaboAnalyst, for example, the integration of diverse omics data promotes a thorough understanding of metabolic pathways and helps identify important biological markers necessary for research on development and disease (Chong et al., 2018). Additionally, the phenomenon of ecological invasions is a key component of biological research and a vital field of study. The introduction of non-native species into unfamiliar habitats has significant ramifications and calls for multidisciplinary management strategies. Examining the origins and effects of these biological incursions, invasion science has become a crucial field that highlights the need to comprehend ecological dynamics and community interactions. As interest in biological invasions increases, new findings are emerging that put conventional ecological theories and practices to the test. The importance of incorporating various scientific viewpoints is shown by this developing discipline, which also highlights how invasive species shape ecosystems and advances our knowledge of ecological resilience (David et al., 2013). When taken as a whole, these discoveries from invasion science and metabolomics highlight the value of multidisciplinary biology research. Fostering cross-disciplinary collaboration and utilizing technological breakthroughs to improve our comprehension of intricate biological interactions are crucial as we look to the future of biological research. In addition to deepening our understanding of the complexities of life, this method lays the groundwork for tackling urgent environmental issues. Future studies can ensure the continued relevance of biology in a world that is constantly changing by acknowledging the interconnection of biological systems and opening the door to creative solutions that support sustainability and biodiversity conservation. We might imagine a thorough comprehension of life that serves both academia and society at large through ongoing investigation and integration of scientific knowledge.

Knowledge Assessment

The chapter includes material designed to review and reinforce each content. It includes Critical Thinking Questions to help test of your understanding of information presented in the chapter and Short answer Questions to review your understanding of the key concepts presented in the chapter.

Critical Thinking Questions

1. **Who is known as the "Father of Modern Biology"?**
   a. Aristotle
   b. Charles Darwin
   c. Gregor Mendel
   d. Louis Pasteur
2. **What is the basic unit of life?**
   a. Atom
   b. Molecule
   c. Cell
   d. Organism
3. **Which branch of biology studies the interaction of organisms with their environment?**
   a. Genetics
   b. Ecology
   c. Physiology
   d. Botany
4. **Which macromolecule is the main source of energy for living organisms?**
   a. Proteins
   b. Lipids
   c. Carbohydrates
   d. Nucleic acids
5. **DNA is primarily responsible for which function in living organisms?**
   a. Energy production
   b. Protein synthesis
   c. Storing genetic information
   d. Regulating body temperature

Short Answer Questions

1. What is biology, and why is it important to study biology?
2. What are the three main domains of life, and how are they different from one another?
3. Define homeostasis and give an example of how it works in living organisms.
4. What is the cell theory, and why is it fundamental to biology?
5. How do autotrophs and heterotrophs differ in the way they obtain energy?
6. What is the scientific method, and how is it applied in biological research?
7. Discuss how biology helps address global challenges such as climate change, disease, and food security.
8. Explain the levels of biological organization from the smallest unit to the largest. Provide examples at each level.
9. Describe the relationship between structure and function in biology, giving specific examples from cells or organs.
10. How has the discovery of genetics shaped our understanding of inheritance and variation among organisms?

Supplementary Materials

Key Terms: A list of key terms is given for quick reference

KEY TERMS FROM THIS CHAPTER

Annotation enrichment analysis	Biological structure	Cell
Cell theory	Cellular structure	Ecology
Ecosystems	Genetics	Human biology
Microbiology	Natural selection	Organism
Plant biology		

Further Resources: Recommendations for additional readings, websites, and multimedia resources.

References

1. Argelaguet, R., Velten, B., Arnol, D., Dietrich, S., Zenz, T., Marioni, J. C., Buettner, F., et al. (2018). Multi-omics factor analysis—A framework for unsupervised integration of multi-omics data sets. *Molecular Systems Biology, 14*. https://doi.org/10.15252/msb.20178124.
2. Bacher, S., Blackburn, T. M., Essl, F., & Genovesi, P. (2017). *Socio-Economic Impact Classification of Alien Taxa (SEICAT)*. https://core.ac.uk/download/286567949.pdf (accessed on 8th March 2025).
3. Barnett, R., Brace, S., Cucchi, T., & Dobney, K. (2013). *Divergent Evolutionary Processes Associated with Colonization of Offshore Islands*. https://core.ac.uk/download/20664364.pdf (accessed on 8th March 2025).

Detailed Table of Contents

CHAPTER 3

CHAPTER 4

CHAPTER 7

Bioarcheology of Identity and Social Life 209

CHAPTER 8

Dental Anthropology and Craniofacial Analysis 243

CHAPTER 11

Ethics and Repatriation in Osteological Research 341

CHAPTER 12

Current Challenges and Future Directions in Osteology 373

LIST OF FIGURES

PREFACE

The human skeleton is not just a support system but also an active participant in locomotion, mechanical force transmission, and metabolism. All joints articulate with function, and all bones provide room for the stresses placed on them during life. Functional anatomy and biomechanics describe how the skeleton transmits forces, how posture occurs, and how variations in shape influence the efficiency of movement. The skeleton also records the passage of time: cellular turnover, healing of microdamage, and aging all leave visible traces. Familiarity with these concepts bioarcheologyenables practitioners to reconstruct skeletal remains across contexts ranging from surgical planning to bioarcheological reconstruction.

Skeletons also bear witness to the hardships of life. Disease, injury, and healing are characterized by alterations in bone surfaces, lesions, and remodeling patterns. Paleopathology employs these signals to reconstruct the past of infectious disease, nutritional diseases, and degenerative diseases in ancient populations. Forensic analysis converts fracture, weapon wounds, and postmortem change to respond to questions of identity and death. Through the incorporation of new imaging and digital techniques into osteological research, new tools enable three-dimensional imaging and quantitative morphometrics and increase our capacity to study bone *in situ* and virtual collections. Ethical concerns and efforts at repatriation further highlight the significance of respectful and systematic methods regarding human remains.

Textbook of Human Osteology Volume 2 builds on the fundamentals to address more complex topics in skeletal function, pathology, and analysis. The work includes new methods of biomechanical assessment and computer modeling. Theory and practical guidance are provided in each chapter, supported by case examples that illustrate key points. Ethical considerations and topical concerns in osteological research are also discussed.

- Chapter 1 presents concepts of functional anatomy and the mechanical behavior of bone under various loading conditions, outlining the reaction of cortical and trabecular tissues to compressive, tensile, and shearing forces.
- Chapter 2 addresses phases of growth, determinants of skeletal maturity, and markers of biological age, describing the chronology of ossification episodes, hormonal influence, and epiphyseal union as a help in age estimation.
- Chapter 3 presents disease manifestations in bone tissue, including infectious lesions, metabolic processes like osteoporosis and rickets, and congenital conditions like cleidocranial dysplasia. The chapter presents criteria for the diagnosis of pathological changes and distinguishes antemortem and postmortem changes. Chapter 4 presents an analysis of trauma by fracture classification, blunt-force and sharp-force patterns

of injury, and methods for linking tool mark or weapon-related trauma to forensic cases. This chapter also guides the interpretation of healing phases to estimate time since trauma.

- Postmortem processes and taphonomic factors that affect preservation and recovery are covered in Chapter 5. Scavenger behavior, soil chemistry, and physical weathering are presented along with excavation techniques for recognizing these processes. Forensic identification techniques, including mathematical models used for stature estimation from long-bone measurements, ancestry determination based on cranial features, and dental comparison, are addressed in Chapter 6.
- Chapter 7 applies bioarcheological methods to examine social identity, diet, and cultural practice through the skeleton. Stable isotope analysis, sites of muscle attachment, and burial treatment patterns are studied as markers of lifestyle and community structure. Chapter 8 describes dental morphology, wear, and craniofacial measurements used in anthropological research, and illustrates how tooth size and enamel defects can provide information about diet, health, and lineage.
- Chapter 9 covers metric and non-metric methods for quantifying population variation within skeletal traits. It covers landmark-based morphometrics, principal component analysis, and trait-scoring systems to compare groups. Chapter 10 introduces imaging and digital methods, such as CT scanning to visualize internal structure and photogrammetry to obtain accurate three-dimensional models. It shows where these might be applied in research and teaching.
- Chapter 11 discusses ethical procedures for the treatment of human remains and repatriation processes. It establishes professional standards, legal frameworks, and community outreach practices that ensure dignity and compliance with cultural heritage legislation. Chapter 12 provides a summary of contemporary challenges, including integrating large databases for comparative analysis, applying machine-learning techniques for pattern recognition, and anticipating future analytical innovations.

This book is for graduate students and professionals from anatomy, anthropology, forensic science, and related biomedical sciences. It will be helpful to researchers conducting skeletal analysis, forensic practitioners seeking modern methodologies, and curators responsible for osteological collections. Interweaving stringent anatomical accuracy with contextual case studies and ethical imperatives, this volume attempts to prepare readers for research and professional careers within the emerging science of human osteology.

FUNCTIONAL ANATOMY AND BIOMECHANICS OF THE HUMAN SKELETON

1

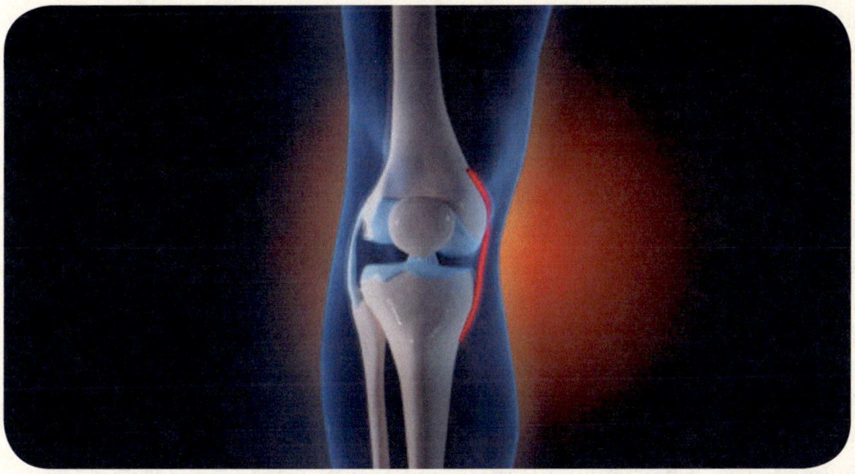

LEARNING OBJECTIVES

After studying this chapter, you will be able to:

1. Describe the structure of the human skeleton
2. Explain the bone development and growth
3. Focus on joints and articulations
4. Discuss the musculoskeletal system interaction
5. Explain the biomechanical principles
6. Understand common skeletal disorders

Introduction

The human skeleton is a hidden framework that, besides supporting the body, also facilitates movement and protects fundamental organs. It is a highly developed interaction between functional anatomy and biomechanics that plays a critical role in how the skeletal system responds to various stresses. The complex system comprises bones, joints, cartilage, and ligaments that play crucial roles in motor function and stability. Functional anatomy investigates how these factors are organized and interact with each other to allow locomotion, while biomechanics provides an analytical framework for investigating the forces acting on them during motion. It is critical to orthopedics, sports science, and rehabilitation because it allows practitioners to treat injuries and optimize physical performance through interventions tailored to each case. Besides, extensive knowledge of biomechanics demonstrates how exercise and the pull of gravity influence the structure and health of bone. Evidence indicates that the human skeleton has an adaptive response to mechanical loads and that regular exercise increases bone density and strength. Disuse or even microgravity environments, however, may lead to severe skeletal degradation, as supported by changes observed in spaceflight studies. These findings demonstrate the importance of dynamic loading for effective skeletal health and for guiding therapeutic interventions to counteract the debilitating impacts of physical inactivity. It is this relationship that gives the impetus to pursue more knowledge on the biomechanics of the human skeleton to understand better how various variables, from exercise protocols to environmental stress, affect skeletal adaptation throughout the course of an individual's life. A combination of advanced imaging modalities, such as high-resolution computed tomography, enhances the understanding of the human skeleton's mechanical and biological characteristics. Such techniques provide three-dimensional reconstruction of skeletal and surrounding soft tissue structures, enabling more precise assessment of their relationships and functions. With the development of accurate anatomical models, researchers can assess biomechanical parameters quantitatively, enhancing the practice of orthopedic surgery and outcomes of treatment. Most importantly, understanding the interactions among different tissues is crucial not only for therapy but also for maximizing sports performance and preventing injuries. As the field continues to expand, the application of such technologies has the potential to enable the creation of novel minimally invasive surgical procedures, musculoskeletal modeling, and other medical treatments designed to maximize human physical capability and rectify skeletal deficiencies.

Definition of Functional Anatomy

Functional anatomy definition involves the study of anatomical structures as they apply to their function and contributions toward the movement and function of the body. Functional anatomy is more concerned with understanding how the various systems, particularly the musculoskeletal system, function normally. Above all, functional anatomy differs from traditional anatomy in that it not only enumerates structures but also concerns the relevance of structures to biomechanical applications. Such a method is most important in clinical domains such as orthopedics, where a thorough understanding of anatomy dictates surgical intervention and rehabilitation protocols. Furthermore, a sense of the interrelated nature of bones, muscles, and connective tissue allows clinicians to predict outcomes based on function and tailor patient care by creating individualized interventions. As functional anatomy remains an evolving field, cutting-edge imaging technology, such as high-resolution computed tomography, is now essential for analyzing anatomical structures. These sophisticated techniques enable precise segmentation and geometrical description of organs, muscles, and neurovascular structures, thereby gaining a better understanding of their functional behavior. These techniques not only enable precise anatomical reconstruction but also allow various applications, such as musculoskeletal modeling, as well as the development of navigated surgical techniques. By generating quantitative data relating traditional anatomy to modern-day biomechanics, such advances improve both teaching and practical application in medicine, eventually enabling improved patient care in complex surgical situations (Audenaert et al., 2010). Beyond that, adding graphical simulations to the teaching of functional anatomy represents the potential for improved medical education and biomechanical modeling. By combining physically and geometrically motivated computations, researchers can create efficient and accurate simulations of muscle movement and deformation. This technique is particularly effective for describing the dynamic interactions required for physical activity and illuminating healthy and pathological patterns of movement. These simulations enhance our understanding of muscle mechanics and enrich the general discipline of functional anatomy with a visual model that can be used to train healthcare providers. Through this, research in functional anatomy is progressively closing the gaps between theoretical and applied content to improve clinical practice and biomechanical research further (Chang et al., 2007) (Figure 1.1).

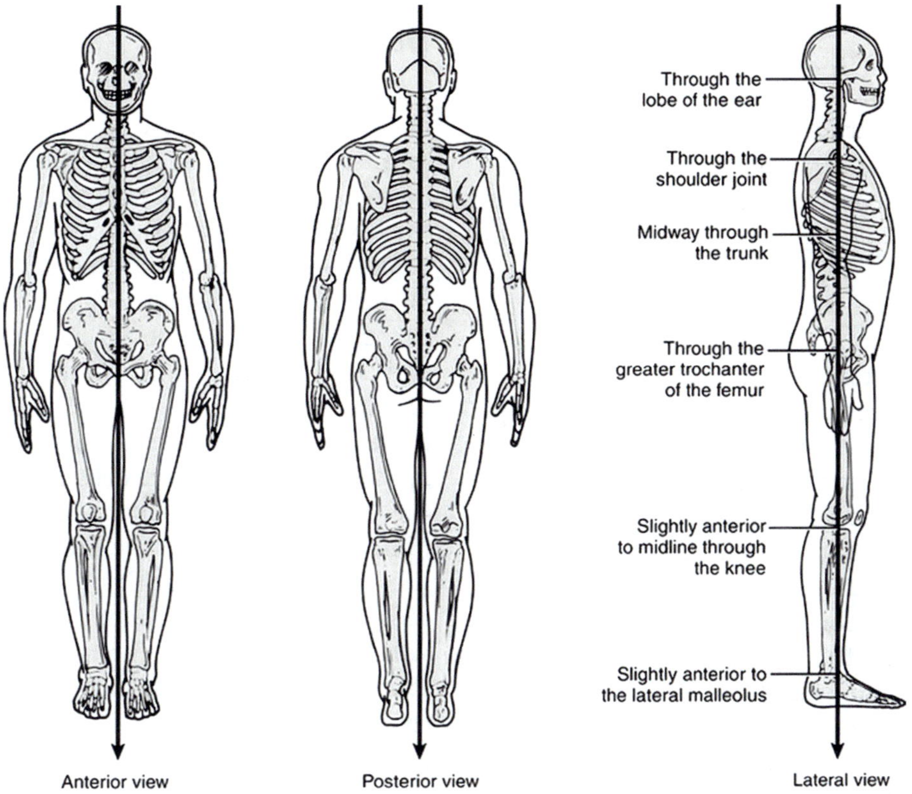

Figure 1.1. The definition of functional anatomy.

Source: https://external-content.duckduckgo.com/iu/?u=https%3A%2F%2Fmusculoskeletalkey.com%2Fwp-content%2Fuploads%2F2016%2F09%2FB978032309104600002X_f02-01-9780323091046.jpg&f=1&nofb=1&ipt=458a4c004c0f48d7f99dc27d5a66a7a5417c55b999ed753b10e1c193b8842111.

Importance of Biomechanics in Understanding the Skeleton

Determining the biomechanics of the human skeleton is important for understanding the complexities of skeletal function and its influence on overall health. Biomechanics interlaces notions of physics with biological constructs, allowing researchers to examine how forces interact within the skeleton during various activities, from walking to lifting to even simple daily functions. By examining the response of bones to these forces, scientists can account for multiple adaptations of the skeletal system to stressors and to aging. This information is not only a prerequisite for the application of effective rehabilitation programs and prevention of injury but also for optimizing athletic performance. Through their intimate knowledge of biomechanics, practitioners can better design interventions that enhance skeletal strength and function, ultimately improving the quality of life for the population with varying ages and activity levels. Finite element analysis (FEA) is now a pivotal tool in biomechanics, particularly for models examining bone structure and mechanical properties. This technique allows researchers to create sophisticated simulations of the intricate shape and physical properties of bone elements. FEA can reveal how anatomical structure variation influences stress distribution and bone deformation in loaded bones. Geometric model variations or simplifications can significantly influence the interpretation of FEA results, so these must be carefully taken into account when interpreting results to understand clinical or evolutionary situations. For instance, FEA-based studies have been successful in examining the relationship between cranial function and structure in different species and in gaining insights into dietary and behavioral specialization. Thus, the use of biomechanics through advanced modeling techniques constitutes an extremely significant bridge between theoretical understanding and applied utility in functional anatomy (Barak et al., 2015). Adding further emphasis on the importance of biomechanics to bone cognition, studies across other species, such as broiler chickens, show that musculoskeletal health can be inadvertently affected by genetic selection. These tests have demonstrated remarkable inertial qualities and alterations in muscle architecture throughout developmental phases. Notably, despite the absence of lameness, underpinning limb pathologies highlighted the intricate coupling between anatomical adaptation and resultant function. Because musculature disproportionately affects the center of mass, these changes may increase muscular stress during functions like standing and locomotion. This lends credence to the need for careful scrutiny of biomechanics when interpreting skeletal structure outside human research, as evidence is contributed to the broader discussion of growth, evolution, and health across species (Codd et al., 2014). By correlating biomechanical theory with comparative and human anatomy, one can gain a better grasp of the skeleton and, hence, more effective methods in many applied fields.

Overview of the Human Skeleton's Role in Movement and Support

The skeleton is an essential support and movement framework, as well as the structural foundation of the body. Composed of 206 bones in an adult human body, it is divided into the axial skeleton—the one that shields vital organs—and the appendicular skeleton, which is mobile. The minute organization allows for the execution of diverse movements, such as walking, running, and jumping—all of which are necessitated by the collective function of bones, joints, and muscles. Types of joints, from synovial to fibrous, are essential to determining the range and type of motion present at each joint, illustrating the skeletons versatility. Also, the skeleton's versatility is highlighted by its ability to vary in response to body stress, which is required for maintaining functionality and mobility over the long term, setting the foundation for the study of biomechanics in human activity.

Within biomechanics, human movement is governed by rules that uncover the complex interaction between bone structure and muscle activity. The skeleton does not merely provide leverage for muscles to contract, but also supports and transmits forces during motion. Muscles are attached to bones through tendons, which enable locomotion through patterns of coordinated contractions and relaxations that move the body. Understanding this interaction is vital to studying how alterations in skeletal integrity, such as fractures or degenerative disease, affect mobility and overall function. Studying these biomechanical principles is vital to establishing rehabilitation methods and interventions designed to optimize movement efficiency while lessening risk of injury. Furthermore, technology-based improvements in motion analysis have expanded our understanding of movement and gait patterns, paving the way for optimal sports performance and improved clinical outcomes through intervention (Baker et al., 2006). Research on bipedalism is used to illustrate the way in which human skeleton evolution has uniquely adapted to support effective locomotion. Not only does the skeleton enable upright posture, but it also makes walking and running more energy-efficient. With evolutionary robotics approaches, scientists are now beginning to simulate the biomechanics of bipedal walking and running and learn about the energetic expenses of different locomotion types. Such simulations can reconstruct the biomechanics of our hominoid ancestors and provide valuable insights into their locomotor patterns in ecological environments (Crompton et al., 2003). This is a paradigm for advancing toward an increasingly integrated understanding of functional anatomy, bridging evolutionary biology with current biomechanics and further elucidating the skeleton's role in supporting and enabling mobility in human locomotion (Figure 1.2).

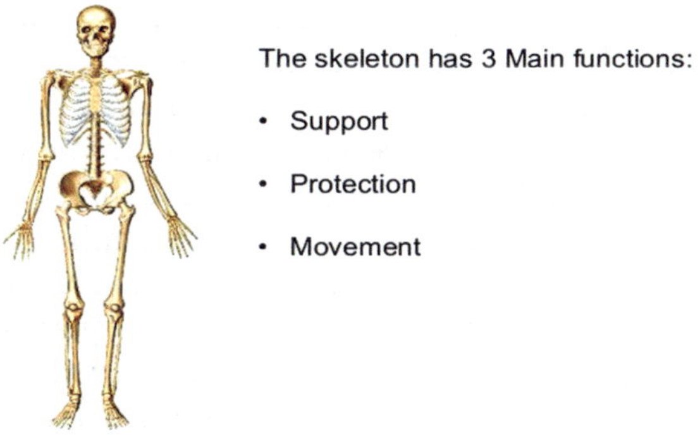

Figure 1.2. The human skeleton.

Source: https://external-content.duckduckgo.com/iu/?u=https%3A%2F%2Fimage.slidesharecdn.com%2Fskeletonpdf-130409033641-phpapp01%2F95%2Fskeleton-pdf-1-638.jpg%3Fcb%3D1365479057&f=1&nofb=1&ipt=2f33f30dd68e31c878aa449a286f890dfb8e43c7275d1756259f3da87e8b74f0.

1.1. Structure of the Human Skeleton

Learning Outcome

1. Composition of bones
2. Classification of bones (long, short, flat, and irregular)
3. Overview of the axial and appendicular skeleton

The human skeletal structure is a remarkable example of evolutionary adaptation that supports basic biomechanical functions. Comprising 206 bones in the typical adult, the skeleton can be divided into two main sections: the axial skeleton, made up of the skull, vertebral column, and rib cage, and the appendicular skeleton, comprising the limbs and pelvic girdle. Maintaining not only the structure of the body but also internally protecting vital organs, while facilitating movement through its joint articulations, is carried out by the bony system. The skeletal structure has advanced, especially regarding limb proportions and joint surfaces, which have evolved to be efficient for bipedal locomotion. To comprehend the multifarious structural components is urgent to ask how they co-operate in order to produce the over-all performance of the human body, and to bring to the fore the tenuous association between form and mobility of the human body. A glance at bone density reveals enormous evolutionary patterns that distinguish contemporary humans from their hominin forebears. Research indicates that modern human beings have lowered trabecular density in the bones relative to their predecessors and other primates and can be explained as a sequence of adaptations due to shifts in lifestyle over time. This lowered bone density may be evidence of lowered reliance on physical exercise that would enhance bone strength in concurrence with increased sedentism and technological advancement. Imaging studies such as peripheral quantitative

CT have provided information on such structural variations, making cross-species comparisons and an improved grasp of functional implications of skeletal adaptation possible. By studying changes in trabecular density, researchers are able to learn about how anatomical structures influence biomechanics and contribute to the general well-being and longevity of modern human skeletal systems (Zipfel et al., 2014).

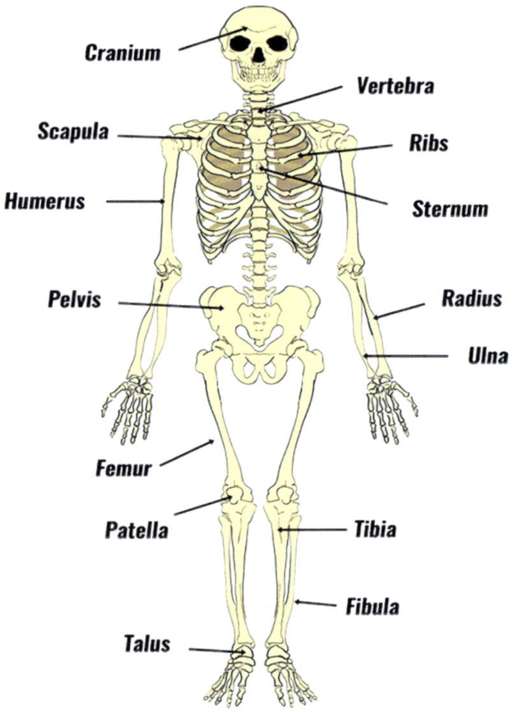

Figure 1.3. The structure of the human skeleton.

Source: https://external-content.duckduckgo.com/iu/?u=https%3A%2F%2Fwww.teachpe.com%2Fwp-content%2Fuploads%2F2019%2F06%2Fgcse-skeleton-bones600.jpg&f=1&nofb=1&ipt=af74f508bf3cf8f41777d37ac27e5179171770e03aa36c1e6b79b779c919ca40.

Furthermore, the study of soft-tissue interactions with the skeleton provides an integrative view of the functional anatomy of the skeletal system. Technical developments in imaging modalities, especially high-resolution computer tomography, have enabled precise muscle and neurovascular relationship analyses over skeletal structures. The three-dimensional approach, in addition to facilitating understanding of joint biomechanics, also emphasizes soft tissue configurations as significant determinants of functional outcomes in orthopedic conditions. Such data are easily translatable to advanced applications, including the creation of musculoskeletal models predictive of performance and injury risk. The marriage of geometric analysis in surgery is educating new methods in minimally invasive and robotic surgery, shedding light on the imperative relationship between anatomical science and clinical practice within biomechanics (Audenaert et al., 2010). By doing so, the design of the human skeleton is more than a supportive and protective framework; it is also a primary element in unravelling the complexities of human movement and health (Figure 1.3).

1.1.1. Composition of Bones

The bones' composition is vital to their functional anatomy and biomechanics. Bones are made up of two main substances: an organic matrix consisting mainly of collagen and inorganic minerals, with hydroxyapatite as the major inorganic mineral. The special combination is what contributes to both strength and flexibility of bones so that they can support different stresses during movement. Tensile strength is provided by the organic part and compressive strength by the mineral composition. Since demands shift in the skeleton, for instance during growth and development or exercise, bone structure can be altered by remodeling and mineralizing processes. The changes occur at the cellular and molecular levels, displaying the dynamic nature of bone tissue as it responds to mechanical stress and metabolic demand, illustrating the form and function dependence of the human skeleton. Aside from hydroxyapatite and collagen, bone also contains a variety of cells, including osteoblasts, osteocytes, and osteoclasts, each playing a specific role in bone formation and integrity. Osteoblasts are responsible for the formation of new bone matrix, while osteoclasts are responsible for bone resorption, and thus regulating the balance of bone mass throughout an individual's life. Osteocytes, the osteoblast-derived bone cells, are mechanosensors that detect mechanical stress and coordinate local remodeling. Cellular activity is critical to bone composition adaptation to environmental forces, including gravity and daily loads. For instance, bone density can be lost during long periods of disuse, as in microgravity found in space, where demineralization results from the absence of gravity-bearing forces, highlighting the adaptive role of bone composition as a response to altered mechanical environments (Arnaud et al., 2025).

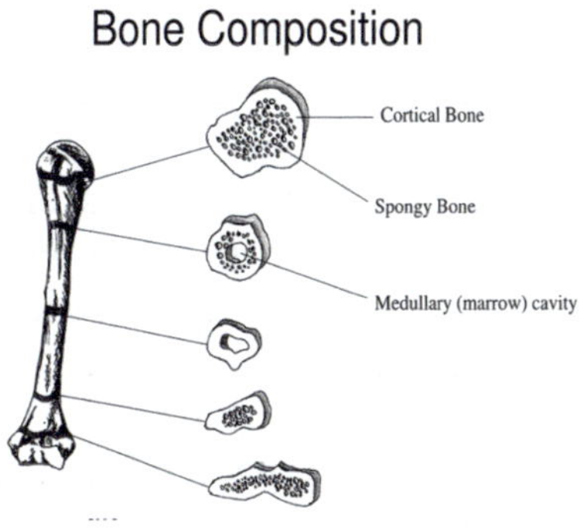

Figure 1.4. The composition of bones.

Source: https://external-content.duckduckgo.com/iu/?u=https%3A%2F%2Fimage1.slideserve.com%2F3147257%2Fbone-composition-l.jpg&f=1&nofb=1&ipt=5491041e2b463a0a6dfd77a587492bf697db7898187a74ad122218889d0f7416.

Applications of bone composition go beyond basic structural mechanics to encompass implications for general musculoskeletal health. For example, research emphasizes the importance of adequate dietary vitamin D and calcium in supporting bone density and averting risk factors for degenerative conditions such as osteoporosis. Alterations in bone structure can lead to severe musculoskeletal disorders; therefore, there is a need to take a holistic approach to bone health. In research on broiler chickens, for example, anatomical alterations can cause a range of leg diseases, illustrating how genetic selection for certain characteristics can unintentionally compromise musculoskeletal integrity (Codd et al., 2014). These observations highlight the importance of understanding the bone's composition, both for functional capacity and for long-term welfare across different species, and thus for informing preventive healthcare measures in both animals and humans (Figure 1.4).

1.1.2. Classification of Bones (Long, Short, Flat, and Irregular)

The classification of bones in the human skeleton can be divided into four groups: long, short, flat, and irregular bones. Long bones, such as the femur and humerus, are long and primarily responsible for the movement and support of limbs. These bones serve as levers to facilitate locomotion and load transmission due to their unique biomechanical properties. Long bone anatomy is made up of four parts: the diaphysis and the two epiphyses, which are crucial for facilitating both strength and flexibility. The geometry of such bones allows them to resist high mechanical stress and to support growth and adaptation to the forces acting on the skeleton during various activities, a phenomenon supported by bone remodeling laws (Czubacka et al., 2017). The short bones, however, are typically cube-shaped and are found mainly in the wrists and ankles. These short bones, for example, the carpals and tarsals, play significant functions in support and stability with a minimal range of movement. Their compactness helps them support weight and absorb shock. The functional significance of short bones is also exhibited by their capacity to facilitate multi-directional movements at the feet and hands in order to enable dexterity and balance. By effectively transmitting force through joints, short bones play a significant role in the overall biomechanics of the human body and, as a result, demonstrate their applicability in daily activities and sports performance (Rockhold et al., 1998). Flat bones encompass an even wider variety of skeletal forms, such as the skull, sternum, and ribs. The bones have a thin, flattened structure with several functions, such as protection and attachment of muscles.

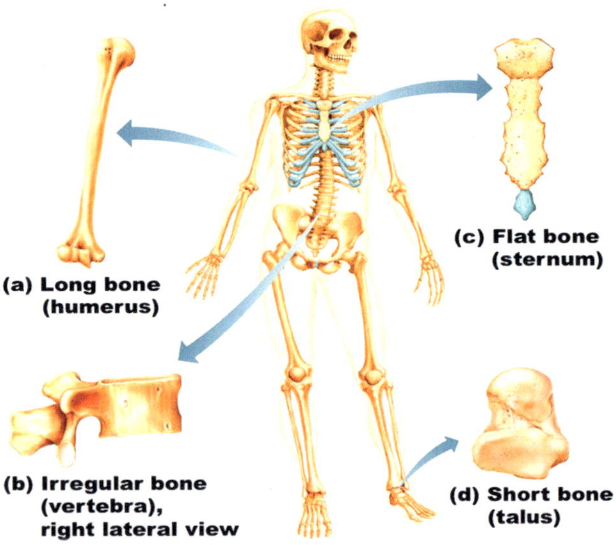

Figure 1.5. The classification of bones in the human skeleton.

Source: https://external-content.duckduckgo.com/iu/?u=http%3A%2F%2Fmsgallagherlhs.weebly.com%2Fuploads%2F3%2F8%2F6%2F9%2F38694679%2F7743270_orig.png&f=1&nofb=1&ipt=deb9a7c7db9df16f19e30d9bc924b1f12b49c4c758b4c9afd97ca23e602a70fc.

The plane structure of these bones facilitates the maximum area for muscular attachment, enabling easy respiration and rotation of the head. Moreover, flat bones protect vital organs such as the brain and the thoracic cavity from mechanical stress. The strength-to-weight ratio of flat bones further affirms their biomechanical importance, as they confer both resilience and flexibility while still supporting the skeletal strength required for various functions at different phases of life (Czubacka et al., 2017). Understanding these categories accentuates the complexity of the human skeleton's functional anatomy and biomechanics, shedding light on each bone type's unique contribution toward providing homeostasis and freedom of movement (Figure 1.5).

1.1.3. Overview of the Axial and Appendicular Skeleton

The human skeleton is composed of two divisions: the axial and appendicular skeletons. The axial skeleton, including the skull, vertebral column, and rib cage, forms the central axis of the body, providing stability and protection for vital organs such as the brain and heart. The sensory organs and the brain are housed in the skull, while the vertebral column supports the head, provides structural support and flexibility to the torso, and protects the spinal cord. Comprising vertebrae that are divided into cervical, thoracic, lumbar, sacral, and coccygeal regions, the axial skeleton plays a crucial role in offering posture as well as movement by functioning together with the musculoskeletal system. Overall, the axial skeleton provides structural stability and a protective casing for vital organs, meeting the principles of functional anatomy. The appendicular skeleton, by contrast, enables the housing of limb bones and girdle bones, i.e., the scapula and pelvis, that attach several limbs to the axial skeleton. Such a partition is significant during locomotion and manipulation of the environment, including the bones that enable an enormous range of motion. The upper limbs are specialized for manipulation and grasping, with maximal action enabled by diverse motions at the joints, while the lower limbs provide stability and support for walking and standing. The femur, tibia, and fibula of the lower limb play key roles in supporting weight and in displaying the biomechanical adaptations required for ambulation on land. Besides, the appendicular skeleton enables complex movements, a sign of the highly impactful evolution of this structure in human evolution, in terms of functionality and flexibility as organisms transitioned from aquatic to terrestrial environments. Interdependence is present in the relationship between the axial and appendicular skeletons in both functional and biomechanical functioning. Through evolutionary mechanisms, specific adaptations have emerged within these skeletal subdivisions, enabling organized and efficient patterns of movement. Through study, it has been found that there are significant morphological differences among species, including an association between vertebral form and ecological and behavioral niches, as observed in felids (Goswami et al., 2018). This functional division illustrates the evolutionary significance of the vertebral column and its association with appendicular elements. Similarly, the transition from aquatic to terrestrial environments has driven innovations in limb shape, further demonstrating the evolutionary trajectories linking axial and appendicular morphologies (Kawano et al., 2014). Such integration of the two divisions not only informs us about mechanical function but also reveals the forces of evolution that have shaped the human skeleton (Figure 1.6).

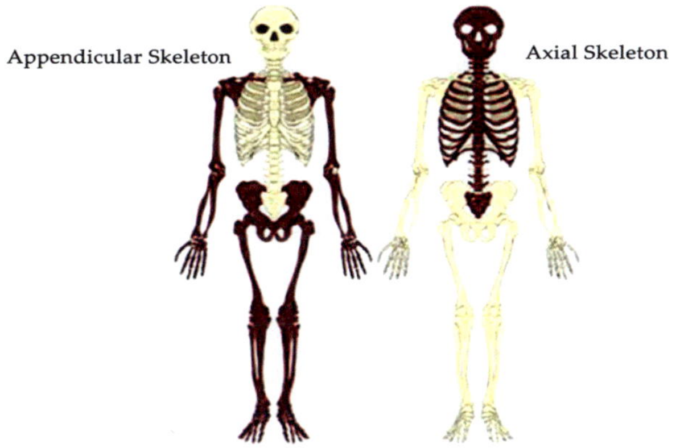

Figure 1.6. Overview of the axial and appendicular skeleton.

Source: https://www.teachpe.com/wp-content/uploads/2019/06/axial800-jpg.jpg.

Test Your Knowledge

1. How is the human skeleton structurally divided into axial and appendicular parts?
2. What are the major types of bones found in the human skeleton?

1.2. Bone Development and Growth

Learning Outcome

1. Process of ossification
2. Factors influencing bone growth
3. Role of hormones in skeletal development

The development and growth of bones are intimately related to the biomechanics and functional anatomy of the human skeleton. During the early stages of life, bones exhibit dramatic alterations according to genetic and environmental factors. Ossification starts in fetal life, wherein cartilage templates sequentially develop into bone. This adaptive process enables the formation of primary ossification centers, leading to the growth of long bones characterized by their trabecular and cortical structure. The biomechanical stress imposed on bones, particularly those that bear weight, also shapes bone strength and density during childhood and adolescence and lays the foundation for skeletal health throughout life. Understanding the biomechanics of bone adaptation is valuable in knowing about patterns of growth and disorders. The relationship between bone density and mechanical loading is evident; strengthened bones through periodic stressing are denser and more structurally sound. Research shows that various musculoskeletal conditions are caused by inadequate mechanical stimuli, leading to reduced bone mineral density and increased fracture susceptibility. For instance, in animal models such as broiler chickens, the connection between a skewed muscle structure and compromised limb function suggests that similar mechanisms might apply to humans, where weakened muscle can affect bone growth and health, particularly during early development (Codd et al., 2014).

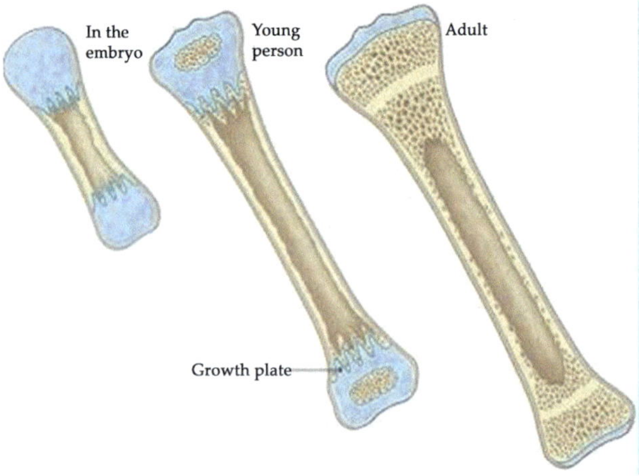

Figure 1.7. The process of bone development and growth.

Source: https://external-content.duckduckgo.com/iu/?u=https%3A%2F%2Fimage.slidesharecdn.com%2Fmainboneformationslide-150925100627-lva1-app6892%2F95%2Fstages-of-bone-formation-1-638.jpg%3Fcb%3D1443175714&f=1&nofb=1&ipt=aa8d8f212605515db0ff3468a88132b6823273a3384a7ca281f4a0b272ad5fbd.

Further analysis of cancellous bone structure provides insights into the skeleton's evolutionary adaptations and mechanical efficiencies. In the course of their development, different species like the non-avian theropods have different cancellous bone architectures that relate to their specific locomotor requirements. These architectural models maximize the bone's ability to resist stresses encountered through mobility. Comparative analysis of the anatomical features of these architectures provides an insight into the biomechanics of movement evolution, linking bone morphology with functional performance. This has implications for our understanding of both human bone development and the treatment of locomotor pathology, as understanding the significance of cancellous architecture can lead to improved interventions to maintain bone health and achieve optimal mobility throughout life (Aamodt et al., 2018) (Figure 1.7).

1.2.1. Process of Ossification

Ossification is central to the development and maintenance of the human skeleton, providing the foundation for functional anatomy and biomechanics. Ossification refers to the development of bone tissue that is executed in two primary mechanisms: intramembranous and endochondral ossification. Intramembranous ossification is the process through which flat bones, such as those in the skull, develop through the direct formation of mesenchymal cells into bone cells.

In contrast, endochondral ossification is the replacement of bone by hyaline cartilage necessary for long bone elongation as well as overall skeleton elongation during development. The dual process of bone accrual reflects not only the complexity of skeletal development but also the role of biomechanical forces in inducing bone strength and density as an individual matures. As ossification proceeds, the effects of genetic and environmental influences are evident, particularly in clinical conditions. Conditions like developmental dysplasia, such as that in Legg-Calvé-Perthes disease, illustrate the contributions of vascularity and skeletal maturity to the process of ossification. Children aged 5–8, who are likely to have a variety of anatomical differences while growing, are susceptible to Perthes disease due to discontinuities in the blood supply to the femoral head. These discontinuities could interfere with normal ossification, resulting in problems in bone structure and function. The determination of these risks illuminates not only the intricacy of ossification but also emphasizes biomechanics as a deciding factor in skeletal health. Studies of such conditions provide insight into the interplay between internal processes and external forces in the formation of bones (Acheson et al., 2016). The heterogeneity of ossification processes also highlights evolutionary compromise in the human skeleton.

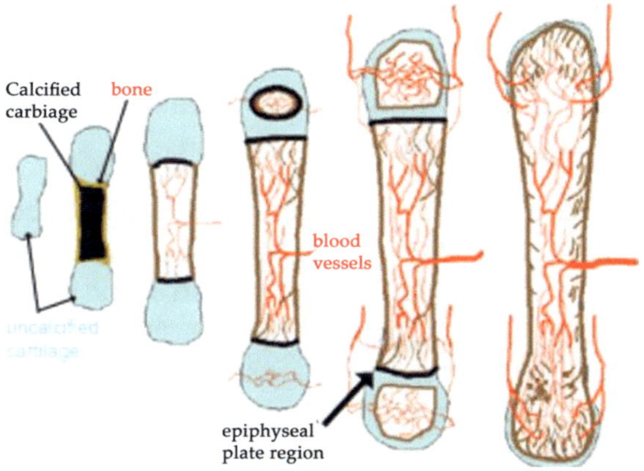

Figure 1.8. The process of ossification.

Source: https://external-content.duckduckgo.com/iu/?u=https%3A%2F%2Fimage1.slideserve.com%2F2879423%2Fossification1-l.jpg&f=1&nofb=1&ipt=2e1db9f89252635e3d1af353689addc7d42faa018b20e2b89e5798df8a9400c5.

Research has shown that variations in ossification timing and process can cause different skeletal morphologies among populations and result in a variety of functional outcomes. For instance, some studies have suggested that anatomical elements of the hand exhibit both primitive and newly evolved traits, providing evidence for the adaptation of the skeletal system over time. This diversity supports ongoing research into how ossification processes are not only enlightening about the individual health of bones but also shaping broader evolutionary patterns in humans. By analyzing these adaptations collectively, knowledge of the functional anatomy and biomechanics of the human skeleton can be discovered, as well as the skeletal disorders themselves and how they may be addressed (Kivell et al., 2016) (Figure 1.8).

1.2.2. Factors Influencing Bone Growth

Bone growth, or ossification, is influenced by numerous factors that collectively ascertain the development and sustenance of the skeleton. One of the predominant influences is mechanical stress, or loading of the bone, which leads to bone growth by activating osteocytes and stimulating osteoblasts. These cells, upon mechanical loading, release signaling molecules that reinforce osteoblast activity, the bone cells responsible for creating new bone. Conversely, the lack of mechanical stress can trigger resorption, wherein osteoclasts break down bone. This alternating mechanism is a reminder of the importance of exercise, as repeated weight-bearing activities can densify and strengthen bones, thereby reducing the risk of osteoporosis and fractures with aging. Understanding the biomechanical forces that influence bone growth is crucial to developing strategies for preserving bone health throughout life. In addition to mechanical stimuli, the nutritional factors play an essential role in the development and formation of bones. Major nutrients like vitamin D and calcium play critical roles in ensuring normal mineralization and maintaining bone mineral density. Calcium is the most essential mineral found in bones, and vitamin D regulates calcium absorption in the intestinal tract and maintains its homeostasis in the blood. Lack of these nutrients can lead to weakened bone and increased susceptibility to fracture and disease, such as rickets in children and osteomalacia in adults. In addition, new evidence also indicated that cancellous bone structural properties are nutrition-dependent, demonstrating unambiguously the influence of nutrition on the biomechanical integrity of bone structures. Quantification of these nutritional contributions is thus necessary for a full appreciation of variables controlling bone growth. Further, genetic susceptibility significantly affects bone growth and total skeletal architecture. Hereditary factors determine bone size, density, and shape, and contribute to a person's susceptibility to various bone diseases. Experiments here have revealed that specific genes regulate bone cell proliferation and differentiation, demonstrating how variations in genes may contribute to differences between groups regarding bone status. Besides, the interaction between genetic and environmental factors, such as exercise and nutrition, elucidates the complexity of bone growth regulation. Moreover, advanced mathematical models have helped elucidate how geometric constraints may determine cell behavior during bone development. Through the integration of results from genetics, biomechanics, and nutrition, a fuller understanding of the factors influencing bone growth is available, leading to healthier development across varied populations (Figure 1.9).

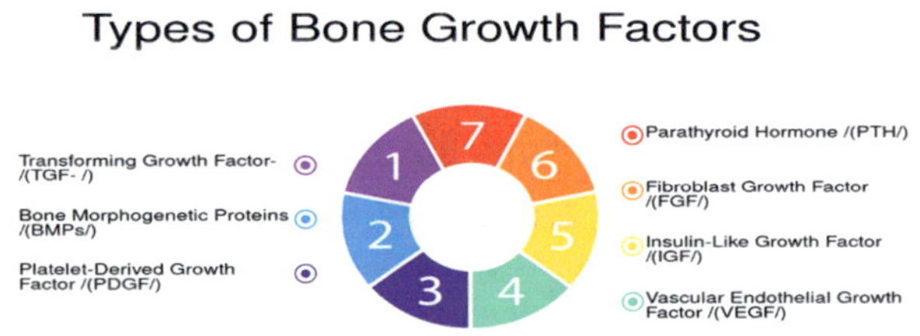

Figure 1.9. Factors influencing bone growth.

Source: https://fastercapital.co/i/Bone-Growth-Factor-Understanding-the-Role-of-Bone-Growth-Factors-in-Orthopedic-Medicine--Types-of-Bone-Growth-Factors.webp.

1.2.3. Role of Hormones in Skeletal Development

Hormones play a crucial role in the complex processes of skeletal growth, impacting both bone development and homeostasis throughout life. Significant hormones involved in skeletal growth are growth hormone, sex hormones, and parathyroid hormone, each making specific contributions to the formation and maintenance of bone tissue. Growth hormone stimulates chondrocyte mitosis, leading to longitudinal growth in epiphyseal plates, whereas sex hormones, particularly estrogen and testosterone, play a significant role during puberty in maturing bone structure and in the ultimate closure of the growth plates. The interplay of these hormones not only determines the size and shape of bones but also their density and ability to withstand mechanical stress, thus defining the functional anatomy of the human skeleton.

A delicate balance of hormones is required to maintain bone health and integrity, as distortion in any one area can lead to catastrophic skeletal disease. For instance, low estrogen levels, typically occurring after menopause, have been reported to accelerate bone resorption, resulting in osteoporosis and susceptibility to fracture. Parathyroid hormone similarly regulates calcium homeostasis and bone remodeling by facilitating osteoclast activity, thereby supporting bone resorption. Such hormones are also needed in excess conditions, e.g., space, where gravity is significantly less.

Research has indicated that changes in hormone responses to weightlessness may be detrimental to skeletal adaptation and health, and stresses the need for effective countermeasures to prevent these effects (Keller et al., 2025; N/A, 2025). Not only are hormones involved in skeletal growth beyond physiological development, but they are also involved in dynamic skeletal adaptation to mechanical and environmental stimuli. Hormones such as glucocorticoids and calcitonin also participate in bone remodeling, underscoring the plasticity of the system. Adaptation occurs based on the physical demands placed on bones, a quintessential example of Wolff's law, which states that bone reacts and adjusts to the loads it experiences. In cases such as prolonged space travel, where astronauts experience reduced mechanical loading and altered hormonal signaling (Keller et al., 2025; N/A, 2025), the ramifications for skeletal development can be drastic. Understanding these hormonal ramifications is critical to developing strategies for maintaining skeletal health, particularly for humans traveling into extraterrestrial environments.

Test Your Knowledge

1. What are the main stages involved in bone development and growth?
2. How do genetic, nutritional, and hormonal factors influence bone growth?

1.3. Joints and Articulations

Learning Outcome

1. Types of joints (fibrous, cartilaginous, and synovial)
2. Range of motion and joint stability
3. Common joint injuries and their implications

The complex interaction among joints and articulations in the human skeleton is responsible for mobility and functional anatomy. Joints are critical areas for movement and flexibility, where bones meet at various points throughout the body. The classification of joints according to type is a reflection of the diversity in structure and function. Synovial joints, which contain a fluid-filled joint cavity, provide extensive motion and are essential for walking, running, and grasping. For instance, the distinctive shape of the human hand, with its finely organized joints, is simultaneously an evolutionary solution for tool use and an intricate biomechanical system for precision grasping. Understanding the structural nuances of joints is critical for understanding how they enable normal function and how pathologies may restrict mobility. In addition, the theory of joint evolution provides excellent insight into human movement biomechanics. Current findings present that recent humans have lower trabecular density compared to nonhuman primates, and this points to a significant change in skeletal structure based on changes in living habits over time. Research has confirmed that this reduction in trabecular density is most evident in limb joints, illuminating an important evolutionary shift toward greater reliance on technology rather than physical adaptation to environmental demands. Not only does this evolutionary explanation further explain functional anatomy, but it also raises questions about the impact of current lifestyle on joint integrity and health. The relevance of this study may help address contemporary issues with joint disorders, further warranting studies on the anatomical and functional development of human joints within a biomechanical environment (Zipfel et al., 2014). Finally, the structure of human joints and their articulations highlights not only functional variety but also a remarkable adaptive quality that synergizes ancient and novel elements. The primate hand, for instance, illustrates this blend, with both well-preserved ancestral forms and specializations to enable fine manipulation. Such factors make the value of a close examination of joint morphology across various primate lineages clear, providing further insights into evolutionary biomechanics. The importance of articulations extends beyond merely affecting movement; they are key indicators of evolutionary history and functional ability. Further, the detailed examination of joint structure will inform future research questions regarding physical activities participation in maintaining joint integrity, ultimately closing the loop between anatomical form and functional use in human motion (Kivell et al., 2016) (Figure 1.10).

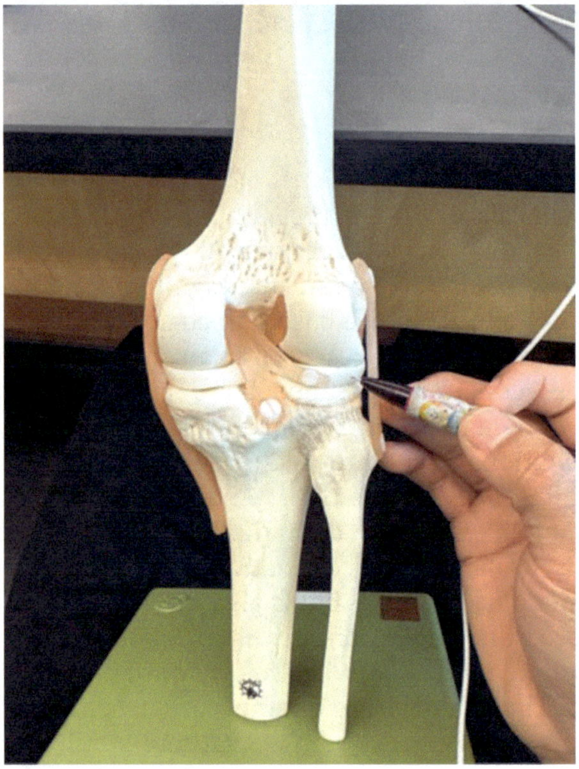

Figure 1.10. Joints and articulations.

Source: https://external-content.duckduckgo.com/iu/?u=https%3A%2F%2Fo.quizlet.com%2FLxRkqZTKpVtcGMQAXQW6Rg.jpg&f=1&nofb=1&ipt=7174f245911df38aba9a33f02b5462e790a6bcca3ca94c70f3b84fa8f049aab3.

1.3.1. Types of Joints (Fibrous, Cartilaginous, and Synovial)

Knowing the various types of joints in the human body helps understand their functional anatomy and biomechanics. Joints are divided into three broad categories: fibrous, cartilaginous, and synovial. Fibrous joints, as the name suggests, are bound together by dense connective tissue and allow minimal movement. A good example of this type is sutures in the cranium, which provide stability and protect the brain. Fibrous joints' stiff framework plays a critical role in enabling the skeleton to retain integrity during biomechanical activities, particularly in locations that require substantial support and protection. The unique orientation of connective tissue fibers in joints prevents movement, highlighting their role in providing a stiff framework for body mechanics. Cartilaginous joints, however, are more flexible without sacrificing stability. These are cartilaginous tissues that connect hyaline or fibrocartilage. One fine example of a cartilaginous joint is the spine's intervertebral discs, which allow slight movement while providing shock absorption and protection of spinal stability. The biomechanical properties of cartilaginous joints play a crucial role in weight transmission and movement, particularly during dynamic functional activity. Research has established that the mechanics of cartilaginous joints change over time in response to the mechanical environment and loading conditions under which they are placed, indicating a dependence of joint remodeling on functional stresses (Giorgi et al., 2015). Therefore, understanding the intricate relationship between the joint structure and function of cartilaginous joints can be used to guide spinal disorder and other musculoskeletal-related therapies. Synovial joints form the most mobile form of joint, and a joint cavity is present that is occupied by synovial fluid, which lubricates and supplies nutrients to the articular cartilage. These joints, such as the knee and shoulder, are highly intricate structures composed of ligaments, tendons, and synovial membranes, each contributing to their stability and mobility. Synovial joint biomechanics are essential because they facilitate movement and load-bearing functions and enable a coordinated approach to dynamic motion. It is known that morphological features of the joint and synovial content can exert a direct effect on the functional outcome of the joint, particularly in the context of aging or trauma (Adams et al., 1993). A comprehensive knowledge of synovial joints thus falls within the broader scope of functional anatomy and biomechanics, highlighting the necessity for ongoing investigation into joint health and its applicability to physical rehabilitation and sports medicine (Figure 1.11).

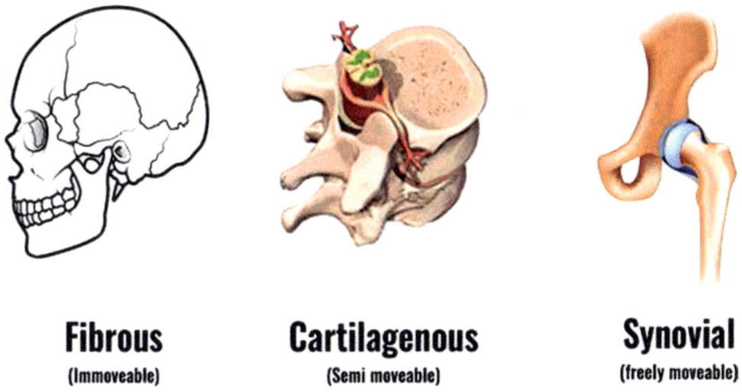

Figure 1.11. The various types of joints in the human body.

Source: https://external-content.duckduckgo.com/iu/?u=https%3A%2F%2Fwww.teachpe.com%2Fwp-content%2Fuploads%2F2019%2F06%2Ftypes-of-joint620.jpg&f=1&nofb=1&ipt=e7121b61dbcf62e448e2af7d65bbafdf25670659e13298019c4decc1adadbfb0.

1.3.2. Range of Motion (ROM) and Joint Stability

The interaction between ROM and joint stability is a simple component of the functional anatomy and biomechanics of the human skeleton. ROM refers to the extent to which a joint can move, which is important for numerous physical movements. Each joint of the human body has a specific range of motion, which is influenced by factors such as anatomical structure, muscular strength, and ligaments. The knee, for instance, can be bent and straightened at hinge joints, while ball-and-socket joints, such as the hip, facilitate broader movement. However, an increased range of movement usually tends to compromise the stability of the joint and reduce injury. Understanding this interaction is essential, as joint stability is required to maintain functional movement patterns and prevent dysfunction during circumstances requiring strength and coordination, and hence highlighting the delicate balance of mobility and stability of human joints. Maximum joint stability is essential to injury and to enhance performance in a variety of activities, from sporting movements to daily function. The limb muscles, ligaments, and joint design largely provide stability. In the shoulder joint, for example, a complex tendon and ligament arrangement stabilizes the humeral head with the shallow glenoid cavity. With an expanded range of movement, for instance, in hypermobile patients, there is a danger of joint dislocation and chronic damage due to poor stabilizing means. In addition, increased differences in joint stability can influence movement biomechanics, with motion of the joints changing gait and posture as a aftermath of joint instability. Therefore, evaluation of individual joint stability is also crucial in terms of consideration both of rehabilitations and sports performance, to preserve maximum range of motion and stability for functional effectiveness. Advances in biomechanical research have better illuminated the intricate interaction between range of motion and joint stability, making way for enhanced rehabilitation methods and performance-enhancing mechanisms. Biomechanics, as a science that integrates engineering principles with the living system, is capable of quantifying the impact of varied ranges of motion on the general health and functioning of joints. Advanced modeling techniques, such as finite element analysis and musculoskeletal modeling, enable researchers to simulate joint behavior under different conditions and predict injury patterns. These studies emphasize the need for rehabilitation programs individualized according to anatomic variations and movement patterns. Notably, as shown by evidence on osseointegration procedures, new techniques are available that can optimize ROM while preserving stability, thereby optimizing functional outcomes in patients with compromised joint stability (Brånemark et al., 2017; Harris et al., 2012). Hence, the interaction of these factors remains at the forefront of efforts to explain human movement and the prevention of injury (Figure 1.12).

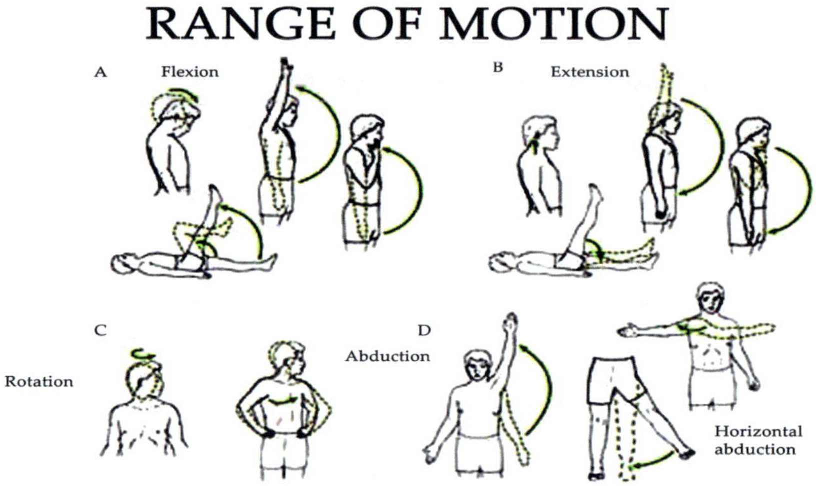

Figure 1.12. The interaction between range of motion (ROM) and joint stability.

Source: https://samarpanphysioclinic.com/wp-content/uploads/2019/02/Range-of-Motion.webp.

1.3.3. Common Joint Injuries and Their Implications

Joint injury is a significant concern in functional anatomy and biomechanics because it has a devastating effect on mobility and quality of life. Overhead sports players, such as baseball players, are two of the most common joint injuries found in the shoulder and elbow. The mechanics of throwing place tremendous stress on these joints, leading to injuries such as ulnar collateral ligament (UCL) sprains and rotator cuff tears. The research has indicated that the kinetic variables, especially elbow valgus torque and shoulder external rotation forces during a pitch, are central to such injuries (Post et al., 2013).

Understanding these biomechanical principles not only helps prevent injury but also enables planning specific rehabilitation interventions to enable affected athletes to return to sport safely. Awareness of joint mechanics is consequently paramount for both practitioners and athletes. The implications of joint injury are far in excess of temporary physical discomfort, impacting functional and psychological status. For instance, knee trauma such as rupture of the anterior cruciate ligament (ACL) can result in chronic instability and increased susceptibility to osteoarthritis, drastically altering the patient's life path. Surgical intervention with intensive rehabilitation is typically required; hence, the importance of mastering in-depth knowledge of knee joint anatomy and biomechanics. Psychological complications, such as fear or anxiety due to re-injury, can also complicate recovery. As noted in research on various groups of sportspeople, the dynamic properties of such injuries play a crucial role in the formulation of effective management interventions (Buckland et al., 2011). Understanding these implications is imperative for healthcare professionals and athletes alike in transcending the challenges that come with joint injuries. Outside of the knee and shoulder, ankle and wrist injuries are also common in other populations, particularly in active groups. Ankle sprains, for example, are extremely common in sports owing to sudden weight changes and bad landings. These injuries can lead to chronic instability if not fully addressed, which can affect both athletic function and activities of daily living. Similarly, wrist injuries, often the consequence of falls or repetitive strain, may lead to compromised grip strength and limited range of motion, particularly in elderly individuals. The variability of these injuries necessitates thorough anatomical and biomechanical knowledge to develop prevention programs and treatment protocols. Through an understanding of the forces that arise in daily activities, clinicians can better predict possible injury and enhance rehabilitation, ultimately benefiting individuals to lead an active life after injury (Post et al., 2013) (Figure 1.13).

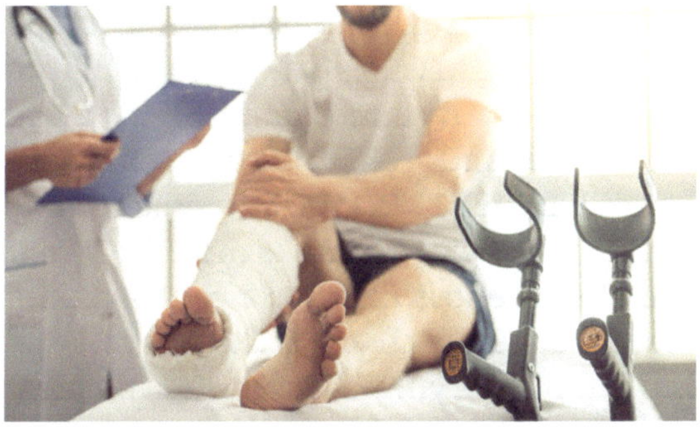

Figure 1.13. Common joint injuries and their implications.

Source: https://external-content.duckduckgo.com/iu/?u=https%3A%2F%2Fanyrates.com%2Fwp-content%2Fuploads%2F2022%2F07%2FAnyRates_HealthCare-780x435.jpg&f=1&nofb=1&ipt=d96a230d736f0fe2621671b3dab74f4da0d23449bb5180ed6bce1fe09deee7ba.

Test Your Knowledge

1. What are the main types of joints and articulations in the human body?
2. How does joint structure influence the range and type of movement possible?

1.4. Musculoskeletal System Interaction

Learning Outcome

1. Role of muscles in movement
2. Tendons and ligaments: structure and function
3. Neuromuscular control of skeletal movement

The human musculoskeletal system is an example of a complex interaction between skeletal and muscular tissues, which is vital for mobility, stability, and overall function. The bones not only provide the structural framework but also serve as levers that act in concert with muscles to facilitate movement. Muscles generate forces acting on bones at more than one joint and produce dynamic interactions that allow for an enormous range of motions from simple joint flexion to sophisticated athletic accomplishments. An understanding sufficient for these interactions emphasizes the importance of biomechanics in studying normal and disease movements. The more scientists discover about the musculoskeletal system's mechanics, with the inclusion of technologies such as musculoskeletal modeling, the more important it is. These instruments allow the analyst to gain insight into torques, forces, and joint mechanics as a whole, which can significantly contribute to our understanding of athletic performance and rehabilitation procedures (Harris et al., 2012). Efficient functioning of the musculoskeletal system is incredibly reliant on the effectiveness of muscle contraction and the compliance of muscle architecture. Muscle fibers exhibit varying characteristics, such as length and organization, that directly influence the development of force and endurance. With increasing life phases or specific body training, changes in muscle architecture might influence the demonstration of strength and mobility. For instance, individuals who undergo resistance training will develop hypertrophy, which alters the mechanical characteristics of muscles responsible for skeletal movement. In addition, dynamic movement between the tendons of muscles and their respective bones is an important aspect of musculoskeletal dynamics, in which the distribution of load is a determinant of joint stability and mobility. Through high-level analysis and modeling, scientists can quantify such changes and enable profound insight into mechanisms of injury and subsequent rehabilitation (Codd et al., 2014). To understand the interaction of the musculoskeletal system, one must examine external factors, such as biomechanics and physiology, across various populations, for example, those with particular health statuses. In studies of broiler chickens, for example, serious musculoskeletal issues have been found, demonstrating how genetic selection for specific traits can compromise health. These findings highlight the broader importance of musculoskeletal health, going beyond human athletes to other animal species subjected to such biomechanical forces. As these studies illustrate, anatomical and physiological development can pose new challenges for locomotion and physical activity. Understanding of these intricate relationships assists researchers and practitioners in designing more effective interventions that will enhance performance and reduce injury, ultimately informing the broader field of functional anatomy and biomechanics (Harris et al., 2012) (Figure 1.14).

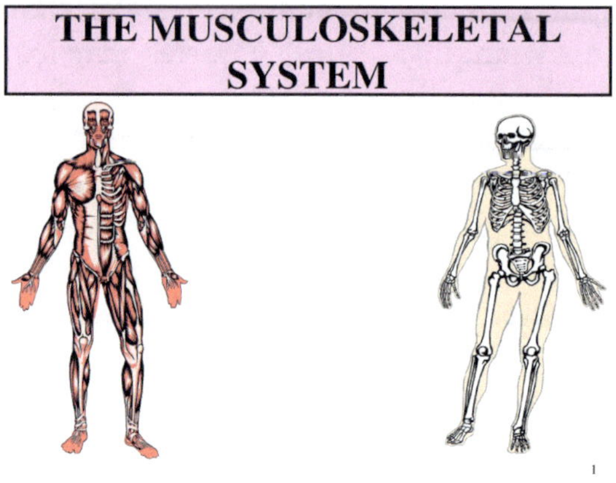

Figure 1.14. The human musculoskeletal system.

Source: https://external-content.duckduckgo.com/iu/?u=https%3A%2F%2Fimage5.slideserve.com%2F9542610%2Fthe-musculoskeletal-system-l.jpg&f=1&nofb=1&ipt=cfb4c25175c07d9539dcce2d54881c664743a48c8b552fd485eb682b08837086.

1.4.1. Role of Muscles in Movement

The role of muscles in movement is at the heart of the understanding of the biomechanics of the human skeleton. Muscles, through contraction and relaxation, generate forces that move and stabilize the skeleton. Skeletal muscles act together with the skeleton, having attachments at more than one place to bones by means of tendons to generate movement in joints. When contracted, a muscle generates a tensile force on a bone to create torque around a joint. This collaboration is not only vital for voluntary movements, such as standing, walking, and lifting, but also for simple involuntary activities, such as maintaining posture. The body's ability to adapt to various physical demands and situations is illustrated by the dynamic interaction of muscles and bones, and the essential role of muscle action in the system's overall function is clearly indicated. The architecture of the skeletal muscle is directly involved in its functional capacity and impacts movement effectiveness and efficiency. Muscles differ in fiber type, which influences their performance under different movement conditions. Fast-twitch fibers are suited to short bursts of power and speed and are involved in basic function during explosive movements, while slow-twitch fibers are resistant to fatigue, optimizing endurance. Moreover, as clarified in current research, structural and compositional changes in muscle with aging lead to decrements in force production and overall physical capacity. Connective tissue hardening and changes in the extracellular matrix are essential contributors to this decrement, affecting muscle recruitment strategy during contraction.

These microscopic alterations can significantly alter biomechanics and reveal subtleties, underscoring the importance of a robust muscular framework in maintaining movement and function with advancing age (Basava et al., 2020). Merging an understanding of muscle function with evolutionary biology can also provide valuable insights into muscle function in human movement. Investigations of extinct species' locomotor mechanics demonstrate how muscle architecture adapts to environmental pressures and provide informative context for contemporary human musculature. For instance, research on cancellous bone architecture demonstrates that muscle position and force output flexibility might be significantly influenced by anatomical variation in response to biomechanical loading. This information not only enhances our understanding of past species locomotion but also shapes modern practices in biomechanics and rehabilitation. The development of methods for modeling the correlation between muscle function and skeletal form underscores the need for an integrated perspective that combines skeletal alignment and muscle activation, thereby enhancing our understanding of the intricate biomechanical interactions that support human walking (Abourachid et al., 2018).

1.4.2. Tendons and Ligaments: Structure and Function

Tendons and ligaments belong to the musculoskeletal system, and each does a unique yet complementary function. Tendons basically connect muscles to bones, facilitating the transfer of muscular forces that enable movement. Their structure is composed of dense connective tissue characterized by collagen fibers oriented to resist tensile forces. This unique architecture allows tendons to resist mechanical stresses associated with most body activities, contributing to overall locomotor efficiency and stability. Ligaments, however, connect bones to other bones within joints to provide stability to joints and restrict excessive movement that could lead to injury. Strength in ligaments is achieved through elasticity, which allows them to absorb and transmit loads without being permanently deformed, thereby maintaining joint stability. The structural heterogeneity between tendons and ligaments is a reflection of their functional demands. For instance, while tendons possess parallel orientation of the collagen fibers, ligaments possess a more complex configuration that can sustain multi-directional loads. New evidence suggests that ligaments are not to be regarded as homogeneously built structures but possess a non-uniformed architecture tuned to their respective demands in terms of loading. This argument is supported by evidence relating to the periodontal ligament, which connects teeth and the jawbone. The fibrous structure of the periodontal ligaments is designed to withstand the fluctuating stresses that accompany activities such as chewing, illustrating a sophisticated adaptation for its peculiar role in the oral cavity. These results support the notion that knee and ankle ligaments are adapted for optimal performance under specific mechanical demands (Naveh et al., 2017). While investigating the biomechanical properties of ligaments, it is necessary to examine their three-dimensional anatomy and the effects of varying loading conditions. For instance, the anatomy study of the ostrich knee joint mentions interesting sesamoid bone and ligament mechanics. Presenting an excess of more than one patella in an ostrich raises questions about evolutionary adaptations that influence knee joint movement and stress transmission. Establishing these associations informs scholars about the mechanobiological attributes of the ligaments and the significant roles they play in maintaining joints stable against various stressors. They not only increase our knowledge about ligament function but also provide an avenue for further study to investigate the evolutionary and adaptive mechanisms behind ligamentous adaptations in other species, towards eventually building an integrated knowledge of the functional anatomy and biomechanics of the human skeleton (Abourachid et al., 2014) (Figure 1.15).

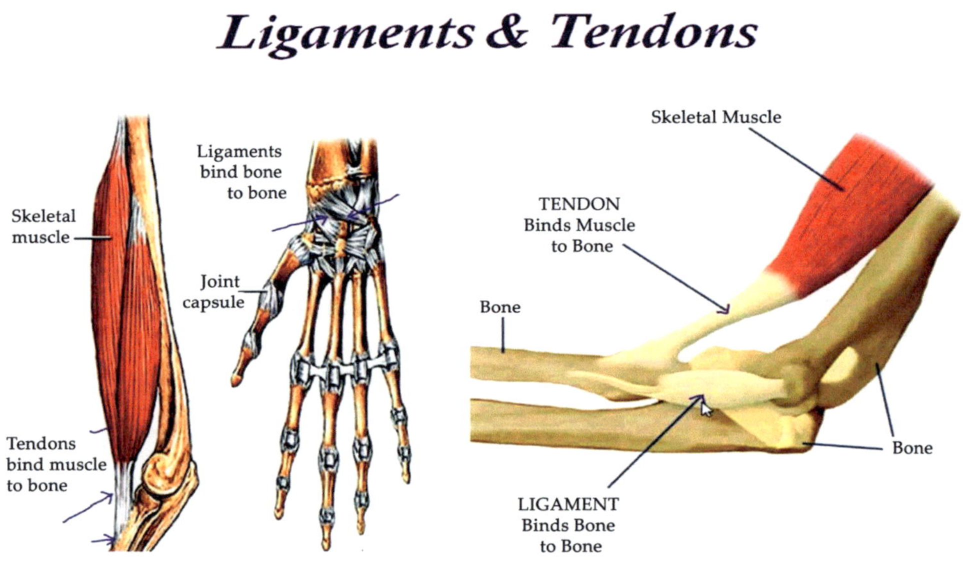

Figure 1.15. Tendons and ligaments: structure and function.

Source: https://external-content.duckduckgo.com/iu/?u=https%3A%2F%2Fs2.dmcdn.net%2Fv%2F9frzN1LICJYTMcE4I%2Fx1080&f=1&nofb=1&ipt=0873beb5a38c5b21fa1f3b043766c7a615975bc92925f4f537809257ac3e59b3.

1.4.3. Neuromuscular Control of Skeletal Movement

The neuromuscular regulation of skeletal movement is at the heart of the challenge of coordinating body function, providing the dynamic system in which muscle and bone work together. The central nervous system is at the center of this control, dynamically regulating muscle activation, synchronization, and inhibition to enable smooth and meaningful movement. Such intricate interaction not only facilitates basic movement but also enables the execution of complex motor tasks, such as sports performance or rehabilitation exercises. Understanding the control mechanisms involved in this neural control is essential for both clinical and sporting applications, particularly where movement patterns have the potential to influence performance outcomes or predispose an individual to injury. As scientists continue to study these mechanisms, new methods emerge that better explain how neuromuscular signals are translated into mechanical advantage, making the interventions used in movement therapy and biomechanics more effective (Baker et al., 2006). Studies on neuromuscular control also involve studies on biomechanical modeling, which attempts to simulate the intricate interactions between nervous impulses and muscle contractions. By employing technologies such as motion capture and electromyography, researchers can collect data on patterns of muscle activity in relation to various skeletal movements. This data serves as the core for developing biomechanical models that simulate human movement, providing insight into how specific muscle groups influence the efficiency and stability of movement. Aside from merely observing movement, such models may incorporate various biomechanical concepts and create an integrated framework for understanding the complexity of human movement. Thus, the application of advanced modeling techniques not only enhances our theoretical comprehension but also enables a finer analysis of neuromuscular control in practice, thereby improving rehabilitation processes and sporting training programs (Harris et al., 2012). Moreover, optimal neuromuscular control is the foundation for injury rehabilitation and prevention strategies in populations such as athletes and rehabilitation patients. Without intact neuromuscular pathways due to injury or neurological disease, resulting dysfunction can lead to aberrant movement patterns and susceptibility to secondary injury. Rehabilitation programs often involve neuromuscular training to restore proper muscle activation and control, enabling safe and effective movement. Techniques such as proprioceptive training and functional movement are designed to reeducate the nervous system, refining communication between brain and muscle. A sound appreciation of neuromuscular control enables practitioners to design specific interventions that not only facilitate recovery but also optimize performance, a key step towards maximizing functional movement in clinical and sporting contexts (Baker et al., 2006).

Test Your Knowledge

1. How do muscles and bones interact to produce movement in the human body?
2. What role do joints, tendons, and ligaments play in musculoskeletal system interaction?

1.5. Biomechanical Principles

Learning Outcome

1. Neuromuscular control of skeletal movement;
2. Newton's laws of motion applied to the skeleton;
3. Analysis of forces acting on bones during activities.

Understanding biomechanical concepts is crucial for examining the human skeleton, particularly in terms of the functional anatomy necessary for stability and movement. Biomechanics examines forces acting upon the skeletal system and how these forces are converted into motion. For instance, gravity is crucial for bone morphology and impacts processes such as biomineralization. In conditions such as microgravity during spaceflight, extensive changes in bone density occur, including demineralization and hypermineralization in several areas of the skeleton, particularly in gravity-dependent bones like the heelbone and skull. Spaceflight and ground-based simulation observations indicate the dynamic adaptation of bones to varied force conditions, highlighting the responsiveness and plasticity of the skeleton to biomechanical forces (Arnaud et al.). Further, clinical gait analysis breakthroughs serve to underscore the importance of understanding biomechanical concepts in practical application. Observations of movement patterns by sophisticated optical systems provide critical insights into the mechanics of walking and running. Current methods focus on accurately measuring kinematic information and the movement of soft tissues in relation to internal bone anatomy, including the same corrections. This degree of accuracy is significant in that it informs clinicians about the specific muscular treatments that can actually remodel biomechanics. Understanding of joint centers and axes of rotation has come to be at the core of the development of individualized treatment plans, enhancing rehabilitation techniques by providing biomechanically founded approaches to intervention (Baker et al., 2006).

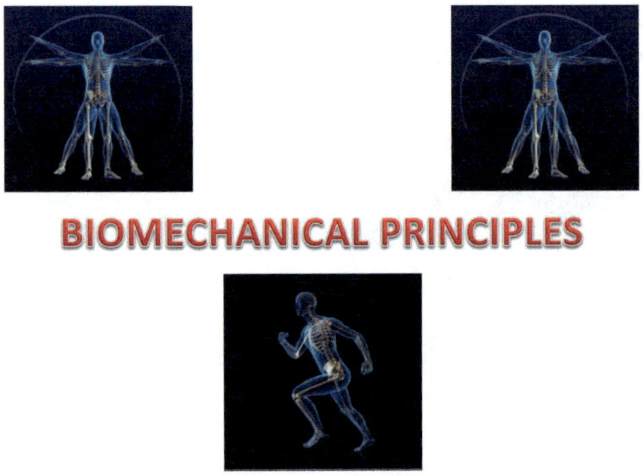

Figure 1.16. The understanding of biomechanical principles.

Source: https://external-content.duckduckgo.com/iu/?u=https%3A%2F%2Fimage1.slideserve.com%2F3193111%2Fbiomechanical-principles-l.jpg&f=1&nofb=1&ipt=d941b670c1462c61b33ba12261f1121dfe7b18cb263c9bcc4b069b7bf5d6ff50.

Ultimately, integrating cutting-edge modeling techniques with biomechanics provides greater insight into the interventions that influence human movement. Where existing deficits in knowledge about the exact processes underlying our gait patterns persist, they are being increasingly filled by research. Subject-specific models that integrate three-dimensional imaging of musculoskeletal anatomy hold promise for radical advancement in clinical gait analysis. Through the simulation of hypothetical interventions, such models can enhance predictive capability, benefitting clinicians in the choice of effective treatment for patients with varying pathologies. This dynamic setting illustrates how biomechanical concepts directly inform clinical practice, providing a pathway to improved outcomes through a biomechanically guided process (Baker et al., 2006) (Figure 1.16).

1.5.1. Newton's Laws of Motion Applied to the Skeleton

Newton's laws of motion applied to the human skeleton provide invaluable insights into biomechanics and functional anatomy. Newton's first law, the law of inertia, describes how objects maintain their position at rest or move uniformly unless a force is exerted upon them by another body. For example, when in a stationary posture, our skeletal system remains firm, requiring muscle contractions to produce movement, such as when standing up from a resting position. This law describes the necessary physical interactions that govern skeletal integrity, with a focus on the function of the muscle-tendon unit, which leverages forces generated by muscle contractions to allow the skeleton to adapt and respond dynamically to external loads or changes in movement. Newton's second law describes how force applied to an object causes it to accelerate in the direction of the force, which has important implications for the human skeleton. This is evident in movements involving rapid acceleration, such as running or jumping, where the significant force produced by the muscles is converted into movement. Biomechanical examination of such movement involves understanding how forces transmitted through the skeleton lead to rotation at the joints and body movement. For example, when there is a forceful quadriceps contraction during jumping, it generates sufficient force to extend the knee and elevate the body, showing the precise application of Newton's second law in sporting ability and daily existence, which must consider both muscle performance and external gravity acting on the body. Besides, Newton's third law, that for every action there exists an equivalent and opposite reaction, is significant in how one can comprehend how the skeleton reacts to its environment. When someone is pushing against the ground while walking or running, the ground pushes back with an equal amount of force in the direction that moves the person forward. This concept is of utmost significance in activities that involve explosive motions, and it highlights the importance of ground reaction forces in both sports and rehabilitation. The biomechanical functional integration also enables clinicians to investigate and predict potential injuries associated with abnormal force distributions, thereby enhancing the efficiency of surgical and treatment measures following muscle or tendon damage (King et al., 2015). The application of these elementary concepts not only serves the research field of biomechanics but also contributes to new practices in interrelated fields, such as space medicine, where customized exercise regimens help reverse the adverse effects of microgravity on the human skeleton (Harris et al., 2025).

1.5.2. Leverage and Mechanical Advantage in Movement

Understanding leverage and mechanical advantage is critical when learning about movement in the context of functional anatomy and human skeletal biomechanics. Leverage is most simply a term describing the in-lever:out-lever ratio. This will determine the effectiveness of a particular force at moving a joint, particularly in limbs. The human body is a complex system of levers, where bones serve as the fixed bars, joints act as fulcrums, and muscles provide the force. For instance, in activities such as lifting and jumping, variations in lever lengths affect the cost and efficiency of energy, and thus impact locomotion biomechanics, as shown in human locomotion efficiency comparisons based on biomimetic models (Crompton et al., 2003). This is key when contrasting biomechanical strategies employed across species and understanding evolutionary adaptations. Additionally, mechanical advantage in relation to certain movements affects the extent of flexibility in the musculoskeletal system under specific conditions. For example, for the craniomandibular region, changes in morphology would affect the functional functioning of Mrs. jaw. Evidence is found in that despite great morphological differences observed among various strains of mice, mechanical advantage in jaw movement remains sustained to a great extent because of adaptive modifications elsewhere in the body's skeletal system, especially on the muscle in-lever length (Baverstock et al., 2014). This is interpreted as a level of plasticity in the mechanical systems of biological organisms that enables efficient functioning, regardless of various morphological adaptations. Therefore, mechanical advantage not only contributes to single movements but also to what evolutionary mechanisms and structural restrictions of anatomy are telling us, and how form and function are interdependent. Leverage and mechanical advantage are valuable in practical contexts, too, in areas like rehabilitation and sport science. Understanding the tenets of these biomechanical principles can aid in the development of effective training regimens that enhance performance while minimizing the risk of injury. Through specific training, athletes can optimize their leverage for particular movements, such as running or jumping, thus increasing their mechanical advantage. Similarly, rehabilitation therapists can apply knowledge of movement mechanics to develop personalized recovery regimens aimed at restoring maximal joint function and muscular economy. This not only recognizes the value of learning leverage in biomechanics but also highlights its potential to facilitate improved movement economy and overall physical functioning in different populations. Its integration can lead to improved success in both clinical and sporting situations, promoting greater insight into the mechanical nature of the human body (Figure 1.17).

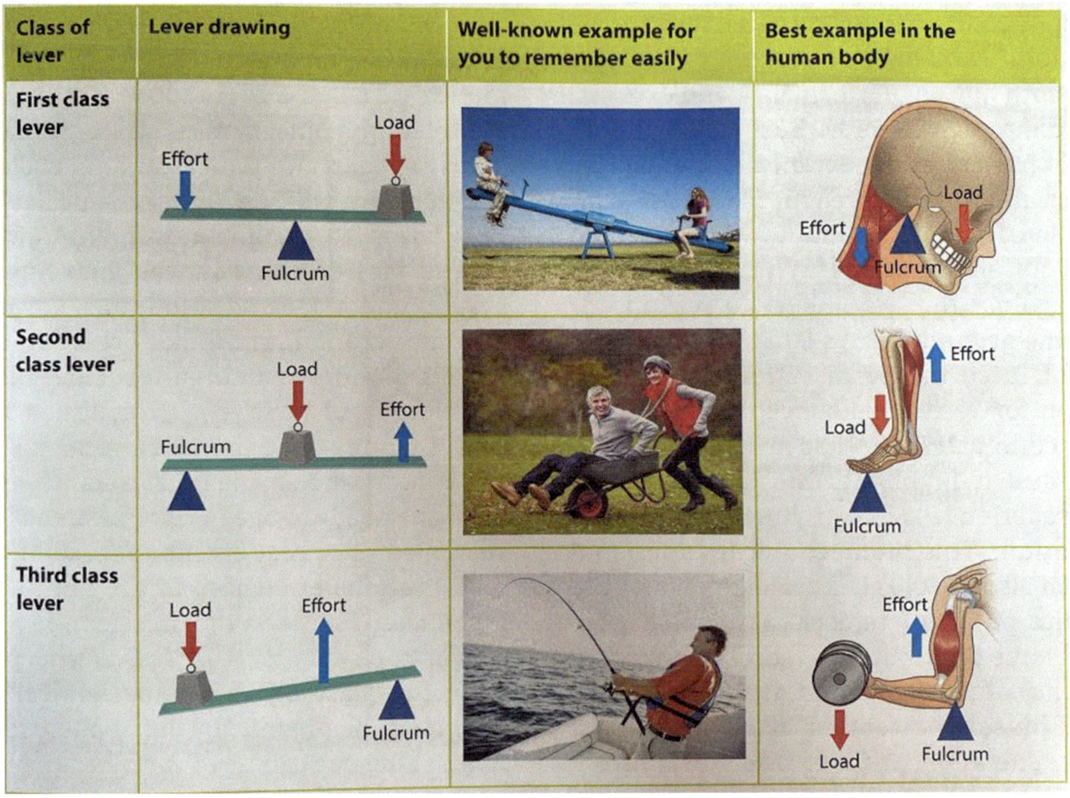

Figure 1.17. Leverage and mechanical advantage in movement.

Source: https://i.ytimg.com/vi/K6RYpUjfMOI/hqdefault.jpg.

1.5.3. Analysis of Forces Acting on Bones During Activities

The human skeleton is subjected to various forces during daily activities, which are essential for maintaining its structural integrity and function. Forces are produced due to muscle contraction, the force of gravity, and external load. Understanding how forces are applied to bone structures involves a complete understanding of biomechanics, the science of examining the mechanics of biological structures with particular reference to movement and load transmission. For instance, during walking or running, ground reaction forces generated by the feet provide upward pressure on the skeletal structure, which in turn influences bone adaptation and remodeling. This dynamic interaction of forces and bone structure is imperative for bone well-being, prevention of injury, and designing effective rehabilitation programs, thus emphasizing the importance of multidisciplinary research in functional anatomy and biomechanics (Harris et al., 2012). For sports or high-impact activities, however, the forces bones experience can be significantly magnified, making it increasingly likely to lead to injury or stress fractures. The proximal femur, for example, is subjected to heterogeneous patterns of loading when it is exposed to high-impact sports. Recent studies utilizing state-of-the-art techniques in biomechanical modeling, including finite element analysis, describe how loads can be responsible for creating mechanical stimuli that initiate bone remodeling events through mechanotransduction pathways. When external loads apply stress to bones, physiological responses are activated, allowing the skeletal system to become stronger and adapt to the forces applied to it. This adaptability is key to understanding bone's response to varying loads, and it highlights the importance of accurately examining stress distribution under different activities (Mathai et al., 2015). Additionally, the importance of variations in load path resulting from surgical interventions, such as total hip arthroplasties, underscores the highly intricate interaction of forces and bone status. Post-surgery patients often experience issues such as stress shielding, where the altered load pattern results in reduced mechanical stimulation of the bone surrounding the implant, which can impact the long-term viability of the graft. Some implants have been shown through experiments to alter stress distribution across the bone, leading to a radical transformation in the patterns of loading around the site of the procedure. Identifying superior implant designs that closely mimic the natural principles of load transmission is essential for avoidingcomplications and improving patient outcomes. Thus, force analysis on bones transcends simple observation and becomes crucial in advancing surgical intervention and improving rehabilitation efforts, as highlighted in today's biomechanical research (Mathai et al., 2015).

Test Your Knowledge

1. What are the basic biomechanical principles that govern human movement?
2. How do forces and levers influence motion and performance in the human body?

1.6. Common Skeletal Disorders

Learning Outcome

1. Osteoporosis and its impact on bone density
2. Arthritis and joint function
3. Fractures: types and healing processes

Skeletal disorders are a crucial area of interest in both clinical and developmental settings, impacting mobility and quality of life. Among the most prevalent skeletal disorders are osteoarthritis, osteoporosis, and other birth deformities. Osteoarthritis, a condition affecting joint cartilage degeneration, results in pain and stiffness that can severely impair physical activity. Conversely, osteoporosis is a disease that involves the reduction of bone density, rendering bones weak and susceptible to fractures. Both diseases highlight the intricacy of skeletal health and the need to know more about the functional anatomy of bones and joints. Knowing it is extremely important because it gives information about how to avoid these disorders and measures to mitigate the effects of these disorders in people's lives. The relevance is drawn across various age groups, and therefore there needs to be an investigation into how such universal skeletal conditions arise and develop at various stages of life. The biomechanics of human movement provides a general framework by which the subject of skeletal diseases can be considered. As investigated in biomechanics, how forces act on the skeleton can give clues to the etiology of conditions like chondronecrosis and angular deformity. For instance, augmented mechanical stress on involved joints has the potential to accelerate degenerative processes, hence accentuating pain and functional deficits. Additionally, the interrelationship between muscle architecture and osseous stability is very critical; unbalance of muscles could lead to pathological loading on bones and joints, thus worsening involved conditions. By understanding the interrelationships between these processes through biomechanical modeling, researchers and clinicians can develop intervention strategies, such as physical therapy or surgical correction, tailored to the individual patient's biomechanical profile. This complex understanding of skeletal disorders is a key reason why a multidisciplinary approach is crucial in developing optimal treatment protocols. New studies in biomechanics focus on the need to investigate how prevalent skeletal disorders develop throughout the stages of development.

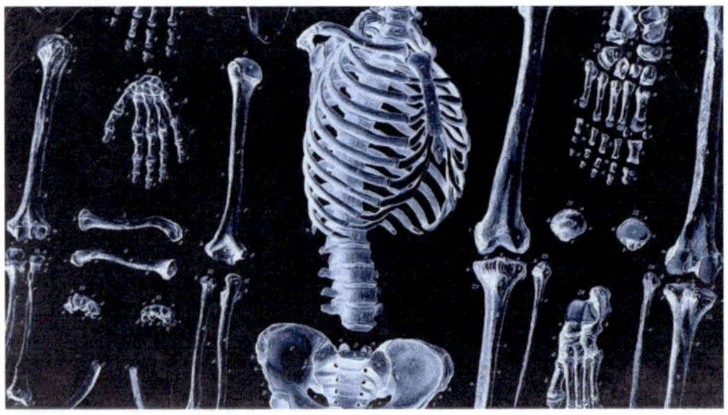

Figure 1.18. Skeletal disorders represent a significant area of concern within both clinical and developmental contexts.

Source: https://external-content.duckduckgo.com/iu/?u=https%3A%2F%2Fi0.wp.com%2Fpost.medicalnewstoday.com%2Fwp-content%2Fuploads%2Fsites%2F3%2F2022%2F03%2Fbone-diseases-engraved-drawing-header-1024x575.jpg%3Fw%3D1155%26h%3D1528&f=1&nofb=1&ipt=f88c8bccfdb503133c94a080fdc2fb38da69bd11a4c871b531e7d028854db3b3.

The analysis of growth-related changes suggests that anatomical and biomechanical changes may influence the expression of disorders in different populations, such as the elderly and athletic groups. For example, accumulation of muscle mass in youths can counterbalance the center of mass, influencing locomotion as well as susceptibility to injury. As stated in recent research, understanding of these alterations during development not only enables the diagnosis of skeletal diseases but also informs prevention. Furthermore, advances in methods and technology, such as finite element analysis, enable a precise examination of biomechanical interactions within the skeleton. Through the combination of findings from biomechanics with clinical understanding, we can enhance our understanding of common skeletal conditions and explore new approaches to improve skeletal health and function in the broader community (Harris et al., 2012; Codd et al., 2014) (Figure 1.18).

1.6.1. Osteoporosis and Its Impact on Bone Density

The mechanical properties of the human skeleton are significantly dependent on bone density, and they are profoundly affected by osteoporotic changes. Osteoporosis is a progressive reduction in bone mass and deterioration in bone tissue, resulting in increased fragility and susceptibility to fractures. Osteoporosis generally goes undetected until a fracture manifests, with the underlying decrease in bone density. Especially trabecular bone, which sustains the majority of the skeletal load, undergoes dramatic changes in osteoporosis. This has been demonstrated in studies to be lower in contemporary humans than in other primates, perhaps a sign of evolutionary adaptation with potential impact on bone health. This reduction in density, particularly in the long bones of the limbs, highlights how evolutionary thinking may have laid the groundwork for contemporary health issues related to bone density (Zipfel et al., 2014). How extensive such changes are is broad-reaching, affecting not only biomechanics but also the quality of one's life as advancing age takes hold. Besides, the biomechanical implications of osteoporosis are substantial, with a higher likelihood of vertebral compression fractures (VCFs). The fractures often occur due to compromised bone quality and geometric deformities of the vertebral body. Reduced bone density in osteoporosis is an indirect cause of these fractures, adding to the risk of future fractures at adjacent vertebral levels. Using image-based finite element analysis (FEA), researchers have shown that osteoporotic spine fragility directly influences its load-carrying capacity, which, in turn, governs stress and strain distribution during mechanical loading. The intricate interactions among osteoporosis, bone density, and mechanical response underscore the need for targeted interventions to ensure proper control and prevention of fracture risk. Such knowledge of the biomechanical modifications caused by osteoporosis may benefit clinical practice to optimize surgical outcomes and improve the patient's quality of life (Mazlan et al., 2016). Considering the severity of osteoporosis's effect on bone density, it is obvious that preventive measures and therapeutic strategies are needed to maintain the skeleton in health, particularly in individuals at higher risk, such as postmenopausal women and the elderly. Interventions such as pharmacological interventions, dietary interventions, and weight-bearing exercise have also been found to be beneficial in reversing bone density loss. Acquiring information on one's risk factors, for example, genetic and lifestyle factors, can also help direct early interventions to preserve bone integrity. Because of the seriousness of maximum bone density in skeletal structural integrity, various approaches integrating prevention and therapy are required. As research advances to uncover the complexities of osteoporosis and its impact on bone density, it is clear that interdisciplinary collaboration is necessary to develop synergistic treatment plans that maintain the functional anatomy and biomechanics of the human skeleton across all ages.

1.6.2. Arthritis and Joint Function

Arthritis profoundly affects joint function, producing pain, stiffness, and decreased mobility. This condition encompasses several different diseases affecting the joints, the two most prevalent being osteoarthritis and rheumatoid arthritis. Osteoarthritis results from breakdown of cartilage and increased friction within the joints, while rheumatoid arthritis results from an autoimmune disease that causes chronic inflammation and joint destruction. Functional anatomy of the joints, as the intricate relationship between bones, cartilage, ligaments, and synovial fluid, is relevant to the pathogenesis of arthritis. With loss of biomechanical function of the synovial joint due to cartilage erosion, pain and disability ensue.

These changes in joint mechanics call for a wide approach to treatment, not just palliation but restoration and preservation of joint function to optimize movement and quality of life. The biomechanics of joint function during arthritis suggest the need to maintain movement patterns that minimize further injury. Joint loads must be regulated to prevent excessive stress on compromised joint structures. Adaptive measures such as altering gait or using assistive devices can be used to reduce excessive pressure and enhance functional mobility, for instance. Biomechanics studies show that understanding the forces that affect joints can be used to develop specific therapeutic interventions, such as physical therapy and surgery. By applying advanced modeling techniques, such as those used in biomechanics research, clinicians can simulate joint behavior under varying conditions to optimize treatment plans that reduce pain while achieving maximum functional outcomes. Such treatments are essential in ensuring independence and an active life for individuals with arthritis. Moreover, research into conditions like Perthes disease informs us about the complex interaction between skeletal maturation and joint function. This disorder of growth hip shows how anatomical and biomechanical factors can predispose a person to long-term joint issues.

The relationship between vascular supply and joint integrity highlights the importance of early diagnosis and treatment. This disease in children has the potential to result in complications, which reflect the relevance of genetic and environmental factors to joint health. Comprehending such conditions in terms of functional anatomy and biomechanics can inform preventive measures and treatment plans. With increasing research, the field of arthritis and allied diseases will continue to move closer toward developing new approaches to address both the symptomology and etiology of joint dysfunction in the human skeleton (Harris et al., 2012; Acheson et al., 2016).

1.6.3. Fractures: Types and Healing Processes

Fractures are a significant concern in human skeletal functional anatomy and are classified into several categories based on their nature and type of injury. Simple (or closed) fractures, where the bone never pierces the skin, and compound (or open) fractures, where the bone pierces through the skin and thus carries a high infection risk, are among the well-known types of fractures. Other types include transverse, oblique, and comminuted fractures, each with a specific break pattern. Understanding these types is essential, as they dictate the treatment method required and the healing process to be expected. Regardless of type, fractures initiate a cascade of biological reactions aimed at restoring skeletal integrity. This biological response is influenced by various factors, including patients' health, age, and the fracture site. Fracture healing isn't always straightforward and generally happens in four phases: hematoma formation, formation of fibrocartilaginous callus, formation of bony callus, and bone remodeling. In the first instance, a hematoma forms at the fracture site, followed by an influx of inflammatory cells that contribute to healing. Subsequently, during the second stage, a fibrocartilaginous callus forms, providing temporary stabilization. This intermediate tissue, composed of cartilage and collagen, bridges the fracture ends. Then, during bony callus formation, the fibrocartilaginous tissue is replaced by a hard bony callus through endochondral ossification. Finally, bone remodeling involves reforming the bone structure and restoring its mechanical function. This multi-step healing process is crucial in returning the bone to its original function and integrity, illustrating the dynamic interaction of cellular and biomechanical parameters in fracture healing. Biomechanical factors dominate fracture healing, since they determine the character and extent of healing. The application of mechanical loads, for instance, may significantly affect the quality and rate of healing.

Advanced monitoring technology, such as intramedullary nails with strain gauges, has in the recent past given a better picture regarding the mechanical conditions of fracture healing *in-vivo*. Real-time measurement of loading conditions and the applied mechanical stimulus to the healing bone is achievable using this innovative approach. By modeling varying loading conditions, researchers gain better insight into the interaction between mechanical forces and biological healing processes, enabling tailored rehabilitation plans for patients. Understanding such biomechanical parameters eventually helps orthopedic professionals to maximize treatment and improve recovery rates in fracture patients (Nemchand et al., 2015; Flores et al., 2017) (Figure 1.19).

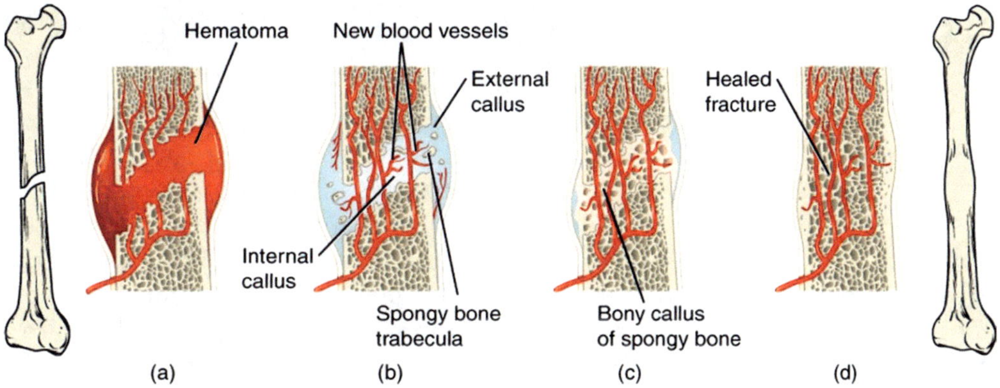

Figure 1.19. Fractures: types and healing processes.

Source: https://s3-us-west-2.amazonaws.com/courses-images-archive-read-only/wp-content/uploads/sites/18/2014/07/19181253/613_Stages_of_Fracture_Repair.jpg.

Test Your Knowledge

1. What are some common skeletal disorders, such as osteoporosis or arthritis?

How do common skeletal disorders affect bone structure and movement?

SUMMARY

It is necessary to understand the complex interplay between skeletal form and its biomechanical functions. The human skeleton is not only a support and protective structural framework but also a dynamic structure that participates in multiple physiological functions. The functional complexity of bone shape, muscle attachments, and joint motion enables multiple types of movement required for daily tasks. From a biomechanical point of view, it is apparent that the skeletal system is shaped for both mobility and stability, thereby demonstrating the evolutionary mechanisms that have enabled human beings to survive in diverse environments. Furthermore, advancements in imaging and modeling technologies, as demonstrated in current research studies, are essential to understanding skeletal biomechanics. The incorporation of high-resolution imaging enables the precise reconstruction of anatomical models, which are of significant importance in areas such as orthopedics and rehabilitation. By using advanced methods to examine the geometrical and anatomical features of bones and related soft tissues, scientists have improved the quantitative understanding of the function of skeletal structures under different loads and conditions (Audenaert et al., 2010). These findings are not only valuable for clinical application but also for the development of surgical technique, providing a foundation for improved patient outcomes. Last, the application of FEA in anatomical studies underscores the importance of accurate modeling in elucidating the mechanics of the skeleton. While FEA is difficult due to the simplifications inherent in model representation, it remains an excellent tool for studying the relationship between skeletal form and function. Evidence demonstrates that slight differences in model geometry can substantially impact predicted bone biomechanical behavior, reinforcing the importance of cautious interpretation (Barak et al., 2015). With ongoing progress in functional anatomy and the biomechanics sciences, ongoing research will be essential to their further refinement, thereby contributing to our integrated understanding of the important role of human skeletons in disease and health.

The human skeleton is a vital framework of the body and a support for movement. The skeleton consists of 206 bones in adult life, and it provides structure and defense for many of the body's vital organs. In its developed form, the skeleton not only facilitates the attachment of muscles but also supports elaborate sets of motion, from the fine dexterity of the hands to the strong locomotion of the limbs. Variation in bone shape and size in response to mechanical loading allows the skeleton to accommodate and optimize function. A case in point is the long limb bones, tailored for leverage and strength, essential for walking on two limbs. This adaptation supports balance and efficient motion, underscoring the skeletal system's contribution to daily functional activities and athletic performance, and reflecting the evolutionary advantage of human adaptability. Apart from its structural support function, the human skeleton is also engaged in blood cell production, hematopoiesis. In the medullary cavities of long bones, bone marrow harbors stem cells that mature into red blood cells, white blood cells, and platelets, all of which play crucial roles in the body. The dual role of the skeleton thus emphasizes an advanced interaction between mechanical and biological processes. Also, the skeletal system's ability to supply mineral homeostasis, in this instance, calcium and phosphorus, is crucial for overall health. The body also uses the skeletal system as a storehouse for minerals, releasing them into the circulatory system when needed, thereby supporting several physiological processes, such as muscle contraction and nerve function, to run smoothly. These functions serve to indicate the importance of the skeleton beyond structural stability. Biomechanics further contributes to our understanding of the functional relevance of human skeletons by investigating how bones and forces interact with structures during movement. FEA has been instrumental in simulating the cranium to investigate how skeletal function and shape correlate and how these components respond to various types of loading (Barak et al., 2015). These types of evaluations show that model simplifications can significantly affect the interpretation of strain patterns within the bony framework. Moreover, comparative studies reveal that musculoskeletal changes during ontogeny can manifest in different locomotor mechanics and muscle structure, as observed in other species such as broiler chickens (Codd et al., 2014). Therefore, understanding the functional sophistication of the human skeleton not only enhances our understanding of human health and performance but also offers ways to treat musculoskeletal disease.

KEY TERMS FROM THIS CHAPTER

- Elasticity
- Appendicular skeleton
- Short bone
- Irregular bone
- Spongy (cancellous) bone
- Epiphysis
- Articulation
- Axial skeleton
- Long bone
- Flat bone
- Compact bone
- Periosteum
- Diaphysis
- Synovial joint

CRITICAL THINKING QUESTIONS

1. Which of the following bones is classified as a long bone?

a. Scapula
b. Femur
c. Vertebra
d. Sternum

2. The primary function of synovial joints is to:

a. Store minerals
b. Provide shock absorption
c. Allow free movement between bones
d. Protect internal organs

3. Which law explains how bone adapts to mechanical stress?

a. Boyle's Law
b. Newton's Third Law
c. Wolff's Law
d. Pascal's Law

4. The knee joint is an example of a:

a. Pivot joint
b. Saddle joint
c. Hinge joint
d. Ball-and-socket joint

5. Which part of the skeleton primarily absorbs compressive forces during standing and walking?

a. Skull
b. Thoracic cage
c. Pelvis and lower limbs
d. Upper limbs

Short Answer Questions

1. What is meant by the term "functional anatomy" in the context of the human skeleton?
2. How does the structure of a long bone contribute to its mechanical function?
3. Describe the role of the vertebral column in weight bearing and movement.
4. What biomechanical advantages do the curves of the spine provide?
5. How do joints enable both stability and mobility in the skeleton? Provide an example.
6. Explain the relationship between bone remodeling and mechanical stress.

Answers to Critical Thinking Questions

1. (b); 2. (c); 3. (c); 4. (c); 5. (c)

REFERENCES

1. Bishop, P. J., Hocknull, S. A., Clemente, C. J., Hutchinson, J. R., Farke, A. A., Beck, B. R., Barrett, R. S., & Lloyd, D. G. (2018b). Cancellous bone and theropod dinosaur locomotion. Part I—an examination of cancellous bone architecture in the hindlimb bones of theropods. *PeerJ*, *6*, e5778. https://doi.org/10.7717/peerj.5778Abourachid, A., Abourachid, A., Adachi, N., Alexander, R. M., Allen, V., Allen, W. L., Allmendinger, R., et al. (2018). Cancellous bone and theropod dinosaur locomotion. Part II—A new approach to inferring posture and locomotor biomechanics in extinct tetrapod vertebrates. https://core.ac.uk/download/161818789.pdf (accessed on 21st July 2025).

2. Abourachid, A., Alexander, R. M., Barnett, C. H., Benjamin, M., Bezuidenhout, A. J., Carter, D. R., Carter, D. R., et al. (2014). Three-dimensional anatomy of the ostrich (*Struthio camelus*) knee joint. https://core.ac.uk/download/36778017.pdf (accessed on 21st July 2025).

3. Acheson, R. M., Acheson, R. M., Adler, R. S., Allen, D. G., Anderson, F. C., Arie, J. P., Atsumi, M., et al. (2016). Skeletal immaturity, rostral sparing, and disparate hip morphologies as biomechanical causes for Legg-Calvé-Perthes' disease. https://core.ac.uk/download/151159396.pdf (accessed on 21st July 2025).

4. Adams, A. M. (1993). Degenerative joint disease and changing subsistence activities in the Arkansas River Valley. https://core.ac.uk/download/492586132.pdf (accessed on 21st July 2025).

5. Alias, M. A., & Buenzli, P. R. (2018). Osteoblasts infill irregular pores under curvature and porosity controls: A hypothesis-testing analysis of cell behaviors. http://arxiv.org/abs/1711.08548 (accessed on 21st July 2025).

6. Arnaud, S. B., & Morey-Holton, E. (2025). Skeletal responses to spaceflight. https://core.ac.uk/download/pdf/42812904.pdf (accessed on 21st July 2025).

7. Audenaert, E., Mahieu, P., Pattyn, C., Van Hoof, T., et al. (2010). Soft tissue structure modelling for use in orthopedic applications and musculoskeletal biomechanics. https://core.ac.uk/download/55761253.pdf (accessed on 21st July 2025).

8. Baker, R. J. (2006). Gait analysis methods in rehabilitation. https://core.ac.uk/download/1665518.pdf (accessed on 21st July 2025).

9. Barak, M. M., Benazzi, S., Berthaume, M. A., Bright, J. A., Bright, L., Chamoli, U., Cox, P. G., et al. (2015). Validity and sensitivity of a human cranial finite element model: Implications for comparative studies of biting performance. https://core.ac.uk/download/151160905.pdf (accessed on 21st July 2025).

10. Basava, R. R., Chen, J. S., He, Q., He, X., et al. (2020). Microstructural analysis of skeletal muscle force generation during aging. https://core.ac.uk/download/286361329.pdf (accessed on 21st July 2025).

11. Baverstock, H. (2014). Craniofacial integration, plasticity and biomechanics in the mouse masticatory system. https://core.ac.uk/download/556179607.pdf (accessed on 21st July 2025).

12. Brånemark, R., & Li, Y. (2017). Osseointegrated prostheses for rehabilitation following amputation: The pioneering Swedish model. https://core.ac.uk/download/323073835.pdf (accessed on 21st July 2025).

13. Buckland, D. M. (2011). Ultrasound imaging of cervical spine motion for extreme acceleration

environments. https://core.ac.uk/download/4432716.pdf (accessed on 21st July 2025).

14. Chang, J., Yang, X., & Zhang, J. J. (2007). Animating human muscle structure. https://core.ac.uk/download/76722.pdf (accessed on 21st July 2025).
15. Codd, J., Hutchinson, J. R., Manchester, P. A., Paxton, H. P., et al. (2014). Anatomical and biomechanical traits of broiler chickens across ontogeny. Part II. Body segment inertial properties and muscle architecture of the pelvic limb. https://core.ac.uk/download/36777728.pdf (accessed on 21st July 2025).
16. Crompton, R. H., Dennis, L. A., & Sellers, W. I. (2003). Predicting the metabolic energy costs of bipedalism using evolutionary robotics. https://core.ac.uk/download/98163.pdf (accessed on 21st July 2025).
17. Czubacka, P., Jaworski, Ł., & Karpiński, R. (2017). The structural and mechanical properties of the bone. https://core.ac.uk/download/249339858.pdf (accessed on 21st July 2025).
18. Flores, A., Machado, J., Marques, A., Marta, A., et al. (2017). Bone immobilization devices and consolidation mechanisms: Impact on healing time. https://core.ac.uk/download/154176088.pdf (accessed on 21st July 2025).
19. Giorgi, M. (2015). Mechanobiological predictions of fetal joint morphogenesis. https://core.ac.uk/download/77001843.pdf (accessed on 21st July 2025).
20. Goswami, A., & Randau, M. (2018). Shape covariation (or the lack thereof) between vertebrae and other skeletal traits in felids: The whole is not always greater than the sum of parts. https://core.ac.uk/download/154748431.pdf (accessed on 21st July 2025).
21. Harris, B. A., & Siconolfi, S. F. (2025). Workshop on countering space adaptation with exercise: Current issues. https://core.ac.uk/download/pdf/42787225.pdf (accessed on 21st July 2025).
22. Harris, G. F., & Slavens, B. A. (2012). *Biomechanics*. https://core.ac.uk/download/213080657.pdf (accessed on 21st July 2025).
23. Kawano, S. (2014). Evaluation of the functional capabilities of fins and limbs for moving on land: Insights into the invasion of land by tetrapods. https://core.ac.uk/download/268633502.pdf (accessed on 21st July 2025).
24. Keller, T. S., & Strauss, A. M. (2025). Bone loss and human adaptation to lunar gravity. https://core.ac.uk/download/pdf/42810351.pdf (accessed on 21st July 2025).
25. King, R. J. (2015). *Doctor of Philosophy*. https://core.ac.uk/download/276265894.pdf (accessed on 21st July 2025).
26. Kivell, T. L., Lemelin, P., Richmond, B. G., Schmitt, D., et al. (2016). *The Primate Wrist*. https://core.ac.uk/download/46164637.pdf (accessed on 21st July 2025).
27. Mathai, B. (2015). Finite element analysis to quantify the effect of surgery in proximal femur. https://core.ac.uk/download/80148540.pdf (accessed on 21st July 2025).
28. Mazlan, M. H. (2016). Biomechanical analysis of osteoporotic spines with diseases using CT-based finite element method. https://core.ac.uk/download/83541263.pdf (accessed on 21st July 2025).
29. N/A. (2025). *Musculoskeletal Discipline Science Plan*. https://core.ac.uk/download/pdf/42808673.pdf (accessed on 21st July 2025).

30. Naveh, G. (2017). Non uniformity: Structural strategy for optimizing functionality in skeletal ligaments. https://open.bu.edu/bitstream/2144/26296/5/Naveh_bu_0017N_13279.pdf (accessed on 21st July 2025).

31. Nemchand, J. L. (2015). Smart implant: The biomechanical testing of instrumented intramedullary nails during simulated callus healing using telemetry for fracture healing monitoring. https://core.ac.uk/download/30339830.pdf (accessed on 21st July 2025).

32. Post, E. (2013). Correlation of shoulder and elbow kinetics with ball velocity in college baseball pitchers. https://core.ac.uk/download/48840818.pdf (accessed on 21st July 2025).

33. Rockhold, L. A. (1998). Secular change in external femoral measures from 1840 to 1970: A biomechanical interpretation. https://core.ac.uk/download/599479349.pdf (accessed on 21st July 2025).

34. Zipfel, B., Richmond, B. G., Ruff, C. B., Cowgill, L. W., Eaton, S., Chirchir, H., Hublin, J. J., et al. (2014). Recent origin of low trabecular bone density in modern humans. https://core.ac.uk/download/30710129.pdf (accessed on 21st July 2025).

GROWTH, DEVELOPMENT, AND SKELETAL AGING

2

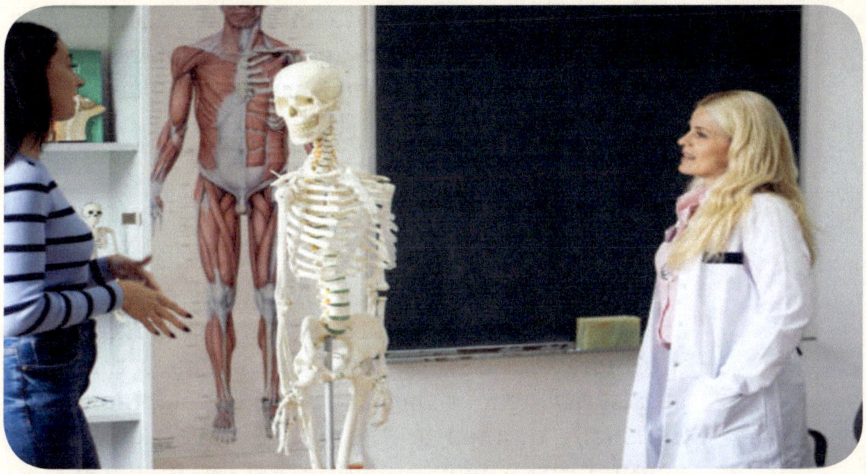

LEARNING OBJECTIVES

After studying this chapter, you will be able to:

1. Discuss the stages of skeletal growth
2. Explain the factors influencing skeletal development
3. Describe the bone remodeling process
4. Know aging and skeletal changes
5. Understand osteoporosis and skeletal aging
6. Focus on prevention and management of skeletal aging

Introduction

The intricate processes of development and growth exert a significant influence on skeletal aging, a process characterized by structural and functional bone alterations. Understanding the correlation is highly critical because it has a direct bearing on people's health and well-being throughout their lifetimes. During growth, characterized by active cell proliferation and differentiation, bones become highly mineralized and denser. As the body continues in early stages of life, the dynamics are significantly altered as the body moves toward later life. The resorption-to-formation ratio becomes increasingly disturbed, leading to most of the skeletal disorders prevalent among elderly subjects. This opening sets the stage for an investigation of the biological and physiologic processes that regulate skeletal aging and highlights the need to address these changes to promote longevity and enhance quality of life. Skeletal aging is inextricably linked to alterations in body composition, namely the cross-talk between muscle mass and fat distribution. More and more studies indicate that sarcopenia, or muscle mass decrease, often occurs concomitantly with augmented body fat deposition, which has significant severe clinical implications for the elderly. Intriguingly, fat redistribution—even to tissues other than fat, such as skeletal muscle—may be detrimental to muscle quality, thereby exacerbating age-associated declines in physical condition and mobility. These shifts in body composition have serious consequences as they are associated with declining physical function and increased risk for disability and death in older individuals.

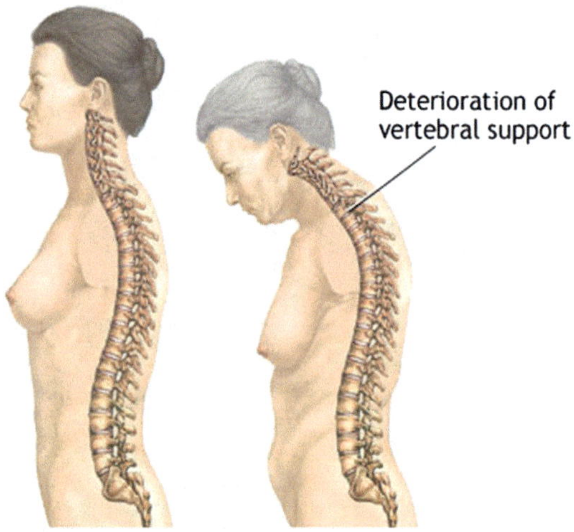

Figure 2.1. The development significantly influences skeletal aging.

Source: https://ssl.adam.com/graphics/images/en/17287.jpg.

Therefore, it is important to understand how these biological processes are interconnected to develop preventive and therapeutic strategies to counteract the unwanted consequences of skeletal aging, as clearly demonstrated by research on muscle quality and its interaction with increased fat mass in aging subjects (Carter et al., 2019). Moreover, regular physical exercise is a key determinant for undoing the adverse effects of skeletal aging on muscle function and metabolic well-being. Exercise cannot be overstressed, as a biological stimulus, its effectiveness has been shown through augmenting skeletal integrity and causing adaptive changes in muscle tissue. Exercise mimetics, or drugs that mimic the physiological effects of exercise, are currently being explored as treatments for age-related muscle and metabolic diseases. Research indicates that such medications can activate pathways in skeletal muscle usually restricted to exercise and hence trigger more profound health benefits in older people. This relationship between exercise, muscle function, and bone health highlights the importance of adding physical activity to interventions that promote more favorable aging trajectories as people move through the various life stages (Handschin et al., 2014) (Figure 2.1).

Definition of Growth and Development

The concepts of growth and development are fundamental pillars in understanding the biological and physiological changes that persist throughout one's life cycle. Development is usually defined as the quantitative rise in amount or weight, manifesting in physical form at various stages of life, particularly at childhood and adolescence. Qualitative changes that result in maturation and organ function are referred to as development, rather than growth. This distinction is essential because it provides an overall view of how people develop physically and mentally. Growth might level off as people get older, but development persists, resulting in improved cognitive function, emotional strength, and social functioning. This distinction is crucial in the aging process, where sustaining growth and development can influence overall health outcomes and well-being. Further, the skeletal aging process is also pivotal in the overall definition of growth and development. Throughout human development, the skeletal system undergoes changes in bone density, mass, and structural integrity. All these changes are inherent results of both growth and development and are influenced by genetic, hormonal, and environmental factors.

The progressive reduction in bone strength results in conditions such as osteoporosis, particularly among older individuals, in which the balance between bone loss and acquisition tilts toward loss. Bone weakening is a sign not only of physical development that has leveled off but also of developmental factors in mobility, independence, and disease susceptibility. It is important to recognize such changes in combating the health conditions of aging, tying back into the definitions of growth and development. Lastly, how the two interact has significant implications for understanding conditions resulting from aging, e.g., sarcopenia, a condition characterized by muscle degeneration and functional loss. As explained, sarcopenia results from the deterioration of muscle mass and function with aging, impacting locomotion and overall health.

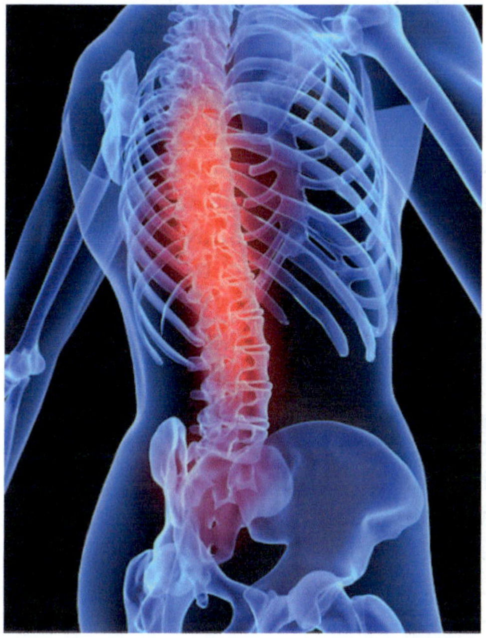

Figure 2.2. The concepts of growth and development.

Source: https://lh4.googleusercontent.com/proxy/GffoCqYsupA4VgGaEU18gx5btWdJZPfQQqiJwDzcLsl-KAZLt6suWjFcKJmPLAZEKTTqlakU40GupmuGZ_0Us2KXwmXHtkH9pyzkbqzQ4GJFiznKRYXt.

The pathophysiology is multifaceted, encompassing both structural changes at the level of individual motor units and qualitative changes in muscle proteins, as addressed in the aging and muscle biology literature (Larsson et al., 2018). The same is true for epidemiological research documenting that the elderly population carries a burgeoning burden of non-fatal disease, supporting the rationale for incorporating growth and development in addressing age-related disease (James et al., 2018). By investigating these interconnected themes, we can foster an enhanced awareness of how growth and development shape skeletal health across the life course (Figure 2.2).

Importance of Skeletal Health

Skeletal health is more than a physical structure; it is part of overall health across the life course. Healthy bones provide the scaffold that facilitates movement and the support for the remainder of the body's physiology, from the protection of organs to the control of hormones. So, skeletal health must be maintained throughout all ages. Skeletal formation is a priority in children and adolescents, as it establishes peak bone mass. Early deficiencies in bone health can lead to fractures and osteoporosis later in life, underscoring the need for proper nutrition and physical activity for proper growth and development. In that regard, awareness of food culture and lifestyle influences that shape bone strength needs to be created so that long-term health is established throughout the life course. The significance of bone health increases with age, as bone diseases are more prevalent. As the population is aging around the world, the burden of musculoskeletal disorders has emerged as a rising public health concern, based on evidence indicating musculoskeletal disorders were among the leading causes of years lived with disability (YLDs) in 2017 (Zhou et al., 2019). Osteoporosis, for instance, affects millions of individuals across the globe and is characterized by brittle bones and an increased susceptibility to fractures and morbidity. Women after menopause are at special risk due to the shift in hormones that directly affects the bone density. The impacts of compromised skeletal health can lead to long-term pain, loss of independence, and increased healthcare costs; hence, the significance of interventions to ensure bone strength in older years. Further, modern epidemiological studies emphasize the importance of targeting modifiable lifestyle and environmental risk factors that influence skeletal health. Dietary modifications, lack of physical exercise, and lifestyle-related factors have been associated with the rising prevalence of bone disease among populations (James et al., 2018). Encouraging weight-bearing exercise on a day-to-day basis, optimizing calcium and vitamin D intake, and reducing risk factors such as smoking can go a long way toward enhancing skeletal well-being. These preventive measures are critical in minimizing the effects of aging on the skeletal system and significantly optimizing the quality of life among the elderly. Public health promotion efforts that enhance awareness and the availability of services such as nutritional counseling and exercise programs can also reinforce individual and collective measures to ensure skeletal health (Figure 2.3).

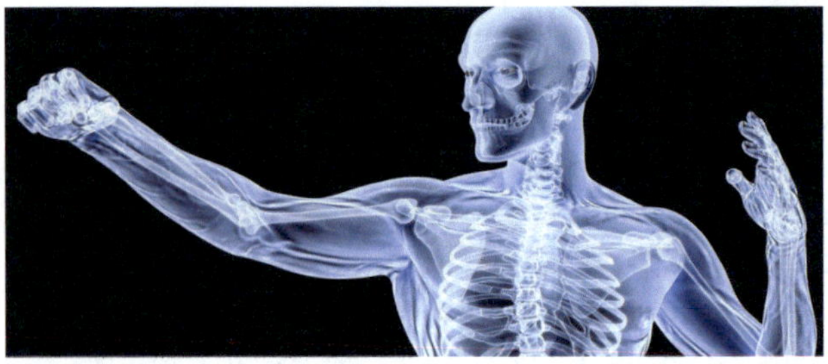

Figure 2.3. The significance of skeletal health.

Source: https://www.dhananjaygupta.com/wp-content/uploads/2018/01/Health-Bones.jpg.

Overview of Skeletal Aging

Skeletal aging is a dynamic biological process that progresses incrementally over the course of life, influenced by numerous interrelated factors. The older one gets, the more dramatically the skeleton alters, with changes in bone density, form, and overall strength. Of the greatest fears of skeletal aging is osteoporosis, characterized by reduced bone density and increased risk of fracture. This reduction is not merely due to aging but is also exacerbated by conditions such as physical inactivity, nutritional deprivation, and hormonal changes. These need to be understood to develop effective interventions that will reverse the impact of skeletal aging, thus allowing individuals to have a better quality of life as they grow older. The weakening of bones with age is also closely linked to various physiological processes, like the balance between formation and resorption of bones. Such processes are generally well-synchronized in healthy young individuals; however, with advancing age, this balance gets lost, in which more bone is resorbed than formed. This shift could be pertinent to the rise in the prevalence of non-alcoholic fatty liver disease (NAFLD) and highlights the complex interplay between metabolic status and skeletal health. NAFLD and other such diseases in the elderly can further accelerate bone mineral loss and muscle wasting, leading to osteoporosis and sarcopenia, respectively (Chiesa et al., 2017). As these interlinked claims of health issues become increasingly salient, understanding their common mechanisms is essential for developing effective treatment modalities. Furthermore, the implications of skeletal aging extend beyond bone health to encompass wide-ranging systemic influences. The connection between skeletal strength and other body systems, such as metabolic function, underscores the utility of a multisystem approach in aging research. Epidemiological studies have implicated that compromised skeletal health may be the cause of increased morbidity and poorer health outcomes in older individuals. It is essential to embrace preventive measures that help maintain bone health at a young age, including proper nutrition that is calcium and vitamin D-rich and regular exercise. By giving these prevention approaches high priority, we can optimize the overall resiliency of the skeletal system to the forces of aging; these measures would not only maximize lifetime health gains but could conceivably prevent the onset of conditions such as NAFLD associated with skeletal aging (Chiesa et al., 2017).

2.1. Stages of Skeletal Growth

Learning Outcome

1. Prenatal skeletal development
2. Childhood and adolescent growth spurts
3. Peak bone mass attainment

The stages of skeletal development are a dynamic interaction of physiological processes that eventually mold the human skeleton from infancy through adulthood. Skeletal development early in life is characterized by a period of acceleration, particularly during infancy and early childhood. During this period, endochondral ossification of the long bones occurs, in which cartilage is replaced by bone tissue. This rapid growth slows considerably as kids enter puberty, when growth plates—epiphyseal plates—begin to open and serve as sites of longitudinal growth. Teen growth height typically peaks in speed due to hormonal changes brought about by puberty, leading to both the acceleration of bone lengthening and the ultimate closure of the growth plates, finally declaring the end of skeletal growth. Following puberty, adolescence introduces new hormonal influences that serve to complete the maturation of the skeletal system. Skeletal expansion typically occurs in late teens through early 20s, characterized by the closure of growth plates and the achievement of peak bone mass—a determinant of long-term bone function. This period of bone development is significant not only for setting height but also for setting a benchmark for bone mineral density. Bone loss and density may become apparent later in life, particularly as physiological aging begins, ultimately leading to conditions such as osteoporosis. Understanding this pathway is imperative to addressing skeletal health and the prevention of age-related bone disease. As people move into midlife and beyond, skeletal aging becomes an increasingly important consideration, with several factors contributing to the progressive loss of bone quality.

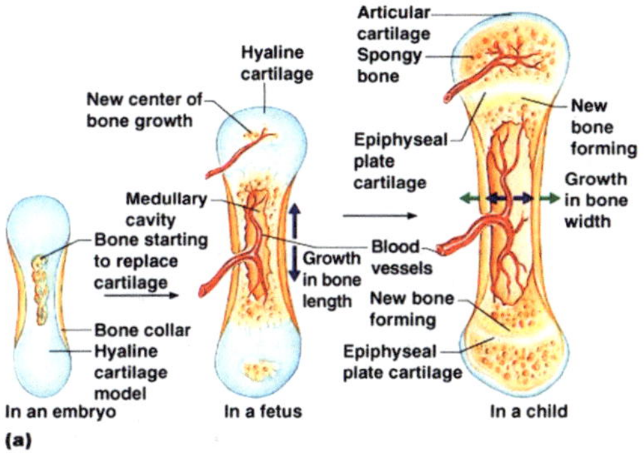

Figure 2.4. The stages of skeletal growth represent a complex interplay of biological processes.

Source: https://external-content.duckduckgo.com/iu/?u=https%3A%2F%2Fslideplayer.com%2Fslide%2F15515727%2F93%2Fimages%2F17%2FStages%2Bof%2BBone%2BGrowth.jpg&f=1&nofb=1&ipt=98bae8ef9d08beee3fc9907bd7f28123209d831bb5e70df6f4de97d107e64469.

The research has shed light on associations between conditions like non-alcoholic fatty liver disease (NAFLD) and skeletal health, highlighting the role of systemic physiological factors in skeletal aging (Chiesa et al., 2017). The relationship among bone density, metabolic status, and aging best illustrates the complexity of the interactions among various body systems. Additionally, the impact of surgical procedures on the skeletal system, such as coronectomy for impacted third molars, best illustrates why bones must be treated gently when the risk of damage is present (Ajbage et al., 2015). These are intricate problems that must be solved to develop effective strategies for maintaining skeletal integrity throughout the lifecycle, ultimately translating into overall health and quality of life (Figure 2.4).

2.1.1. Prenatal Skeletal Development

Fetal skeletal development is important for establishing a foundation for long-term well-being and physical function. During the early first trimester, skeletal formation begins with mesenchymal cells that later develop into chondrocytes and osteoblasts, the cells that form cartilage and bone, respectively. The initial stage of development is sensitive to environmental factors and maternal well-being. For instance, exposure to harmful chemicals or radiation may disrupt this delicate process to result in congenital malformations or growth restrictions. For example, prenatal exposure to chemotherapy has been found to potentially influence skeletal growth, such as in intrauterine growth restriction, which may result in shorter birth lengths and weights and make the fetus vulnerable to skeletal deficiencies later in life (Özlem Terzi et al., 2025). As the skeletal growth enters the second trimester, ossification continues to develop a firmer bony structure in place of the cartilage-based scaffold. The phase is characterized by the formation and appearance of primary ossification centers in the diaphyses of long bones, facilitating bone growth and elongation. Skeletal dysplastic disorders might occur as a result of abnormalities during this phase that could result in postnatal deformities or functional impairments. In addition, the interplay between prenatal determinants and bone health remains of great interest, as prenatal stressors can affect health trajectories during childhood and adolescence. Evidence emphasizes that adverse prenatal exposures, such as maternal undernutrition or psychosocial stress exposure, can have detrimental effects on musculoskeletal ontogeny and development and lead to increased chances of developing chronic disease in adulthood (Scheffler et al., 2021). Finally, the third trimester is also a crucial time for bone formation as the fetus approaches term. In utero movements and positions mechanically load bones and cause an increase in bone mineralization and density, essential for preparing the infant's skeleton for the stresses of life outside the uterus. An understanding of how in utero forces influence skeletal development is paramount to establishing at-risk groups. For instance, infants exposed in utero to systemic drugs or ionizing radiation may have skeletal abnormalities or developmental delay. Prenatal exposure to chemotherapy illustrates the long-term consequences on bone health; infants may have different dysplasias of the skeleton, which necessitate long-term follow-up and early intervention (Özlem Terzi et al., 2025). Together, these findings highlight the importance of prenatal care in enabling optimal skeletal development, thereby influencing growth and aging patterns throughout a lifetime (Figure 2.5).

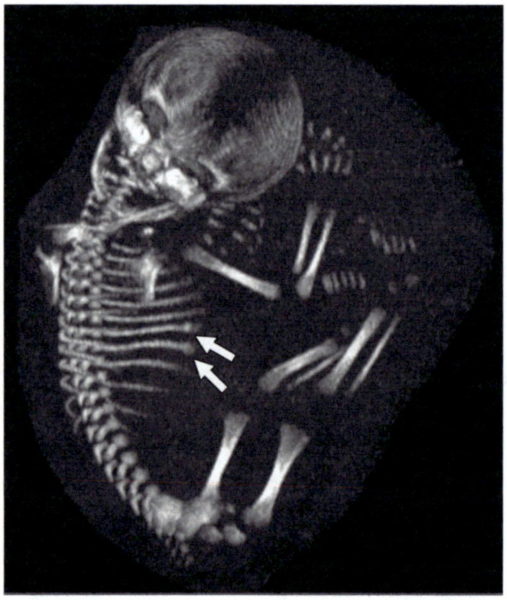

Figure 2.5. The process of prenatal skeletal development.

Source: https://ajronline.org/cms/10.2214/AJR.17.19337/asset/images/large/05_17_19337_10c.jpeg.

2.1.2. Childhood and Adolescent Growth Spurts

The process of growth spurts in childhood and adolescence is a ubiquitous pattern of human development, characterized by abrupt increases in height and weight at different ages. During early childhood, it is slow but uniform, with active physical change in children. Actually, research has shown that differences in long bone growth, such as the tibia and fibula, are influenced by nutrition, hormones, and genetics (Belcastro et al., 2022). As babies grow into toddlers, the size of their limbs starts to develop, particularly in relation to getting more agile. These morphological alterations not only signify the physical expansion of the body that keeps pace with motor development but also prepare for further growth spurts encountered during later stages of life. Adolescence is a transitional stage marked by the most intense growth spurts, which are closely related to hormonal changes during puberty. This period of development is characterized by accelerated growth velocities, leading to intensified bone extension and maturation. These growth spurts are a function of an interaction between sex-specific hormones, such as testosterone and estrogen, that regulate both skeletal growth and the function of the growth plates. These studies note that, to a high degree of precision, tibial and fibular growth measures, in aggregate, are strongly correlated with age and mark the universality of this developmental milestone across sexes (Belcastro et al., 2022). This growth also corresponds to significant physical capacity and psychosocial transformation, impacting personal development and social standing during these young years. The growth spurts that occur during childhood and adolescence have significance that transcends the physical, since they occur before significant changes in bone aging. It is important to be aware of the timing and nature of these growth phases to identify potential health concerns related to bone development. During these growth spurts, adolescents and children are particularly prone to injury because their bones are developing rapidly and may not yet have reached full structural strength. Also, the patterns of growth observed in childhood play a crucial role in predicting skeletal aging, as variations in growth spurts can dictate bone density and health later in adulthood. The trajectory set during these early growth phases dictates physical fitness outcomes and susceptibility to age-related skeletal diseases, demonstrating the significance of monitoring growth during these formative phases (Figure 2.6).

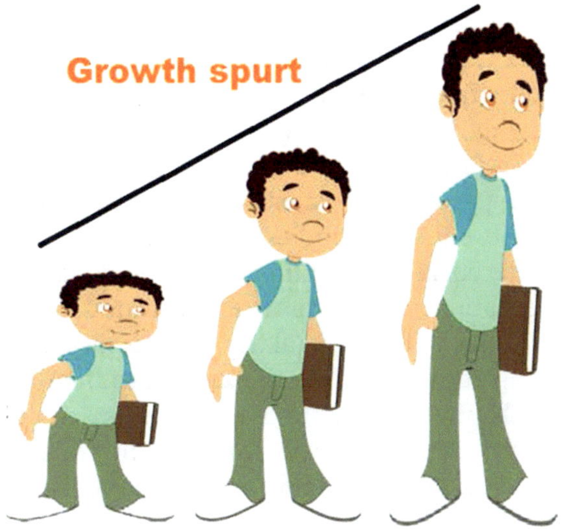

Figure 2.6. The process of childhood and adolescent growth spurts.

Source: https://study.com/cimages/multimages/16/hnet.com-image_23119211150329182962.png.

2.1.3. Peak Bone Mass Attainment

Peak bone mass achievement represents a crucial milestone in skeletal maturation, with far-reaching implications for long-term bone health and osteoporosis prevention in old age. This process usually occurs in adolescence and early adulthood when bone formation outruns resorption, leading to a peak skeletal density and strength. Factors affecting the attainment of this include genetics, hormonal status, dietary nutrient intake, and lifestyle. The roles of calcium and vitamin D, in particular, are established; adequate consumption of these is needed for optimal bone mineralization. Also, weight-bearing activities during growth spurts contribute to the establishment of peak bone mass, as bone development is enhanced through mechanical loading that induces osteoblast activity. Thus, interventions to promote the adoption of healthy lifestyle habits during formative periods can have a long-term impact on skeletal integrity and overall health outcomes in aging populations (Hathaway-Schrader et al., 2019). Moreover, the process of attaining peak bone mass is not merely a matter of genetics or biochemical function but is heavily influenced by environmental factors as well. Lifestyle and dietary intake during the growing years make a critical difference. As an example, child and adolescent activity levels are directly correlated with bone density; denser, more robust bones tend to be found among individuals who are regularly engaged in weight-bearing activities. Also, the assimilation of food that has phytonutrients that contribute to bone strength can accelerate direct mineralization processes. According to evidence, adherence to a healthy diet is associated with optimizing the skeletal system's capacity to reach peak bone mass (Tieland et al., 2017). Thus, encouraging the provision of an environment that facilitates active lifestyles and well-balanced dietary practices during development is important for achieving healthy, robust bones in adulthood. As women and men enter aging and then adulthood, it is crucial to preserve the peak bone mass attained to prevent age-related skeletal illness. Osteoporosis is a significant factor in this condition, where there is reduced bone density and increased susceptibility to fractures. Bone loss usually accelerates after menopause in women due to decreased estrogen levels, necessitating screening and maintenance of skeletal health throughout life. This loss with age is compounded by lifestyle problems of inactive lifestyles and dietary deficiencies, which can further contribute to skeletal decline. Therefore, understanding the interaction between peak bone mass attainment and later-life bone health enables health interventions to reduce the burden of osteoporosis and improve quality of life among the elderly (Hathaway-Schrader et al., 2019).

Test Your Knowledge

1. What are the main stages of skeletal growth from infancy to adulthood?
2. How does skeletal growth change during childhood and adolescence?

2.2. Factors Influencing Skeletal Development

Learning Outcome

1. Peak bone mass attainment
2. Genetic factors
3. Nutritional influences

The intricate process of bone development is regulated by numerous factors and is largely controlled by genetics in determining unique growth patterns and bone morphology. Genetic tendencies contribute to the timing of growth plate activity and hormonal control, which directly determines the maturation of the skeleton. Research has shown that certain genes can alter the timing and character of skeletal development, providing a solid genetic foundation for structural organization. For example, differences in the secretion of growth hormone may cause deviations in height and skeletal alignment throughout adolescence. This genetic influence is not confined to rates of skeletal growth but also extends to bone density and the formation of patterns thereof, which may manifest in conditions such as malocclusion, where dental misalignments reflect interactions between genetics and the environment that affect overall skeletal development. Environmental influences like these play an equally important role in determining skeletal growth and health, with nutrition an essential part. Appropriate intake of essential nutrients, such as vitamin D and calcium, is crucial for maintaining optimal bone mineralization and growth. Inadequate consumption during periods of critical growth could lead to undesirable consequences, such as growth retardation or skeletal deformity, which may further exacerbate functional impairment. The interplay between dietary habits and genetic vulnerabilities is evident in research establishing associations between nutritional status and outcomes related to skeletal well-being. For instance, some diets can influence the expression of genes involved in bone growth and density. Therefore, it is clear that uniform access to a healthy diet is essential for human beings, particularly during the child and adolescent growth spurts when the skeletal system undergoes remarkable alterations, underscoring the importance of an all-encompassing approach to skeletal health that involves both genetic and environmental factors. Aside from diet and genetics, socio-cultural factors play an important role in determining the complexities of skeletal development. These are lifestyle, exercise, and social body image and health ideals that may affect an individual's growth pattern. Physical activity, particularly weight-bearing activities, is important in stimulating bone growth and bone strength throughout one's lifespan.

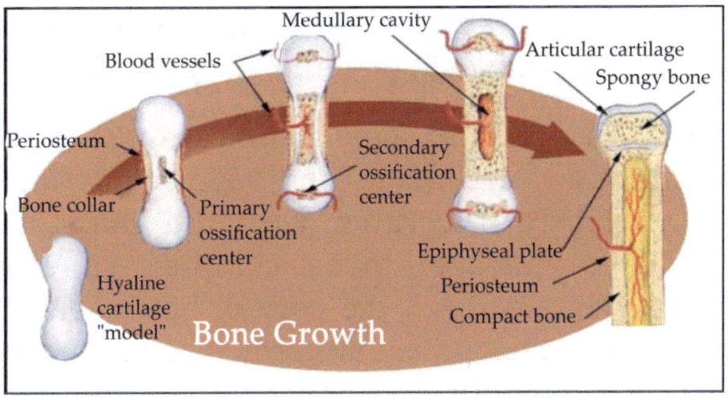

Figure 2.7. The intricate process of skeletal development.

Source: https://www.mheresearchfoundation.org/sitebuilder/images/illu_bone_growth-740x379.jpg.

Further, cultural attitudes to health can dictate dietary habits and active or passive lifestyles, which, in turn, influence bone health. Children, for instance, raised in cultures where sports and outdoor recreation are encouraged tend to have stronger bones than children with more sedentary lifestyles. Additionally, research shows that the perception of body image in society can go on to affect unhealthy eating habits or exercise patterns, thereby affecting skeletal development as well as overall health.

The integration of these various socio-cultural determinants highlights the intricate process of skeletal growth within the broader context of growth, development, and aging (Figure 2.7).

2.2.1. Genetic Factors

Genetic impact on development and skeletal aging is significant, with the potential to determine individual differences in skeletal form and function. Genetic factors influence bone growth and remodeling cycles, and polymorphisms in genes with significant effects can alter skeletal health throughout life. A notable characteristic of such genetic impacts is epigenetic mechanisms, in which gene expression is controlled without altering the DNA sequence itself. For example, mechanisms such as DNA methylation, histone modifications, and microRNAs play significant roles in regulating muscle and bone gene expression, impacting overall skeletal health.

Since skeletal muscle constitutes such a substantial percentage of body weight and is so closely integrated with the skeleton, one must unravel these complex genetic interactions to reach the core of how skeletal aging and development are brought about, thus emphasizing the importance of further studies in this vital area (Adamo et al., 2015). Moreover, the interplay between androgen receptor (AR) gene polymorphisms and muscle growth exemplifies how genetic factors can converge with hormonal influences to regulate growth patterns. Gene changes within the AR gene, namely the CAG repeat number, are likely to affect muscle mass and function, though in complex ways. Studies have shown that greater numbers of CAG repeats are associated with higher circulating testosterone levels, but this does not necessarily translate into greater muscle mass or strength. This intricacy highlights the interrelatedness of lifestyle, hormonal, and genetic variables, which cumulatively influence skeletal growth and aging. Investigating these interactions is relevant, as understanding the nuances of how genetic vulnerabilities interact with environmental factors can lead to targeted interventions that improve skeletal health and arrest age-related loss (Bogaert et al., 2014). In light of an aging population, understanding the genetic basis of skeletal aging is increasingly important for facilitating preventive therapies and optimizing health throughout the life course. Genetic susceptibility manifests in skeletal diseases in multiple ways, not only in bone density but also in fracture risk and osteoporosis. Coordination between the effects of genetics and extrinsic stimuli, i.e., diet and exercise, is important in determining skeletal resilience as one ages. For instance, the complex regulation of bone remodeling by numerous genetic pathways underscores the importance of ongoing studies to unravel gene-environment interactions. By understanding these genetic processes, researchers can improve skeletal health and facilitate adaptive processes during aging, ultimately resulting in improved quality of life for the elderly (Adamo et al., 2015) (Figure 2.8).

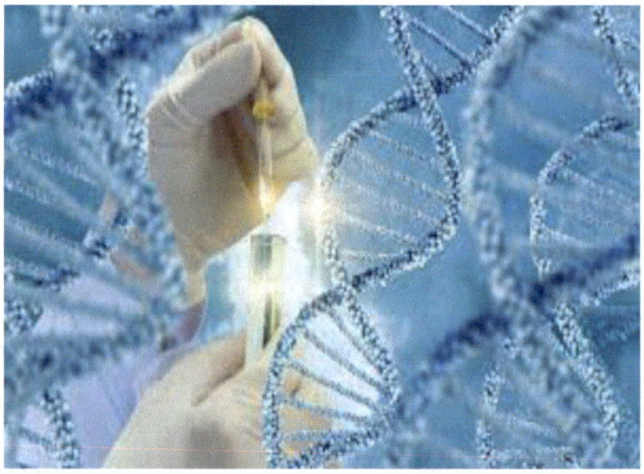

Figure 2.8. The impact of genetic factors on growth and skeletal aging.

Source: https://encrypted-tbn0.gstatic.com/images?q=tbn:ANd9GcSTIj5fiJrUY8ai5waiLoerp92qX9xkbC7Mhg&s.

2.2.2. Nutritional Influences

Nutritional effects are crucial to determining patterns of growth throughout development and to influencing bone health and aging in a significant way. The developmental years, with their dietary demands, lay the foundation for long-term health. Inadequate nutrition during these formative years may lead to stunted growth, reduced bone density, and an increased risk of health problems in later life. For instance, studies have shown that caloric intake and the quality of nutrition influence bone maturation, as deficiencies disrupt bone structure and integrity. These nutritional-skeletal outcome linkages underscore the importance of dietary vigilance during development, because the repercussions of suboptimal nutritional choices can span a lifetime, affecting not just growth patterns but also susceptibility to degenerative conditions later in life. Recent experimental research on nutritional deprivation sheds light on the physiological mechanisms underlying these outcomes. A study on the effects of nutritional deficiency in European starling nestlings proved that caloric intake and effort invested in food procurement were accountable for cellular senescence and inflammation. The study revealed that a suboptimal diet with high begging activity increased markers of DNA damage, indicating a multifaceted interplay between nutrition and developmental stressors. This link underscores that the nutritional environment plays an important role in the development and growth, with disturbed intake being seen in long-term adverse outcomes on health. These findings extend to how avian models may be reflected in humans, where early-life inflammatory events resulting from nutritional deficiencies at critical developmental stages can predispose to later complications, including osteoporosis and other aging-related conditions (Andrews et al., 2017). Moreover, the importance of nutritional impact becomes evident in the context of processes of skeletal maturation. A study examining the timing of knee joint development reveals significant heterogeneity in nutritional and environmental-influenced skeletal age. In early childhood, periods of rapid growth are marked by extensive morphological changes, which are strongly influenced by adequate nutrition. These findings suggest that adequate dietary balance is not only essential for the continuation of immediate growth but also for the maximal development of the skeleton. As children progress through various phases of growth, the nutritional considerations in skeletal age estimation highlight the subtle dynamic relationship between diet and growth mechanisms. The interaction between environmental factors and skeletal growth underscores the need for ongoing research to explore how diet can be used to combat age-related skeletal decline in adulthood (Gallagher et al., 2015).

2.2.3. Environmental Impacts

The interaction between environmental factors and skeletal aging represents a significant determinant of growth and development as it has a notable influence on bone health. Toxic ecological substances, such as particulate matter and heavy metals, are responsible for inducing adverse effects on skeletal health. Toxic exposures may alter bone density and be a causative factor in age-related bone disease, such as osteoporosis. It has also been observed that the inflammatory reaction induced by environmental toxins accelerates the degeneration of bone cells, further stimulating skeletal aging. This association highlights the imperative of a healthy, hygienic environment for maintaining bone health throughout life, calling for a multidisciplinary approach to addressing public health issues intertwined with environmental quality. Lifestyle factors connected with the environment, as well as with pollutants, are significant determinants of skeletal growth. Sedentary lifestyles were a consequence of urbanization, adversely affecting bone health across all population groups. Decreased physical activity that is critical for bone health is often everyday in urban settings where the populace is locked indoors due to safety concerns or lack of green spaces. Furthermore, modern living conditions and eating habits in urban settings could put people at risk of inadequate intake of essential nutrients, such as vitamin D and calcium, which are necessary for optimal bone growth and maintenance. Reducing these lifestyle determinants through public policy and community planning can create environments that support active living and healthy eating, thereby contributing to better skeletal well-being in the population. The publication of the World Health Organization's (WHO) new physical activity guidelines and sedentary behavior indicates the importance of regular exercise in enhancing skeletal health, especially with age. People of all ages, including the elderly, are encouraged to engage in moderate-to-vigorous exercise to counter the ill effects of a sedentary lifestyle. These recommendations are based on growing evidence that physical activity not only improves overall health but also directly enhances bone strength and density. Reducing sedentary behavior and muscle-strengthening exercises are the most important prevention strategies against skeletal aging and concomitant complications. The integration of these physical activity guidelines into community initiatives can provide essential frameworks for encouraging more healthy environments and promoting the skeletal health of individuals at all stages of life, as specified in the WHO's global physical activity strategy (Bull et al., 2020) (Figure 2.9).

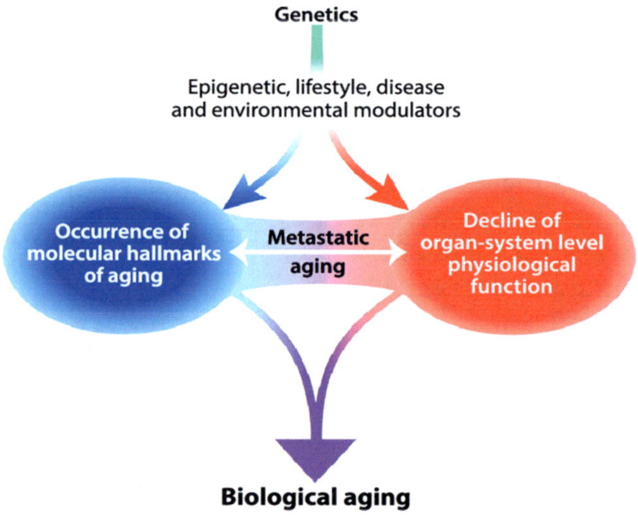

Figure 2.9. The interaction between environmental factors and skeletal aging.

Source: https://www.researchgate.net/publication/317189504/figure/fig1/AS:614002795221023@1523401082554/Biological-aging-is-a-multifactorial-process-The-molecular-hallmarks-of-aging-and.png.

Test Your Knowledge

1. What genetic and hormonal factors influence skeletal development?
2. How do nutrition and physical activity affect skeletal growth and development?

2.3. Bone Remodeling Process

Learning Outcome

1. Role of osteoblasts and osteoclasts
2. Hormonal regulation of bone remodeling;
3. Impact of physical activity on bone health

Bone remodeling is an active, continuous physiological process that plays a crucial role in maintaining skeletal health throughout an individual's life. Bone remodeling is a coordinated action of two major cell types: osteoblasts, which are involved in bone building, and osteoclasts, which are responsible for bone resorption. Surprisingly, bone remodeling is necessary not only during development, when the skeleton is adding mass and strength, but also in adulthood, where it sustains the skeleton by replenishing old bone tissue and repairing micro-damage caused by ordinary activity. Equilibrium in the remodeling process is required; any imbalance can lead to diseases such as osteoporosis, characterized by reduced bone density and increased susceptibility to fractures. Thus, understanding the bone remodeling process's complexity is key to understanding how circumstances such as aging and disease can alter the integrity of the skeleton, as well as overall health. Research has uncovered that systemic factors, including hormones, nutrition, and mechanical loading, have a very significant effect on the bone remodeling process. For instance, hormonal changes, particularly estrogen and testosterone levels, are essential for regulating osteoblast and osteoclast function. Furthermore, dietary components, particularly calcium and vitamin D, are essential for the proper functioning of these cells. Mechanical loading, generated by weight-bearing exercise, also triggers bone formation, indicating the contribution of exercise towards ensuring bone density. Equilibrium among these influences is essential as a person grows older; the remodeling process itself begins to slow down, leading to diminished bone mass and increased risk of fracture. Thus, interventions that augment diet and promote exercise can have a pivotal role to play in preventing the effects of skeletal aging and improving the longevity of bone status. Bone remodeling and the aging process have also been of considerable research interest, with new findings indicating areas of intersection between skeletal health and other systems in the body.

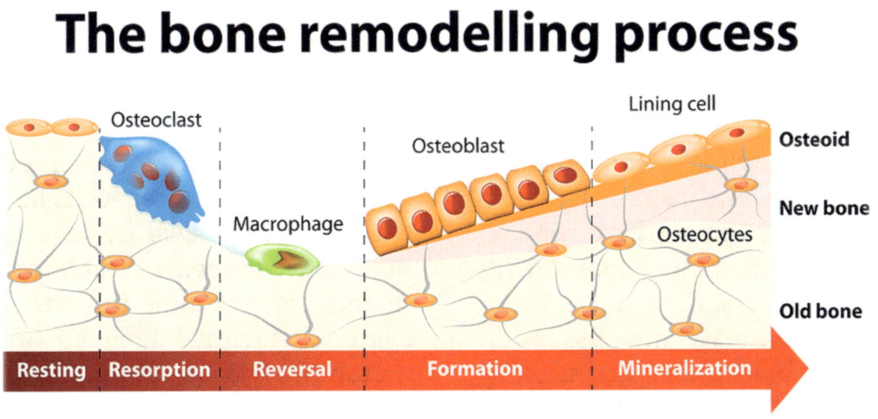

Figure 2.10. The process of bone remodeling.

Source: https://external-content.duckduckgo.com/iu/?u=https%3A%2F%2Fbonebalance.co.uk%2Fwp-content%2Fuploads%2F2021%2F04%2FBone-remodelling-process.png&f=1&nofb=1&ipt=959787ffec9cf2cff587749ff6ada24d4ca0e88081e09362c83c6c7450df313a.

Bone health, for example, has been described in studies to have more overt links to the occurrence of conditions like non-alcoholic fatty liver disease (NAFLD), which is further influenced by factors such as obesity as well as insulin resistance (Chiesa et al., 2017). Of interest is the association of NAFLD with osteoporosis, as this points to an underlying common pathophysiological mechanism due to the process of aging, inflammation, and metabolic deregulation. Finally, the very process of aging can independently contribute to decreased lean body mass and bone mineral density, thereby further increasing the risk of skeletal sequelae with age (Chiesa et al., 2017). Thus, understanding the interactions between these systems is crucial for designing efficient strategies to maintain skeletal health during the aging process. Through targeted research and intervention, health outcomes and quality of life can be improved among the elderly (Figure 2.10).

2.3.1. Role of Osteoblasts and Osteoclasts

The activities of osteoclasts and osteoblasts are at the heart of the dynamic process of bone remodeling, which is necessary to maintain healthy skeletons throughout an individual's lifetime. Osteoblasts are cells responsible for bone matrix production that mineralize to contribute to bone strength. Osteoblasts originate from mesenchymal stem cells and are vital in the growth and repair stages of bone, making a significant contribution to the achievement of peak bone mass during growth. Osteoclasts, on the other hand, are of monocyte/macrophage lineage and possess the function of resorbing bone tissue and thereby, maintaining bone density and structure. There should be a balance between these two cell types; an excess of osteoclast activity can lead to conditions such as osteoporosis, characterized by bone fragility and increased susceptibility to fractures. Knowledge of this balance is critical for addressing skeletal aging, in which bone remodeling efficacy generally declines, leading to structural deficits. Further intricacy in bone biology comes from the activity of many regulatory molecules, including hormones, cytokines, and signaling molecules, that regulate the activities of osteoblasts and osteoclasts. For instance, parathyroid hormone and calcitonin regulate calcium homeostasis by modulating the activity of these bone cells. Furthermore, new evidence indicates that galectin-3 is produced by osteoclasts and osteoblasts and significantly affects their activity. Galectin-3 was identified as a modulatory molecule in the osteogenic lineage, promoting cell survival and differentiation, and thus implicated in bone disease and health (Fantauzzi et al., 2017). Therefore, this communication, encouraged by these regulatory molecules, emphasizes the fine homeostasis of appropriate bone remodeling and the implication that it has in maintaining skeletal integrity in synchronization with one's progressing age. The aging process profoundly affects osteoblast and osteoclast function, altering bone density and strength. With increasing age, the functioning of osteoblasts becomes less while osteoclast activity remains unchanged or increases, resulting in net loss in bone mineral density. This imbalance not only encourages diseases like osteoporosis but may also affect the overall design and function of the skeleton. Moreover, the activity of galectin-3 is particularly noteworthy in this context, with its participation in the osteogenic differentiation of the mesenchymal stem cells having relevance to vascular health also (Ajbage et al., 2015). The dialogue between osteoblasts and osteoclasts in this context aims to further elucidate how systemic factors, such as inflammation and metabolic status, can contribute to skeletal aging. By investigating these correlations further, researchers can develop targeted therapies that can maintain bone strength in older persons and reduce the risk of fracture (Figure 2.11).

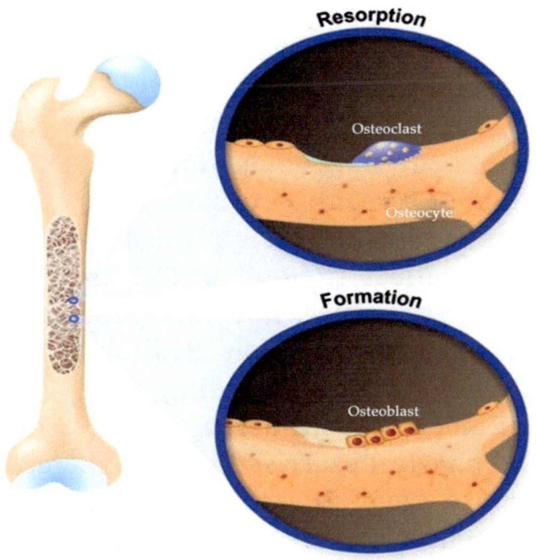

Figure 2.11. The roles of osteoblasts and osteoclasts are integral to the dynamic process of bone remodeling.

Source: https://external-content.duckduckgo.com/iu/?u=https%3A%2F%2Fi.ytimg.com%2Fvi%2FTau2aedWoWM%2Fmaxresdefault.jpg&f=1&nofb=1&ipt=920352c5d68152654366f5204aab761bf4afc5153909322b5ef8ea46443b65cb.

2.3.2. Hormonal Regulation of Bone Remodeling

The hormone control of bone, distributed by bone remodeling, is the prevailing factor in the skeleton's health at all life stages, particularly development and senescence. Basic hormones such as parathyroid hormone (PTH), calcitonin, and sex steroids closely control the function of bone-forming osteoblasts and bone-resorbing osteoclasts. PTH, for instance, indirectly stimulates osteoclasts through osteoblasts to enhance calcium mobilization into circulation. Conversely, calcitonin inhibits osteoclast activity, thereby reducing bone resorption. Understanding these hormonal interactions is crucial not only for comprehending the basic biology of bone remodeling but also for treating skeletal aging pathologies, such as osteoporosis, where hormonal imbalance can accelerate bone loss and weakness. In recent years, the role of osteocytes, once an overlooked aspect of bone physiology, has emerged as a significant factor in hormonal control. They are mechanosensors that detect mechanical loads and hormonal stimulation, thereby synchronizing bone remodeling. Osteocytes release regulatory proteins such as RANKL and sclerostin, which significantly impact osteoclast and osteoblast function, respectively. In their optimal working condition, osteocytes regulate an equilibrium remodeling process, which is essential for skeletal growth and maintenance. Dysregulation of osteocyte function often exacerbates bone diseases, making them key mediators in the hormonal bone disease framework (Bellido et al., 2015). This new perspective highlights the utility of high-level investigation into the therapeutic potential of targeting osteocyte signaling mechanisms to enable healthier aging bones. The interaction between hormonal regulation and bone remodeling is most evident in aging. In this case, hormonal changes have a direct impact on bone status. For instance, loss of estrogen in postmenopausal women brings about a dramatic increase in menstrual bone loss, raising the risk of fractures. Such a transition not only highlights the role of sex hormone protection in skeletal stability but also reflects the complex balance among many hormones during the aging process. In addition, challenges inherent in the aging of the skeleton, such as increased fragility and vulnerability to fracture, are potentially circumvented by the identification and possibly the modulation of these hormonal processes. As we sort out the intricate web of these interrelations, the promise of targeted hormonal therapy can be an innovative path to improving outcomes for victims of manifestations of skeletal aging (Ajbage et al., 2015). This is still a research area of significance as the world grapples with an increasingly aging population.

2.3.3. Impact of Physical Activity (PA) on Bone Health

Engaging in consistent physical activity is vital for bone health and development across the lifespan. The relationship between PA and BMD is particularly significant during childhood and adolescence when the skeletal system experiences accelerated growth. Weight-bearing, high-impact activity, such as jumping, running, and resistance training, acts on bone to stimulate growth and increase BMD. Evidence suggests that boys have stronger linear associations between PA amount and BMD at weight-bearing sites compared to girls. Hence, intervention is warranted to promote such activity in both sexes. Since optimal bone health acquired during childhood can postpone osteoporosis and other fractures in adulthood, it is essential to maximize sports participation during growth phases to achieve optimal skeletal stability (Ouyang et al., 2025). But the subtleties of the physical activity's influence on bone status are more complex than mere involvement. Variation in PA volume, intensity, and type can create differential effects on skeletal outcomes across sexes. Specifically, while boys show linear increases in BMD with increasing levels of PA, girls appear to have some nonlinear threshold levels that must be met to gain similarly. For example, girls have demonstrated an effective amount of PA of approximately 15,000 monitor-independent movement summary units per day. Boys and girls also show intensity-based thresholds, indicating a limit beyond which further increases in BMD are negligible. The sensitive acknowledgment of sex-specific reaction underscores the need for targeted physical activity recommendations for particular needs to optimize bone health in formative years (Ouyang et al., 2025). The broader significance of physical activity to health must also respond to the contemporary challenge offered by rising rates of childhood obesity, as collated by. The sedentary behavior and excessive watching of screens by contemporary children add to the risk of obesity, which in turn may adversely affect skeletal health and growth. Physical inactivity is not only pathogenic for impaired bone health but also for a plethora of other disorders, including cardiovascular disease and metabolic derangement. Promoting regular physical exercise becomes increasingly critical to reversing these harmful trends. Recommendations are made that children aged 6-12 years receive at least 60 minutes of physical exercise daily. The inclusion of successful family and community-based interventions can promote active settings where children achieve the level of physical activity necessary to provide healthy skeletal development and guard against obesity and resulting complications (Figure 2.12).

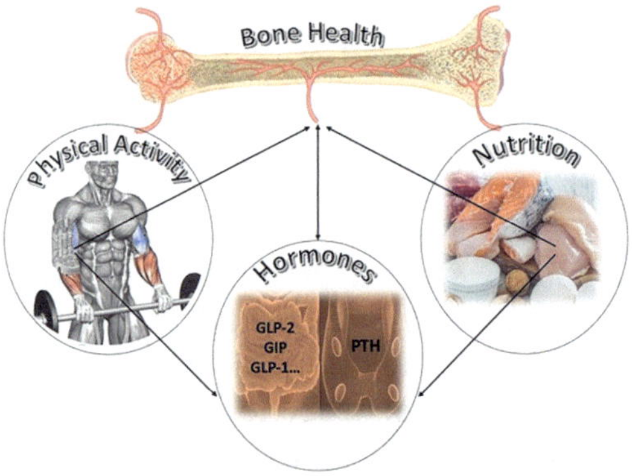

Figure 2.12. Engaging in regular physical activity.

Source: https://www.frontiersin.org/files/Articles/704647/fendo-12-704647-HTML/image_m/fendo-12-704647-g001.jpg.

Test Your Knowledge

1. What are the main steps involved in the bone remodeling process?
2. How do osteoclasts and osteoblasts coordinate to maintain bone health during remodeling?

2.4. Aging and Skeletal Changes

Learning Outcome

1. Decrease in bone density
2. Changes in bone structure
3. Increased risk of fractures

Aging also strongly influences skeletal changes that contribute to certain health problems, particularly in the elderly. As age advances, bone tissue structure remodeling becomes increasingly out of sync. This is coupled with bone resorption, the process by which bone is dissolved, as well as loss of bone-building. Subsequently, bone density loss increases the risk of fractures, osteoporosis, and fractures. The interaction with endocrine changes, particularly the loss of estrogen in women following menopause and testosterone in older men, exacerbates this process. Skeletal muscle mass, a key determinant of bone strength, also declines with age, further compromising bone health. Understanding these changes is essential for developing strategies to sustain bone health throughout the aging process. In addition to hormonal changes, genetic and environmental factors also play a role in the skeletal changes that occur during aging. Genetic predispositions can influence a person's susceptibility to osteoporosis, impacting bone rates of turnover as well as skeletal stability. Additionally, lifestyle factors such as diet, physical exercise, and exposure to sunlight can exacerbate or reduce such changes. A diet low in one or both of the two key nutrients, calcium and vitamin D, has adverse skeletal effects, as they are crucial for bone integrity. On the other hand, regular physical exercise, and indeed weight-bearing exercise, has been shown to enhance bone density and overall skeletal strength. Thus, promoting a good lifestyle can be a preventive measure against a decrease in skeletal function with an increase in age. Interventions ranging from dietary modifications to physical exercise may be decisive in maintaining bone strength. Complex cellular and molecular events of skeletal aging have been reported to occur with aging. As an illustration, it is coupled with increased bone inflammation that is brought on by inflammatory cytokine and immune cell elevation causing the disruption of the normal bone remodeling balance. This inflammatory condition can lead to modification in the function of osteoclasts and osteoblasts, the two cell types implicated in bone resorption and bone formation, respectively. Furthermore, the accumulation of oxidative stress, which rises with age, has been reported to compromise osteoblastic function and increase bone loss. The intricate interplay among aging, inflammation, and oxidative stress is crucial for the formulation of targeted interventions to counter skeletal alterations associated with aging. By addressing such underlying causes, it may be possible to lessen the adverse skeletal consequences of aging and consequently enhance the quality of life among the elderly population (Lin et al., 2024; Caspersen et al., 2025).

2.4.1. Decrease in Bone Density

Reduced bone density is an essential aspect of skeletal aging that poses severe health risks, particularly the high incidence of fractures. As one ages, particularly in postmenopausal women, bone resorption exceeds bone formation. Such a disparity lowers bone mineral density (BMD), a direct assessment of bone strength. Longitudinal studies have demonstrated that peak bone mass achieved during growth is the strongest predictor of reducing the consequences of bone loss with age. The significance of achieving greater peak bone mass becomes evident as individuals reach advanced ages, when decreased BMD increases the risk of fragility fractures, thereby raising morbidity and mortality risks for skeletal health. Evidence shows the significance of exercise in combating bone density loss, particularly when initiated at early stages of life. Participating in weight-bearing activity throughout growth not only helps establish peak bone mass but also lays the foundation for skeletal function that can be maintained into older age. There is evidence that exercise will reverse the decline in bone density that is commonly seen with aging. Moderate-intensity exercise programs, especially during youth, have been shown to elicit favorable changes in bone architecture and mineral density, translating into increased resistance to subsequent bone loss throughout life. By mitigating the adverse effects of aging on bone density, exercise emerges as an important intervention to maximize skeletal health and reduce the risk of fractures, which can irreversibly diminish quality of life.

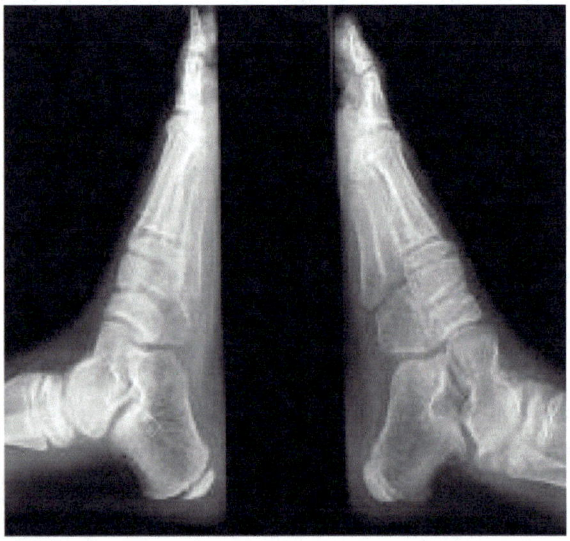

Figure 2.13. The aging process significantly influences skeletal changes.

Source: https://www.researchgate.net/profile/Jan-Berger-4/publication/26742607/figure/fig1/AS:310043565150210@1450931554965/Decreased-bone-density-over-the-left-ankle-and-hind-foot.png.

Additionally, integrating nutritional interventions and physical training is needed to maximize bone health throughout an individual's life. Adequate intake of calcium and vitamin D complements the skeletal benefit of exercise, maximizing the positive effects on bone density and structure. Research identifies diet and exercise interactions during developmental stages as crucial for raising peak bone mass, thereby impacting bone density trajectories in aged populations. With an increased risk of fragility fractures among aging populations, awareness of the interactions between lifestyle factors and skeletal health is imperative. Successful intervention techniques integrating exercise and diet thus present a promising avenue to combat bone density decrease, facilitating healthier aging and improved skeletal integrity across the lifespan (Karlsson et al., 2008a; Karlsson et al., 2008b) (Figure 2.13).

2.4.2. Changes in Bone Structure

Understanding the changes in bone structure throughout a lifetime is relevant to understanding the broader implications of growth, development, and skeletal ageing. Bone accretion outnumbers bone resorption during childhood and adolescence, and there is a net gain in bone mass and density. It is critical to the acquisition of maximum bone mass, typically reached in early adulthood. However, with advancing age and the transition into middle age and beyond, the equilibrium tips inappropriately towards bone resorption, with a resultant severe effect on structure. The role of specific genes such as Tet1 and Tet2 has been emphasized in recent literature to play an important function in regulating the bone marrow stromal cell (BMSC) functions, such that their deregulation can result in alterations in the bone structure that occur in aging. This underlines the need to explore genetic effects as potential modifiers of skeletal health across life stages. Aging does not merely reduce the volume of bone but also its quality, transformation dependent upon a range of intrinsic and extrinsic variables. Investigations have indicated that histological bone characteristics, such as trabecular structure, deteriorate with age, resulting in a less stable skeletal structure.

Specifically, Tet1 and Tet2 knockout mouse studies show profound reductions in trabecular bone volume and alterations in osteogenic differentiation, underscoring the intricate interaction between genetic factors and bone health. Furthermore, reduced osteoblast populations in these models reflect compromised bone regeneration and repair, a risk factor for fractures and related conditions. The interaction between compromised osteogenic capacity and augmented adipogenesis invites questions about the metabolic changes that accompany aging, underscoring the importance of consolidating an adequate understanding of these transitions in bone morphology throughout the life cycle. Besides alterations in cellular and molecular kinetics, the neurovascular morphology encasing bones also changes with aging and affects both bone health and the repair processes. The spatial distribution of calvarial nerves has been found to diminish systematically with age, with considerable heterogeneity being observed among the various areas of the skull. Quantification of TUBB3+ nerve density indicates an early loss in some areas, consistent with vascular changes reflected in vessel fractions. These alterations in the neurovascular terrain can impede the bone's capacity to modify in response to mechanical stressors, thereby culminating in a loss of structural solidity and systemic skeletal function. The addition of the neurovascular interaction dimension adds a level of sophistication to understanding bone structural changes with age, highlighting that skeletal health is not merely dependent on cellular activity but also on the interplay between nerves and blood vessels within the surrounding tissue, which further affects therapeutic interventions against age-induced bone loss.

2.4.3. Increased Risk of Fractures

As individuals undergo different stages of life, the vulnerability to fractures increases significantly, particularly as a part of the aging process. The reasons for this are multifaceted, and among them the alterations in the bone density and structure play pivotal roles. Bones respond to various mechanical stresses during development and growth, but with advancing age there is a loss of bone mass along with alterations in the internal structure of the bones. These changes can contribute to conditions such as osteoporosis, in which bones lose density, become porous, and weak, increasing the risk of fractures. Furthermore, hormonal changes, particularly among postmenopausal women, are also a significant contributor to this process of breakdown. Understanding the physiological basis of these changes provides critical context for the increase in fractures with age, underscoring the need to prevent bone health decline throughout life. In addition to age-related changes, some disease conditions also increase the risk of fracture. For instance, diseases such as acromegaly, in which there is excessive secretion of growth hormone (GH), are associated with increased prevalence of vertebral fracture despite normal bone mineral density (BMD). Research has shown that patients with the disease experience adverse effects on skeletal architecture due to increased GH levels, resulting in impaired bone strength. Studies comparing transgenic mice with elevated serum GH levels to their nontransgenic controls reveal striking differences. The infected mice have trabecular thinning and volume loss, along with a deleterious alteration of cortical BMD and thickness, leading to an impairment of bones' mechanical properties. These findings highlight the multifactorial nature of the risk factors and the complex relationship between hormonal balance, bone density, and fracture susceptibility (Chavassieux et al., 2015). Moreover, the risks of fractures are not reserved for adults but also include those in children and adolescents who have their own vulnerabilities to withstand throughout development and growth. In younger groups, the impact of dietary deficiencies, such as calcium and vitamin D, may compromise bone strength and growth. Deficient intake or absorption of these essential nutrients may result in suboptimal bone mineralization and increase a person's risk of fracture during physically active years. Similarly, certain lifestyle factors, including physical inactivity and excessive screen use, can have a detrimental effect on bone health by reducing weight-bearing activity, which is essential for stimulating bone development. With recent studies indicating that a significant percentage of the population does not meet recommended dietary intakes for bone health, healthy lifestyle choices should be encouraged to avoid the increased risk of fracture that persists across all phases of life (Ajbage et al., 2015) (Figure 2.14).

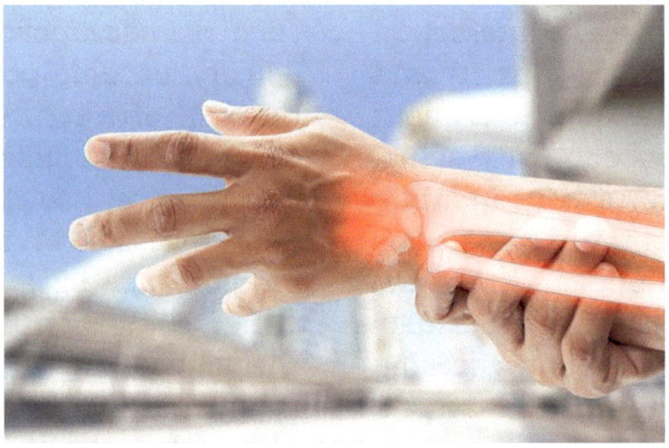

Figure 2.14. Increased risk of fractures.

Source: https://mydoctor.kaiserpermanente.org/mas/Images/thumbnail_large_news-research-hiv-bone-fractures_tcm88-2403710.jpg.

Test Your Knowledge

1. What structural changes occur in the skeleton as a result of aging?
2. How does aging affect bone density and joint function?

2.5. Osteoporosis and Skeletal Aging

Learning Outcome

1. Definition and prevalence of osteoporosis
2. Risk factors for developing osteoporosis
3. Consequences of untreated osteoporosis

The interaction of osteoporosis and skeletal aging is significant, as both conditions are the cause of bone health decline with age. Osteoporosis is characterized by low bone quality and density, leading to a greater risk of fractures, particularly in older individuals. Aging is a physiological process that is the cause of various changes in the physiology of the body, such as changes in bone remodeling, which is the balance between bone resorption and bone formation. Under such circumstances, dietary deficiencies and hormonal changes are the most critical factors. Specifically, estrogen deficiency in postmenopausal women has been linked to accelerated bone loss, underscoring the importance of sex hormones for skeletal health. There is a need to comprehend these interactions so that ways and means can be planned to reverse the impact of osteoporosis and improve the quality of life in individuals experiencing skeletal aging. Moreover, the role of metabolic disorders such as diabetes significantly complicates the osteoporosis and skeletal aging scenario. It is evidence that adolescents with type 1 diabetes mellitus (T1DM) have lower total body bone mineral density (TBBMD) and other critical indicators when glycemic control is poorer (Elżbieta Wierzbicka et al., 2018). It underscores the delicate interplay between general metabolic health and bone health. Poor metabolic control may also increase the risk of osteoporosis and, in turn, frailty and other complications in older age.

The implications of the findings are that active management of metabolic conditions can be key to preserving bone health during critical growth periods. By controlling glycemia, health care professionals can potentially ward off the adverse effects of diseases that cause skeletal aging and enhance bone growth in susceptible groups. Apart from metabolic disease, environmental factors are also involved in bone health, including osteoporosis and aging. Heavy metal poisoning is an example here, where the use of metals such as lead and cadmium has been shown to have adverse effects on bone density and skeletal health (Jaishankar et al., 2014). Exposure to these metals can disrupt metabolic processes and amplify oxidative stress, further destabilizing bones. Aging of the population leads to an increased prevalence of osteoporosis-related fractures; hence, awareness of the interplay between biological and environmental factors on bone is needed. It is thus crucial that exposure to heavy metals is dealt with through public health interventions in the general framework of controlling osteoporosis and its role in bone aging, emphasizing a coordinated effort to improve bone health across the lifespan (Figure 2.15).

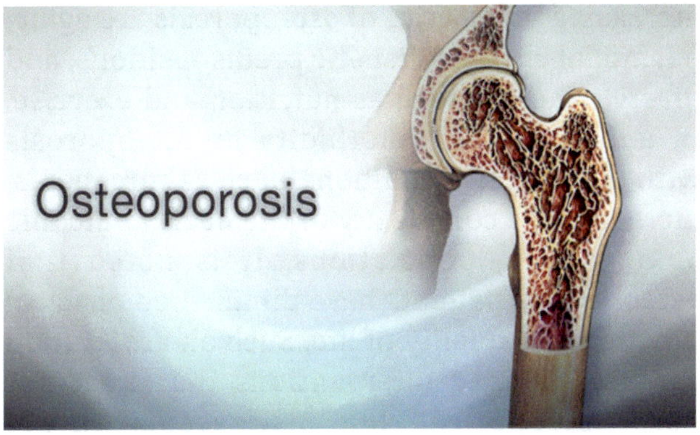

Figure 2.15. The relationship between osteoporosis and skeletal aging.

Source: https://ssl.adam.com/graphics/Multimedia/en/23780/23780ed.jpg.

2.5.1. Definition and Prevalence of Osteoporosis

Osteoporosis is a bone disease characterized by decreased bone density and weakened bone structure, making the bones more fragile and prone to fracture. The condition is typically not identified until a fracture has occurred, and it is an important public health issue, particularly among older people. It is generally diagnosed by dual-energy X-ray absorptiometry (DEXA) scans that measure bone mineral density (BMD) relative to the standard population. With aging, the healthy process of bone remodeling, in which bone is resorbed and replaced with fresh bone, becomes deranged, leaning toward bone loss. Accordingly, osteoporosis is classified by the World Health Organization (WHO) using defined T-score cut-points below -2.5, emphasizing early detection and treatment in skeletal health care, particularly in relation to growth, development, and aging. The epidemiology of osteoporosis is startling, with millions of people worldwide being affected, mostly postmenopausal women and elderly men. Research reveals that nearly 30% of women over the age of 50 will experience fractures due to osteoporosis during their lifetime, depicting the widespread impact of the disease on public health. The causes of the increasing prevalence of osteoporosis are aging, hormonal changes, genetic predispositions, and lifestyle factors such as nutrition and exercise. In addition, the comorbidity of osteoporosis with other aging conditions, such as sarcopenia, increases the complexity of the health outcome among aging populations. It is noted that osteoporosis patients have diminished physical function and quality of life. Such an association calls for holistic interventions that treat not only osteoporosis but also accompanying musculoskeletal disorders in order to improve the health outcome of aging populations. The multifactorial nature of osteoporosis underscores the need for targeted interventions and preventive strategies to reduce its impact. Physical fitness is also a basic preventive and therapeutic factor against osteoporosis, as weight-bearing exercise strengthens bones and reduces the risk of fractures. As is noted by evidence, regular physical activity can do a lot to reverse some of the adverse effects of aging, including less muscle mass and strength, which are typically compounded by osteoporosis. Further, public health campaigns for developing awareness on the need for bone health include advocating for dietary changes with the addition of calcium and vitamin D and adequate physical activity. Despite the overall perception that physical activity raises the risk of injury among active elderly, it has been shown in research that participating in regular physical exercise is beneficial without an equivalent increase in risk of injury among this age group (Baker et al., 2015). It is therefore significant to understand the definition and prevalence of osteoporosis for the encouragement of an all-encompassing dimension of health encompassing growth, development, and skeletal aging.

2.5.2. Risk Factors for Developing Osteoporosis

The understanding of risk factors for osteoporosis development is crucial in the context of skeletal growth, development, and aging. Osteoporosis is characterized by decreased bone density and increased fragility, such that individuals are at risk of fractures. Multiple risk factors for osteoporosis include age, gender, genetic factors, and lifestyle. As one grows older, especially in post-menopausal women, bone resorption exceeds bone formation, leading to a net loss of bone mass. Additionally, genetic susceptibility plays a major role, with some populations demonstrating a higher prevalence of osteoporosis because inherited characteristics that influence bone density are more common in these populations. Hence, these internal risks should be identified to develop prevention programs and educate people about the need to keep their skeletal systems healthy throughout their lives. In addition to internal factors, external influences such as diet and exercise also significantly influence susceptibility to developing osteoporosis. A poor diet that is calcium and vitamin D-deficient might compromise bones because these nutrients are essential for bone mineralization. Research has shown that individuals whose diets are high in processed foods and low in nutrient-dense vegetables and fruits may begin losing bone density at an early age. Further, physical inactivity is highly linked with reduced bone mass. Resistance and weight-bearing exercises performed regularly stimulate bone growth and reduce the risk of osteoporosis. By incorporating physical activity into one's lifestyle and following an adequately balanced diet, one can play an active part in , maintaining bone density, and resistance to osteoporosis. The interplays among osteoporosis and other health diseases further complicate the risk factor picture. For instance, patients with metabolic disease and obesity are at higher risk for developing osteoporosis because increased adiposity and insulin resistance adversely affect bone health. Research shows that such conditions cause a decrease in bone mineral density over time and contribute to skeletal degradation with advancing age. Osteoporosis is not limited to affecting the bones alone; it may trigger a cascade of events concerning the other systems of the body, such as the liver and muscle function. The intricate interconnections among these systems underscore the importance of addressing osteoporosis risk factors with an integrated strategy, as outlined in later epidemiological studies. With multidimensional strategies that address multiple factors in health, it is possible to mitigate the adverse effects of osteoporosis (Ajbage et al., 2015; Chiesa et al., 2017) (Figure 2.16).

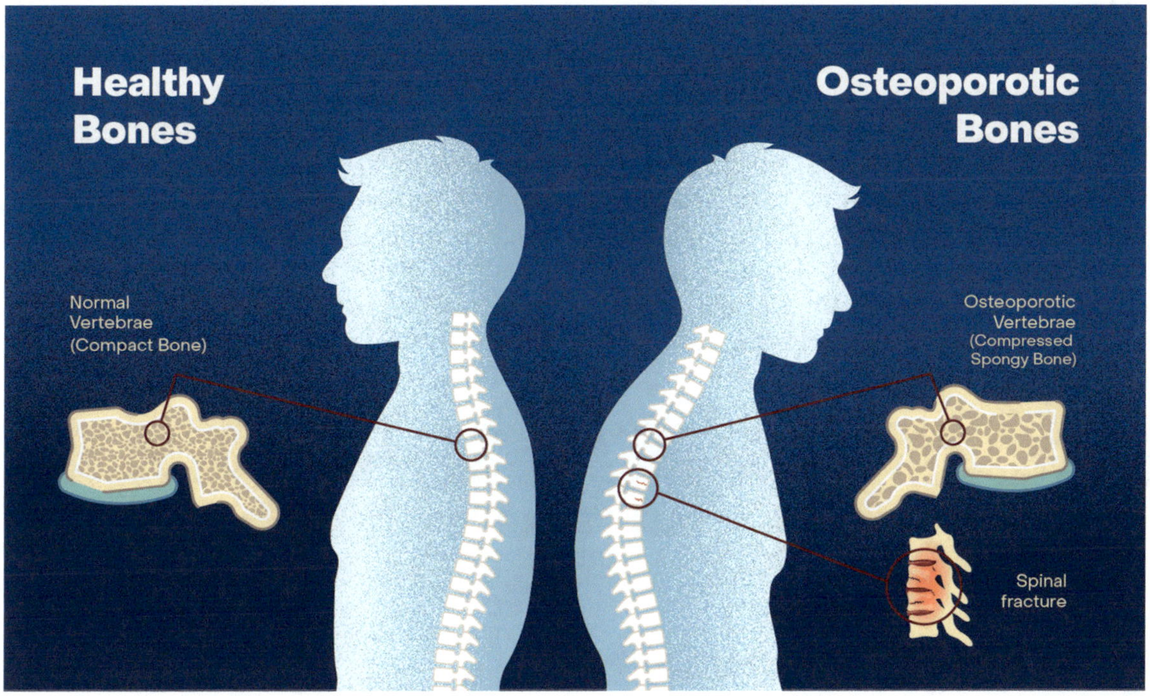

Figure 2.16. The risk factors for developing osteoporosis.

Source: https://spinehealth.org/wp-content/uploads/2024/01/Osteoporosis-01-2.png.

2.5.3. Consequences of Untreated Osteoporosis

Untreated osteoporosis can have severe physiological and psychological consequences, primarily among the elderly. As bone density declines, individuals become increasingly susceptible to fractures from even minor falls or injuries. These fractures, especially at the hip, spine, and wrist, can result in long-term disability or reduced mobility, severely impairing quality of life. Additionally, the likelihood of complications, such as surgical interventions to repair fractures, also rises with deteriorating bone quality. Aside from physical consequences, the psychological significance of osteoporosis should not be downplayed; patients experience increased levels of depression and anxiety with loss of function and loss of independence. Thus, it is the systemic origin of osteoporosis that makes early diagnosis and proper management techniques imperative to minimize its cascading outcomes on physical as well as mental health. The association between undiagnosed osteoporosis and general systemic health conditions is fundamental. According to research, it has been proven that osteoporosis occurs in conjunction with other chronic conditions such as cardiovascular disease and diabetes, which are highly common among elderly people. It has been proven through research that oral health is associated with bone health, and diseases like periodontitis can increase osteoporosis risk, particularly among the elderly. At this point, it is important to maintain oral and skeletal integrity to prevent future systemic disease. These links highlight the multifaceted relationship between osteoporosis, overall health, and the importance of comprehensive healthcare policies that address osteoporosis and its complications. Failure to treat osteoporosis increases the risk of these interrelated diseases, leading to a compromise in the overall well-being of the patients. Prevention in osteoporosis is important to the prevention of long-term complications and improvement of outcomes. This can include lifestyle interventions such as diet therapy to strengthen bone density through calcium and vitamin D intake, and weight-bearing exercise to promote bone growth. Pharmacological agents are also used to retard or even reverse bone loss, significantly reducing the risk of fracture. Engaging the health professionals in regular screenings and assessments can also enable early intervention, resulting in an improved prognosis for high-risk individuals. If osteoporosis is not treated, its effects extend beyond the patient, significantly contributing to healthcare systems through the added costs of injuries. Therefore, detection and treatment of osteoporosis become crucial in enhancing quality of life and healthy aging, ultimately causing a reduction in healthcare spending due to untreated conditions of skeletal aging.

Test Your Knowledge

1. How does osteoporosis contribute to skeletal aging and increased fracture risk?
2. What age-related factors accelerate bone loss leading to osteoporosis?

2.6. Prevention and Management of Skeletal Aging

Learning Outcome

1. Importance of a balanced diet
2. Role of exercise in maintaining bone health
3. Medical interventions and treatments

Prevention and management of skeletal aging are becoming more recognized as a vital part of overall health care in elderly individuals. Physical exercise is an essential tool for its promotion to maintain normal growth, development, and physiological function. Evidence indicates that approximately 80% of American teenagers and adults do not engage in adequate physical activity, thereby compromising not only skeletal health but also overall health, including improved sleep and mood, as well as reduced risk of chronic disease (Piercy et al., 2018). Weight-bearing activities, such as walking, jogging, and resistance training, performed regularly stimulate bone remodeling and enhance muscular strength, both of which are critical for preventing osteoporosis and fractures associated with aging. So, engagement in formal sport not only combats the effects of aging on the bone but also contributes towards general health advantages. Besides physical training, nutrition therapy also plays a critical role in controlling skeletal aging. The calcium and vitamin D diet plays a crucial role in maintaining bone density and preventing fractures. Calcium, which is the primary material of bone structure, should be adequately consumed during life, especially during the maximum growth and aging periods. Vitamin D facilitates calcium absorption and plays a significant role in maintaining normal bone mineralization. However, many populations are deprived of these nutrients to a large degree due to diet and lifestyle changes. The Global Burden of Diseases, Injuries, and Risk Factors Study 2016 also illustrates rising age-related health burdens, underscoring the need for improved dietary strategies within a comprehensive management plan for bone health (Vos et al., 2017). Expanded public health initiatives in nutrition education may help individuals make the right dietary choices that enhance skeletal health. In addition, the inclusion of lifestyle modification in regular health screening can significantly affect the prevention and control of skeletal aging.

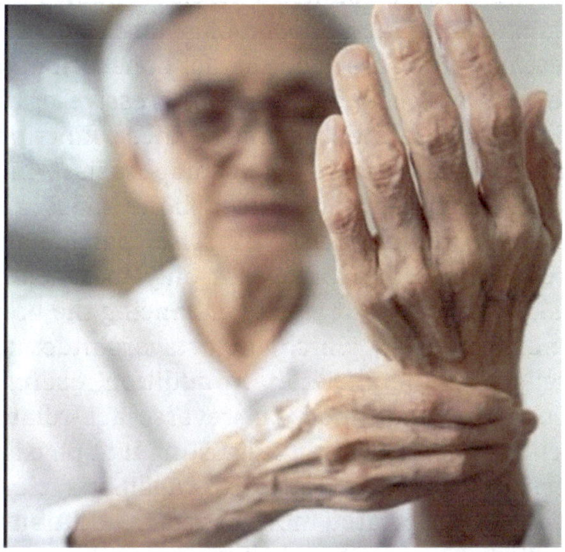

Figure 2.17. The prevention and management of skeletal aging.

Source: https://www.frontiersin.org/_rtmag/_next/image?url=https%3A%2F%2Fwww.frontiersin.org%2Fimage%2Fresearchtopic%2F48505&w=3840&q=90.

With populations growing old and disabling diseases becoming more common, healthcare systems need to combat such diseases as osteoporosis and degenerative joint diseases. Routine screening of bone status can enable early detection of abnormalities and prompt intervention, thereby reducing the burden of skeletal disorders. Apart from that, running special educational campaigns can raise awareness of bone health and encourage individuals to take proactive measures, such as regular exercise and a healthy diet. Since the demand for age-related healthcare services continues to increase, an integrative approach through lifestyle modifications, nutritional supplements, and preventive medicine will play a pivotal role in mitigating the impact of skeletal aging on individuals and society as a whole (Figure 2.17).

2.6.1. Importance of a Balanced Diet

A balanced diet is key to achieving maximum growth and development, particularly at junctures in life such as childhood, adolescence, and even adulthood. Such nutrient foods provide the body with vital vitamins, minerals, and macronutrients for physical growth and mental processes. For instance, proteins are necessary for muscle growth and repairing tissues, whereas calcium and vitamin D are necessary for maintaining bones, increasing bone density and strength. Malnutrition at this stage can lead to stunted development and increased vulnerability to adult-onset diseases. Thus, the consumption of varied food groups not only ensures meeting nutritional demands but also lays the foundation for healthy aging. This preventive lifestyle approach to diet can effectively treat most of the skeletal ageing diseases, where diet and lifestyle influence still remain a factor for musculoskeletal integrity well into old age. Along with physical growth, proper diet enhances mental wellbeing and intellect significantly throughout an individual's lifespan. The gut-brain axis also plays a part in this dynamic interplay, with a better diet directly affecting gut microbiota composition. An extensive array of and very nutritious diet has been found to promote a healthy microbiota profile, which is essential to brain health (Cryan et al., 2019). Short-chain fatty acids produced by probiotic gut flora have been suggested to be responsible for a better mood and reduced rates of cognitive disorders. Therefore, food habits developed during this time have long-range effects not only on physical but also mental health stability, and thus potentially reduce the impact of neurodegenerative diseases. With the growing incidence of age-related cognitive impairment, it is important to quantify the role of an adequate diet in supporting brain function and enabling cognitive resilience against the challenges of aging. In addition, the role of an equal diet extends to preventing inflammation and oxidative stress, both of which are major drivers of skeletal aging.

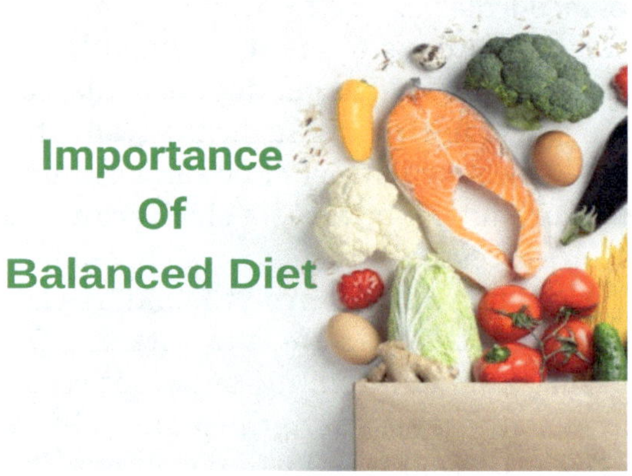

Figure 2.18. Importance of a balanced diet.

Source: https://dolclinic.com/wp-content/uploads/2020/10/Importan-Balanced-Diet.png.

Greater intensities of oxidative stress have been associated with numerous chronic diseases that compromise bone structure, including osteoporosis and arthritis (Sharifi-Rad et al., 2020). Fruits and vegetables, being rich in antioxidants, can counteract these adverse effects, thereby preserving skeletal integrity. By their neutralization of free radicals, these foods intervene directly in the biological processes which control bone repair and remodeling. Secondarily, low intake of processed foods reduces the pro-inflammatory burden of dietary substances. With a scientific understanding of nutrition, the intricate relationship between food composition, reduced oxidative stress, and skeletal system health indicates the pivotal role of balanced nutrition in maintaining longevity and enhancing the quality of life during aging (Figure 2.18).

2.6.2. Role of Exercise in Maintaining Bone Health

Exercise plays a significant role in maintaining bone health throughout life, particularly in growth, development, and skeletal aging. Weight-bearing and resistance exercise enables the dynamic regulation of osteoblast and osteoclast activities, which are necessary for bone formation and loss, respectively. With progressive aging, it is the age-related decline of these functions that leads to diseases like osteoporosis, which is characterized by reduced bone mass and increased fracture risk. Exercise, particularly in early life, contributes not only to reaching peak bone mass but also to enhancing the bone mineral density, which imparts architectural strength to the skeleton. In addition, exercise throughout adulthood can reverse age-related declines in bone health, suggesting that physical activity plays a protective role against skeletal aging and associated morbidities. In addition to the skeletal benefits, exercise also has broader implications for general physical health, which has a bearing on bone health. Greater muscular strength and improved balance resulting from continuous exercise reduce the risk of falls, a frequent cause of fractures for older adults. The incorporation of resistance exercise programs is shown to result in considerable improvements in muscular strength that underlie the musculoskeletal and, by extension, the bones. Furthermore, exercise and nutritional interventions have also been seen to hold promise in the prevention of sarcopenia, which is integrative muscle wasting that often coexists with aging and affects bone health indirectly. Despite evidence indicating that tissue-specific exercise regimens can lead to beneficial changes in muscle and bone function, this evidence underscores the need for a multidimensional intervention to maintain skeletal integrity across the lifespan (Burton et al., 2010).

Emerging evidence supports the role of specific nutritional interventions, in addition to exercise, as having a key role to promote bone health. Some supplements, including creatine, have been shown to enhance muscle strength and mass, with positive effects on bone density, particularly in susceptible groups at risk of muscle wasting. The combined effects of exercise and supplementation have been shown to yield dramatic improvements in muscle function and bone density, thereby reducing fracture risk and enhancing quality of life. In cancer patients, where muscle wasting and reduced bone health are prevalent, exercise interventions, coupled with nutritional support, have been found to reverse these changes, confirming the potential of exercise as an intervention in clinical practice. In this regard, the focus on constant exercise coupled with the proper type of nutritional interventions turns into a necessary step towards a betterment of peak bone accrual and, in turn, overall functioning among aging populations (Fairman et al., 2018).

2.6.3. Medical Interventions and Treatments

Aging significantly affects bone health, with frequent cases of diseases such as sarcopenia, progressive loss of muscle mass and strength. Effective medical treatments are necessary to reduce these effects and enhance the quality of life among elderly people. Recent studies indicate that there are different causes of sarcopenia, including hormonal imbalance, inflammation, and malnutrition. Despite research on pharmacological treatments, outcomes have been largely poor, while some treatments have demonstrated notable efficacy. One likely line of treatment has been angiotensin-converting enzyme inhibitors, but the need for more intensive randomized controlled trials is also apparent. Lastly, resistance training is the most potent intervention against sarcopenia, although patients often lack the motivation or physical stamina to undertake high-intensity exercise programs. Strategically integrating different treatment modalities can provide a multipronged approach to skeletal aging and well-being. Nutritional interventions also play a significant role in counteracting age-related muscle loss and preserving skeletal health. The importance of adequate nutrient intake, particularly protein, has been emphasized to preserve muscle mass throughout the aging process.

In older age, a typical reduction in appetite and alterations in metabolism contribute to inadequate nutrition and exacerbate muscle degeneration. Supplementation protocols, such as creatine (Cr), have been of interest due to their ability to increase lean body mass and maximize physical function. When added to structured exercise programs, such interventions might promote substantial improvements in muscle strength and overall function. Clinical evidence demonstrates the potential of such nutritional interventions, which can contribute to adaptations to physical activity, especially in those at risk for muscle loss. Thus, properly planned diets that take into consideration the specific needs of the elderly can do much to counteract the adverse effects of aging on the skeleton. In addition to physical and nutritional therapy, psychosocial factors and combined treatment approaches play a central role in elucidating the complexity of aging and physical decline. The mental status of the elderly has a definite influence on their adherence to health-related measures, including exercise and dietetic interventions. Interventions that involve social support and behavioral therapies can bring about active participation in health care among individuals. Creating environments that facilitate physical activity and healthy food intake can increase motivation and compliance. Further, addressing mental health can improve health outcomes for the aging population. As multidisciplinary strategies gain momentum, there is consensus that a synergistic approach that integrates physical, dietary, and psychosocial dimensions is crucial for effective intervention and treatment in the regulation of growth, development, and skeletal aging. This integrative model not only enhances quality of life but also fosters resilience to aging change.

Test Your Knowledge

1. What lifestyle practices help prevent or slow skeletal aging?
2. How can early management strategies reduce the risk of age-related skeletal disorders?

SUMMARY

Skeletal aging occurs inextricably with the general processes of growth and development. With advancing age, skeletal muscle undergoes significant changes that impact its function and composition. Insight into these changes is vital to designing interventions to reverse the negative influences of aging on skeletal well-being. Of particular interest is the decrease in muscle mass and regenerative function, which diminishes physical performance and increases vulnerability to a variety of health issues. By examining the processes underlying these changes in skeletal muscle with advancing age, researchers are better able to understand the mechanisms underlying both declines in muscle quality and communication between muscle and fat. In so doing, this understanding provides potential access to new strategies to facilitate muscle resistance and overall health in the elderly. Moreover, recent findings portray sarcopenia not just as a mere consequence of decreased muscle mass, but rather as a complex interface between muscle quality and altered body composition. The accumulation of adiposity, particularly in skeletal muscle, then emerges as a major complicating factor in this scenario. Since studies have emphasized that not all fat is damaging, but excess can lead to negative effects on muscle contractility and overall function by increased lipotoxicity. The interdependence between muscle wasting and fat accumulation highlights the importance of a comprehensive, more selective perspective of skeletal aging beyond measures of muscle mass. Addressing these factors in intervention programs would optimize the effectiveness of interventions, ensuring both the quantity and quality of muscle as humans age. In this way, understanding the complex dynamics of growth, development, and skeletal change associated with aging reveals pathways to optimize health outcomes in older adults. Emphasizing the retention of muscle mass and functional integrity provides a holistic approach to resolving the effects of aging. Far more research is needed to uncover the mechanisms underlying muscle-fat interactions, particularly in the context of inflammation and metabolic health. These results not only provide an improved understanding of skeletal aging but also have significant roles to play in the development of effective interventions that enhance the quality of life in elderly individuals. Finally, maintaining skeletal health is a core aspect of encouraging active, independent living late in life, thereby ultimately benefiting society as a whole.

The intricate interaction of growth, development, and aging of the skeleton is a complex process akin to a multifaceted network of biological determinants that not only shapes physical height but also impacts overall well-being. At each stage of life, from infancy to senescence, the skeleton undergoes significant adaptations. These adaptations are based on a myriad of genetic, environmental, and dietary factors that converge to determine bone density, anatomy, and physiology. Notably, the mechanisms that drive these changes are increasingly recognized to involve the microbiota-gut-brain axis, which plays a vital role in regulating many physiological processes, including bone health. An appreciation of this axis underscores the emerging perspective that the health of one's bones can be closely linked to gut health and, consequently, to mental health, thereby portraying a multiaxial model of skeletal aging (Cryan et al., 2019). With the progress of skeletal aging, a higher incidence of some degenerative diseases is seen, which highlights the need to lay sound healthcare plans. In particular, the development of musculoskeletal disorders further highlights the necessity for targeted interventions aimed at preserving mobility and preventing disability in older people. Trends in morbidity and mortality offer proof of heavy disease burden, particularly in the elderly, which adds further justification to give priority to preventative health interventions. The latest findings show that increased longevity is often accompanied by an increase in chronic conditions such as osteoarthritis and osteoporosis, underscoring the need to optimize integrated care opportunities. Solving the issues posed by bone aging enables healthcare systems to enhance the quality of life of older adults, ensuring that physical obstacles do not overshadow their longevity (Zhou et al., 2019). In addition, the role of lifestyle factors, in turn, cannot be too strongly emphasized. A consistent exercise regimen, dietary modification, and stress management are significant factors in maintaining skeletal integrity and preventing deterioration with age. Weight-bearing exercises, for instance, directly impact bone density, whereas adequate calcium and vitamin D intake increase bone mineralization. Furthermore, recent evidence emphasizes the role of the microbiota-gut-brain axis in regulating exercise and diet behavior, as it does for cognition and emotional health. Therefore, a coordinated approach involving physical, dietary, and mental health is required for individuals at all stages of the life cycle, particularly as they face the complexities of bone aging. Highlighting this multi-dimensional framework can encourage a more holistic perspective of growth and development across the lifespan (Cryan et al., 2019).

KEY TERMS FROM THIS CHAPTER

- Endochondral Ossification
- Skeletal Maturation
- Chronological Age
- Skeletal Age Estimation
- Epiphyseal Fusion
- Bone Maturation
- Skeletal Age
- Epiphyseal Closure
- Degenerative Changes
- Epiphyseal Plate
- Bone Remodeling
- Biological Age
- Pubertal Growth Spurt
- Growth Plate
- Chronological Age
- Pubertal Growth Spurt
- Intramembranous Ossification
- Osteoporosis

CRITICAL THINKING QUESTIONS

1. **Which of the following bones is the last to complete its ossification?**
   a. Clavicle
   b. Femur
   c. Sternum
   d. Tibia
2. **Which of the following best describes the pattern of skeletal development?**
   a. Distal to proximal
   b. Posterior to anterior
   c. Proximal to distal
   d. Cranial to caudal
3. **What type of ossification is responsible for the development of flat bones like the skull?**
   a. Endochondral ossification
   b. Intermembranous ossification
   c. Periosteal ossification
   d. Subchondral ossification
4. **The pubic symphysis is often used in aging adult skeletons because:**
   a. It is unaffected by age
   b. It has predictable age-related changes
   c. It fuses early in life
   d. It only changes in females
5. **The appearance and fusion of ossification centers is most commonly used to estimate:**
   a. Sex
   b. Stature
   c. Age-at-death
   d. Ancestry

Short Answer Questions

1. Define endochondral and intramembranous ossification. How do they differ in terms of bone formation?
2. What role do growth plates (epiphyseal plates) play in skeletal development, and how are they used in age estimation?
3. Explain how dental eruption is used to estimate age in subadult skeletons.
4. Describe two morphological changes in the pelvis that can be used to estimate age-at-death in adult skeletons.
5. Explain the importance of the medial clavicular epiphysis in age estimation.

Answers to Critical Thinking Questions

1. (a); 2. (d; 3. (b); 4. (b); 5. (c)

REFERENCES

1. Moresi, V., Marroncelli, N., Coletti, D., & Adamo, S. (2015). Regulation of skeletal muscle development and homeostasis by gene imprinting, histone acetylation and microRNA. *Biochimica Et Biophysica Acta (BBA) - Gene Regulatory Mechanisms, 1849*(3), 309–316. https://doi.org/10.1016/j.bbagrm.2015.01.002Ajbage, J. O., Heijsters, G., Politis, C., Salem, A., et al. (2015). Coronectomy of deeply impacted lower third molar: Incidence of outcomes and complications after one year follow-up. https://core.ac.uk/download/55765860.pdf (accessed on 21st July 2025).
2. Aljameel, S. S., Althumairy, L., Albassam, B., Alsheikh, G., Albluwi, L., Althukair, R., Alhareky, M., et al. (2023). Predictive artificial intelligence model for detecting dental age using panoramic radiograph images. *Big Data and Cognitive Computing, 7*(8). https://www.semanticscholar.org/paper/f0b51bd1082d25e6eed35b2b2ca96d60e101b621 (accessed on 21st July 2025).
3. Almonacid-Fierro, J. G. A. (2022). The pandemic of childhood obesity: Challenges and possibilities from physical activity. *Health Promotion Perspectives, 12*, 229–230. https://www.semanticscholar.org/paper/185ed590bc54f5d8353491f7877dbeea3256bc59 (accessed on 21st July 2025).
4. Andrews, C., Bateson, M., Bedford, T., Kolenda, C., et al. (2017). Early-life adversity accelerates cellular ageing and affects adult inflammation: Experimental evidence from the European starling. https://core.ac.uk/download/80696879.pdf (accessed on 21st July 2025).
5. Baker, J. R. (2015). The prevalence and risks of injury for masters' athletes: Current findings. https://core.ac.uk/download/211331646.pdf (accessed on 21st July 2025).
6. Belcastro, M. G., Marchi, D., & Pietrobelli, A. (2022). The relationship between bipedalism and growth: A metric assessment in a documented modern skeletal collection (Certosa Collection, Bologna, Italy). https://core.ac.uk/download/534234897.pdf (accessed on 21st July 2025).
7. Bellido, T., & Delgado-Calle, J. (2015). Osteocytes and skeletal pathophysiology. https://core.ac.uk/download/84831375.pdf (accessed on 21st July 2025).
8. Bogaert, V., De Naeyer, H., De Spaey, A., Derave, W., et al. (2014). Genetic variations in the androgen receptor are associated with steroid concentrations and anthropometrics but not with muscle mass in healthy young men. https://core.ac.uk/download/55845621.pdf (accessed on 21st July 2025).
9. Bogin, B., & Smith, B. H. (2000). Chapter 11. Evolution of the human life cycle. http://deepblue.lib.umich.edu/bitstream/2027.42/134403/1/Bogin%20%26%20Smith_2000_Evolution%20of%20the%20Human%20Life%20Cycle%20rd.pdf (accessed on 21st July 2025).
10. Bull, F., Al-Ansari, S. S., Biddle, S., Borodulin, K., Buman, M. P., Cardon, G., Carty, C., et al. (2020). World Health Organization 2020 guidelines on physical activity and sedentary behavior. *British Journal of Sports Medicine, 54*, 1451–1462. https://doi.org/10.1136/bjsports-2020-102955 (accessed on 21st July 2025).
11. Burton, L. A., & Sumukadas, D. (2010). Optimal management of sarcopenia. https://core.ac.uk/download/20453974.pdf (accessed on 21st July 2025).
12. Carter, C. S., Justice, J. N., & Thompson, L. (2019). Lipotoxicity, aging, and muscle contractility: Does fiber type matter? https://open.bu.edu/bitstream/2144/40625/7/carter_justice_thompson_Lipotoxicity_paper_04302019.pdf (accessed on 21st July 2025).

13. Caspersen, I. D., Fritzbøger, A. F. Ø., Petersen, J., Birkebæk, N., Christensen, A. M. R., Schou, A. J., Kristensen, K., et al. (2025). Effect of testosterone treatment during puberty in boys with Klinefelter syndrome (The TIPY Study): Protocol for a nationwide randomized, double-blinded, placebo-controlled study. *BMJ Open, 15*. https://www.semanticscholar.org/paper/0c7cc7092d375c5778d799b2e87960a757379447 (accessed on 21st July 2025).

14. Chavassieux, P., Chenu, C., Hopkinson, M., Javaheri, B., et al. (2015). Excessive growth hormone expression in male GH transgenic mice adversely alters bone architecture and mechanical strength. https://core.ac.uk/download/36778145.pdf (accessed on 21st July 2025).

15. Cherry, K., Jazwinski, S. M., Kim, S., Myers, L., et al. (2018). Body composition, IGF1 status, and physical functionality in nonagenarians: Implications for osteosarcopenia. https://core.ac.uk/download/188830392.pdf (accessed on 21st July 2025).

16. Chiesa, C., Donini, L. M., Lenzi, A., Pacifico, L., et al. (2017). Non-alcoholic fatty liver disease connections with fat-free tissues: A focus on bone and skeletal muscle. https://core.ac.uk/download/98335830.pdf (accessed on 21st July 2025).

17. Conboy, I. M., Conboy, M. J., Etienne, J., Liu, L., et al. (2020). Skeletal muscle as an experimental model of choice to study tissue aging and rejuvenation. https://core.ac.uk/download/323080532.pdf (accessed on 21st July 2025).

18. Cryan, J. F., O'Riordan, K. J., Cowan, C. S. M., Sandhu, K. V., Bastiaanssen, T. F. S., Boehme, M., Codagnone, M. G., et al. (2019). The microbiota-gut-brain axis. *Physiological Reviews, 99*, 1877–2013. https://doi.org/10.1152/physrev.00018.2018 (accessed on 21st July 2025).

19. Devi, H. S. C., Manda, A., Priya, C. P., Datla, P. V., Kandikatla, P., Babu, N. H., & Alla, R. K. (2023). Correlation of sagittal skeletal malocclusion and growth patterns between digital and conventional dermatoglyphics. *Uttar Pradesh Journal of Zoology*. https://www.semanticscholar.org/paper/dc64ffba0a0c3b127889e0e8ad2f56a2f2e2dc86 (accessed on 21st July 2025).

20. Fairman, C. M., Galvão, D. A., Hart, N. H., Kendall, M., et al. (2018). The potential therapeutic effects of creatine supplementation on body composition and muscle function in cancer. https://core.ac.uk/download/213607833.pdf (accessed on 21st July 2025).

21. Fantauzzi, C. B., Iacobini, C., Menini, S., Pugliese, G., et al. (2017). Role of galectin-3 in bone cell differentiation, bone pathophysiology and vascular osteogenesis. https://core.ac.uk/download/141696866.pdf (accessed on 21st July 2025).

22. Gallagher, J., Hackman, L., & Schaefer, M. (2015). Variability of developmental timings of the knee in young American children as assessed through Pyle and Hoerr's radiographic atlas. https://core.ac.uk/download/30663211.pdf (accessed on 21st July 2025).

23. Handschin, C., & Svensson, K. (2014). Modulation of PGC-1α activity as a treatment for metabolic and muscle-related diseases. https://core.ac.uk/download/33298388.pdf (accessed on 21st July 2025).

24. Hathaway-Schrader, J. D., Steinkamp, H. M., Chavez, M. B., Poulides, N., Kirkpatrick, J. E., Chew, M. E., Huang, E., et al. (2019). Antibiotic perturbation of gut microbiota dysregulates osteoimmune cross talk in postpubertal skeletal development. *American Journal of Pathology, 189*, 370–390. https://doi.org/10.1016/j.ajpath.2018.10.017 (accessed on 21st July 2025).

25. Horenberg, A. L., Ren, Y., Zeng, E. Z., Rindone, A. N., Pathak, A. P., & Grayson, W. L. (2025). 3D imaging reveals changes in the neurovascular architecture of the murine calvarium with aging. *Bone Research, 13*. https://www.semanticscholar.org/paper/3915e6d6d8c14a0f5959

58a10d210f36d927ac3f (accessed on 21st July 2025).

26. Jaishankar, M., Tseten, T., Anbalagan, N., Mathew, B. B., & Beeregowda, K. N. (2014). Toxicity, mechanism and health effects of some heavy metals. *Interdisciplinary Toxicology, 7*, 60–72. https://doi.org/10.2478/intox-2014-0009 (accessed on 21st July 2025).

27. James, S. L., Abate, D., Abate, K. H., Abay, S. M., Abbafati, C., Abbasi, N., Abbastabar, H., et al. (2018). Global, regional, and national incidence, prevalence, and years lived with disability for 354 diseases and injuries for 195 countries and territories, 1990–2017: A systematic analysis for the Global Burden of Disease Study 2017. *The Lancet, 392*, 1789–1858. https://doi.org/10.1016/s0140-6736(18)32279-7 (accessed on 21st July 2025).

28. Karlsson, M., Nordqvist, A., & Karlsson, C. (2008). Physical activity increases bone mass during growth. *Food & Nutrition Research, 52*. https://www.semanticscholar.org/paper/c0bdddb3e9a8b70a29edebf57c84b06da89adfed (accessed on 21st July 2025).

29. Karlsson, M., Nordqvist, A., & Karlsson, C. (2008). Sustainability of exercise-induced increases in bone density and skeletal structure. *Food & Nutrition Research, 52*. https://www.semanticscholar.org/paper/8cd97de3dbd0b77970d3e86591e126e2e39c76a1 (accessed on 21st July 2025).

30. Lai, J. C., Tandon, P., Bernal, W., Tapper, E. B., Ekong, U. D., Dasarathy, S., & Carey, E. J. (2021). Malnutrition, frailty, and sarcopenia in patients with cirrhosis: 2021 practice guidance by the American Association for the Study of Liver Diseases. *Hepatology, 74*, 1611–1644. https://doi.org/10.1002/hep.32049 (accessed on 21st July 2025).

31. Larsson, L., Degens, H., Li, M., Salviati, L., Lee, Y. I., Thompson, W. J., Kirkland, J. L., et al. (2018). Sarcopenia: Aging-related loss of muscle mass and function. *Physiological Reviews, 99*, 427–511. https://doi.org/10.1152/physrev.00061.2017 (accessed on 21st July 2025).

32. Lin, Y., Li, Y., Liang, G., Yang, X., Yang, J., Hu, Q., Sun, J., et al. (2024). Single-cell transcriptome analysis of aging mouse liver. *The FASEB Journal, 38*. https://www.semanticscholar.org/paper/5aa9d39e5012ad8154a1e1b0729c01fe6f593ba2 (accessed on 21st July 2025).

33. Ouyang, S., Cao, D., Yin, Y., Ma, F., & Ren, G. (2025). Sex differences in physical activity dose-response effects on site-specific bone mineral density during childhood and adolescence. *Scientific Reports, 15*. https://www.semanticscholar.org/paper/ebb5fdc3e423b297d6b48f991d75ad35251e43eb (accessed on 21st July 2025).

34. Piercy, K. L., Troiano, R. P., Ballard, R., Carlson, S. A., Fulton, J. E., Galuska, D. A., George, S. M., et al. (2018). The Physical Activity Guidelines for Americans. *JAMA, 320*, 2020–2020. https://doi.org/10.1001/jama.2018.14854 (accessed on 21st July 2025).

35. Scheffler, A., Rogol, M., Iancu, T., Hanć, T., Moelyo, A., Suchomlinov, A., Lebedeva, L., et al. (2021). Growth during times of fear and emotional stress. *Human Biology and Public Health*. https://www.semanticscholar.org/paper/2c2d5eb4d109fe7ac59de2f6aeb0ea3810211b88 (accessed on 21st July 2025).

36. Sharifi-Rad, M., Kumar, N. V. A., Zucca, P., Varoni, E. M., Dini, L., Panzarini, E., Rajković, J., et al. (2020). Lifestyle, oxidative stress, and antioxidants: Back and forth in the pathophysiology of chronic diseases. *Frontiers in Physiology, 11*. https://doi.org/10.3389/fphys.2020.00694 (accessed on 21st July 2025).

37. Smith, N., Cakouros, D., Ryan, F. J., Lynn, D. J., Paton, S., Arthur, A., & Gronthos, S. (2025).

DNA hydroxy methylases Tet1 and Tet2 regulate bone aging and BMSC metabolism through the IGF-1/mTOR signaling axis. *Stem Cells*. https://www.semanticscholar.org/paper/45c363dd72a2cc3ba6e98e8d3d4996e89eb2038f (accessed on 21st July 2025).

38. Terzi, Ö., & Hatipoğlu, S. (2025). Infant patient exposed to chemotherapy and radiotherapy in the womb: Letter to editor. *Medical Science and Discovery*. https://www.semanticscholar.org/paper/0dffc8e4e1da212323df0335c3ee26ce14350b31 (accessed on 21st July 2025).

39. Tieland, M., Trouwborst, I., & Clark, B. C. (2017). Skeletal muscle performance and ageing. *Journal of Cachexia, Sarcopenia and Muscle, 9*, 3–19. https://doi.org/10.1002/jcsm.12238 (accessed on 21st July 2025).

40. Vos, T., Abajobir, A. A., Abate, K. H., Abbafati, C., Abbas, K., Abd-Allah, F., Abdulkader, R. S., et al. (2017). Global, regional, and national incidence, prevalence, and years lived with disability for 328 diseases and injuries for 195 countries, 1990–2016: A systematic analysis for the Global Burden of Disease Study 2016. *The Lancet, 390*, 1211–1259. https://doi.org/10.1016/s0140-6736(17)32154-2 (accessed on 21st July 2025).

41. Weissenfluh, N. G. (2019). Periodontitis and the elderly: An overview of the disease and its impact on an aging population. https://core.ac.uk/download/213463617.pdf (accessed on 21st July 2025).

42. Wierzbicka, E., Świercz, A., Płudowski, P., Jaworski, M., & Szalecki, M. (2018). Skeletal status, body composition, and glycemic control in adolescents with Type 1 diabetes mellitus. *Journal of Diabetes Research, 2018*, 1–14. https://doi.org/10.1155/2018/8121634 (accessed on 21st July 2025).

43. Zhou, M., Wang, H., Zeng, X., Yin, P., Zhu, J., Chen, W., Li, X., et al. (2019). Mortality, morbidity, and risk factors in China and its provinces, 1990–2017: A systematic analysis for the Global Burden of Disease Study 2017. *The Lancet, 394*, 1145–1158. https://doi.org/10.1016/s0140-6736(19)30427-1 (accessed on 21st July 2025).

PALEOPATHOLOGY AND SKELETAL DISEASE

3

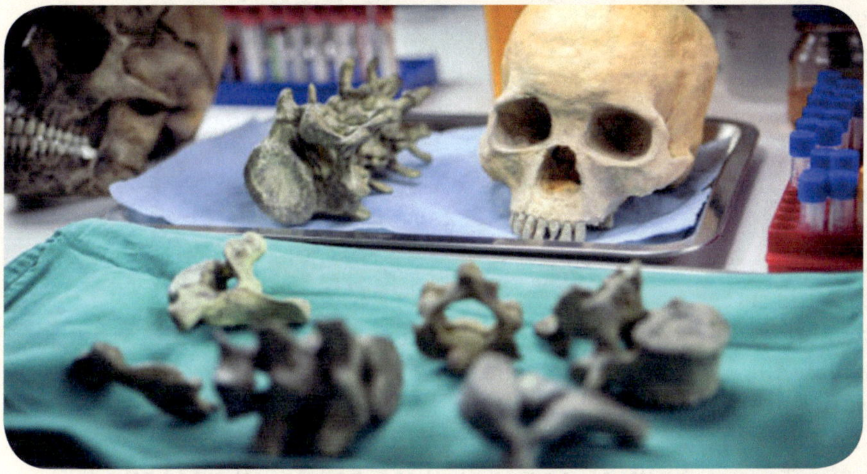

Introduction

Paleopathology, a multidisciplinary field of research that examines disease records in ancient human and animal skeletons, offers crucial insights into the history of disease and health development. By exploiting osteoarchaeological techniques, researchers can analyze skeletal records to reconstruct earlier conditions of health, for instance, the occurrence of skeletal disease and its expression. This evaluation allows for a more comprehensive understanding of how various environmental, cultural, and biological factors influenced health among ancient populations. The application of contemporary diagnostic techniques, in conjunction with traditional examination methods, provides a comprehensive approach to diagnosing conditions such as osteoarthritis and other musculoskeletal disorders. This new focus reflects the growing recognition that skeletal remains are a rich repository of historical health data, thus bridging the gap between medical history and archaeology. Paleopathology not only sheds light on the frequency and progression of disease in extinct populations,

LEARNING OBJECTIVES

After studying this chapter, you will be able to:

1. Describe the methods of paleopathological research
2. Explain the common skeletal diseases identified in paleopathology
3. Discuss the role of environment in skeletal health
4. Identify case studies in paleopathology
5. Understand the intersection of paleopathology and modern medicine
6. Learn about ethical considerations in paleopathological research

but it also highlights the multifaceted interaction between human behavior and health outcomes. For instance, lifestyle habits such as nutrition, physical activity, and occupational exposures can leave a distinctive mark on the skeleton, as evidenced by entheses and the cross-sectional geometry of long bones. Some recent research has emphasized the importance of embracing the small-data paradigm to maximize the interpretive value of small samples, particularly within biologically and culturally similar groups. Through this, researchers can superimpose contextual conditions, such as age and sex estimates, over their data to better understand the implications of specific pathologies. Paleopathology is therefore an important window into the biological reactions of ancient humans to ecological and social stressors, expanding knowledge of their lives. The addition of paleopathological data adds a richer story to human adaptation and resilience under fluctuating ecological conditions. Skeletal data reveal patterns of health that illuminate researchers regarding the population's health in the past. Findings from research indicate that residential changes to suboptimal surroundings may be linked to declining health, and therefore linking disease patterns in the skeleton to environmental factors. Of specific interest is a collaboration across numerous localities within the Western Hemisphere that revealed heterogeneous health among pre-Columbian populations. This range of data highlights the significance of paleopathology in depicting long-term patterns of health and their implications for societal change, including the effects of European conquest and changes in population size. Lastly, paleopathology offers fascinating insights into how humans have adapted to environmental pressures and lifestyle changes, and a model for future research into skeletal disease and its correlation with demographic change (Becker et al., 2019; Steckel, 2025) (Figure 3.1).

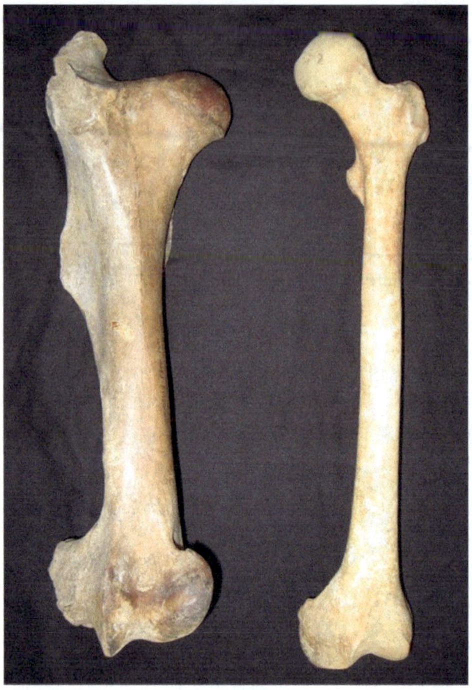

Figure 3.1. The study of paleopathology in skeletal disease.

Source: https://media.springernature.com/lw685/springer-static/image/chp%3A10.1007%2F978-3-030-44600-0_53-1/MediaObjects/118056_0_En_53-1_Fig2_HTML.jpg.

Definition and Scope of Paleopathology

Paleopathology is a specialist discipline that examines evidence of disease in previous populations by analyzing skeletal remains and archaeological materials. The discipline applies to a multi-disciplinary endeavor, borrowing truth from anthropology, medicine, and archaeology to describe the quality and extent of disease incidence and morbidity that afflicted previous societies. This field seeks to reconstruct the patterns of health and disease among populations and individuals, providing an interpretive context for understanding how environmental and social processes affected health in the past. As an ongoing and developing field, paleopathology has evolved significantly, leading to methodologies designed to enhance the identification of disease in human remains and putting finds into broader histories. Paleopathology extends beyond mere identification of disease, involving a profound analysis of its social and cultural context. Through the embrace of technological and research innovations, paleopathologists can analyze the impact of disease on individual health, population demography, and societal structure. For instance, changes in population trends and settlement patterns are often associated with disease outbreaks and their subsequent effects on mortality.

The field is also concerned with the application of consistent terminology to promote clarity and converse better among researchers. As identified, finding an agreed-upon vocabulary for these changes is meant to reduce confusion and enable better comparisons among studies towards a better understanding of human health in the past (Assis et al., 2016). The evolution of paleopathology also replicates broader scientific advances, taking on an interdisciplinary approach that develops its critical framework. Scientists from diverse backgrounds, including the biomedical sciences and social theory, ask different questions that refine our understanding of skeletal disease and what it can reveal about the history of human beings. Technology, for example, has been pivotal in refining paleopathology as a research discipline, from imaging technology that discloses interior structures non-invasively, through to biochemical protocols that simplify the examination of disease markers. With these advances, however, ethical issues must also be addressed to achieve responsible research. As the field advances, ongoing debate over such ethical issues will be instrumental in maintaining the integrity and value of paleopathological research (Grauer et al., 2022) (Figure 3.2).

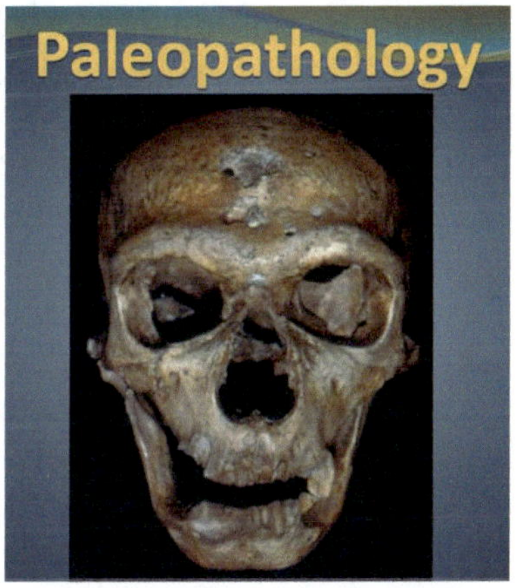

Figure 3.2. Paleopathology.

Source: https://cdn.slidesharecdn.com/ss_thumbnails/09-week9-230609135821-f9cdbbb4-thumbnail.jpg?width=640&height=640&fit=bounds.

Historical Development of the Field

The history of paleopathology, the examination of ancient diseases through the study of human and animal remains, has progressed considerably since its inception. Initial research was primarily visual inspection of bone remains for signs of illness, such as those related to trauma or starvation. However, with the progress in the field, researchers began using progressively sophisticated approaches, including radiography, computed tomography, and histopathological analysis, which allowed them to learn more about skeletal disease. This shift towards an increasingly interdisciplinary study paved the way for groundbreaking discoveries in terms of disease prevalence and types that afflicted ancient populations, giving way to profound human health stories over the passage of time. The evolution of molecular techniques has further revolutionized paleopathology, particularly for the study of diseases that were not straightforward to diagnose based on traditional methods. The application of ancient DNA (aDNA) analysis and metagenomics techniques not only elucidated the genetic signatures of pathogens but also enabled researchers to explore the coevolution of humans and disease, as observed in studies on tuberculosis (Ileana et al., 2020). This disease has a long history, with evidence traced in human bones dating back to Neolithic times. By tracing such diseases' evolutionary history, paleopathologists can reveal patterns of adaptation, migration, and interactions with the environment that shaped historical human populations and health. Along with these advancements, ongoing advances in bioinformatics are complementing researchers' abilities to cross-validate data and enhance approaches to studying ancient pathogens (Giovannangelo et al., 2025). Comparative evaluation of taxonomic pipelines for aDNA shows that applying multiple analytical frameworks can yield more authentic results, ultimately improving our understanding of the health issues faced by ancient human communities. All these developments are highly relevant to reassembling the health narratives of less well-represented populations, thereby improving our understanding of humanity's common past. As techniques in paleopathology grow more advanced, the field holds the potential to assist in answering some of the most basic questions about past diseases and their relations to society, thereby improving our understanding of the human past.

Importance of Studying Skeletal Diseases in Ancient Populations

Skeletal diseases of ancient populations must be analyzed in order to uncover the health and habits of previous societies. Through the study of skeletons of individuals from different epochs, researchers can access a rich source of data on the rates of diseases, nutritional intakes deficiency, and overall conditions of being well. The skeletal record can serve as a database to examine how environmental influences impact human health, for instance, diet, activity, and social organization. For instance, according to research documents, the lack of evidence in past studies impedes our understanding of patterns of human well-being over the timescale of millennia. However, skeletal analyses can provide insights into such trends by revealing patterns of health conditions within a location, as seen in joint ventures in the Western Hemisphere. This technique provides valuable background information for measuring long-term health trajectories and social responses to environmental change, hence enhancing our knowledge of human adaptation. Skeletal disease can also further inform us about the social and economic mechanisms of ancient societies. Bone pathologies also uncover not only individual health but also social conditions such as population, wars, and the movement of people. Some diseases, for example, can uncover the pressure within communities when dealing with adversity posed by changes in the environment or availability of resources. The examination of skeletal disease can tell us a great deal about how early humans adapted to their environments, particularly their diets, which are important not only for physical health but also for the organization of society. Toward this end, studies have indicated that even early humans suffered from nutritional problems as the discovery of ancient hominin cranial remains with signs of anemia attests. These findings mark the complexity of ancient diets and their significance in understanding human growth over time, and illustrate significant interdependencies between health and environment. Aside from intellectual interest, the examination of skeletal diseases in ancient populations has broad significance for contemporary public health initiatives. Understanding past health trends provides us with a template for making sense of current trends in health disparities. By learning how past populations responded to environmental pressures, we can better inform our response to such issues today, particularly in populations under the same ecological pressures. For instance, learning how nutritional deficiencies were manifested in past populations may illuminate long-term health conditions common in today's societies.

When data on skeletal condition are collected over a range of time intervals, they provide an overall picture of human health evolution and define avenues for further research and intervention. Through these studies' findings, past and present become connected to illustrate the ongoing role of paleopathology in explaining human health over the centuries (Figure 3.3).

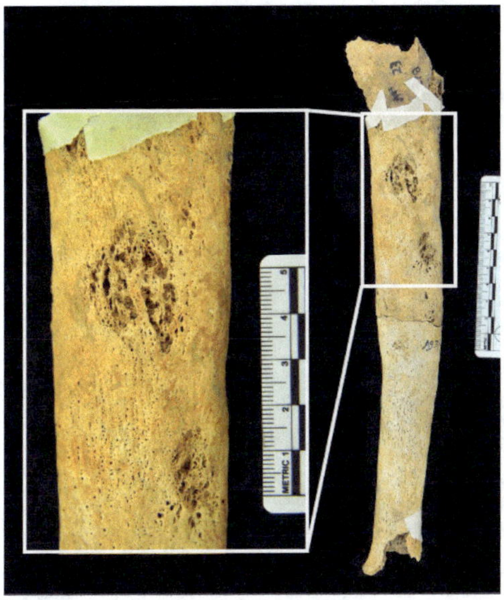

Figure 3.3. The study of skeletal diseases in ancient populations.

Source: https://stri.si.edu/sites/default/files/styles/lightbox/public/ancient_diseases_photo_2.jpg?itok=f1A64Vyu.

3.1. Methods of Paleopathological Research

Learning Outcome

1. Osteological analysis techniques
2. Imaging technologies in paleopathology
3. Bioarchaeological approaches to skeletal remains

The investigation of paleopathological research includes numerous methodologies, each contributing especially to our knowledge of skeletal disease in past populations. One of the basic methods is the analysis of skeletal remains for signs of pathological changes, which may indicate the presence of particular diseases, trauma, or lifestyle-related stresses. Scientists employ macroscopic examination routinely to establish overt change, such as lesions or distortions that are indicative of health state. Technological advancements greatly enhance the method. For example, X-ray imaging and computed tomography (CT) allow for high-contrast visualization of internal anatomy, yielding information that can be missed with routine investigation alone. These imaging methods allow skeletal remains to be studied non-invasively, leading to a better knowledge of the skeletal pathology while maintaining the integrity of the archaeological finds and advancing the subject matter in ways that earlier methods were unable to do. Another important methodology employed in paleopathology is biomolecular analysis, which examines ancient DNA, proteins, or isotopes to provide contextual evidence on the health and diet of past populations. Stable isotope analysis, for instance, now plays a focal role in studies of the diet and nutritional status of individuals within archaeological samples. By analyzing the isotopic composition of bone remains, researchers can draw conclusions about diet, migration, and social status in ancient societies. The technique not only supplements evidence from skeletal analyses but also situates it within broader environmental and social contexts. Moreover, combining dietary knowledge with skeletal lesion data provides a more holistic picture of disease and health prevalence in past populations. Such a multidisciplinary approach demonstrates the complexity of human health and emphasizes the need to integrate methodologies in paleopathological studies. Lastly, the integration of modern imaging technologies, such as Reflectance Transformation Imaging (RTI), is a significant advancement towards the documentation and analysis of skeletal pathologies. RTI allows the capture of high-resolution surface data that can enhance visibility for subtle skeletal changes critical to disease. These imaging techniques have proved particularly useful in perinatal skeleton and other delicate specimen research, where traditional methods might be cumbersome or even destructive. up. The combination of RTI and conventional methods opens the way for a more nuanced examination of skeletal lesions and their impact on population health. As evidenced from some of the studies, such as those on the bioarcheology of children in the Baltic region, these cutting-edge methodologies create new paths for analyzing and interpreting skeletal remains, in turn enhancing our understanding of people's lives in the past (Peterson et al., 2016; Morrone et al., 2022) (Figure 3.4).

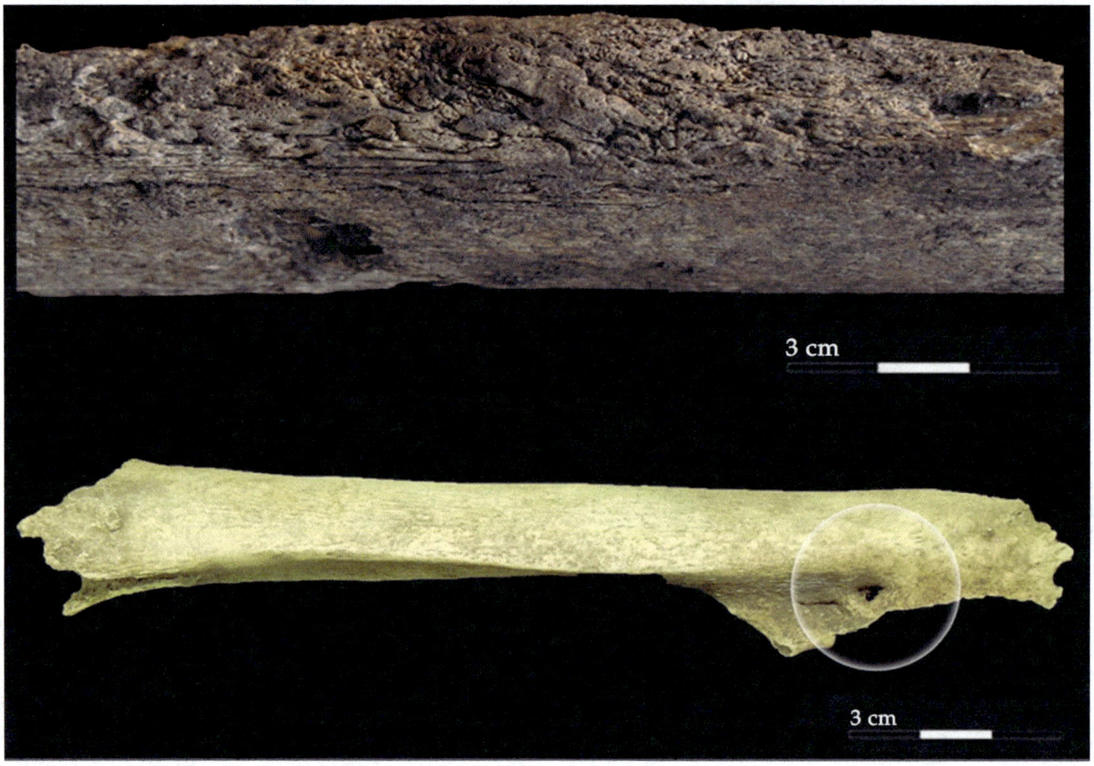

Figure 3.4. The exploration of paleopathological research encompasses a variety of methodologies.

Source: https://external-content.duckduckgo.com/iu/?u=https%3A%2F%2Fstatic.cambridge.org%2Fbinary%2Fversion%2Fid%2Furn%3Acambridge.org%3Aid%3Abinary%3A20200819025857167-0815%3AS104566352000005X%3AS104566352000005X_fig2.png%3Fpub-status%3Dlive&f=1&nofb=1&ipt=a22c10c264a86dd8073e1e01b48973ec149eda012697e6827eae5c317cdfdcd5.

3.1.1. Osteological Analysis Techniques

Paleopathology requires strong osteological analytical techniques capable of properly interpreting sicknesses in the skeletons and their implications for ancient people. Such techniques involve various methods that allow researchers to evaluate and document skeletal remains, leading the way to understanding the health and way of life of the past. Macroscopic analysis, radiographic study, and histological examination are some of the techniques that gather important information regarding the presence and evolution of diseases like osteoarthritis and osteoporosis. By accurately defining and delineating these conditions, researchers can relate skeletal changes with factors such as age, sex, and lifestyle. Including the incorporation of advanced imaging techniques also facilitates an assessment of skeletal integrity, which provides more understanding of how biomechanical stress impacts skeletal well-being over time. Thus, such approaches not only enhance the comprehension of the individual condition but also shed light on broader sociocultural and environmental contexts (Becker et al., 2019). In recent times, the need for multidisciplinary intervention of osteological investigation has emerged, particularly in responding to the complexity of skeletal disease. This interdisciplinary convergence enables the synthesis of evidence from anthropology, biomechanics, and medicine to improve understanding of skeletal determinants of health in past populations. In studies of conditions such as entheses and long-bone cross-sectional geometry, researchers emphasize a small-data protocol that focuses on well-preserved skeletal remains of biologically and culturally relevant populations. Such a methodological strategy facilitates a comprehensive evaluation of abnormalities, allowing for correlations among patterns of bodily movement and skeletal variation. Researchers have increasingly focused on establishing standardized testing protocols to ensure the maximum possible reliability of the evidence, which is essential for making cogent inferences about past populations and their adaptive variation to environmental stress (Becker et al., 2019). Osteological analysis techniques also play a crucial part in the investigation of osteoporosis and related skeletal diseases in ancient populations. The understanding of osteoporosis as a multifaceted disorder presupposes a delicate assessment of various factors, including age, menopausal state, and lifestyle, before death. By applying scientific techniques, scientists can identify diachronic patterns and variations in bone health, providing a diachronic perspective on how alterations in society—such as diet and occupation—have influenced skeletal integrity throughout history. By careful analyses of bone material, scientists integrate biomedical and historical perspectives on the history of osteoporosis, both among modern populations and ancient civilizations. This framing emphasizes the profound impact that socio-cultural conditions have had on skeletal health, linking past to contemporary biomedical discussion of osteoporosis (Figure 3.5).

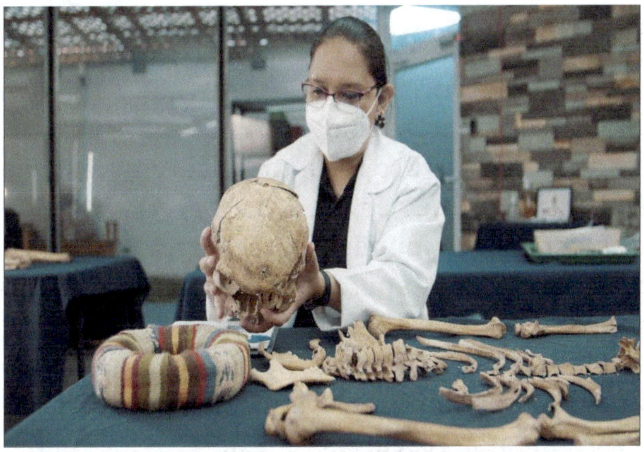

Figure 3.5. The study of paleopathology requires robust osteological analysis techniques.

Source: https://external-content.duckduckgo.com/iu/?u=https%3A%2F%2Fi.ytimg.com%2Fvi%2FcmSU7_eCt9E%2Fmaxresdefault.jpg%3Fsqp%3D-oaymwEmCIAKENAF8quKqQMa8AEB-AHUBoAC4AOKAgwIABABGEkgZShlMA8%3D%26rs%3DAOn4CLBmjWlOSPjffW0XW6qI_lvXCyBh9w&f=1&nofb=1&ipt=4514eb47a6452bc144486671863da6bb28655804d227174f2f16842e87ecdf12.

3.1.2. Imaging Technologies in Paleopathology

Imaging technologies have revolutionized the practice of paleopathology, enabling scientists to examine ancient skeletal evidence without invasive sampling. X-ray imaging, computed tomography (CT), and magnetic resonance imaging (MRI) allow researchers to visualize internal structures without disrupting the specimens. These technologies enable more refined inspection of skeletal pathology, allowing detection of disease and conditions that may not be discernible by conventional methods. The application of CT scans, for instance, has been particularly valuable for revealing subtle details of bone shape and pathological changes, such as lesions or deformities, thereby allowing a better understanding of skeletal disease in past populations. Integrated multidisciplinary methods are the solution to addressing the intricacy of diseases like cancer in fossil bones.

Studies currently suggest that signs of cancer in the archaeological record are scarce, leading to the proposal that carcinomas in the past were fewer than they are today. But this concept is founded on a narrow range of methodologies, operates primarily through coarse bone appearances, and may overlook small pathological details. By employing current imaging technologies alongside traditional assessments, researchers can provide more comprehensive information on ancient neoplastic diseases and thereby enrich the history of human health (Gardner et al., 2020). Also, the cross-pollination of paleopathologists and imaging specialists has much potential for future research. The necessity of consensus-based knowledge in unraveling complex mummy cases highlights the significance of multidisciplinary cooperation. An example is research on an ancient Egyptian mummy that referred to the successful utilization of multi-disciplinary diagnostic teams that integrated radiological and paleopathological contributions (Beckett R et al., 2019). This type of collective endeavor not only illustrated the diversity of possible diagnoses but also pointed up the shortcomings in any one line of approach. By creating standards through interdisciplinary discourse, the field of paleopathology can adopt a more reflective perspective on the skeletal diseases that have victimized human beings over the course of centuries, and thus achieve a broader appreciation of health and disease in ancient individuals.

3.1.3. Bioarchaeological Approaches to Skeletal Remains

Bioarchaeological analyses of skeletons provide contextual meaning to disease and health in human populations through paleopathology. Besides enabling researchers to identify the various conditions of the skeleton, the analytical techniques illuminate the mundane lives of inhabitants of ancient societies. By thorough documentation of osteoarthritis, entheses, and cross-sectional geometry variation in long bones, scientists are able to quantify the biomechanical stress endured by individuals.

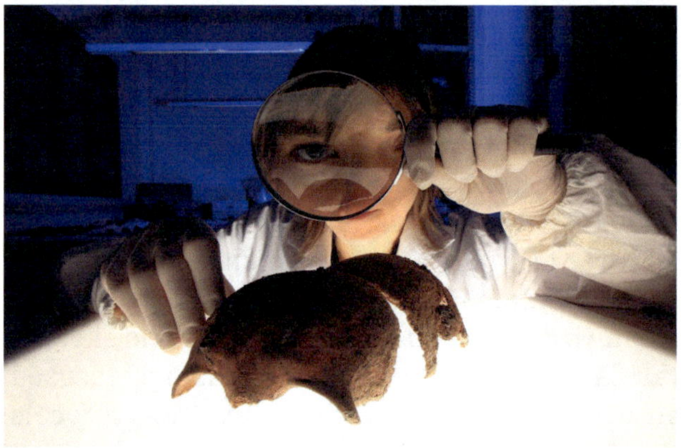

Figure 3.6. Bioarchaeological approaches to skeletal remains.

Source: https://external-content.duckduckgo.com/iu/?u=https%3A%2F%2Fbigea.unibo.it%2Fen%2Fresearch%2Fresearch-groups%2Fevolutionary-anthropology%2Fbioarcheological-approach-to-the-study-of-human-evolution%2F%40%40unibo.tiles.richtext%2F4c02ff6a841a48778fb3430ff8999a33%2F%40%40images%2Fb15b6c82-2854-421f-a9bf-0a7c84fc2078.jpeg&f=1&nofb=1&ipt=9a7559e

84c064fbb06a59f3699cf615f085a01eb94429d
e2b0807f3e75810e94.

This approach is complementary to the policy underlined in recent scholarship, requiring accurate description and definitions of skeletal disease to build a robust dataset. bioarcheologists Within the framework of small data, bioarcheologists can examine abnormalities incrementally and limit their judgments, thereby building a fuller picture of ancient populations and environmental adaptations (Becker et al., 2019).

Analytical frameworks applied within the discipline of bioarcheology today utilize sophisticated statistical techniques extensively to counteract scalability issues that may arise in analyzing skeletal materials. For instance, the application of Generalized Estimating Equations (GEE) allows researchers to draw meaningful correlations between articular surfaces from individual specimens. This has yielded insightful information, such as in studies on the Tiwanaku state population, where researchers noted eminent differences in elbow joint osteoarthritis across groups. The use of GEE, bioarcheological in addition to presenting more advanced outcomes from bioarcheological data, also maintains the integrity of the dataset by addressing issues of data independence (Bass et al., 2019). By means of these new methodologies, scholars can build an informed picture of skeletal health that is respectful of the heterogeneity of individual and collective patterns in ancient populations. The integration of bioarcheological data with clinical information further underscores the implications of skeletal studies for reconstructing historical diseases.

By focusing on multidisciplinary research that integrates osteological evaluations with current pathophysiologic knowledge, researchers can place skeletal findings in contemporary medical contexts. Such collaborations allow the examination of the impact of levels of physical activity, occupation, and environmental circumstances on alterations in the skeleton over time. New technologies, such as CT imaging and motion capture, enable new solutions for the analysis of skeletal remains. This multidisciplinary strategy deepens the history of skeletal disease and health, fostering dialogue between ancient practice and modern interpretation, ultimately shaping the future of paleopathology and skeletal disease research (Becker et al., 2019) (Figure 3.6).

Test Your Knowledge

1. What methods are commonly used in paleopathological research to identify disease in ancient skeletal remains?
2. How do imaging and comparative analysis contribute to paleopathological investigations?

3.2. Common Skeletal Diseases Identified in Paleopathology

Learning Outcome

1. Osteoarthritis and its implications
2. Tuberculosis and its effects on the skeleton
3. Treponemal diseases and their historical significance

Paleopathology skeletal disease analysis is crucial for measuring the incidence and manifestations of conditions within ancient populations. Osteoarthritis is among the most common skeletal diseases, resulting from cartilage deterioration and underlying bone changes, most often exacerbated by mechanical stressors. The osteoarthritic anatomical changes, such as eburnation and osteophyte formation, have been clearly documented in osteological evidence from a wide range of archaeological sites. A paleopathological interpretation of osteoarthritis pathogenesis not only helps identify the physical stressors faced by ancient human populations but also implies evolutionary accommodations to their environments. More focus on integrative methods, such as those advocated by contemporary research, attempts to further differentiate the correlation between skeletal health and lifestyle factors in the past, ultimately providing us with a better picture of the evolution of such conditions throughout history (Gardner et al., 2020). Osteomyelitis and tuberculosis are also frequently encountered in paleopathological descriptions and illustrate the impact of infectious disease on human health during different ages. Osteomyelitis, a bacterial infection of bone, may result in large skeletal changes recognizable in archaeological populations. The lesions of this disease commonly represent not only individual health difficulties but also broader epidemiological patterns within populations. Tuberculosis, another debilitating infection illness, has a unique skeletal expression, most commonly in the type of spinal lesion referred to as Potts disease. By examining the prevalence and distribution of such conditions among ancient populations, researchers are able to better understand the social and environmental conditions that led to the origin of infectious diseases. Further study of such conditions provides better explanations of the robustness of ancient populations and their resilience in the face of health crises (Gardner et al., 2020). Pathologies that result from trauma constitute a significant element of paleopathological studies in addition to infectious and degenerative diseases. Fractures and bone deformities resulting from traumatic accidents provide valuable insights into the lifestyles and activities of prehistoric populations. The presence of healed fractures in skeletal remains not only indicates the physical challenges an individual faced but also the medical knowledge of the period. Moreover, analysis of skeletal trauma, coupled with data on occupational hazards and social conflict, gives us insight into broad cultural and environmental contexts that affect human endeavors. As more researchers adopt interdisciplinary approaches, such as combining biomechanics and epidemiology, the study of skeletal trauma is advancing. This new approach has the potential to extend our understanding of how ancient populations managed survival in their own environments (Becker et al., 2019).

3.2.1. Osteoarthritis (OA) and Its Implications

Investigation of OA in bone samples is crucial to extend our understanding of the meaning of this degenerative condition within past populations. Osteoarthritis, characterized by cartilage degradation and bone changes, significantly affecting mobility and quality of life. In paleopathology, the presence of OA may also inform us about the health and lifestyle of ancient people. For instance, various studies show that OA prevalence may differ across populations depending on occupation or environmental stress. Moreover, diagnosing OA as present or absent may not capture variations in joint health, thereby complicating the interpretation of skeletal data. Therefore, the application of state-of-the-art statistical methods, such as Generalized Estimating Equations (GEE), can help resolve such scalar issues and enable researchers to interpret OA more effectively within bioarcheological contexts (Bass et al., 2019). The evidence from skeletal remains, especially those of Homo antecessor, demonstrates the broader implications of osteoarthritis. The morphological aberration in the left patella of this species reveals an osseous overgrowth referred to as an osteophyte. These lesions, often a response to joint instability or trauma, can lead to OA due to abnormal loading of the knee joint. This finding is one way traumatic events can manifest as osteoarthritic changes in bones over time, providing us with valuable insights into the health and longevity of early humans. Paleopathological study through holistic approaches can elicit the association between trauma, joint health, and lifestyle and thus enhance our understanding of the adaptation of prehistoric humans to musculoskeletal stressors (Bermúdez de Castro et al., 2016). Osteoarthritis in paleopathology not only tells us about the health of the person but also about the wider social and environmental contexts of past populations. The differential OA levels in disparate skeletal samples can infer varied activity patterns and occupational loads that are indicative of subsistence economies, social structure, and even environmental burdens faced by ancient people. Beyond individual instances, OA's implications also point to population-level changes in well-being over millennia as markers of resilience or adaptive responses to environmental adversity. By combining the study of OA with statistical analysis, researchers can construct a more accurate representation of skeletal disease and its importance to human evolution, thereby contributing to our understanding of health in the ancient and modern world (Bass et al., 2019) (Figure 3.7).

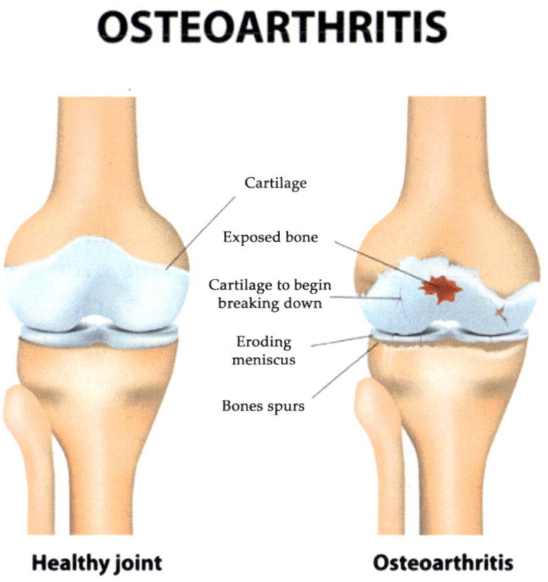

Figure 3.7. The study of osteoarthritis (OA) in skeletal remains.

Source: https://external-content.duckduckgo.com/iu/?u=https%3A%2F%2Fwww.orchardhealthclinic.com%2Fwp-content%2Fuploads%2F2020%2F09%2Fcomparison-of-healthy-joint-and-joint-with-osteoarthritis.png&f=1&nofb=1&ipt=330bee993ac51a2418bb3a9b6d4f90be79f823c1c18169c445307dc1170a2977.

3.2.2. Tuberculosis (TB) and Its Effects on the Skeleton

The pathological effects of TB on the human skeleton are particularly significant, as evidenced by its ubiquity in the past and its mnemonic in paleopathological studies. TB primarily affects the respiratory system, but also affects the skeleton to create conditions such as Potts disease that particularly affect the spine. This form of tuberculosis is characterized by the formation of abscesses that can destroy spinal elements, often producing spectacular deformities and disabling consequences in affected individuals. The osteoarchaeological record produces proof for TB's skeletal dynamics, where paleopathologists are capable of utilizing a variety of macroscopic examination, radiography, and molecular techniques to identify the illness among ancient populations. These techniques have enabled the diagnosis of TB in various skeletal individuals, supporting the importance of knowing the disease's evolutionary trend in addressing the health of humans over time. Paleopathological information, particularly from Transdanubian populations, indicates geographic and temporal tendencies in skeletal TB frequency among previous societies. An extensive investigation of a large sample of human osteoarchaeological material from the region has revealed that such cases were prevalent from the 9th through the 13th century alone. The association of microscopic evidence with advancements in molecular methods has enabled the successful identification of Mycobacterium tuberculosis DNA in skeletons exhibiting signs of the disease, thereby confirming its historical presence. The findings also show the diversity of TB prevalence and suggest that lifestyle and environmental factors may have contributed to its pattern among populations. This information is significant for understanding the socio-economic and health problems faced by ancient societies, and it adds to our understanding of the history of the disease as well as the pathological reactions triggered in infected skeletal remains—moreover, paleopathology of such osteediseases as TB carries important differentials in differential diagnosis, specifically overlapping pathology. The development of osteolytic lesions in subjects raises the issue of how to diagnose neoplastic diseases as opposed to infectious disorders like tuberculosis, where the precision of an accurate paleopathological diagnosis becomes critical. For instance, even though TB can produce lesions similar to those observed in certain skeletal remains, accurate delineation requires optimal examination of lesion patterns and characteristics. This is especially the case for comprehensive studies where the integrity of the skeleton is of utmost concern during differential diagnosis. Further research, directed towards developing diagnostic techniques, is essential to enhance our ability to recognize and categorize such conditions with accuracy, ultimately helping us better understand skeletal disease in the ancient population and providing informative insights into the long-term impact of tuberculosis in human history (Figure 3.8).

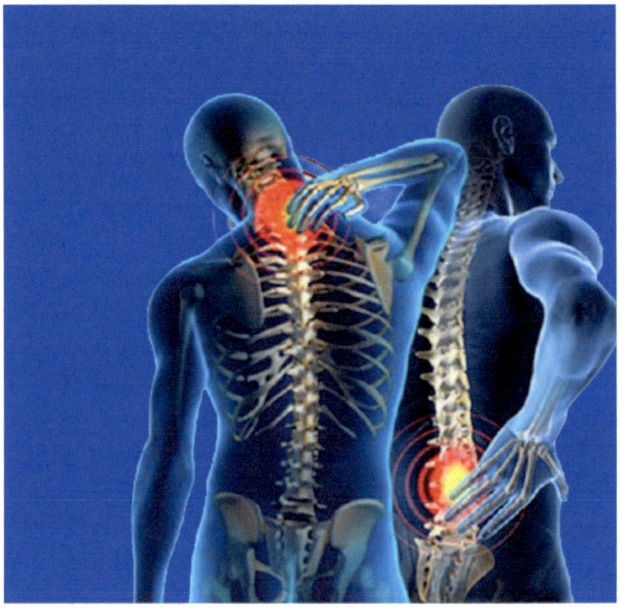

Figure 3.8. The pathological effects of tuberculosis (TB) on the human skeleton.

Source: https://www.spinesurgeonindelhi.com/img/services/spinal-tb.png.

3.2.3. Treponemal Diseases and Their Historical Significance

A study of treponemal diseases, including syphilis, yaws, bejel, and pinta, provides us with a valuable vantage point from which to consider human health and social structure over time. Treponemal diseases, caused by the bacterium Treponema pallidum, have had a fundamental influence on societies since their appearance, particularly on population and mobility. Bioarchaeological evidence demonstrates that treponemal disease has had a persistent impact on populations, influencing morbidity and mortality profiles. For example, the prevalence of diseases like yaws has been inextricably associated with environmental and sociocultural factors, demonstrating how early-life health experiences can predict disease expression in adulthood. This awareness is vital in crafting contemporary public health initiatives to eradicate such diseases, as seen with the World Health Organization's efforts to control yaws in developing nations (Mathena et al., 2013). Syphilis's historical introduction to Europe in the late 15th century was a turning point, and it fueled widespread debate regarding its onset and the consequent sociopolitical implications. Anthropological, historical, and medical perspectives have come together to consider how treponemal diseases affected not only personal health but also significant transformations in society. Studies of the coevolution of human populations with Treponema organisms have revealed intricate associations between the diseases and ancient population movements, trade networks, and cross-cultural exchange. These networks facilitated the spread of treponemal disease, underscoring the necessity of contextualizing these diseases within the worlds of interaction and their very different impacts across populations and geographic regions (Akrawi et al., 2020). The importance of paleopathological investigation in understanding the treponemal diseases cannot be overstated. It not only broadens our understanding of the biological manifestations of infection through skeletal diagnosis but also contributes to our understanding of the sociocultural determinants of disease and health. By adopting enhanced diagnostic criteria and uniform methods for recording skeletal lesions, researchers can build a clearer picture of the historical prevalence and distribution of treponemal diseases. Applying biogeochemical analysis to identify diet is one aspect of this research, as is examining how environmental and socioeconomic factors affect disease expression. Focusing therefore on the social determinants of health, including age, sex, and class, enables the effects of treponemal diseases over centuries in populations to be understood more effectively (Akrawi et al., 2020).

Test Your Knowledge

1. What are the most common skeletal diseases identified through paleopathological studies?
2. How do paleopathologists distinguish between disease-related changes and normal skeletal variation

3.3. The Role of Environment in Skeletal Health

Learning Outcome

1. Treponemal diseases and their historical significance;
2. Impact of diet on skeletal diseases;
3. Influence of climate and geography.

A natural setting forms the core basis of skeletal health and influences variables such as diet, activity levels, and exposure to infectious agents. Paleopathological studies have shown how skeletal diseases often correspond to the life experience of ancient people, which in turn is closely related to their environmental context. For instance, the availability of diverse food sources directly affects bone density and growth patterns across groups. In agricultural populations, the change to farming altered the content of foods, often leading to deficiencies of key nutrients like calcium and vitamin D, and thereby affecting skeletal integrity. Furthermore, environmental stressors like the terrain and the weather affected physical activity and the likelihood of sustaining injuries, and thereby the skeletal pattern over generations. Understanding these relationships is crucial, as they can shed light on how skeletal health might be mitigated or enhanced through adaptive responses to environmental change. Another consideration of the role of the environment in skeletal health is occupation- and lifestyle-related biomechanical stressors. In populations that engage in much physical labor, for instance, those engaged in agriculture or construction work, specific skeletal adaptations are evident. The study of osteoarthritis and entheses reveals how repetitive strain and heavy load-bearing can lead to degenerative conditions characterized by joint wear and abnormal bone growth. By evaluating the prevalence of such conditions in relation to environmental demands, one can examine the adaptive responses of skeletal systems to mechanical forces. More recent methods have underscored the importance of precise sampling and detailed documentation of occupational behavior to create a more lifelike picture of how environmental factors shape skeletal form and health.

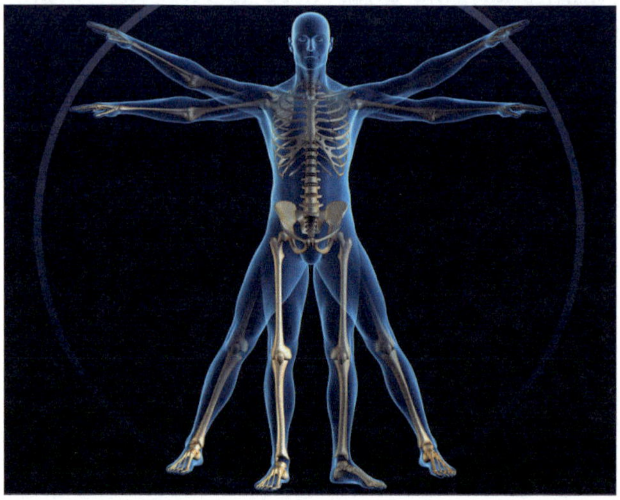

Figure 3.9. The environment plays a crucial role in shaping skeletal health.

Source: https://nutraceuticalbusinessreview.com/article-image-alias/bone-and-joint-health-in-a.jpg.

This is in accordance with the slight data movement, whose focus is to thorough investigation of localized samples, thereby allowing for a better appreciation of the environmental-skeletal transformation interface across cultures and eras (Becker et al., 2019). Finally, the interaction between the environment and bone health cannot be explained without knowledge of the role of disease and pathogens. Previous experience with infectious disease and its correlation with skeletal abnormality can illustrate the strong role played by determinants of environmental health. Paleopathology studies have confirmed that some expressions of bone, e.g., lesions or deformities, tend to occur as responses to infection at the systemic level. By merging archaeological data with contemporary conceptions of health, scientists are better able to perceive the selective pressures that operated on diseases endemic to the milieus provided. With continued research into the historic frequency of conditions like tuberculous osteitis or syphilitic lesions, it becomes clear that environmental factors, like sanitation and population, have a direct relationship between disease dynamics and, consequently, bone fitness (Gardner et al., 2020). The environment is thus both an impetus and a safeguard for skeletal well-being, not only affecting physical adaptation but also the long-term evolution of disease (Figure 3.9).

3.3.1. Impact of Diet on Skeletal Diseases

The interaction between diet and skeletal diseases provides valuable insight into paleopathological studies, particularly regarding how dietary inadequacies affect bone fitness. Dietary intake dictates not only the physiological state of human beings but also their bone structure. For example, insufficient absorption of essential nutrients such as calcium and vitamin D can lead to low bone density, osteomalacia, and osteoporosis. Such diseases manifest as deformities or distortions of bone structure, and thus identifying them is important for archaeological human bones. Augmenting our understanding of ancient diets through isotopic analysis might shed light on past nutritional patterns and their impact on skeletal disease, thus adding to the broader picture of the health of ancient populations. Dietary findings might also differentiate groups, illuminating the way in which different diets influenced the distribution of some skeletal diseases across different populations, as already seen in the study of carcinoma in ancient societies (Gardner et al., 2020). Careful observation of food habits also allows researchers to infer links between lifestyle changes and the development of skeletal diseases using historical timelines. For instance, the transition from hunter-gatherer groups to agricultural groups experienced a radical decrease in dietary variation, something that might have had long-term impacts on skeletal health. Agricultural diets, which were starchy staple-based, may not have met nutritional needs to support optimal bone function, suggesting a connection between diet and the fold of disease, such as osteoporosis and arthritis. Exams of entheses and cross-sectional geometries of long bones can also delineate these changes and elucidate how a shift in diet influenced levels of physical activity and, consequently, the strength of the skeleton.

By targeting these various dietary influences, scientists can construct a clearer picture of how dietary change affected the health of ancient people and led to distinctive patterns of skeletal disease (Becker et al., 2019). Additionally, information regarding the effect of diet on skeletal diseases facilitates intense controversies about the determinants of modern health outcomes that are the products of ancestral foodways. Contemporary diets stray from the conventional pattern of use, and diet-related diseases, such as skeletal illness, rise. These contemporary analogies place great importance on learning from past dietary patterns and disease relationships. With the help of paleopathology resources, such as rigorous skeletal analysis alongside epidemiological data, writers can learn lessons from the past that can shape today's public health initiatives. Through multidisciplinary collaborative research integrating investigations in nutrition, anthropology, and osteology, researchers can best learn how food choices influence skeletal health from generation to generation. The interdisciplinary study provides evidence on which to tackle current skeletal disorders through the lens of diets and life expectancy in the past (Gardner et al., 2020) (Figure 3.10).

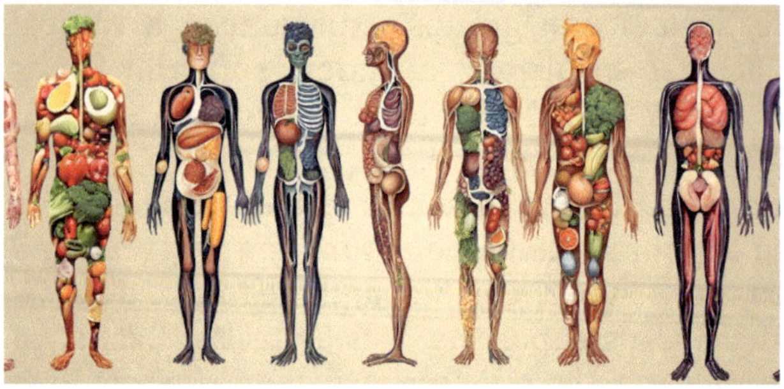

Figure 3.10. Impact of diet on skeletal diseases.

Source: https://longevity.stanford.edu/lifestyle/wp-content/uploads/sites/31/2023/10/Blog-Photos-4.png.

3.3.2. Influence of Climate and Geography

The relationship between geography and climate profoundly influences the incidence and manifestation of skeletal disease over time. Geographic locations shape human habitation, resource availability, and infectious agent transmission, thereby profoundly influencing health. For instance, in areas with warmer temperatures, certain pathogens, such as Coccidioides immitis, flourish, leading to more cases of valley fever among residents. This fungal infection thrives in arid environments, illustrating how geography dictates the specific health concerns of the populations. Such climatic knowledge of the factors influencing skeletal disease provides worthwhile information about ancient populations, including the migration pathways and conditions of existence, which helped in the transmission of the diseases and thus the larger issue of the interdependence of the environment and human health as explored in paleopathology and skeletal disease research (Darling et al., 2014). For ancient urbanization, geography's role is even more important. Settlements founded in rich valleys or on navigable rivers tended to have population densities that enabled the transmission of infectious diseases, particularly Mycobacterium tuberculosis. This disease's connection to urbanism highlights the dynamic between demographic pressure and bone health. Where populations are high, close living conditions lead to higher contact rates, thereby increasing the probability of transmission. Besides that, urbanization is typically accompanied by changes in living patterns, such as poverty and overcrowding, which increase the incidence of skeletal disease. Geographical conditions thus not only control the patterns of disease but also the shape of human societies themselves, as reflected in demographic trends and health patterns that may be traced in archaeological collections (N/A, 2018). Furthermore, population movements in response to geographic and climatic change shape the epidemiology of paleopathological evidence. Examination of ancient Egyptian Akhetaten skeletal remains, for example, indicates biological affinity and diversity profiles that mirror migration and settlement within specific geographic contexts. Studies of the South Tombs cemetery indicate that individuals would originate from diverse sources, with climatically influenced migrations within the Nile Valley. This movement led to a founder effect, in which a population has reduced genetic variation due to restricted gene flow into a new society. Such a reference to the influence of geography and climate on population dynamics is valuable for understanding the trend in health in ancient times. They assist us in understanding how the environment affects the epidemiology of skeletal illness and promote further exploration of the relationship among climate, geography, and healthcare outcomes within the scope of paleopathology (N/A, 2018).

3.3.3. Social Factors Affecting Health and Disease Prevalence

Where social determinants intersect with healthcare outcomes provides a valuable outlook through which skeletal illness prevalence can be studied in paleopathology. Health is significantly influenced by historical and cultural contexts, determining populations' biological responses to environmental risks. In ancient populations, whether social hierarchy or occupation controlled exposure to physical demands and dietary resources ultimately determined skeletal health. For instance, working populations will have higher levels of osteoarthritis, illustrating an evident connection between lifestyle and incidence of skeletal disease. Becker et al. (2019) highlight the necessity to document and examine variations in bone health because biomechanical stress and physical activity differences occur in different social environments. Their examination of these historical backgrounds allows for more complex explanations of the skeletal conditions, such as entheses and osteoarthritis, opening the door to the understanding of inequalities in health among disparate social groups. In addition, paleopathological studies of the onset and development of diseases like osteoporosis inform about the broader determinants of socio-economic status for health. In the majority of ancient cultures, social setting and lifestyle dictated access to nutrition and medicine, and hence skeletal integrity. As noted in recent research, osteoporosis is a multifactorial disease that is linked to several social determinants like gender, age, and lifestyle (Curate et al., 2014). The effect of menopause, for instance, is most pronounced in women who are past menopause, who have an increased risk of bone fragility and consequent fractures. Such demographic notes highlight how conditions in the past, both sociocultural and otherwise, may be used to account for the etiology of bone loss and contrasted with modern populations. By assessing skeletal diseases through this socio-historical lens, one can better understand how past and present societal structures contribute to health disparities. Ultimately, the evaluation of skeletal diseases through paleopathology is enriched by an immersive understanding of social factors, which, in turn, reveals a complex web of health determinants. The interaction among lifestyle behaviors, environment, and sociocultural practices leaves an indelible imprint in the ancient population's skeletal record. Scientists are able to deconstruct the nuances of disease etiology and how they are managed acutely to sociocultural conditions through a small data strategy. Becker et al. (2019) elucidate the importance of identifying osteoarthritis and related conditions as biological responses to such social settings, with it being suggested that collaborative efforts by researchers can be used to clarify such associations further. Such influences, through proper understanding, not only help explain the skeletal well-being of ancient societies but also inform current public health strategies to minimize such disparities in modern societies (Figure 3.11).

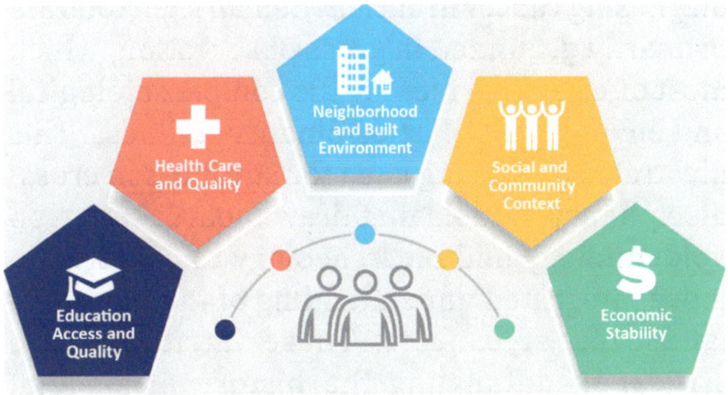

Figure 3.11. Social factors affecting health and disease prevalence.

Source: https://www.cdc.gov/public-health-gateway/media/images/images/sdoh/SDOH-icons.png.

Test Your Knowledge

1. How do environmental factors such as nutrition, climate, and physical activity influence skeletal health?
2. What role does living environment play in the development of skeletal disorders?

3.4. Case Studies in Paleopathology

Learning Outcome

1. Analysis of skeletal remains from ancient Egypt
2. Examination of skeletal diseases in prehistoric Europe
3. Insights from Native American skeletal remains

Case studies in paleopathology play a crucial role in understanding the link between diseases of the skeleton and the ancient population. By analyzing skeletons, scientists can uncover information about health, lifestyle, and environmental factors that affected individuals over time. The fact that little evidence of cancer was found in ancient groups contrasts sharply with prevalence rates today, hypothesizing that present environments play a key role in the formation of cancer. Notably, modern methods for diagnosing cancer in ancient human skeletons are primarily grounded in gross observation, which most often fails to identify the complex biological and environmental determinants of illness. This illustrates a pressing need for advances in cross-disciplinary models that draw bioarcheologyon epidemiology and bioarcheology to construct a more integrated understanding of the historical landscape of cancers. These intricacies are critical in untangling the history of skeletal disorders across time and cultures, ultimately giving impetus to the science of paleopathology (Gardner et al., 2020). Further research into osteoarthritis and related conditions provides significant insight into the ancient populations' biological responses to bodily stressors and lifestyle choices. The strategies employed in ongoing research focus on a 'small data' approach, in which detailed descriptions of skeletal abnormalities are examined within biologically and culturally comparable samples. It is feasible to carefully examine the influence of age, sex, and occupation on the skeletal responses to biomechanical loads. By analyzing these conditions with the aid of a robust framework of osteological and clinical studies, researchers have begun developing established assessment approaches. Like comparative analyses, such methodologies have played a significant role in revealing important trends in the incidence and expression of osteoarthritis across populations, relating mechanical load and physical activity to skeletal deformity. Therefore, such analytical methods play a key role in revealing the dynamic interaction between ancient lifestyles and skeletal maladies (Becker et al., 2019).

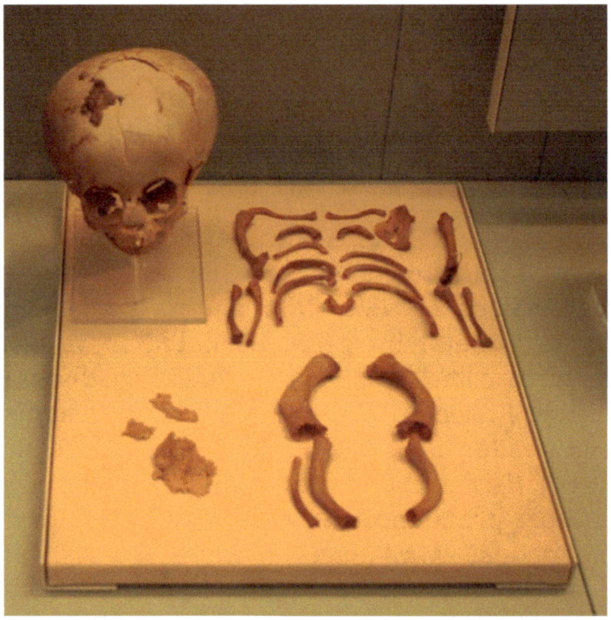

Figure 3.12. The exploration of case studies in paleopathology.

Source: https://bonesdontlie.wordpress.com/wp-content/uploads/2013/01/screen-shot-2013-02-01-at-7-34-26-am.png.

The application of newer imaging technologies, such as CT scans and motion-tracking systems, to paleopathological analysis is an area of research with significant promise for the future. These technologies enable non-invasive testing that yields more precise data on the physiological processes underlying bony modification. Osteologists and pathologists, in collaboration, could offer insights into disease processes at a more basic level, revealing how bone diseases manifest and progress over time. Further, collaboration with extant populations to contrast skeletal health and biomechanics between generations can yield valuable contextual information. Not only does this enhance the current pool of knowledge, but it also emphasizes how historical patterns of disease relate to modern public health issues. Finally, the continued exploration of these techniques will make valuable contributions to paleopathology, bridging gaps between ancient and modern knowledge of skeletal illness (Becker et al., 2019) (Figure 3.12).

3.4.1. Analysis of Skeletal Remains from Ancient Egypt

Analysis of skeletal remains from ancient Egypt provides invaluable information about the health and diseases that afflicted its inhabitants. By examining the physical remains, researchers can identify many skeletal pathologies that indicate the stressors to which the populations were subjected. Even conditions as prevalent as osteoarthritis and periodontal disease have been discovered, typically in relation to diet, environmental factors, and hierarchy. Skeletal data point to the fact that, despite sophisticated medical care documented in Egyptian texts, individuals were suffering from debilitating conditions unmentioned in written accounts during their lifetimes. In addition, the analysis of such remains helps to position illness, not just in individualistic terms, but also as a community-level disease and a reflection of broader socio-economic realities within ancient Egyptian society. Notably, paleopathological examinations have observed instances of specific infectious diseases among Egyptian populations. Bony remains have proven helpful in tracing traces of disease like tuberculosis and leprosy, with significant implications for the epidemiology of these diseases in antiquity. For example, the presence of lepromatous leprosy in skeletons provides a timescale for the introduction and dissemination of the disease in the region. The evidence contradicts earlier speculations about the prevalence of specific diseases among ancient people and underscores the need for a wide-ranging approach to examining skeletons. Through gross inspection and advanced analytical techniques, researchers are progressively unfolding the disease histories embedded in these ancient bones and thereby enriching our comprehension of disease dynamics in the past (Robbins et al., 2009). Furthermore, the implications of cancer and other neoplastic diseases that emerged in skeletal data also need to be investigated further and critically appraised. The evidence indicates that the frequency of the diseases reported in antiquity was much lower than in contemporary populations. This has led people to speculate about cancer being more frequently caused by modern environmental and lifestyle determinants. But methods traditionally applied in paleopathological studies, primarily skeletal-based, may lack the weak tumoral evidence that requires a multidisciplinary strategy combining archaeological methods with contemporary genomics and epidemiology (Gardner et al., 2020). Therefore, even though skeletal analysis is crucial for reconstructing the health landscape of ancient societies, further refinement of methodologies is required to fully comprehend the pathologies that afflicted them and their historical significance.

3.4.2. Examination of Skeletal Diseases in Prehistoric Europe

Analysis of prehistoric European skeletal diseases provides insight into the nature of life for ancient individuals and their state of health. Applying rigorous methods, scientists have attempted to determine various skeletal conditions, including osteoarthritis and other biomechanical stress-induced alterations. Highlighted in recent studies, examining these conditions using a small-data approach allows scientists to derive meaningful conclusions while ensuring that the samples are well preserved for the bones. It underscores the need to include age and sex estimates in analyses, as demographic factors play a significant role in influencing the occurrence and manifestation of skeletal disease. Moreover, understanding the pathogenesis of such diseases helps us better appreciate the biological adaptations of early human beings to their environment, thereby providing scope for further study into the interplay between way of life factors, health, and socio-cultural activity in prehistoric Europe (Becker et al., 2019). The scarcity of paleopathological information on neoplastic conditions, e.g., neoplasms in ancient humans, is highly prejudicial to research on skeletal conditions. The scarcity is often not only a result of the preservation quality of the skeleton but also of the relative difficulty in detecting and diagnosing them in ancient man. For instance, differential diagnosis is made difficult by the common features of most neoplastic lesions, which conceal the true diagnosis. Researchers have extensively used advanced techniques, such as radiological and computed tomography scans, to analyze skeletal remains further. However, as neoplastic disease research progresses, reproducible indicators and sound methods must be developed to enhance the diagnostic process. These developments offer scope for future work that can elucidate the incidence of malignant and benign lesions in archaeological contexts, towards improved comprehension of prehistoric European health (Cunha et al., 2013). In addition to qualitative analyses of skeletal remains, incorporating biomechanical assessments offers an integrated perspective on the comprehension of prehistoric European skeletal diseases. By examining burial contexts and considering the range of occupational activities ancient individuals engaged in, researchers can correlate changes in the skeleton with movement patterns and work intensity. Careful analysis of long bone cross-sectional geometry and enthesis changes is valuable information on physical activity intensity, which can tell us about socio-economic and cultural dynamics in ancient societies. This multifaceted approach not only assists in documenting specific skeletal ailments but also informs broader interpretations of prehistoric European responses to stress and adaptability. By combining osteological data with the analysis of social archaeology, these analyses emphasize the essential interaction between human health and environmental interaction as constituting the skeletal record of ancient societies (Becker et al., 2019) (Figure 3.13).

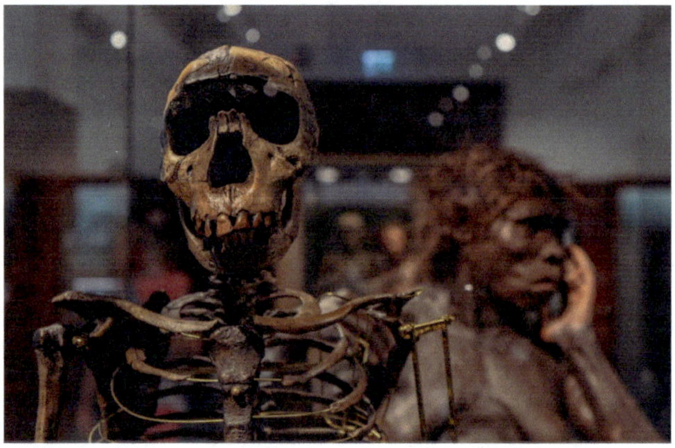

Figure 3.13. Examination of skeletal diseases in prehistoric Europe.

Source: https://images.ctfassets.net/cnu0m8re1exe/tkkCAt1jtHhsXD9Ywejzb/047cdd24ca295b196120de3e05e6b318/ancient-human-skeleton-in-museum.jpg?fm=jpg&fl=progressive&w=1200&h=800&fit=fill.

3.4.3. Insights From Native American Skeletal Remains

Studies of Native American skeletal remains have yielded immense information relevant to the understanding of paleopathology. These remains are drawn from diverse populations across different temporal and geographical contexts and provide essential artifacts for estimating health, disease prevalence, and the lifestyles of indigenous people. Different studies have demonstrated radical representations of skeletal diseases such as osteoarthritis and tuberculosis, both environmentally and socially determined. For instance, the observation of wear patterns on joints has been able to reveal the physical burden imposed on individuals through labor-intensive lifestyles or communal obligations, giving insight into health inequalities through subsistence strategies. Therefore, the bone record not only tells us about past states of health, but also allows a competent assessment of how past conditions have shaped disease patterns in the populations. The role of osteological data in helping to explain patterns of osteoporosis and bone trauma in Native American populations cannot be overstated. Through paleopathological analysis, scientists have identified distinctive patterns of bone density loss and fragility fractures that run counter to prevailing biomedical paradigms, which tend to discount the influence of cultural and environmental variables on health outcomes. Pathological analysis of these fossil remains suggests a dynamic relationship among diet, social standing, and disease prevalence. Later advances in biomedical techniques enhance our capacity to discern these patterns, not just to isolate individual cases but also to identify larger trends among populations. Skeletal evidence, as such, is an important instrument through which we can read the socio-cultural processes that configure health and illness among Native American populations (Curate et al., 2014). Furthermore, ethical concerns under which Native American skeletal remains are researched demand a thoughtful approach to the research strategy of paleopathology. The field has evolved to encompass multidisciplinary methodologies that integrate anthropological, archaeological, and biomedical perspectives to better understand skeletal disease. Of particular interest, researchers must engage with Native American people to ensure that scientific research is respectful of the cultural context and contemporary significance of these remains. Since the discipline grapples with its own historical origins and disagreement regarding exhumation and examination of human skeletons, scientific investigation must be weighed against respect for indigenous belief and narrative. That mix of interest enhances our understanding of skeletal disease while reinforcing the role of Native American contributions in the destiny of paleopathology (Grauer et al., 2022) (Figure 3.14).

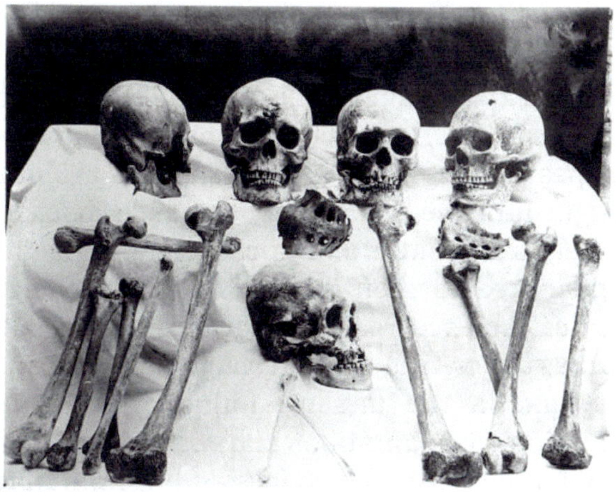

Figure 3.14. Insights from Native American skeletal remains.

Source: https://cdn2.picryl.com/photo/1930/12/31/the-bones-of-cliff-dwellers-ca1900-chs-2076-a9b21c-640.jpg.

Test Your Knowledge

1. How are case studies used in paleopathology to understand ancient diseases and injuries?
2. What insights can individual skeletal case studies provide about the health and lifestyle of past populations?

3.5. The Intersection of Paleopathology and Modern Medicine

Learning Outcome

1. Lessons learned from ancient diseases
2. Relevance of paleopathology in understanding contemporary health issues
3. Contributions to forensic science and anthropology

The intersection of paleopathology and contemporary medicine offers a unique perspective on the historical understanding of diseases, particularly those that have impacted human populations over centuries. By examining the skeletal remains of ancient civilizations, paleopathologists can identify remnants of diseases that plagued these populations, such as tuberculosis, syphilis, and leprosy. Analysis of the past through this type of analysis provides insight into the development of such diseases, the environmental and social conditions that contributed to their spread, and how ancient medical science reacted. Advances from such studies are critical to modern medicine because they aid in the understanding of pathogen evolutionary adaptations and resistance within populations. Also, the understanding stimulates studies on improving existing healthcare practices that can be formulated to combat similar diseases encountered in the modern world, thus indicating the utility of diseases in the past in informing present medical practice. Further research into the implications of finding ancient diseases is the challenges and results encountered by paleopathological research. The development of new metagenomic and bioinformatics methods has revolutionized the identification of pathogens in degraded ancient DNA samples and has enhanced our understanding of health patterns in the past. New studies show that the use of multiplexed taxonomic pipelines such as Kraken2 leads to more effective pathogen detection, significantly improving historical epidemiology. By analyzing samples from populations such as the Casas Grandes, researchers have begun to discern patterns in disease and health that demonstrate the effects of farming on human well-being. This body of research not only contributes to the reconstruction of past modes of life but also offers a conceptual framework for interpreting the development of afflictions that still impact human populations today, thus bridging the gap between ancient customs and modern medicine (Giovannangelo et al., 2025). Furthermore, child health, examined as a field grounded in paleopathology, has dire implications for anthropology and medicine today. The data obtained from the study of the non-adult skeleton highlight the salient points of past growth, diet, and social roles. This general overview, particularly in regions where the bioarcheological record is under-researched, enables the researcher to understand the subtleties of past societies in ways that intersect with contemporary pediatric medicine. For instance, studies on diet patterns and health inequalities illustrate how experiences in the early years influence long-term health outcomes. This evidence of systemic ill health in previous populations can inform modern public health efforts to prevent disease and improve nutrition in children (Morrone et al., 2022). Such a link between paleopathology and modern medicine, therefore, continues to enrich the discussion across time and culture regarding health.

3.5.1. Lessons Learned from Ancient Diseases

The paleopathology study of ancient diseases gives important insights into human health and the dynamics of disease in the past. Through the examination of skeletal remains, researchers can identify several pathologies, such as lesions associated with tuberculosis or treponemal diseases, that inform us about how these diseases impacted the population. These findings not only inform modern medical environments but also reflect the socio-environmental contexts of their time and display how disease and health are inextricably linked with social organization. The prevalence of certain diseases in ancient populations, for instance, is frequently a function of agricultural practices, housing conditions, and migratory patterns. Understanding these linkages allows present researchers to consider the ways in which present-day health crises may mirror past health patterns, thereby providing insights that inform more effective public health measures and instructional programs today. Moreover, within the field itself, the evolution of methodologies has broadened the scope of paleopathological studies by taking in perspectives from other fields of science. As detailed in the paleopathology's historical record, the field's evolution is marked by an increasing application of technologies and an increasing interdisciplinarity. Skeletal analysis now requires the talents of not only anthropologists and archaeologists but also members of the medical community, along with biochemical sciences. This collaborative framework advances the study of ancient diseases by providing more detailed interpretations and facilitating an understanding of complex interactions among human hosts and pathogens. Their contemporary application, hence, can complement preventive healthcare practices to enable professionals to anticipate and neutralize prospective healthcare problems with historical contexts (Grauer et al., 2022). Their associated ethical considerations in paleopathological analysis cannot be disregarded either. With the overlap between archaeology, history, anthropology, and medicine (Esteban et al., 2019), there is a responsibility to treat remains with respect and care. This responsibility to advance scientific knowledge while respecting the cultural significance of human remains pushes investigators to balance the desire for knowledge with ethical considerations. Lessons derived from past disease research will therefore need to move beyond scientific discoveries to include reflections on how these experiments are conducted. Ethical procedures will be necessary to preserve the heritage of those being studied and to acknowledge their role in advancing health knowledge within the grand narrative of human history. In encouraging such moral engagement, the field of paleopathology can thrive by recalling previous generations who struggled with disease and thereby ultimately raising our understanding of health today (Figure 3.15).

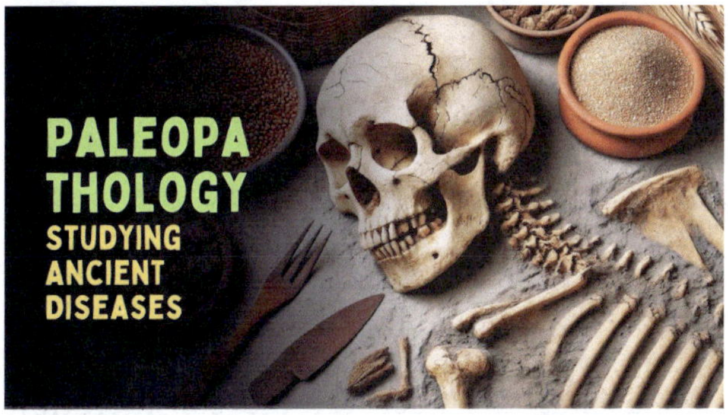

Figure 3.15. Lessons learned from ancient diseases.

Source: https://external-content.duckduckgo.com/iu/?u=https%3A%2F%2Fi.ytimg.com%2Fvi%2FZOUmbQYuu2s%2Fmaxresdefault.jpg&f=1&nofb=1&ipt=15aa4ff9b3a0821f40695fbc41ef4583348606d77aa99dec5880ae6a5c9937d0.

3.5.2. Relevance of Paleopathology in Understanding Contemporary Health Issues

Paleopathology offers an important understanding of present health issues by providing a historical perspective to the investigation of diseases of the skeleton. Modern medicine concentrates on observing disease within the context of populations in the modern era; however, paleopathology encourages an enduring understanding with a focus on how diseases such as osteoarthritis have evolved across the centuries and responded to environmental as well as to lifestyle conditions. By studying ancient populations' skeletal remains, scientists can track patterns of disease manifestation, enabling a better understanding of the effects of social behaviors and biomechanical stress on health. This kind of research clarifies the links between physical activity and the long-term development of joint diseases and informs existing health policies aimed at preventing musculoskeletal disorders in the current environment. The persistence of such health conditions over time justifies the applicability of paleopathological analysis to human skeletal health today, and they may be helpful in disease prevention and control. Furthermore, integrating paleopathological data with biocultural frameworks enhances understanding of the effects of social context on health and disease. In particular, the discipline of bioarcheology has been successful at examining the juncture between cultural practice and biological health and in emphasizing the need for the consideration of factors at both the societal and individual level. Utilizing models bioarcheologysuch as Tilley's "bioarcheology of care," researchers can analyze caregiving practices among ancient individuals and document how social support networks played a role in health management. This interdisciplinarity insists that health is not only a biological issue but one heavily influenced by society, identity, and culture. Information derived from skeletal remains in conjunction with archaeological and anthropological data can be used to explain how caregiving in the past influences current health interventions and ultimately contributes to an overarching picture of health in various settings. The techniques used in paleopathology and bioarcheology also play a significant role in informing our understanding of health problems in the contemporary world. Advances in analytical techniques and statistics are increasingly allowing researchers to consider the quality of evidence on conditions like osteoarthritis and their prevalence among different populations. For example, studies of the interaction between exercise and skeletal change are yielding significant evidence of the influence of lifestyle on health. In addition, fine control of age and sex during skeletal study enables findings to be interpreted in their correct context and pertinent to current scenarios. Although scholars stress the need for interdisciplinary research, the integration of osteology, pathology, and clinical studies is the essence of the comprehension of health's complexity in contemporary times. By rigorous technique, paleopathology supplies a basic approach to dealing with contemporary health concerns by highlighting the fact that skeletal diseases are always present chronically throughout the course of history and carry implications to the future.

3.5.3. Contributions to Forensic Science and Anthropology

In anthropology and forensic science, paleopathology is a key cross-disciplinary field that assists to a large extent in interpreting skeletal diseases and their significance for identification and investigation. Through thorough observation of pathological conditions, researchers can gain invaluable information about the persons under investigation, including their health, lifestyle, and presumed causes of death. Forensic anthropologists apply the identification of non-normal conditions to differentiate individuals from one another and reconstruct how they met death. This is not only crucial for providing distinctiveness in forensic use but also for enhancing understanding of past populations and their responses to disease. The subtle functions of pathology, particularly the recognition of normal and abnormal patterns, are significant during the verification of forensic anthropological findings and play a central role in foul play, age estimation, and other forensic applications (Ubelaker et al., 2014). Genetic analysis tracing back to bioarcheology is a significant advancement in identifying disease and understanding its impact on previous people. The study at the Tomb of the Shroud is an excellent illustration of this development, whereby the analysis of the bones and associated artifacts revealed the presence of diseases such as Mycobacterium tuberculosis and Mycobacterium leprae. These discoveries not only revealed the presence of these specific diseases within these ancient groups but also established a genetic link suggesting family ties among those persons interred in the tomb. Moreover, the presence of disease-molecular screening enhances our knowledge of how diseases such as leprosy operated in historical contexts. The data is fundamental in forensic science and anthropology as they provide the epidemiology of the disease and broader implications for human organization and health (Donoghue et al., 2009). Paleopathology, in its study of skeletal disease, thus plays a dual role within the interfaces of forensic science and anthropology. It is used to uncover the intricacies of disease presentation in human remains while providing crucial information for forensic investigations. By applying the recognized pathological conditions, forensic anthropologists can provide critical interpretations that extend beyond individual cases, informing us about the health patterns of past populations, structures of society, and even environmental conditions. Such broad analysis not only fills out the narrative of historical identities but also provides current ramifications for understanding how disease evolves and affects communities. Finally, these findings complement the richness of forensic science and anthropology, constructing a more complex picture of human history through the lens of health, disease, and death (Ubelaker et al., 2014) (Figure 3.16).

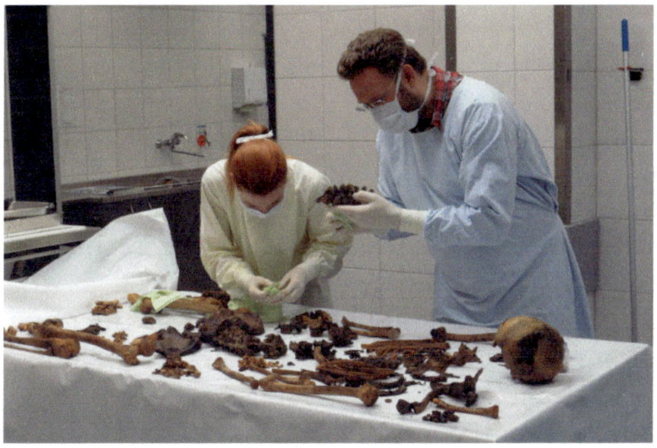

Figure 3.16. Contributions to forensic science and anthropology.

Source: https://external-content.duckduckgo.com/iu/?u=https%3A%2F%2Fd2f0ora2gkri0g.cloudfront.net%2Fbkpam2194568_2d68a797bec948e6a6e1919224f998f1.jpg&f=1&nofb=1&ipt=148c490c06f390d8571d8e14a1e8645ef600c8a7e4cb7c2e9d6066a7bf71bd84.

Test Your Knowledge

1. How does paleopathology contribute to our understanding of disease patterns in modern medicine?
2. In what ways can the study of ancient skeletal remains inform current diagnostic and treatment practices?

3.6. Ethical Considerations in Paleopathological Research

Learning Outcome

1. Treatment of human remains in research
2. Cultural sensitivity and respect for ancestral populations
3. Legal implications of excavating and studying skeletal remains

Ethics in paleopathological research are intricate and vital to the integrity of the discipline. Scientists handling old bones are confronted with complex issues regarding the respectful treatment of human remains, as well as the implications of their findings. The question of informed consent is one of the primary ethical challenges, particularly where ancient populations whose cultural context is not readily available are involved. This lack of direct representation demands greater sensitivity to the dignity and rights of these individuals, as highlighted in the discussion of the moral place of scientists within their discipline. Furthermore, researchers must be sensitive to the potential impacts their results may have upon living descendants or culture groups associated with the remains. Responding to these issues ensures that paleopathology is practiced with respect and appreciation for the past, informing a more compassionate approach to interpreting and representing diseases of the skeleton (Grauer et al., 2022). The interpretation of evidence in paleopathology also has important ethical implications, especially when interpretations made from skeletal remains influence our knowledge of past populations. Scholars must balance scientific inquiry with the sociocultural narratives that may arise through their research. For example, articulating the widespread incidence of diseases like tuberculosis among ancient peoples not only sheds light on past health crises but also stirs controversy over the information conveyed and interpreted throughout society. While reporting on conditions that may have sociocultural impacts, such as those found in studies of childhood tuberculosis in northern Italy, authors must exercise caution. Stereotypes and negative stigmas about particular diseases should not be reinforced, recognizing that what they learn has the potential to reinforce biases inadvertently, should it be reported without heed (Pangrazzi et al., 2023). Moreover, the use of advanced technology in paleopathological research makes it even harder to take ethical concerns into account. Techniques such as genomic analysis and imaging provide us with greater information regarding the past populations, but also raise questions of privacy and ownership of biological data. The potential for genetic information to be used for ill or health status to be misinterpreted is a challenge that must be addressed with strict ethical guidelines. With the pace of technological advancement, setting and adhering to strong ethical guidelines is even more critical. Ensuring all research conducted is respectful of the cultural significance of remains, promotes collaborations among descendant communities, and maintains open disclosure about methodology and implications is paramount. This multimodal approach not only enhances the quality of research but is part of an expansive, respectful study of human health complexities over time (Grauer et al., 2022).

3.6.1. Treatment of Human Remains in Research

The treatment of human remains in paleopathological studies involves a range of ethical, methodological, and scientific considerations that underscore the importance of context and sensitivity. Proper treatment of bone remains typically begins with excavation under rigidly controlled conditions to preserve archaeological integrity. When recovered, scholars must be respectful in their analysis, often in collaboration with descendant peoples, in order to honor cultural values and historical records. This approach instills a culture of respect among individuals, aim of not just increasing scientific knowledge but also acknowledging the humanity of the people represented in these remains. Management of human remains is then turned into an interdisciplinary exercise that marries anthropology, ethics, and science, thereby enriching the analysis of skeletal disease and providing meaningful insights into discourse on the state of ancient health. When treating skeletal disease, the investigator faces the challenge of accurately interpreting ancient illness in the context of contemporary medical insight. Earlier paleopathology relied primarily on gross observation of bones, thereby limiting knowledge of diseases such as cancer in the archaeological record. Recent studies have maintained that cancer was quite unusual in the past, and environmental and lifestyle factors have been recognized as major predictors of disease expression. However, according to research initiatives, the methods of studying cancer in ancient humans must be advanced and incorporate interdisciplinary integration, utilizing methodologies from bioarcheology, epidemiology, and cancer genomics. By developing improved methods for analyzing skeletal remains, scientists aim not just to diagnose disease but also to understand precisely its pathogenesis and epidemiological patterns, thereby bridging knowledge gaps and remapping historical patterns in health (Gardner et al., 2020). Furthermore, evaluating specific skeletal states, such as osteoarthritis and entheses, is pivotal to understanding biomechanical adaptation and stress reactions in earlier populations. Investigations pursue a minimal-data approach, using well-preserved skeletal remains to allow a comprehensive assessment of age, sex, and abnormality descriptions. By adhering to strict methodologies and collaborating among osteologists and pathologists, scientists ensure maximum precision in their findings. Advances in statistical analysis and biomechanics have enabled scientists to make meaningful correlations between body movement and bone change, thus advancing a more advanced understanding of disease in the past. This fine-grained analysis of how human bones are used not only advances paleopathology research but also underpins broader questions about the interactions among lifestyle, environment, and health across human history (Becker et al., 2019).

3.6.2. Cultural Sensitivity and Respect for Ancestral Populations

The study of paleopathology necessitates an informed attitude characterized by cultural sensitivity and respect for ancestral populations. Researchers and scholars need to appreciate that ancient people's remains are not so much scientific artefacts as documents of communities whose histories are alive and diverse. Coming to indigenous communities with humility is required to value the complex interplay between their ancestors' well-being and today's health concerns. Cultural assessments are also accommodative, allowing indigenous people to influence research agendas and design, particularly when such studies are used to reveal how environmental disruptions, as documented in Mailer et al. (2013), have impacted Native American health in the past. Through collaborative research partnerships, scientists gain an appreciation not only for skeletal disease but also for the broader socioeconomic and cultural contexts that shape these groups' experiences of health. Paleopathology's available technologies, such as metagenomic analysis of ancient DNA (aDNA), yield unique insights into past patterns of health and disease. However, the ethical issues involved must not be exaggerated. The protocols for the recovery and analysis of aDNA from ancestors' remains must be guided by a commitment to preserving the cultural importance these remains hold for contemporary groups. Scholars have an obligation to enact ethical protocols for the recovery that place foremost the interests and concerns of descendant communities. As exemplified by the research results on the Casas Grandes peoples by Giovannangelo et al. (2025), establishing trust and equitable partnerships with indigenous populations can enrich scientific discovery without derailing cultural heritage. Thus, it is the meeting of the two in ensuring research unfolds without eroding the dignity of those whose histories it seeks to recover that matters. Moreover, cultural sensitivity is not merely required in the proximate scientific context but also informs broader narratives about health inequities faced by indigenous peoples in the modern period. Addressing historical injustices—e.g., those perpetrated through the desecration of indigenous food systems, as reported in Mailer et al. (2013)—is critical to achieving health equity in modern contexts. Researchers are not merely documenting past health statuses but also illuminating how those statuses relate to today's differences.

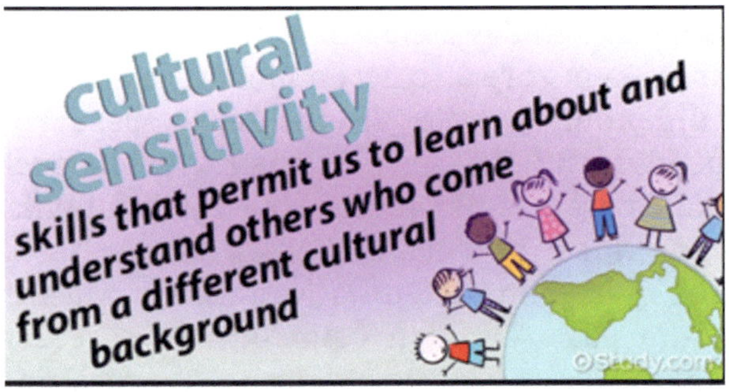

Figure 3.17. Cultural sensitivity and respect for ancestral populations.

Source: https://study.com/cimages/multimages/16/cultural.png.

Community-based research enables this connection by allowing researchers to partner with indigenous communities to build understanding together. Doing so, paleopathology can not only teach us in academic discourse on skeletal disease, but also guide initiatives aimed at confronting disparities in health among ancestral populations today. This kind of convergence of inquiry and respect can lead to more holistic, ethically grounded approaches to the study of the health of the human species through an evolutionary lens (Figure 3.17).

3.6.3. Legal Implications of Excavating and Studying Skeletal Remains

Excavation and analysis of skeletal remains raise significant legal issues regarding data collection and the ethics of working in archaeology and bioarcheology. From local to international law, legal frameworks control what is to be done with human remains as a means of balancing scientific research with dignity owed to the dead and to their inheritors. All but a few have strict control measures that include permits prior to excavation and the assurance that any research has been conducted openly and in consultation with local people. Legal protection in this form is particularly required where there are Indigenous communities because ancestral remains are to be dealt with in accordance with culturally defined principles that tend to prioritize repatriation and ceremonial reburial over scientific analysis. In addition, skeletal remains are usually protected by numerous legal protections for heritage preservation. For example, archaeological sites containing human remains are commonly designated as cultural heritage sites, so they require greater caution in excavation procedures. This legal safeguard encourages scientists to consider the ethical dimensions of their findings, that is, how those findings relate to the larger picture of human biology and health, for instance, findings related to paleopathology. A big part of this discussion is the balance that scientists must maintain between advancing scientific knowledge and staying within legal bounds, so that artifacts unearthed are handled with dignity and respect. Failure to comply with legal stipulations can lead to legal sanctions, including fines and a loss of research reputation, which can ultimately impact academic progress. The study of skeletons, although legally limited, has the potential to provide important insights into ancient human populations, particularly regarding health and disease patterns. As is evident in the Kallithea Laganidia cemetery example, analysis of skeletal remains enables researchers to explore demographic information, disease rates, and cultural stratification among ancient people. However, legalities surrounding research of this type necessitate an ethical approach to academic practice. to prioritize acquiring the appropriate permits, collaborating with descendant populations, and promoting disposition processes in accordance with cultural beliefs. Redressing these legal and ethical nuances enhances the validity and integrity of research findings and strengthens the academic literature base in paleopathology and skeletal disease. Prioritizing ethics within the law helps researchers ensure their research is respectful of both the scientific community and the populations from whom these remains are derived, thereby establishing a relationship of respect and trust.

Test Your Knowledge

1. Why is it important to handle ancient human remains ethically in paleopathological research?
2. What ethical guidelines govern the excavation, study, and display of skeletal remains in paleopathology?

SUMMARY

Paleopathology is an important bridge between historical medical knowledge of states of health and modern-day medical knowledge. Through careful examination of bones, scientists have started reconstructing the intricacies of diseases that plagued earlier populations. In the context of significant advances in methodology, from the application of interdisciplinary approaches like bioarcheology and epidemiology to sampling and statistical methods, there is a lingering compelling need for more research into conditions like cancer and osteoarthritis. New research shows that conditions previously thought rare may actually require further study, particularly when more diverse skeletal evidence is available. Therefore, developing a better understanding requires innovative methods that tend to transcend conventional paleopathological techniques to ensure data obtained are both robust and representative of diverse populations (Gardner et al., 2020). Second, the limitations of current methods underscore the need to develop our methods and broaden our analytical frameworks. As recently noted, a dependence on gross observation is insufficient to describe the entire gamut of skeletal diseases. By adopting a narrow data viewpoint that emphasizes meticulous description of specific conditions such as osteoarthritis and entheses, scientists can more effectively assess biological responses to early lifestyle factors and environmental stresses. Such a nuance would not only make results more robust but also extend our understanding of the pathogenesis of these conditions in human antiquity. Greater scrutiny and a deliberate focus on methodological accuracy can lead to conclusions that reinterpret our knowledge of skeletal disease and its relevance to human health over time (Becker et al., 2019). Lastly, the future of paleopathology relies on integrative work that draws on multiple disciplines and new technologies. Through interdisciplinary collaboration among osteologists, pathologists, and other specialists, scientists can design comprehensive methods that merge advanced imaging technology with biomechanical modeling. These advances are of central significance to understanding the nuances of skeletal illness in relation to high levels of physical activity and other predictors of human health. An emphasis on collaborative research that makes use of both ancient information and modern scientific techniques will not only broaden our understanding of skeletal ailments but also enrich the history of human health. Such research can yield more detailed, contextually informed data on how shifts in the environment and in way of life have impacted the incidence and expression of skeletal illness (Becker et al., 2019).

Paleopathology is useful when it comes to disease and health in the past, as attested by recent developments in osteoarthritis (OA) in the' estimation of skeletons. GEE-based studies have been proven capable of harmonizing scalar problems that have been a bane in traditional techniques. A seminal study on 1,195 Tiwanaku state adults (AD 500-1,100) is a prime example. By bilateral investigation of the elbow joint and associated articular surfaces in individual specimens, scientists identified significant differences between core and colony Tiwanaku populations in OA prevalence. This nuanced method not only preserves data intact but also provides more informative insights into specific patterns of movement, underscoring the premium on robust statistical modeling in bioarcheological analysis. These findings highlight the dynamic relationship between disease and social processes in ancient populations, which is needed to understand present health conditions within skeletal analysis (Bass et al., 2019). In addition to arthritis, paleopathological evidence is increasingly interpreted as neoplastic disease, discussing the complexities of lesion identification in ancient skeletons. A research conducted on a 71-year-old man, whose skeleton is included in the Coimbra Identified Skeletal Collection, identified several osteolytic lesions, specifically on the skull. The methods used—macroscopic, radiological, and computed tomography—demonstrate the technological progress that enables the analysis of skeletons. But the research also highlights differential diagnosis difficulties, specifically the inability to separate metastatic tumors from multiple myeloma. The findings suggest that a broader categorization, "neoplastic condition," may be optimal, which harmonizes with the reasoning in clinical and paleopathological literature. This must be investigated further to enhance diagnostic accuracy and retrieve strong indicators, which may lead to greater insight into cancer frequency and severity in the past (Cunha et al., 2013). Overall, research into osteoarthritic changes and neoplastic disease in skeletons contributes to the greater narrative of health in ancient groups. By integrating advanced statistical approaches and diagnostic methods, paleopathologists are better able to construct more robust interpretations of skeletal information. They contribute to a greater understanding of how sociocultural factors and environmental pressures have influenced the prevalence of certain illnesses over time. As the pool of paleopathological research grows, it not only sheds light on the medical past of populations but also fuels debates over existing health inequities and disease change. This convergence of ancient pathology and modern public health perspective testifies to the continued relevance of paleopathological studies in creating a deeper understanding of human disease and health across time, demonstrating the subtle interdependence between past and current medical concerns (Bass et al., 2019; Cunha et al., 2013).

KEY TERMS FROM THIS CHAPTER

Paleopathology
Bone lesions
Healed fracture
Osteomyelitis
Leprosy (Hansen's disease)
Arthritis
Rheumatoid arthritis
Rickets
Scurvy
Skeletal remains
Trauma
Periostitis
Tuberculosis (skeletal)
Syphilis
Osteoarthritis
Osteoporosis
Osteomalacia
Anemia (cribra orbitalia)

CRITICAL THINKING QUESTIONS

1. **What is the primary focus of paleopathology?**
   a. Genetic ancestry analysis
   b. Reconstruction of past environments
   c. Study of ancient diseases in human and animal remains
   d. Dating of archaeological sites
2. **Which bone changes are commonly associated with rickets?**
   a. Porotic hyperostosis
   b. Bowing of long bones
   c. Vertebral compression fractures
   d. Ankylosis of joints
3. **The skeletal manifestation known as "saber shin" is typically associated with which disease?**
   a. Tuberculosis
   b. Syphilis
   c. Osteoarthritis
   d. Leprosy
4. **Periosteal reactions on long bones most commonly indicate:**
   a. Degenerative joint disease
   b. Infectious or inflammatory processes
   c. Traumatic injury
   d. Congenital deformities
5. **Which of the following conditions is caused by vitamin C deficiency?**
   a. Osteoporosis
   b. Rickets
   c. Scurvy
   d. Osteopetrosis

Short Answer Questions

1. What is paleopathology, and how does it contribute to our understanding of ancient populations?
2. Explain the difference between antemortem, perimortem, and postmortem skeletal lesions.
3. Describe how tuberculosis can be identified in skeletal remains. Which bones are typically affected?
4. What are the characteristic skeletal features of syphilis in the tertiary stage?
5. How can nutritional deficiencies like rickets and scurvy be detected in bones?
6. Discuss the osteological changes observed in cases of leprosy.

Answers to Critical Thinking Questions

1. (c); 2. (b); 3. (b); 4. (b); 5. (c)

REFERENCES

1. Baker, B. J., Crane-Kramer, G., Dee, M. W., Gregoricka, L. A., Henneberg, M., Lee, C., Lukehart, S. A., Mabey, D. C., Roberts, C. A., Stodder, A. L. W., Stone, A. C., & Winingear, S. (2020). Advancing the understanding of treponemal disease in the past and present. *American Journal of Physical Anthropology*, *171*(S70), 5–41. https://doi.org/10.1002/ajpa.23988Assis, S., Cardoso, F. A., Henderson, C. Y., Jurmain, R., et al. (2016). In search of consensus: Terminology for entheseal changes (EC). https://core.ac.uk/download/42143591.pdf (accessed on 21st July 2025).
2. Bass, W. M., Brothwell, D. R., Buikstra, J. E., Dieppe, P., Felson, D., Gagnon, C. M., Gagnon, C. M., et al. (2019). Evaluating elbow osteoarthritis within the prehistoric Tiwanaku state using generalized estimating equations (GEE). https://core.ac.uk/download/323311271.pdf (accessed on 21st July 2025).
3. Becker, S. K. (2019). Osteoarthritis, entheses, and long bone cross-sectional geometry in the Andes: Usage, history, and future directions. https://core.ac.uk/download/323311202.pdf (accessed on 21st July 2025).
4. Beckett, R., Caramella, D., Conlogue, G., Garvin, G., Natale, G., Nelson, A., Saleem, S., et al. (2019). Diagnosis by consensus: A case study in the importance of interdisciplinary interpretation of mummified remains. https://core.ac.uk/download/162426281.pdf (accessed on 21st July 2025).
5. Bermúdez de Castro, J. M., Gracia-Téllez, A., Martinón-Torres, M., Martín-Francés, L., et al. (2016). Evidence of trauma in a ca. 1-million-year-old patella of *Homo antecessor*, Gran Dolina-Atapuerca (Spain). https://core.ac.uk/download/79528962.pdf (accessed on 21st July 2025).
6. Bernert, Z., Donoghue, H. D., Fóthi, E., Hajdu, T., et al. (2011). New skeletal tuberculosis cases in past populations from Western Hungary (Transdanubia). https://core.ac.uk/download/19085581.pdf (accessed on 21st July 2025).
7. Buzic, I., & Giuffra, V. (2020). The paleopathological evidence on the origins of human tuberculosis: A review. https://core.ac.uk/download/534218941.pdf (accessed on 21st July 2025).
8. Cunha, E., Marques, C., & Santos, A. L. (2013). Better a broader diagnosis than a misdiagnosis: The study of a neoplastic condition in a male individual who died in early 20th century (Coimbra, Portugal). https://core.ac.uk/download/pdf/144051457.pdf (accessed on 21st July 2025).
9. Curate, F. (2014). Osteoporosis and paleopathology: A review. https://core.ac.uk/download/pdf/151538188.pdf (accessed on 21st July 2025).
10. Darling, M. I., & Donoghue, H. D. (2014). Insights from paleomicrobiology into the indigenous peoples of pre-colonial America–A review. https://core.ac.uk/download/19779615.pdf (accessed on 21st July 2025).
11. Donoghue, H. D., Fratpietro, R., Gibson, S., Greenblatt, C. L., et al. (2009). Molecular exploration of the first-century tomb of the shroud in Akeldama, Jerusalem. https://core.ac.uk/download/1687724.pdf (accessed on 21st July 2025).
12. Esteban, J., Fernández, P. L., & Franco, A. (2019). Paleopathology of soft tissues: What mummies can reveal. https://core.ac.uk/download/477977215.pdf (accessed on 21st July 2025).

13. Gardner, E. (2020). Cancer in ancient human populations: Methods and practice in bioarcheology and paleopathology. https://core.ac.uk/download/323062037.pdf (accessed on 21st July 2025).
14. Gidna, A., Mabulla, A., Arriaza, C., Musiba, C., Uribelarrea, D., Barboni, D., Baquedano, E., et al. (2012). Earliest porotic hyperostosis on a 1.5-million-year-old hominin, Olduvai Gorge, Tanzania. https://core.ac.uk/download/pdf/19726080.pdf (accessed on 21st July 2025).
15. Giovannangelo, V. L. (2025). Comparative bioinformatic methodologies in paleogenetic pathogen identification in the Casas Grandes. https://core.ac.uk/download/657666498.pdf (accessed on 21st July 2025).
16. Graff, E. (2011). Mycenaean occupants of ancient Kallithea: Understanding a population's health, culture, and lifestyle through bioarcheological analysis. https://core.ac.uk/download/144145505.pdf (accessed on 21st July 2025).
17. Grauer, A. (2022). Introduction. https://core.ac.uk/download/614446076.pdf (accessed on 21st July 2025).
18. Mailer, G. (2013). Decolonizing the diet: Synthesizing Native-American history, immunology, and nutritional science. https://core.ac.uk/download/484257191.pdf (accessed on 21st July 2025).
19. Mathena, S. A. (2013). Developing a multistage model for treponemal disease susceptibility. https://core.ac.uk/download/480812860.pdf (accessed on 21st July 2025).
20. Morrone, A. (2022). *Vaikuse LAPSED: LÕUNA-EESTI KESK- JA VARAUUSAEGSETE LASTE TOITUMISE JA TERVISE MULTIDISTSIPLINAARSED UURINGUD ARHEOLOOGLISE AINESE PÕHJAL*. https://core.ac.uk/download/541335832.pdf (accessed on 21st July 2025).
21. N/A. (2018). *The Amarna South Tombs Cemetery: Biocultural Dynamics of a Disembedded Capital City in New Kingdom Egypt*. https://core.ac.uk/download/195380021.pdf (accessed on 21st July 2025).
22. Ouellette, L. (2014). *The Bioarcheology of Care*. https://core.ac.uk/download/61661236.pdf (accessed on 21st July 2025).
23. Pangrazzi, C., Tonina, E., & Larentis, O. (2023). Osteological evidence of possible tuberculosis from the early medieval age (6th–11th century), Northern Italy. https://core.ac.uk/download/576881431.pdf (accessed on 21st July 2025).
24. Peterson, M. K. (2016). Egyptian mummy CT scan analysis and a comparison of Midwest Museum practices for the Grand Rapids Public Museum. https://core.ac.uk/download/144152588.pdf (accessed on 21st July 2025).
25. Robbins, G., Gray, K., Schug, M., Mohanty, R. K., Tripathy, V., Misra, V. N., & Shinde, V. S. (2009). Skeletal evidence for leprosy in India by the second millennium B.C. https://core.ac.uk/download/pdf/288249.pdf (accessed on 21st July 2025).
26. Steckel, R. H. (2025). *The Best of Times, The Worst of Times: Health and Nutrition in Pre-Columbian America*. https://core.ac.uk/download/pdf/6646131.pdf (accessed on 21st July 2025).
27. Ubelaker, D. H. (2014). Contributions of pathological alterations to forensic anthropology interpretation. https://core.ac.uk/download/268589417.pdf (accessed on 21st July 2025).

TRAUMA ANALYSIS IN FORENSIC AND BIOARCHAEOLOGICAL CONTEXTS

4

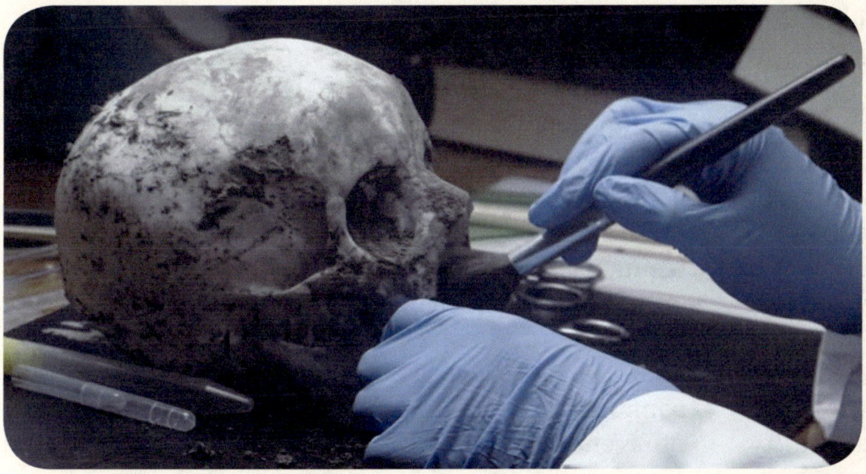

LEARNING OBJECTIVES

After studying this chapter, you will be able to:

1. Discuss the historical perspectives on trauma
2. Explain the types of trauma
3. Understand forensic applications of trauma analysis
4. Evaluate bioarcheological applications of trauma analysis
5. Describe the methodological approaches
6. Focus on ethical considerations

Introduction

As human osteology evolved, the subdisciplines of bioarcheology and forensic anthropology became increasingly pivotal in understanding how trauma has affected individuals and groups throughout history. Both make use of methods aimed at reconstructing life courses, with trauma analysis as a primary resource in unearthing physical and sociocultural expressions of violence, health, and mortality. The integration of bioarcheological and forensic anthropological methods not only enables the analysis of individual cases but also allows the construction of broader narratives about past groups. Additionally, this dual trajectory enriches our knowledge of how historical trauma has impressed itself on skeletal populations, as comparative study can shed light on present societal trends, cultural patterns, and stressor effects over time. In examining the methodological approaches in these disciplines, focus moves away from mere identification and documentation of injuries to the skeletal system and more toward a complex examination of causation and significance of trauma. Bioarchaeologically developed methods have become extremely useful in forensic practice, particularly for analyzing commingled remains and determining individual histories from fragmented bone material. The application of measurement techniques, as demonstrated in research on the reassociation of tali and calcanei, serves to demonstrate the capability of quantitative measures to confirm qualitative interpretations of trauma (Buikstra et al., 2018). By its nature, analytical procedure can provide not only information about the biological context of traumatic skeletons but also about the sociocultural contexts that underlie these skeletal markers. Investigation of frailty in skeletal remains is also a critical component of trauma analysis, emphasizing the importance of conserving health stress in previous populations. Current frailty estimation procedures, while bioarcheological predominantly focused on bioarcheological assemblages, will need to be extended to forensic contexts to effectively evaluate the effects of traumatic events on an individual. The modified skeletal frailty index (SFI+) demonstrates how researchers are increasingly bridging these two domains by offering more nuanced analyses of the embodied stressors faced by military veterans (Frazier et al., 2022). This double vision not only enhances our comprehension of the effects of individual trauma but also invites a more holistic understanding of how cultural and social determinants affect bodily health and resilience in the long run. The integration of these approaches ultimately facilitates a richer dialogue of the human experiences embedded in skeletal remains, contributing to forensic investigation and bioarcheological accounts.

Definition of Trauma in Forensic and Bioarchaeological Contexts

Trauma's connotations extend beyond mere physical harm, affecting interpretations of past contexts and life histories. In forensic anthropology, trauma is usually examined from an incidentality perspective, where researchers are trying to identify patterns of damage to the skeleton in the hope of inferring that such was due to accidents, crime, or natural factors. Such analysis serves to reconstruct events at the moment of an individual's death, hence aiding legal investigations. For example, the presence of particular fracture patterns or lesions can indicate malintent or accidental events, severely impacting the explanation of mortality in differing contexts, as illustrated in research measuring the rate of trauma over time. Through integration of biological and cultural models, forensic practitioners are better equipped to understand the complex interactions between health, environment, and socio-political conditions that affect trauma presentation on the human body. In bioarcheological research, trauma is examined through a broader socio-cultural perspective, emphasizing the daily lives of individuals in their own time and place. Researchers are more likely to establish connections between patterns of violence, social differentiation, and environmental conditions and explain how these factors play a part in the prevalence of trauma in a population. In a seminal piece of work, the violent history of the Peruvian central coast was used to show how crises of a socio-political nature and resource competition created differential patterns of trauma along both gender and social class lines. Interventions used encompassed both physiological harm and sociocultural processes, both affecting the full spectrum from elite to subaltern. Such a result is used to underscore the fact that trauma is not merely physical but also an outcome of multifaceted societal processes. These multifaceted relationships give us a glimpse into how previous populations both navigated and migrated within their worlds, shaping the health consequences that ensued. The development of indexes such as the modified SFI+ presents an elaborate means for assessing trauma in both forensic and bioarcheological contexts. This index enables more precise assessment of markers of stress, enabling researchers to isolate greater or lesser degrees of health and fragility within skeletal tissue. In one seminal study, the SFI+ application produced differences in trauma markers in military veterans compared to civilians that were detectable, illustrating how the individual's experience of stress might affect skeletal health profiles. Analytical techniques like these have important implications for forensic anthropology, with contextual underpinnings for trauma being known to inform both cause-of-death determination and interpretation of individual life history. Positioning the analysis of trauma within such macro-level frameworks allows scholars to build a more comprehensive picture of the embodied histories of past populations, providing scope for future interdisciplinary study to bridge the gap between skeletal analysis and cultural interpretation (Figure 4.1).

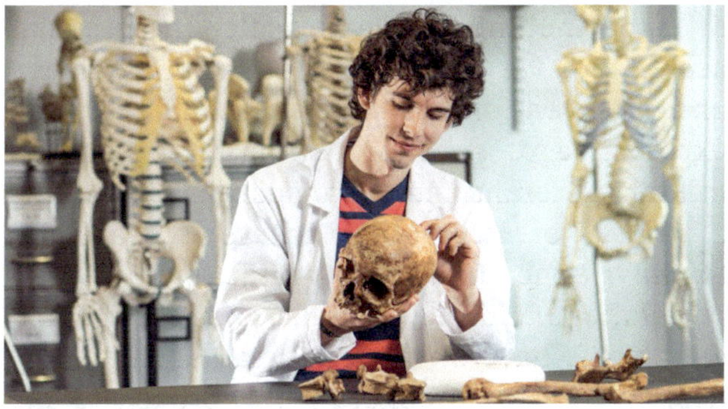

Figure 4.1. The trauma in forensic and bioarcheological contexts.

Source: https://www.bournemouth.ac.uk/sites/default/files/styles/b_16_9_desktop/public/assets/images/anthropology-facility-4.jpg?itok=367bjqHW.

Importance of Trauma Analysis in Understanding Human History

A close reading of human history necessitates a critical examination of trauma that has been endured by populations in the past. Trauma studies in forensic as well as bioarcheological contexts prove that skeletal trauma and stress markers provide crucial information regarding the living conditions of individuals and groups. For instance, an application under a modified SFI+ enables scientists to compare diverse biomarkers of illness and stress across populations, i.e., military and non-military, to explain differences in living and health outcomes influenced by lifestyle factors and cultural habits. The findings indicate how the analysis of skeletal trauma and frailty enables researchers to chart the complex interplay of social forces and individual histories, enhancing our understanding of health inequities and mortality risks in ancient populations (Frazier et al., 2022). Moreover, trauma analysis is crucial in approximating social dynamics and cultural practices throughout human history. In Roman Britain, for instance, examination of decapitation burials provides a breathtaking sophistication in the social attitudes towards violence and death. The presence of such burials in a range of contexts suggests that the activities were not exceptional or punitive but an integral part of the structure of Late Roman culture. By applying scientific methods to osteological profiles and burial context, researchers argue for a nuanced reading of identity conveyed through mortuary practice. Analysis not only clarifies our understanding of funerary practice but also improves our perspective on how ancient communities negotiated the intersection of trauma, identity, and community (Christie et al., 2023). By understanding the significance of analyzing trauma, historians and archaeologists can learn about the myriad ways in which trauma has shaped human history. Through examination of the physiological manifestations of trauma in bones, a tale is uncovered that transcends mere mortality levels or archaeological material. Instead, it speaks to the resilience and ingenuity of human populations faced with hardship. By bioarcheologyintegrating interdisciplinarity that draws on bioarcheology, forensic anthropology, and cultural studies, trauma analysis supports a deeper understanding of people's lives across different eras. This type of understanding does not merely humanize history but also offers valuable lessons for contemporary arguments about the impact of violence, social inequality, and cultural resilience in present populations, thereby increasing our knowledge of humanity's past as a whole (Figure 4.2).

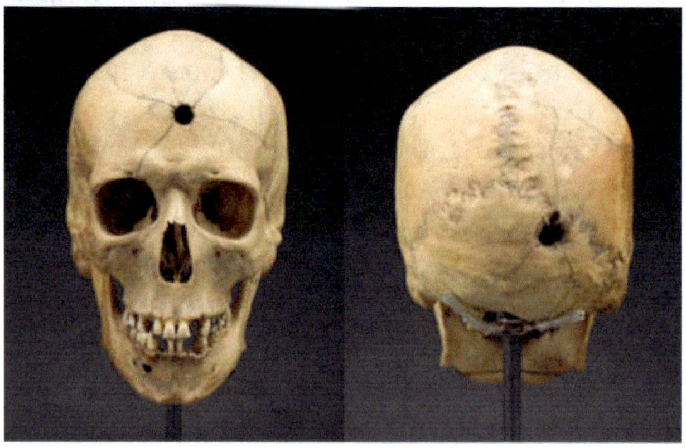

Figure 4.2. An in-depth understanding of human history necessitates a critical examination of trauma experienced by past populations.

Source: https://files.mtstatic.com/site_7339/53508/0?Ex pires=1750861619&Signatu re=iskOUcd~Q0rZflzJFnff fuLRV9wTT9MfidXkteN ZPXRvzHIr4j52l6n 5VHNvd6LEVGlehRvIRK nn5VOue4IN3qZBUXAJ rDz29iEHhwPKHTjnogFERg7huLLDVWU0akaN veP777Fk12inY2XVIkt7~rjQu26ICJVIXwLhiRM MAFo_&Key-Pair-Id=APKAJ5Y6AV4GI7A555NA.

Overview of Methodologies Used in Trauma Analysis

The methods applied in bioarcheological forensic and bioarcheological investigations of trauma are central to demystifying the intricacies of human experience and interaction in the past. One of the prevailing approaches is to analyze skeletal remains with meticulous attention to determine trauma types, including fractures and surgery, from a comprehensive bioarcheological examination. For example, one investigation in the Quebrada de Humahuaca region of Argentina used nonparametric statistical testing to contrast interpersonal violence patterns within a sample of 153 skulls. This analysis differentiated between antemortem and perimortem fractures, cut marks, and trophy skulls and produced significant information on social dynamics and the health stressors encountered by these groups. This close examination enables researchers to construct accounts of past violence and its implications for community organization, and to suggest the broader cultural background in which the skeletal remains are situated (Botta et al., 2014). In addition to classic skeletal analysis, more recent forensic methods have emerged, particularly within the field of health assessment through skeletal frailty indices. These are designed to quantify physiological stress markers in human skeletons—literally, frailty assessment is now an integral measure of health dynamics in both bioarcheology and forensic anthropology. Recent studies have highlighted the importance of using modified skeletal frailty indices that account for varying degrees of skeletal damage and intervention histories to make the lived experience of specific populations, such as military veterans, more transparent. Examining a variety of stress biomarkers, researchers acknowledge nuanced variation between populations and the influence that culture and way of life have on skeletal health. This study design provides a generative approach to the reading of complete life histories embedded in skeletal remains, ultimately increasing our understanding of frailty and health stressors within historical populations (Frazier et al., 2022) detailed assessment of trauma calls for a multi-aspect methodology that is based on classical and new methods. The intersection of biometrics of stress with archaeological context enables researchers to create intersubjectivities between skeletal evidence and broader social narratives. For example, the delineation of particular patterns of trauma—such as antemortem injury prevalence—cannot only define individual histories but also the larger context of violence and survival within a population. In addition, analysis of regional differences in exposure to trauma, as observed in the above-cited Quebrada de Humahuaca study, provides comparative insight into sociocultural processes. Thus, integrating these diverse methods enables intricate interpretations of human behavior over time, underscoring the fundamental interconnectedness of health, trauma, and socio-environmental conditions in forensic and bioarcheological science.

4.1. Historical Perspectives on Trauma

Learning Outcome

1. Evolution of trauma analysis in forensic science
2. Historical case studies illustrating trauma analysis
3. The role of trauma in understanding past societies

Historical research of trauma, particularly in bioarcheological contexts, provides significant lines of evidence regarding how past populations lived and responded to physical and social stressors. The cyclical occurrences of conflict, disease, and environmental stress, as evidenced by archaeological investigations, are immortalized in the human bones found at excavations. These remains will often display pathologies indicative of trauma, like fractures and signs of infectious disease, which are the physical record of historical populations' lived experiences. By examining skeletal trauma systematically, researchers can reconstruct the patterns of trauma from violence and stress endured by individuals and populations and aid in a multidimensional understanding of their sociocultural dynamics. This model mirrors contemporary forensic anthropological practice as trauma analysis begins to expand to incorporate both historical and forward-looking scientific approaches, recognizing the continuity of human suffering across diverse contexts (Frazier et al., 2022). Further, the evolution of trauma interpretation within bioarcheology is noted in the movement away from artifact-based analyses and towards increased focus on human remains. Academics are now looking at the potential of skeletal analysis in revealing pertinent information about trauma's social impact, particularly war and regular violence. In Croatia, for instance, the vast osteological archive contains numerous samples that reveal the complex interaction between bodily health and social violence in prehistory. Through advances in bioarcheological methods, incorporating mixed research approaches and multidisciplinary collaboration is needed in understanding the complex context of trauma. Historical analysis not only informs today's practice but also forms the basis of the superiority of skeletal evidence in broader arguments about health and social structure, and that yesterday still impacts today's perception and policy on trauma (Adamić et al., 2015).

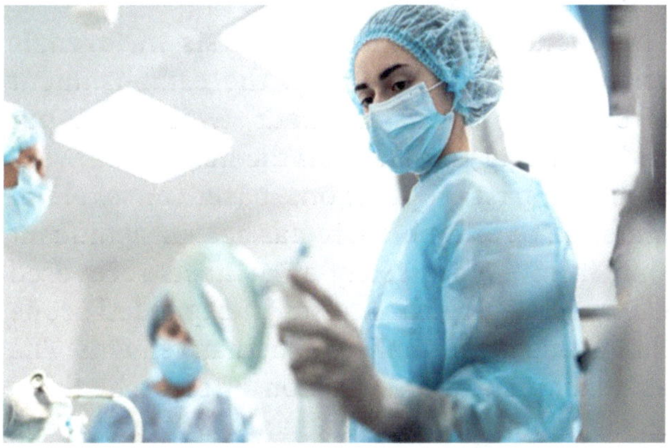

Figure 4.3. The historical exploration of trauma.

Source: https://images.law.com/contrib/content/uploads/sites/401/2020/11/Healthcare-worker-Article-202011241642.jpg.

Unpacking further the methods of trauma analysis mirrors the variety of frameworks applied to comprehend skeletal data. For example, the measurement of frailty using indices such as the modified skeletal frailty index (SFI+) accounts for various individual health statuses, demonstrating the combined impact of environmental stress and cultural lifestyle on skeletal wellbeing. Comparative results in military and civilian cohort studies demonstrate how trauma experience is manifested in different skeletal indicators, which inform forensic and bioarcheological assessment. Context is the central theme in these questions, as the application of biocultural models provides a deeper understanding of how military culture may affect health outcomes among veterans. The dynamic interplay between historical trauma and its material manifestations through human remains makes bioarcheology a critical research theme to develop modern trauma thinking further and to guide subsequent research aimed at enhancing knowledge on the human condition (Frazier et al., 2022) (Figure 4.3).

4.1.1. Evolution of Trauma Analysis in Forensic Science

The evolution of trauma analysis in forensic science is interlinked with the establishment of bioarcheological methods, which have put an increasing emphasis on the health and well-being of past populations based on skeletal material. Over time, there has been a significant shift from a focus solely on artifacts recovered from archaeological sites to an expanded scope that includes the analysis of human remains. The establishment and evolution of bioarcheology, as a branch of physical anthropology, have enabled greater insight into the traumatic injuries and diseases suffered by residents of ancient societies. As scientific techniques improve, researchers have now begun to obtain valuable evidence from human remains that not only comments on personal health but also on social behavior, particularly in contexts affected by endemic war and other stressors, such that detailed investigation of trauma in historical populations is now possible (Adamić et al., 2015). In recent years, trauma research has moved once again, though more toward understanding social dynamics among prehistoric groups. For instance, studies on Neanderthals have revealed a high degree of complexity in their responses to injury and healing, suggesting that they cared for one another and implying strong social connections among them. This shift in perception presents a different picture from the earlier presumption regarding Neanderthals' indifference towards suffering. By studying healed patterns of trauma, researchers have argued that Neanderthal medicine was professional and comprehensive, indicating higher societal complexity.

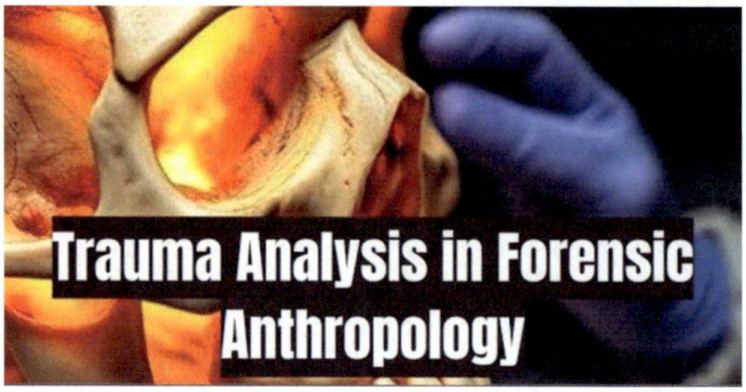

Figure 4.4. The evolution of trauma analysis in forensic science.

Source: https://i.ytimg.com/vi/8s6P4hFhhu8/sddefault.jpg.

Secondly, the use of bioarcheological data within forensic science allows the investigation not only of bodily trauma but also of its social dimension, thereby filling in the story of past human health (Hitchens et al., 2018). Trauma analysis within forensic science is now at the forefront of constructing an extended bioarcheological narrative that accounts for the intersection of society's structures and health. Through methods such as osteological assessment and advanced imaging, forensic scientists can unlock strata of information related to previous trauma that align with broader historical trends. The growing recognition of the importance of skeletal analysis provides fertile ground for studying how environmental and social factors have previously influenced health outcomes. This evidence not only contributes to forming a brief picture of human behavior's history but also serves as a crucial source for contemporary use by the medical and psychological professions, sharpening our understanding of trauma both as a physical and social entity as time passes (Adamić et al., 2015) (Figure 4.4).

4.1.2. Historical Case Studies Illustrating Trauma Analysis

The relevance of trauma analysis in both bioarcheological and forensic contexts is clearly illustrated by several historical case studies that illustrate the interplay between the skeleton and cultural stress experience. One such insightful case is the investigation of skeletal frailty in military veterans, where a new skeletal frailty index (SFI+) was proposed to assess the embodied stressors individuals experience. This new approach revealed lower frailty in the veteran group than in civilians and demonstrates the complex dynamics of lived experience within military culture. The use of severity scales rather than flat binary measures provides greater analytical rigor, enabling researchers to detect subtle differences in health indicators across groups. These findings illuminate how social interventions and roles affect physiological outcomes and, therefore, enhance our understanding of trauma as biocultural and physiological within historical populations (Frazier et al., 2022). Equally intriguing is the study of non-adult skeletal remains, which have long been pushed to the margins in historical accounts. Recent efforts to enhance child voice in bioarcheology have been promising, revealing rich information about community health, coping strategies during crises, and responses to crises. The analysis of the skeletons of children can help explain how we form and interpret trauma in a social context and thus enhance a broader understanding of population resilience. The intricacies of trauma in childhood are also in a position to clarify further intergenerational stressors that persist over time to delineate patterns of vulnerability in the young that can inform health and social agendas today. For future directions, these studies also call for methodological creativity in the Baltics, where children's bioarcheology has been less examined, and for an appreciation of integrating a holistic approach to trauma (Morrone et al., 2020). Incorporating trauma analysis into previous case studies not only reevaluates the understanding of previous communities but also upends contemporary narratives by extending the possibilities of who and what are considered significant in archaeology. By exploring the embodiment of stressors in skeletal remains, researchers can probe deeper into meanings related to health inequalities, societal functioning, and cultural beliefs. The emphasis on minute skeletal trauma analysis also further clarifies the intricate psychological and emotional contexts that accompany physical trauma. These results are of greater than mere historical interest; they emphasize the significance of recognizing the complicating blending of trauma in constructing human experiences throughout history. The developing discourse on these findings seeks not only to confirm the lived experiences of oppressed groups but also to reinforce our analytical frameworks for comprehending trauma in a socio-historical setting (Frazier et al., 2022; Morrone et al., 2020).

4.1.3. The Role of Trauma in Understanding Past Societies

Knowledge of the effects of trauma within ancient societies is essential to understanding how they built their hierarchies and social dynamics. Researchers have managed to determine that skeletal evidence can provide information about interpersonal violence, which is a crucial aspect showing underlying tensions among communities. For instance, studies among populations from Quebrada de Humahuaca present the prevalence of trauma caused by interpersonal violence, with a significant proportion of victims in evidence of survival after having been exposed to traumatic situations. Such data, for example, the epidemiology of cranial trauma by population, imply violence trends within society that cross both age and gender and indicate a widespread cultural tolerance of violence throughout the Late Regional Development Period. Such analysis not only illuminates the individual experience but also the social organizations and relations of power present in ancient societies (Botta et al., 2014). An examination of trauma also informs us about social inequalities that may have taken place in past populations. In sites such as Kaman-Kalehöyük, evidence of health inequality coupled with documented trauma illustrates the effect of the socio-political environment on community wellness. Remains from this site reveal not only the presence of traumatic injury but also indicators of biological stress consistent with lower socio-economic status for some groups. The dynamics of rates of violence and population health profiles suggest that modifications in the social organization impacted population health and safety, creating increased exposure for marginalized communities. Thus, bioarcheological data point to the ubiquitous intersection of trauma, health, and socio-economic status, highlighting the subtle nuances of everyday life in ancient communities (Anderson et al., 2017). The implications of trauma analysis extend beyond individual health to offer a better understanding of the socio-political climate of ancient communities. Through the identification of healed and unhealed wounds, we can infer not only how individuals were exposed to violence, but also how the community responded to violence. The occurrence of perimortem trauma, such as weapon wounds, indicates that some populations experienced periodic episodes of violence, perhaps linked to raids or warfare on a systemic level. The evidence compels academics to reconceptualize descriptions of cultural behavior and group security, as it documents a climate in which violence structured society. Besides, when correlating evidence of trauma with history, researchers can study how populations accommodated to, resisted, or promoted patterns of violence, gaining clues about the agency and resilience of past societies (Anderson et al., 2017; Botta et al., 2014) (Figure 4.5).

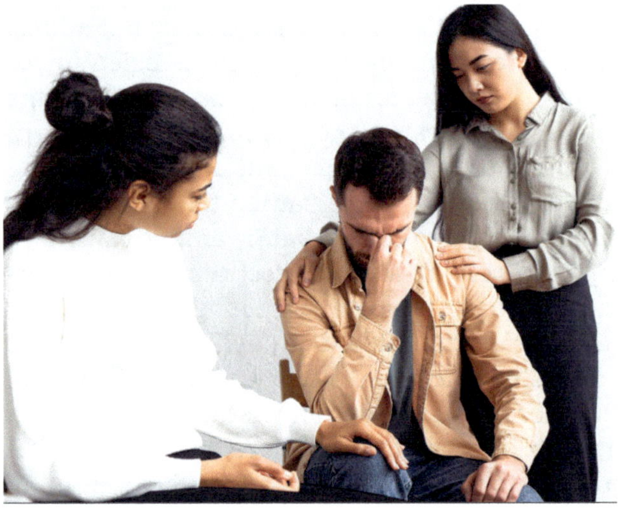

Figure 4.5. The role of trauma in understanding past societies.

Source: https://theremedymn.com/wp-content/uploads/2023/05/1-e1685084907292.jpg.

Test Your Knowledge

1. How have historical perspectives on trauma evolved across different civilizations and time periods?
2. What evidence do skeletal remains provide about trauma and injury in past populations?

4.2. Types of Trauma

Learning Outcome

1. Blunt force trauma and its implications
2. Sharp force trauma and its identification
3. Environmental trauma and its effects on skeletal remains

Trauma analysis, particularly in bioarcheological and forensic contexts, tends to display complex patterns of social life and interpersonal violence. One common type is blunt force trauma, which is often revealed by skeletal analysis. For instance, the presence of orbital blowout fractures provides information on the mechanical forces involved in violent confrontation. While these fractures are predominantly evaluated in the context of current clinical practice, their presence in skeletons necessitates a biocultural explanation of the behaviors and circumstances that may have conceivably resulted in such trauma. By applying standardized techniques, such as the new scoring system used to measure these fractures, investigators can better estimate the occurrence and effects of interpersonal violence in earlier populations and, in turn, glimpse their social interaction and conflict patterns (Ornot et al., 2024). In addition, the effects of social changes, for example, those caused by military campaigns, can profoundly influence the type of trauma at archaeological sites. The Roman conquest of Britain, say, initiated revolutionary changes in settlement and agricultural patterns and communal attitudes towards the dead and burial. One analysis of decapitation burials in this time reveals the complexity of trauma. It suggests that certain types of punishment or violence were practiced, but may not have resulted in their depiction. Instead, specific burial treatments may suggest ritual activities or social deviance. This requires context-sensitive analysis, with grave furnishings and osteological profiles read within broader social contexts (Christie et al., 2023). Trauma analysis must thus be undertaken in a nuanced fashion responsive to the intersections among culture, violence, and identity. In addition to interpersonal forms of trauma, skeletal analysis may also be applied to identify the types of collective trauma faced by populations. Contextual trauma, which is caused by chronic societal stressors such as war, disease, or climatic shifts, is more likely to leave its mark on both population and individual levels. One such example would be the long-term effects of the violent conflict that arose with Roman occupation, which are reflected in skeletal evidence of stress, malnutrition, or other disease-related issues. These traumas overlap with visible evidence of violence, which assists in better comprehending how complex forms of stress were handled and responded to by ancient societies. Thus, trauma analysis transcends mere categorization of injuries, dealing with broader implications for survival within communities and continuity of culture in the face of pervasive adversity (Figure 4.6).

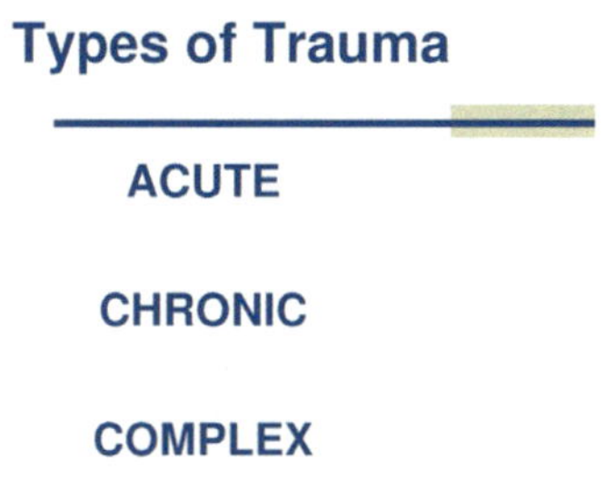

Figure 4.6. Types of trauma.

Source: https://external-content.duckduckgo.com/iu/?u=https%3A%2F%2Fimage.slideserve.com%2F1438528%2Ftypes-of-trauma-l.jpg&f=1&nofb=1&ipt=3d68af1a07d8b4feeff62d6a6e36dacf9dd413957d91943738876549d35db4cb.

4.2.1. Blunt Force Trauma and Its Implications

The study of blunt force trauma provides deep insight into sociocultural trends and patterns of violence over time. When examining skeletal remains within various archaeological contexts, bioarcheologists generally look for evidence of interpersonal violence in the form of cranial trauma. An example representative study in the Quebrada de Humahuaca context is a good illustration of the fact that the study of 153 skulls from some sites, such as Los Amarillos and La Huerta, provides high rates of interpersonal violence-related trauma. The investigative techniques enabled researchers to distinguish between antemortem and perimortem fractures, and this provided critical information regarding survival prospects and the characteristics of inflicted injuries. This exercise of learning about trauma not only reveals personal health outcomes but also mirrors broader societal features, such as conflict, stability, or social organization in the periods at issue, and demonstrates that trauma can be a good indicator of historical human behavior and cultural practice (Botta et al., 2014). In addition, blunt force trauma has been studied in ways that extend beyond survival analysis alone; it bears implications for the study of social stratification and prevention of violence in modern-day contexts. In particular, examining cranial trauma from a neurosurgical perspective or a bioarcheological perspective provides a new vehicle for linking patterns of injury to demographic markers like sex, age, and geographical place. It has been found that the prevalence of trauma may vary significantly between populations. For example, the regional variation across the three sites of Quebrada de Humahuaca illustrates how social and environmental conditions can shape the dynamics of violence experienced by different groups. Such a dense dataset of injuries facilitates close examination of how warfare, cultural practice, and social complexity each contribute towards the formation of human interactions and the potential for violent conflict (Botta et al., 2014). In modern forensic uses, recognition of blunt force trauma also enriches the field's methodology for diagnosis and analysis. Orbital blowout fractures, caused by blunt force strikes, present a specific challenge in correlating skeletal information with clinical diagnoses. The translation of clinical parameters for these fractures into a skeletal evaluation matrix underscores the importance of adapting methodologies for archaeological research. Studies that bioarcheological develop scoring systems based on visible features of injuries have broad applicability to both forensic and bioarcheological contexts. Through extensive study of bones with modern study protocols, researchers can establish standardized procedures that improve accuracy and previsibility in trauma pattern assessment. This multidisciplinary dialogue between forensic and bioarcheological analyses further informs our understanding of human violence across time, enabling more sophisticated discussions of past behaviors and modern implications (Figure 4.7).

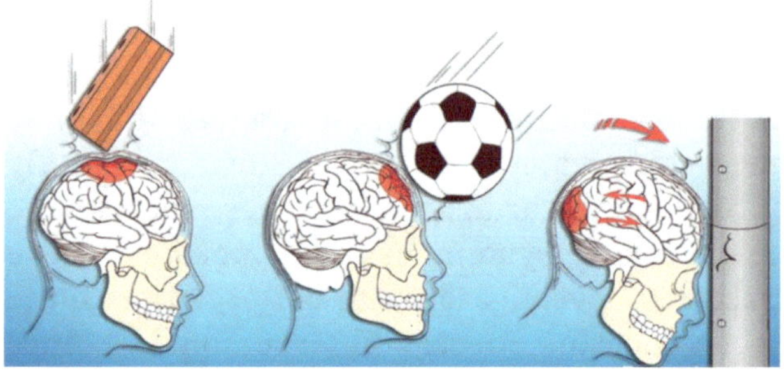

Figure 4.7. The analysis of blunt force trauma reveals significant insights.

Source: https://external-content.duckduckgo.com/iu/?u=https%3A%2F%2Fstudy.com%2Fcimages%2Fvideopreview%2Fvideopreview-full%2Fgb8bi4t5yh.jpg&f=1&nofb=1&ipt=b82a844468b2dadd4f3b883b0fca893fff0a282f7a8bb3cdda50ad28c594848a.

4.2.2. Sharp Force Trauma and Its Identification

Sharp force trauma identification within both forensic and bioarcheological contexts presents multifaceted challenges and opportunities for examination. It calls for a detailed examination of skeletal remains to expose traces of wounds that may determine historical patterns of violence. In the collection at Smith's Knoll, precise examination revealed evidence of sharp force trauma on various bones, particularly ribs and long bones, which are vital in describing under what conditions individuals died. Sharp force trauma, being clean and precise, is more likely to reflect planned violence, be it by blades or other bladed instruments. The nuances of such injuries, coupled with the relative comparisons between historical and bioarcheological data, give strength to the interpretative process that goes into developing understanding about the mechanisms of trauma in both past and contemporary populations. Ultimately, such analysis provides acute observations on interpersonal violent conflict recorded in prehistory and history. Compounding the sharp force trauma further is the differential in weapons used in such trauma. History, as recorded, and archaeological evidence tend to reflect that typical patterns are found with various weapons. The analysis above from the Smiths Knoll differentiated injuries likely inflicted by bayonets from those inflicted by swords, not only indicating the nature of violence but also potential tactics employed in ancient warfare. The same applies to other archaeological findings, like Late Roman Britain decapitation burials, which suggest diverse culturally constructed definitions of violence. The ritualistic aspect of decapitation, as testified in skeletal material, shows that sharp force trauma is not merely a signifier of homicide but can comprise more extensive social or cultural practices. By the association of archaeological information to systematic osteological analysis, scientists can obtain a deeper insight into the society's values towards death and violence in specific periods, as testified to both in the Smiths Knoll assemblage and Late Roman Period research. In light of such discovery, incorporation of sharp force trauma analysis into forensic and bioarcheological research creates avenues for understanding diverse roles encompassed by violence across human history. The potential for bridging traumas to skeletal remains with socio-cultural dynamics prevailing during this time augments the importance of prioritizing context in trauma analysis. As seen in both Smith's Knoll assemblage and decapitation burial analysis, sharp force injury is not only a war legacy but has narrative significance proportionate to broader societal practice. Using such an integrated methodology combining osteological analysis with contextual history, it is possible to build a balanced picture of the representation of trauma in earlier material culture. Such rigorous examinations are an enriching contribution to the existing controversy over violence in archaeology, shedding light on human experience in the manifestation of sharp-force injury and on the relevance of analyzing trauma (Figure 4.8).

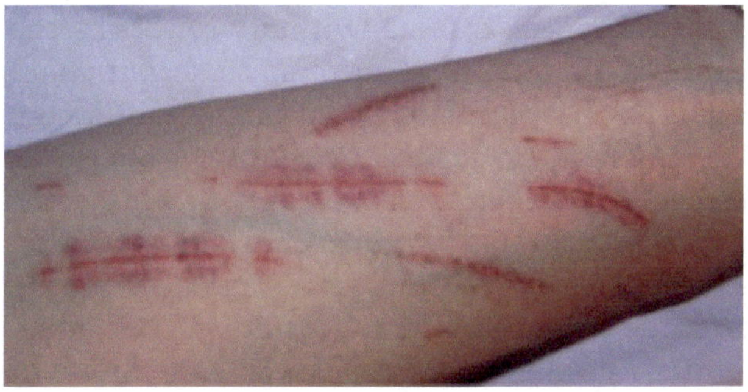

Figure 4.8. The identification of sharp force trauma presents intricate challenges.

Source: https://external-content.duckduckgo.com/iu/?u=https%3A%2F%2F08f043fb5b.clvaw-cdnwnd.com%2F65cf06e22b1051f5df11dfe70b7dd6da%2F200000162-df3d0e03be%2Fself_inflicted_wrist_cuts.JPG&f=1&nofb=1&ipt=3998965ea45372513be9e2ecc21b1e0ff5de3280fb949e97a36e109ce88d61c1.

4.2.3. Environmental Trauma and Its Effects on Skeletal Remains

Environmental trauma and its interaction with environmental factors substantially influence skeletal analysis in forensic and bioarcheological contexts. Environmental trauma can result from a variety of etiologies that can range from natural disasters, demographic stress, and anthropogenic impacts. This resulted in skeletal trauma that can change bone morphology, create stress markers, and lead to trauma-suggestive pathologies. As researchers examine these bone remains, it is increasingly clear that the environment in which humans lived—such as geographic location, resource availability, and social dynamics—can provide important clues about the nature of the environmental trauma they experienced. For instance, groups who reside in locations threatened by seismic activity can have characteristic bone injury patterns, and this can provide information on environmental trauma interaction in daily life. The application of statistical methods of high sophistication, such as Generalized Estimating Equations (GEE), allows the bioarcheologists to assess environmental trauma without reducing the complex pattern of conditions that contribute towards the placement of remains within the bones. The approach helps scientists avoid scalar issues that can arise in assessing osteoarthritis or other traumas in bone analysis, providing a holistic overview of data across all scales, from demographics to the health of individual joints. Using GEE, research can uncover important differences in traumatic injury and health profiles between populations, showing how environmental stressors influence skeletal markers across contexts. Such a robust statistical method then becomes important to forward trauma analysis in bioarcheology, allowing for greater insight into how environmental factors influence health over time, as seen in analyses of varied populations across varied geographical contexts. Through particular case studies, for example, those in Canyon de Chelly, it is seen how environmental trauma intersects with the phenomenon of violence among populations living close to historically strife-prone locations. The skeletal material examined from this area suggests a high incidence of trauma across individuals, especially when compared to their equivalents in surrounding cultural regions. These findings emphasize the likelihood that pressures from the wider environment—competition over resources and cultural conflict—accentuated the circumstances of violence. Furthermore, the study highlights the manner in which older individuals were more likely to show signs of trauma, maybe exhibiting a pattern of societal organization where such trauma patterns mix with demographic and health variables, once again demonstrating the complex effects of environmental trauma on the skeletal population in an extensive bioarcheological context (Tegtmeyer et al., 2017; Bass et al., 2019).

Test Your Knowledge

1. What are the main types of trauma identified in osteological and clinical studies?
2. How can different types of trauma be distinguished based on skeletal evidence?

4.3. Forensic Applications of Trauma Analysis

Learning Outcome

1. Role of trauma analysis in criminal investigations
2. Techniques used in forensic trauma analysis
3. Case studies highlighting forensic trauma analysis outcomes

The subtleties of trauma analysis within forensic contexts provide valuable information on people's lived experiences, particularly in assessing health and biomarkers for stress. From the examination of skeletonized remains, researchers can obtain helpful information on the physiological effects of trauma. This is most evident when using modified indices, such as the skeletal frailty index (SFI+). The application of SFI+ offers an implied assessment of trauma as it employs a larger number of stress indicators beyond presence or absence, where more is known about the health profile of a person. These types of measurements are statistically relevant in distinguishing between groups like military veterans and civilians, thereby opening the doors to understanding the ways in which contextual influences operate on frailty and overall health outcomes in forensic anthropology (Frazier et al., 2022). This analytical strategy further explores the analysis of skeletal data in a legal setting, offering critical perspectives on individuals' life histories. Understanding the applications of forensic trauma analysis extends to critical assessment of the impact on society, e.g., how warfare is conveyed in skeletal human remains. The comparison of trauma patterns between bioarcheological contexts sheds light on extreme variations in health and trauma among populations over time periods. When bioarcheologists analyze collections, for instance, the osteological materials from Croatia, they provide a past context that can prove beneficial for forensic investigation in the present (Adamić et al., 2015). The focus on traumatic and pathological examples within these collections offers an opportunity to bridge archaeological evidence with existing forensic applications, with the possibility of generating evidence for current debates on health and legal definitions of trauma. Through this interdisciplinary understanding, the congruence of forensic anthropology and bioarcheology is laid bare, wherein holism emerges as a driving factor in the interpretation of skeletal trauma.

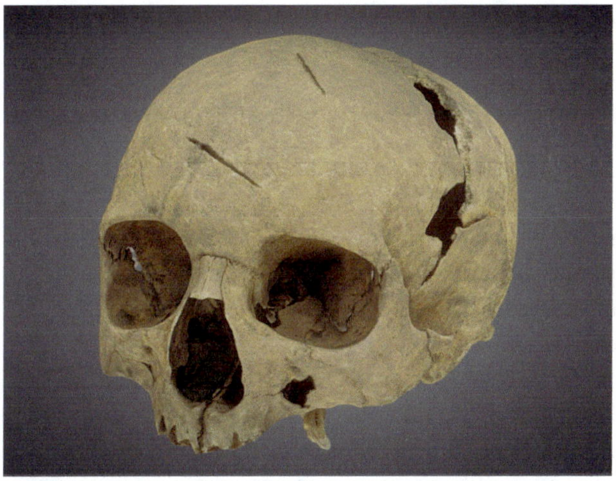

Figure 4.9. The intricacies of trauma analysis within forensic contexts.

Source: https://external-content.duckduckgo.com/iu/?u=https%3A%2F%2Fsocialsci.libretexts.org%2F%40api%2Fdeki%2Ffiles%2F129122%2Fimage21-10.png%3Frevision%3D1&f=1&nofb=1&ipt=6a9ea39c8d168a972fcdf7c124103e2e8b146e33f315376192c8d231264c15f4.

Overall, the interdisciplinary insights that emerge from the analysis of trauma have far-reaching implications for both forensic anthropology and bioarcheology. When forensic scientists and bioarcheologists collaborate, they can enhance trauma assessment accuracy, leading to more sound legal verdicts and a better understanding of past health trends. Both should collaborate, particularly with researchers attempting to add more complexity to how stressors are measured quantifiably. The recent trends toward the use of increasingly complex indices, including SFI+, reflect a changing way of thinking about the influences of trauma, and thus contribute to richer forensic and bioarcheological explanations (Frazier et al., 2022). By highlighting the interconnectivity of individual health histories with broader societal patterns, these analyses continue to guide and refine methodologies, ultimately toward an enhanced, rigorous understanding of human lives over time (Figure 4.9).

4.3.1. Role of Trauma Analysis in Criminal Investigations

In a criminal investigation, trauma analysis is a crucial tool to unravel the cause of death. By rigorously examining bone remains, forensic practitioners can distinguish between different types of injuries and potential causes. The distinction is not anecdotal but scientific and may reveal patterns of violence or neglect. One strong example is provided by research conducted in the Quebrada de Humahuaca region, where bioarcheological evidence indicated a high frequency of interpersonal violence trauma in a sample that consisted of 153 skulls from multiple archaeological sites. The contrast between antemortem and perimortem fractures revealed the chances of survival of victims after serious injury, demonstrating how trauma analysis broadens our understanding of past social life and conflict, deepening our insights into violent acts and their impact on society (Botta et al., 2014). The synthesis between new technologies, such as micro-computed tomography (micro-CT) and three-dimensional printing (3D printing), has revolutionized the course of trauma analysis in forensic science. These technologies allow for detailed visualizations of skeletal trauma that would otherwise be hard to quantify with precision. For instance, utilizing micro-CT, one can aid in the alignment of severed skeletal components, analyze tool marks, and provide a three-dimensional perspective of complex cases of dismemberment. This high-resolution method not only aids in recovering the tactics used in violence but also maximizes the probative value of the results in court cases. Use of such technologies is a classic example of how trauma analysis has evolved to involve sophisticated resources, thereby improving the accuracy of investigations and the reporting of results in trials (Baier et al., 2017). Understanding the importance of trauma analysis in criminal investigations is basic to the development of comprehensive legal and forensic systems. While investigators apply means to control for contextual variables such as age, sex, and regional patterns of trauma, they can construct more nuanced narratives than bare static facts. Illuminating the patterns of violent interactions and their manifestation on the body, trauma analysis makes the forensic science and the legal process more robust. As with the analysis of trauma in the context of Quebrada de Humahuaca, broader implications regarding values and practices in society necessitate interdisciplinary debate among archaeologists, forensic scientists, and social historians. Such endeavors place the significance of trauma analysis as a required tool in the reconstruction of multifaceted histories of violence, thus better informing us about human behavior in both historical and modern contexts.

4.3.2. Techniques Used in Forensic Trauma Analysis

The analytical techniques employed in forensic analysis of trauma are diverse and well-designed for thorough examination of skeletal remains. Of these, transition analysis (TA) stands out as it applies a multidimensional perspective to biological age estimation from skeletal morphology. TA entails integrating data from the public symphysis, iliac auricular area, and cranial sutures to obtain an overall perspective on the mechanisms of skeletal aging. However, studies have indicated that there is variation in the accuracy of TAs among populations. For instance, estimates from the Hamann-Todd Collection yielded a mean absolute error of 11.6 years, with considerable variation by ancestry, demonstrating the inconsistency of traditional methods in producing uniform results across different demographic groups. These factors underscore the need to continue refining forensic techniques to enhance their adaptability across contexts and populations, in line with broader objectives in trauma analysis (Simon et al., 2020). In forensic science, systematic examination of trauma is highly critical for legal reasons, particularly to determine the cause and timing of injuries. Techniques such as histological analysis and three-dimensional imaging have gained popularity because they enable close assessment of bone microstructure and overall architectural integrity. Modern imaging methods can visualize internal anatomy without causing specimen damage, making it more straightforward to distinguish perimortem from postmortem trauma. Furthermore, bioarcheological integrating bioarcheological data enhances our understanding of historical trends in health and trauma rates in past populations. By examining skeletal remains within archaeology contexts, researchers are better positioned to place trauma within broader socio-historic situations, revealing how incidents like war and disease have impacted overall population health over time (Adamić et al., 2015). In addition, the interdisciplinary connections established between forensic trauma analysis and bioarcheology reveal fertile areas of research and approach. The robust osteological collections, as in the case of Croatia's abundant heritage, are valuable resources that provide insights into past pathological and traumatic cases. The collections are of valuable use in the reformulation of existing forensic practice based on comparative datasets that reveal the psychosocial impact of trauma over time. Continuous study of modern and ancient remains encourages further understanding of the effects of environmental and cultural factors on the manifestation of trauma. Consequently, as forensic practice evolves bioarcheological through the integration of bioarcheological insights, the field will benefit greatly, undertaking improved trauma analysis that not only aids contemporary justice but also leaves a historical record (Adamić et al., 2015) (Figure 4.10).

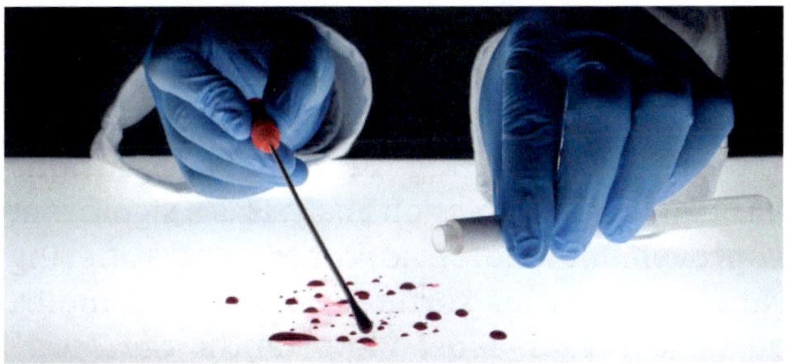

Figure 4.10. The methodologies employed in forensic trauma analysis.

Source: https://external-content.duckduckgo.com/iu/?u=https%3A%2F%2Fwww.precisa.com%2Fwp-content%2Fuploads%2F2021%2F09%2Fforensics-1-1024x472-1.jpg&f=1&nofb=1&ipt=e2cc7f1c313d0d1a5595e99a4c6ae05d4370fda2b5fd45f6f7dbb17f43733857.

4.3.3. Case Studies Highlighting Forensic Trauma Analysis Outcomes

Forensic trauma analysis of skeletal remains is crucial in assessing the socio-cultural dynamics of previous populations, particularly in relation to interpersonal violence. Case studies from regions such as Quebrada de Humahuaca in Argentina illustrate the prevalence of interpersonal violence indicated in bioarcheological evidence. A comprehensive analysis of 153 cranium remains from three sites revealed a high frequency of trauma, comprised mainly of antemortem injury indicative of survival following violence. Furthermore, both genders were equally represented, and differences between sites pointed to geographical factors influencing trauma manifestation, with the Yacoraite site recording the most frequent record of injuries. These findings not only shed light on the physical consequences of social violence but also fuel debates on the broader implications of violence in these early societies (Botta et al., 2014). Further along in forensic trauma analysis, another case study is on methodological enhancement in the identification of individuals from commingled remains. In the present research, the lengths and widths of some ankle bones in a sample of 197 individuals were meticulously measured to allow precise reassociations between calcanei and tali. Formulating 12 precise equations through linear regression analysis is a significant improvement in forensic anthropology, offering valid methods for sorting remains in complex burial contexts. Most importantly, the study concluded that bilateral asymmetry and sex did not affect the method's effectiveness, thereby advancing its application in forensic settings (Buikstra et al., 2018). This, therefore, points to the ancient significance of adherence to strict methodology in the proper interpretation of trauma and identification crucial in the solving of cases of unreported historical violence. In aggregating findings from various forensic trauma examinations, it is evident that the implications are much closer to each other than any single case; they reflect long patterns of behavior, health, and conflict at the societal level. The interaction of trauma evidence with the cultural context in which it arises facilitates a better understanding of past human experience. For instance, the cyclical patterns of violence in the Quebrada de Humahuaca region cry out for explanation by the social orders that generated such violence. Moreover, the mechanical explanation demonstrated in the example of commingled remains broadens the use of forensic anthropology by using statistical precision to optimize identification. Collectively, these case studies encompass the multi-disciplinary nature of trauma analysis, bringing together archaeology, forensic science, and anthropology to illuminate the complex stories woven into human existence over time (Botta et al., 2014; Buikstra et al., 2018).

Test Your Knowledge

1. How is trauma analysis used in forensic investigations to determine cause of injury or death?
2. What skeletal features help forensic experts differentiate between ante-mortem, peri-mortem, and post-mortem trauma?

4.4. Bioarchaeological Applications of Trauma Analysis

Learning Outcome

1. Understanding health and disease through trauma analysis
2. Trauma as a reflection of social and cultural practices
3. Case studies from bioarcheological sites

When considering the nuances of bioarcheological applications, researchers typically emphasize the significance of trauma analysis in their reconstruction of the quotidian lives of ancient peoples. The technique extends beyond mere identification of lesions on the bones and moves toward a more comprehensive understanding of social organization, health, and mortality among the ancient groups. By employing more advanced statistical methods, bioarcheologists can properly examine patterns of injury and trauma in bone remains and illuminate social and environmental pressures endured by the person.

It is through this process of layered analysis that a better appreciation for the interrelation of specific traumas and demographic variables such as sex, age, and social status is realized, and a clearer picture of life and death in the past is obtained. One of the significant advances in trauma analysis is the use of Generalized Estimating Equations (GEE) to address scalar problems typically encountered when analyzing osteological data. By supporting population-averaged statistical models, GEE enables researchers to correlate multiple articular surfaces within a single specimen, yielding a robust, unbiased dataset. For instance, when studying the elbow joints of individuals from the Tiwanaku state, this technique identified significant differences in osteoarthritis prevalence, thereby indicating differences in physical activity and population lifestyle. These findings underscore the strength of GEE in further refining the use and interpretation of trauma and the meaning of trauma within the bioarcheology paradigm, paving the way for more substantial and more comprehensive research in the field (Bass et al., 2019). The integration of trauma analysis with demographic estimation techniques also bioarcheological strengthens bioarcheological research. Transition analysis (TA), the integration of data among different areas of anatomy, enhances the accuracy of age estimation, a critical aspect in making sense of trauma patterns in ancient populations. By comparing TA-estimated ages with known skeletal ages and the examination of variability among demographic groups, researchers can cast light on the relationship between trauma, aging, and health disparities of the past. Such observations not only enhance the practice for age estimation but also shed light on how trauma influences survival and the health of people over a period. The combination of better statistical uses and demographic analysis is, thus, a big leap forward in the study of bioarcheological trauma analysis since it is possible to interpret skeletal remains and contexts better (Simon et al., 2020) (Figure 4.11).

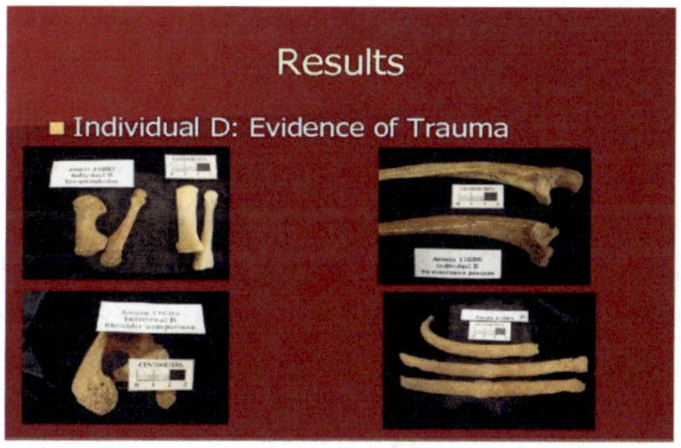

Figure 4.11. Case studies highlighting forensic trauma analysis outcomes.

Source: https://external-content.duckduckgo.com/iu/?u=https%3A%2F%2Fpresent5.com%2Fpresentation%2F8f4aaf53e04402e21e8fc158673d5158%2Fimage-9.jpg&f=1&nofb=1&ipt=235ece68c7755d22be928cf37eebeedb7122c50e4492f6d5041424d8c0bbce14.

4.4.1. Understanding Health and Disease Through Trauma Analysis

At the meeting point of health and disease from a trauma analysis perspective, the skeletal remains are at the forefront in both the forensic and bioarcheological fields. The study of trauma to bones not only reveals historical instances of physical injury but also serves as a marker of social and environmental stressors experienced by individuals and groups. Trauma patterning is used in forensic anthropology to reveal bioarcheologythe circumstances surrounding the death of an individual, while in bioarcheology, it informs a broader context of patterning of health and society in previous times. This addition of trauma analysis to health assessments allows researchers to develop comprehensive explanations of the living conditions, resilience, and vulnerabilities of past populations with an emphasis on the complex interactions between individual experiences and shared health consequences. The utilization of modified indices to assess skeletal frailty provides further depth to understanding trauma-related health. By comparing various biomarkers of stress and trauma, researchers can differentiate between slight variations in health profiles of different groups, i.e., civilians and ex-servicemen. For example, a study employing the skeletal frailty index (SFI) and its variant (SFI+) has shown striking differences in the preservation and health condition of the skeletons between these groups. The significance of the findings is to highlight the importance of locating health within cultural practices and social expectations. With a trauma-informed perspective, the SFI+ describes how individuals embody their experience—preparing for bodily markers of health and frailty that reflect overall trends of stress and resilience in their unique sociocultural contexts (Frazier et al., 2022). Extending the relationship between trauma and health, skeletal studies at archaeological sites reveal the profound impact of sociopolitical dynamics on population health. For instance, trauma with and without healing in skeletal remains from Kaman-Kalehöyük reveals interpersonal violence that directs toward history more than an acute process, indicating systemic health issues based on conflict in society. The prevalence of high rates of antemortem trauma and signs of nutritional stress indicates the adverse effect that socioeconomic inequalities have on community health in the Middle Bronze Age. Such an analysis not only contributes to a more profound understanding of daily life in ancient societies but also offers a significant observation regarding the lasting effects of violence and insecurity on social structure and individual health (Anderson et al., 2017).

4.4.2. Trauma as a Reflection of Social and Cultural Practices

Considering the complex dynamic between trauma and cultural practice reveals that the somatic manifestation of social conflict can offer insight into historical background. One example is the burial practice during the Late Roman Period of Britain, especially decapitation burial, which carries a range of meanings depending on social practice. The variation of burial rites indicates sophisticated social sentiments regarding violence and death, and how these inform us about the tension between individuality and communal norms. Such archaeological findings point to the imperative of understanding these rituals not merely as punitive actions but as culturally pertinent forms that articulate sociopolitical systems en masse. Methodological application of bioarcheological techniques allows scholars to determine patterns that highlight the lived experiences of the individuals, bringing into focus the operation of trauma in mediating identities in the socio-cultural fabric of Roman Britain (Christie et al., 2023). Further, the study of violence in the Peruvian central coast indicates how trauma is a vital indicator of social stratification and the consequence of environmental as well as political instability. The diachronic analysis of trauma across shifting eras reveals correlations between the incidence of sociopolitical crises and violence. It reveals that significant incidents, such as drought or the emergence of a warrior elite, can exacerbate tensions within society and initiate further aggression and repeated performances of trauma. This study reveals how different social classes, especially men engaged in military labor, are becoming more susceptible to violence, illustrating the bigger picture of struggle over resources and social inequality. Concurrently, the fact that females also suffer equally high rates of suffering during heightened periods of violence also makes our understanding of trauma as a social process more complex (Dulanto et al., 2016).

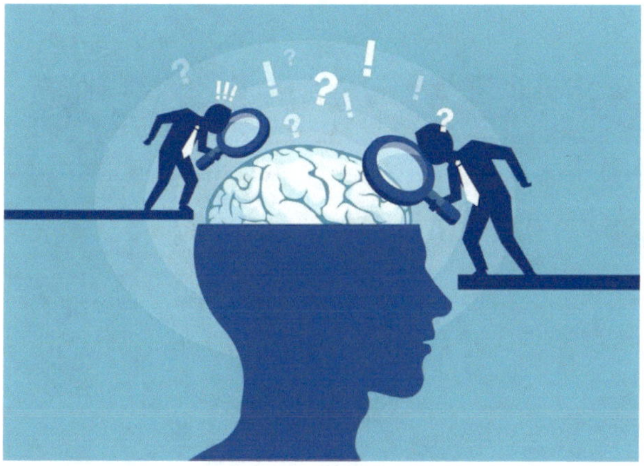

Figure 4.12. Trauma as a reflection of social and cultural practices.

Source: https://media.licdn.com/dms/image/v2/C5612AQGzj8J1UzA_6A/article-cover_image-shrink_720_1280/article-cover_image-shrink_720_1280/0/1643011632765?e=2147483647&v=beta&t=EX_8Zow62sc-VKzhHmbPnjd21u1cYskQ3vLeqMu4gpA.

Both the case studies of Roman Britain and the Peruvian coast highlight intersectional overlap in the confluence of trauma and cultural practices, illustrating the capacity of the two to inscribe historical narratives. By studying the funerary practices and bones of ancient humans, scientists commendably employ trauma as an important tool to challenge social dynamics. This highlights the importance of contextualization—showing how aspects specific to particular societies, such as power dynamics, resource distribution, and environmental concerns, shape experiences of trauma. Thus, these analyses not only contribute to knowledge on historical violence but also intervene in broader debates on how past narrative histories of trauma can be applied in the present in order to learn from the past and better understand cultural resilience and social adaptation in periods of crisis (Christie et al., 2023; Dulanto et al., 2016) (Figure 4.12).

4.4.3. Case Studies from Bioarchaeological Sites

Intriguing discoveries about the complexity of interpersonal violence surface while analyzing bioarcheological sites, as evident in case studies from the Quebrada de Humahuaca area in Argentina. The area, which is characterized by its disordered social life during the Late Regional Development Period (1250–1430 AD), is introduced with elevated trauma prevalence due to interpersonal violence. Analysis of a sample of 153 skulls from three sites—Los Amarillos, La Huerta, and Yacoraite—found high frequencies of trauma to the cranial bone. The analysis differentiated between antemortem and perimortem fractures, revealing patterns indicative of survival and the dynamics of combat. There were high rates of trauma in the groups, which meant that this violence was part of the community structure, a reflection of broader sociopolitical tensions at the time, as suggested by differential rates of trauma among the sites (Botta et al., 2014). The evidence that was revealed in Yacoraite, which had the highest frequency of trauma, sheds light on the geographic diversity of social acts and community responses to violence. This unequal distribution of trauma and prevalence of trophy skulls at La Huerta presents a fascinating explanation of cultural violence practice. The uniformity of trauma among males and females and across various age groups indicates that violence was widespread in all spheres of life within these communities, or as a method of conflict resolution, or upgradation of status following conflict. In addition, statistical methods employed in the study verify the role of bioarcheological data in fully understanding the nature of interpersonal violence, presenting a whole-picture interpretation of historical human interaction and its consequences (Botta et al., 2014). bioarcheological Beyond displaying violent patterns, bioarcheological contexts also enable the critical examination of human remains within mixed assemblages. The improvement process in re-associating skeletal remains, such as tali and calcanei, highlights the importance of precise sorting of commingled human remains. Using linear regression, researchers have derived robust equations to improve the precision of these associations between individuals. Such accuracy is also crucial in forensic and bioarcheological contexts, as it is central to reconstructing ancient populations' social relationships and health conditions. Finally, both case studies from sites such as Quebrada de Humahuaca and novel sorting techniques illustrate the ever-evolving field of bioarcheology. Bioarcheology is a valuable means by which to examine trauma, violence, and how their consequences affected previous groups of people.

Test Your Knowledge

1. How is trauma analysis used in bioarchaeology to interpret violence, accidents, and lifestyle in past populations?
2. What can patterns of skeletal trauma reveal about social behavior and occupational activities in ancient communities?

4.5. Methodological Approaches

Learning Outcome

1. Radiological techniques in trauma analysis
2. Histological methods for examining trauma
3. Integrative approaches combining multiple methodologies

Methodology is in the limelight of modern bioarcheology to generate trustworthy and legitimate results in the study of trauma. Modern statistical procedures, such as Generalized Estimating Equations (GEE), have been proposed to address the scalar problems prevalent in osteological studies. For instance, GEE has been demonstrated to work by relating articular surfaces across individual specimens to provide a comprehensive dataset with less bias, thereby revealing significant differences in trauma patterns among groups, such as the Tiwanaku population (Bass et al., 2019). This approach not only provides the added subtlety of the data involved but also ensures that the complex interrelations of the various joint surfaces are more accurately reflected, allowing more precise interpretations of the conditions of ancient biology and culture. The demographic reconstructions of skeletal analysis are further complicated by the built-in problems of estimating age. Its reliance on a limited number of skeletal elements may overlook dramatic variations in aging rates across anatomical regions. The transition analysis (TA) is a multifactorial approach that integrates data from the public symphysis, iliac auricular area, and cranial sutures to improve age estimation. However, studies indicate that TAs accuracy may be significantly disparate based on the demographic population in question, as indicated by the varying absolute errors of different populations in the Hamann-Todd Collection (Simon et al., 2020).

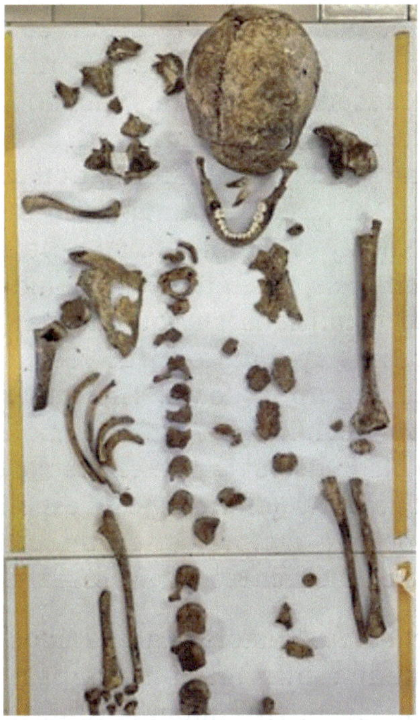

Figure 4.13. In contemporary bioarcheology, methodological approaches.

Source: https://upload.wikimedia.org/wikipedia/commons/thumb/5/54/Bioarcheology_Laboratory%2C_picture_made_by_me.jpg/250px-Bioarcheology_Laboratory%2C_picture_made_by_me.jpg.

The differences highlight the need for additional methodological models in forensic anthropology to better reflect the diverse characteristics of skeletal remains. Conjoining varying methodological approaches not only enhances the specificity of trauma analysis but also entails a greater understanding of historical populations' experiences. The use of a combination of statistical and analytical approaches helps researchers navigate the intricacies of trauma and demographic reconstructions comfortably. By employing sophisticated data analytics frameworks, researchers can obtain insights into movement trends, lifestyle factors, and health conditions among ancient populations. Therefore, such a collaboration of bioarcheologists with forensic specialists is essential in addressing the multi-aspectual nature of trauma analysis in furthering knowledge on how ancient societies dealt with environmental and social stressors. Such interdisciplinary engagement is set to shift future research into the spheres of health, trauma, and cultural practices within a historically contextualized framework (Figure 4.13).

4.5.1. Radiological Techniques in Trauma Analysis

The complexity of trauma examination in forensic and bioarcheological contexts has motivated the use of advanced radiological techniques, which yield unprecedented information regarding skeletal material. Such techniques, such as X-ray, computed tomography (CT), and magnetic resonance imaging (MRI), facilitate the non-destructive examination of bone integrity and structural flaws. For instance, in forensic settings, radiologic techniques allow for the detection of patterns of trauma, including fractures and soft tissue injury, to reveal critical information about the circumstances of a person's death. Utilizing these technologies, forensic anthropologists can construct detailed histories of injuries that may be indicative of accidental or intentional violence, thereby enriching the legal situation. The application of radiological analysis to forensic investigations is a shift in paradigm toward increased scientific grounding in the study of trauma dynamics. Similarly, in bioarcheology, radiological techniques introduce a unique point of view by which researchers are able to address historical populations, namely those vulnerable, such as children. As one is reminded of in recent scholarly work, the skeletal remains of non-adults might give helpful information about their socio-environmental surroundings and health conditions, despite being previously omitted from archaeological debates (Morrone et al., 2020). Radiological analysis allows exploration of growth patterns, deficiencies, and trauma, thereby providing information on the adaptation mechanisms of ancient societies. By preserving these skeletal remains and analyzing their biological signatures, radiological methods enable researchers to uncover the typically secondary histories of young people in past societies and thus hear their voices more distinctly within the archaeological record. This abundant knowledge contributes to broader discussions of resilience and vulnerability in past contexts, recovering multifaceted interactions between individuals' lives and communities' experiences. The use of radiological techniques extends beyond simple typing and identification, as they are key to resolving complex identification issues. Forensic anthropology confronts the commingling and disarticulation of remains, which pose serious challenges that necessitate more sophisticated methodologies for determining individuality and demographic affiliations (Meier-Augenstein et al., 2020). Anthropologists may make their observations more accurate by combining radiological tests with osteological and genetic methods. This will correct for uncertainties inherent in skeletal assessment. Contrasting radiological data with other scientific analyses, such as isotope and DNA analyses, will provide a multidisciplinary approach to the demographic characteristics and geographical origins of skeletal populations. These integrated approaches not only increase the strength of inference from human remains but also contribute to promoting methodologies in the analysis of trauma in both forensic and bioarcheological contexts. The interdisciplinary approach emphasizes the importance of integrating advanced technologies into the reconstruction of lives and of positioning trauma within the broader landscape of history.

4.5.2. Histological Methods for Examining Trauma

The technicalities in analyzing trauma have been highly improved with the application of histological procedures, by which researchers can specialize extensively on the microscopic constitutions of traumatized tissue components. Histological methods entail cutting thin sections of bone and soft tissue samples to study cellular and subcellular alterations that may be caused by trauma. The microscopic difference between traumatized and normal tissues can yield critical information about the timing and nature of trauma. Such specificity is particularly valuable for application in forensic analysis, when the precise information about the conditions surrounding a person's trauma can be applied towards reconstructing events leading up to death. The integration of histological examination into trauma research begins to bioarcheological elucidate the complex interactions between biological responses and environmental factors, thereby enhancing forensic and bioarcheological research.

In bioarcheology, histological methods provide dual benefits: information on past human action and on environmental conditions that may have affected survival. By examining bone microstructure, scientists can observe evidence of changes in bone material associated with trauma, stress, and illness. The information is significant for establishing how specific traumas impacted individuals over the course of their lifetimes and for shaping broader trends in life and death in ancient populations. For instance, examination of bone remodeling after healing can show how frequent violence or accidents were in society. Alongside this, these methods provide a more subtle understanding of the construction of socio-cultural trauma, demonstrating how societies respond to injury and accommodate what is occurring (Domett et al., 2014). Histology not only enhances our knowledge of trauma at the individual level but also poses challenges and limitations that researchers must navigate. While histological methodologies offer the potential for groundbreaking advances, they also require a judicious approach to specimen procurement and preparation. Contamination and sample degradation can lead to misinterpretation. Moreover, histological analysis can account for some aspects of trauma, but cannot represent the complexity of human existence or the socio-cultural settings in which trauma occurs. Thus, more truly interdisciplinary approaches are required that bring together histological data with archaeological, historical, and anthropological knowledge. Not only does such a holistic strategy extend our understanding of trauma in both bioarcheological forensic and bioarcheological contexts, but also the strengths and weaknesses inherent within any one single analytical approach (Domett et al., 2014) (Figure 4.14).

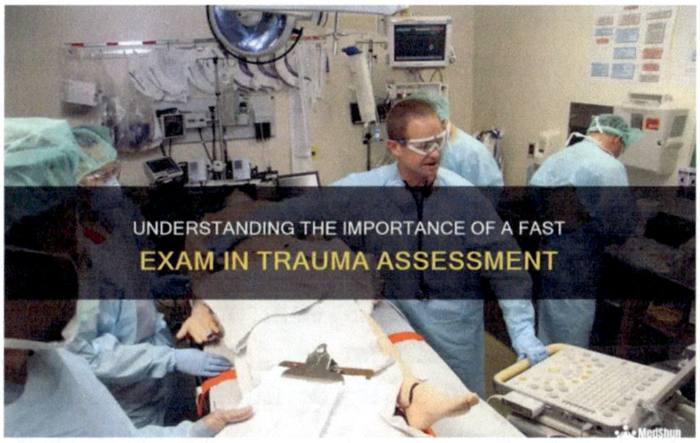

Figure 4.14. The intricacies of trauma analysis benefit significantly from the incorporation of histological methods.

Source: https://external-content.duckduckgo.com/iu/?u=https%3A%2F%2Fmedshun.com%2Fimages%2Fresources%2Fwhat-is-a-fast-exam-in-trauma_20240419205809.webp&f=1&nofb=1&ipt=4acbe34b118093ddf04e713947341c16f734b746d51e5d5968569d320bb0af7b.

4.5.3. Integrative Approaches Combining Multiple Methodologies

Research on trauma in forensic and bioarcheological analysis is enriched by an integrative approach that combines quantitative and qualitative methods. The multidisciplinary approach clarifies the interplay between environmental, social, and cultural conditions and bodily trauma in populations. Blending both osteological research and contextual historical data enables researchers to craft a comprehensive account of the lived experience of the communities. For instance, the skeletal remains of Canyon de Chelly reveal demographic profiles and patterns of trauma that illuminate not only personal statuses of health but also societal processes and conflicts writ large (Tegtmeyer et al., 2017). Through an integration of skeletal analysis and ethnographic data, scientists are better equipped to situate violent histories of these individuals within larger contexts, developing a more informed conceptualization of trauma in the context of ancient social organization. By integrating contemporary imaging techniques with traditional skeletal analysis, a deeper investigation of the manifestation of trauma is possible. Technologies such as three-dimensional imaging and radiology offer non-invasive techniques for viewing internal pathologies that are not external on the surface. This integration of methodologies can reveal patterns of trauma and indicators of health within populations, contributing to a more nuanced conceptualization of community resilience and vulnerability. For example, the analysis of non-adult skeletal remains has gained greater emphasis, highlighting the importance of understanding children's roles within their populations (Morrone et al., 2020). Their skeletal evidence can stress community health and adaptive outcomes, and contribute key knowledge about the effects of trauma on societies. Thus, the successful incorporation of bioarcheological multidisciplinary approaches not only supports forensic science but also enhances bioarcheological interpretations. Interdisciplinary approaches that unite fields promote collaboration among disciplines such as archaeology, anthropology, and forensic science. Sharing ideas and methods across disciplines results in a more consolidated study of trauma, facilitating researchers in posing complex questions that a single disciplinary approach might overlook. Conjoining social theory with bioarcheological research, for instance, can help explain structural inequalities and their impact on individuals' health outcomes. By cross-fertilizing various methodologies, researchers can connect the physical evidence to the sociocultural context, which enhances a more profound comprehension of trauma's role in human history. In the long term, continued work on integrative methodologies will not only further enhance existing methods but also expand the range of usability for trauma analysis in forensic and bioarcheological applications, paving the way for new future studies.

Test Your Knowledge

1. What are the key methodological approaches used in scientific or osteological research?
2. How do different methodological approaches affect data collection and interpretation?

4.6. Ethical Considerations

Learning Outcome

1. Ethical implications of studying human remains
2. Consent and the treatment of remains in research
3. The impact of trauma analysis on descendant communities

The complexity of trauma analysis within forensic and bioarcheological contexts inherently raises some ethical concerns that must be taken seriously. Researchers who conduct the analysis of violence and trauma in the past generally use experimental methods in an effort to replicate injury patterns, providing evidence for past contexts. Nevertheless, this approach is troublesome in terms of the implications of human replication, even in the controlled environment of a lab. For researchers, it is essential to balance the pursuit of knowledge with empathy toward the people whose remains are being studied. The potential trauma done to communities linked to the remains and the endured history embodied should be avoided with care, and caution should be exercised not to overload scientific investigation at the expense of the memory and dignity of the victims of trauma (Fibiger et al., 2023). This is compounded by increasing scrutiny of human remains acquisition, particularly in bioarcheology. The repatriation demands African remains and artifacts within Euro-American holdings foreground the need for challenging ethically re-examining research norms. Researchers must confront the injustices and adverse eugenicist tendencies that have accompanied the study of human remains as part of the colonial past. Greater respect for provenance and cultural context is required as researchers reflect on their positions in relation to the societies from which these remains derive (Apoh et al., 2020). Ethically robust research must incorporate the voices of descendant communities, respecting their rights to reclaim their heritage and stories, thereby creating a paradigm grounded in reconciliation and respect for one another (Apoh et al., 2020). Finally, ethical thought transcends acquisition and analysis into presentation and interpretation of findings from the study of traumas. While presenting data, researchers must be cautious not to sensationalize it so as to further victimize the communities under study with the traumas they are investigating. An ethical framework calls for transparency in method and sensitivity to the nuances of historical trauma, so findings enhance our knowledge of past societies without dehumanizing the people depicted in the data. Through the adoption of an integrated approach that entails interdisciplinary collaboration and engagement with indigenous communities, researchers can facilitate an enhanced ethics and sense of accountability in discussion within forensic and bioarcheological contexts, eventually enhancing intellectual knowledge and cultural sensibility (Apoh et al., 2020; Fibiger et al., 2023) (Figure 4.15).

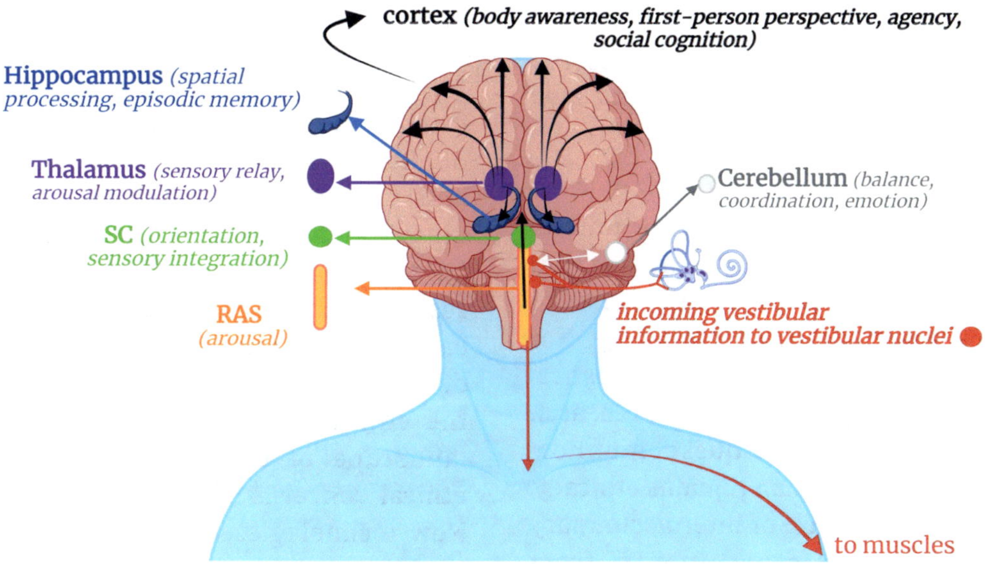

Figure 4.15. The multifaceted nature of trauma analysis.

Source: https://www.frontiersin.org/files/Articles/1015749/fnins-16-1015749-HTML/image_m/fnins-16-1015749-g001.jpg.

4.6.1. Ethical Implications of Studying Human Remains

In recent ethical discussions about the consequences of analyzing human remains, the complexity of historical context cannot be overlooked. Bioarchaeological methodology often recreates colonial histories victimizing marginal groups, and thus, concerns regarding consent and property arise. Analysis of remains acquired through colonial mechanisms or illicit means requires ethical reflection. As scholars advocate for the repatriation of remains to their homelands, it is important to examine how this activity relates to the contemporary debate over cultural rights and scientific responsibility. Case studies, such as those in Ghana, may be used to determine the inherent cultural value placed on human remains in a critically balanced framework. Such dialogue is required to set ethical guidelines that respect the dignity of the deceased without preventing scientific inquiry (Apoh et al., 2020). The role of forensic anthropology in the study of trauma adds complexity to the ethics of working with human remains. By applying techniques borrowed from other scientific disciplines, scientists seek to enhance the accuracy of human skeletal identification. While these scientific successes resolve legal and humanitarian issues, they raise immediate ethical concerns about how the deceased are treated. Forensic examination of remains has to balance revealing agonizing histories with sensitivity toward the individuals whose remains are examined. Ethical standards increasingly require practitioners to consider the opinions of descendants and concerned communities when performing forensic examinations. By forming partnerships with indigenous stakeholders and prioritizing openness, forensic anthropologists can fulfill their responsibilities in the sensitive nature of their work. In so doing, not only do they preserve the dignity of human persons, but this also sustains the significance of ethical consideration in the scientific milieu (N/A, 2022).

As the controversy continues to unfold, it is increasingly evident that ethics should be incorporated in the very practices of both bioarcheology and forensic anthropology. Not only is the issue to detect historical injustice, but also to face it by applying modern research techniques. In addressing the question of how to conduct research on human remains ethically, there must be a promotion of interdisciplinary dialogue that incorporates inputs from anthropology, ethics, and law. Such terminology must focus on the voices of marginalized groups impacted by research processes, advocating for inclusive models that aim for mutual respect and understanding. Ethical demands cannot be secondary but rather should lead the investigative procedures at all stages. Since these disciplines develop alongside changing societal norms, there is an ethical window for professionals to chart the ethics of stewardship of the living through regard for the legacies of the subjects under study (Apoh et al., 2020; N/A, 2022).

4.6.2. Consent and the Treatment of Remains in Research

The ethical management of human remains in forensic and bioarcheological study is of utmost concern because it is inextricably linked with a variety of societal and cultural values surrounding death and dignity. Researchers are increasingly aware of the importance of obtaining informed consent from donors or kin, particularly in human remains research aimed at understanding past populations. This is further significant when investigating trauma with a biocultural approach, where understanding the lived realities of these individuals takes precedence.

The field of forensic anthropology, for instance, finds it challenging to deal with the implications of having to work with remains and has to balance scientific inquiry with dignity and respect for the dead and surviving family members. Incorporating designs that are respectful and dignified into research protocols can provide access to an integrated model of understanding trauma without sacrificing the ethical basis for examining remains. The landscape of consent also complicates the ethical concerns surrounding human remains. New technologies, such as 3D printing, upend traditional thinking about consent, as seen in recent studies on public attitudes toward the use of 3D-printed human remains in court cases. Overall, respondents said they would agree to such uses in demonstrations during trials as a potentially more powerful replacement for photographs. However, these feelings are closely tied to the understanding that consent from the next of kin would be paramount before any reproduction or study of remains. This speaks to the thin line between technological advancement and ethical responsibility on which academics must walk the regulations—or, in this instance, lack thereof—on the creation and application of 3D prints. The emphasis on ethical usage is crucial to guaranteeing that such practices reflect respect for human dignity in furtherance of lawful academic and legal objectives (Carew et al., 2023). Furthermore, the concerns regarding frailty, trauma, and consent further highlight the requirement for ethical frameworks in human remains research. Forensic environments particularly benefit from the utilization of tuned indices, including the skeletal frailty index, which accounts for both indicators of physiological health and the impact of an individual's respective culture. As illustrated by assessments of such indicators in populations, these assessments can provide important information about an individual's lived experience and stressors, particularly among veterans. The receiving analysis of such indices should also consider the overtones of traumatic histories intertwined with bodily remains. Researchers should be careful to present these reports truthfully, ensuring that their reports treat the involved people and families with respect. By practicing ethically and engaging in ongoing dialogue about consent and ethical treatment, the profession can comprehend trauma in a way that respects the dignity of working with human remains (Frazier et al., 2022).

4.6.3. The Impact of Trauma Analysis on Descendant Communities

The analysis of trauma through forensic and bioarcheological methodology can directly affect descendant communities, particularly those suffering historical injustices. By revealing the traumas of their ancestors, such analyses deepen understanding of collective suffering and resilience. Recovery of this past for descendant populations tends to have double meanings: validation of their ancestors' suffering and healing capacity. Knowing about specific traumatic events—whether through colonization, slavery, or other practices of oppression—has the potential to generate a new sense of identity and community cohesion among members. By so doing, analysis of trauma not only emphasizes the continuity of effects of past atrocities in the historical record but also underscores the need for recognition and therapeutic action in the present cases. Analysis of trauma also encapsulates the complexity associated with the repatriation of human remains and cultural artifacts. As Apoh et al. (2020) highlight, controversies surrounding the repatriation of African remains obtained during colonial periods highlight ethical considerations intertwined with bioarcheological inquiry. Repatriation to descendant communities is not symbolic but is a powerful agent for renegotiating past histories that have disemancipated their being. Interacting with the tangible objects of ancestors provokes more intense emotional reactions and requires acknowledgment of lost cultural transactions over centuries. The intricate interplay between trauma, exploitation, and recovery of stories provides a space in which descendant communities can begin redoing histories on their own terms with collective acknowledgment of ancestry.

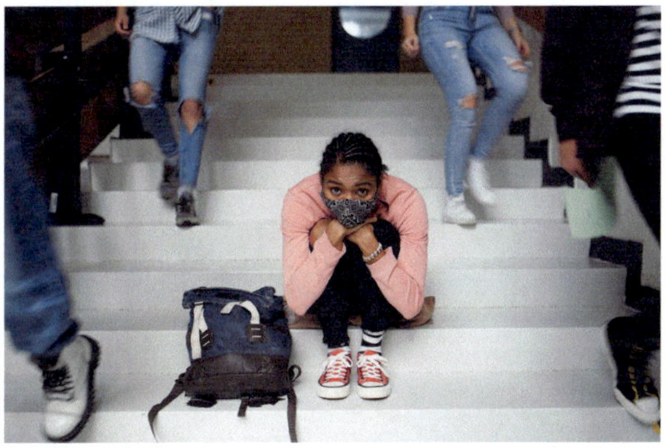

Figure 4.16. The impact of trauma analysis on descendant communities.

Source: https://external-content.duckduckgo.com/iu/?u=https%3A%2F%2Fblog.ahwendowment.org%2Fhubfs%2Fblog%2FUnderstanding-the-Effects-of-Trauma-in-Individuals-and-Communities.jpg%23keepProtocol&f=1&nofb=1&ipt=8fd0b1e7b76d2af3701d5c233beb89d06af600e043f4c5e6a34c08b9a62be9eb.

Finally, the applications of trauma analysis are to understanding social health disparities that have persisted across generations. As depicted in Graham et al. (2014), oral health disparities across populations can illuminate the long-term consequences of structural disparities founded upon historical trauma. By analyzing these differences in health bioarcheological ly, descendants could trace how health and resource accessibility were influenced by social structures. Such an understanding promotes advocacy and informs contemporary health initiatives to enhance the continued aftermath of discrimination. Trauma analysis then enables descendant communities to receive the information they need to meet present challenges and to encourage a culture-informed trajectory of healing and reconciliation (Figure 4.16).

Test Your Knowledge

1. Why are ethical considerations important in research and professional practice?
2. What principles guide ethical decision-making in scientific studies?

SUMMARY

The significance of trauma analysis, in both forensic and bioarcheological contexts, offers an enriched understanding of past human lives and demonstrates the complex interaction between bodily violence and social architecture. By studying bones, researchers can detect patterns of injury that may be indicative of society's ills of warfare, family violence, and epidemic disease. This interdisciplinary pursuit not only brings our understanding of ancient societies to life but also reveals to us how these ancient traumas can influence modern societal trends. Additionally, as is clear in the various research being conducted in bioarcheology, the information gathered from skeletal analysis may be used to better comprehend health inequalities in the modern era, thereby highlighting the need to research past trauma to resolve current issues. Additionally, the approach established in bioarcheological research has introduced new dimensions to the understanding of trauma and its effects. With the development of specialized techniques to study skeletons, researchers are now able to determine a particular trauma and its associated pathologies that were not seen previously. As evident from recent studies, continued research on populations that have been subjected to endemic warfare presents itself as proof of the effect of historical trauma on health status and thus provides significance to present health issues. The Croatian Academy of Sciences and Arts' osteological collection, for example, is a treasure trove, enabling researchers to situate physical trauma within broader social and historical contexts, further consolidating the practice of trauma analysis in reconstructing complex life histories (Adamić et al., 2015). Additionally, fetal paleopathology offers a fresh avenue of research into trauma analysis in bioarcheology, enriching maternal and infant health in past communities. This new field of study addresses the limitations surrounding the jargon and methods employed to characterize historic infant skeletal populations, revealing important information about the wholesale impact of societal trauma among mothers and their children. In analyzing experiences that affected fetal health, researchers broaden the trauma studies discourse and contribute to the general knowledge of pathways of health across generations. Such collaborative endeavors facilitate interaction between archaeologists, anthropologists, and medical professionals to continually uncover such intricate connections and underscore the role of historical traumatic narratives in shaping modern society's health outcomes (Lewis et al., 2017).

The study of trauma analysis reveals the profound intersections of forensic anthropology and bioarcheology, particularly in understanding past social existence and the health of individuals. In a landmark study of cranial remains from Argentina's Quebrada de Humahuaca, researchers examined various forms of trauma to assess interpersonal violence among ancient populations. Analysis of a sample of 153 skulls from three different sites—Los Amarillos, La Huerta, and Yacoraite—found a high rate of antemortem fractures, i.e., most of the individuals had survived trauma. This indicates an ongoing state of social conflict towards the close of the Regional Development Period, and it informs us about the lives of populations in the past. Most importantly, trauma consistency within sex and age groups means that violence among individuals crossed demographic groups, though with geographic variation in trauma frequency implying localized responses to social stressors (Botta et al., 2014). To complement these insights on interpersonal violence, analysis of trauma also extends to an understanding of physiological stressors through bioarcheological models. An influential study of frailty among skeletal remains illustrates how trauma may manifest in various forms typical of health conditions in populations. Scientists found many biomarkers of stress by employing a skeletal frailty index modified and listed antemortem fractures as one of the main areas of investigation to evaluate trauma. It was found that military persons exhibited different degrees of frailty compared to civilians, and this contributes to existing knowledge regarding the impact of social experience and social roles on bone health. Findings underscore the value in thinking not only about the physical dimensions of trauma but also the sociocultural aspects of it in forensic contexts, thereby enhancing interpretive models used in trauma analysis (Frazier et al., 2022). In addition, the principal conclusions of trauma analysis highlight the importance of interdisciplinary approaches that synthesize methods from forensic anthropology and bioarcheology. This integration enhances trauma analysis by enabling researchers to situate findings within broader sociopolitical, cultural, and environmental contexts. Trauma analysis through numerous lenses—such as physical injury patterns, risk of mortality, and indicators of health—depicts the multidimensionality of human distress and organization among past populations. It also highlights the potential uses in modern forensic environments of that data, when an understanding of patterns of injury can indicate not only a case but also a pattern of violence and health disparity. This interdisciplinary convergence, therefore, indeed lays the groundwork for a more advanced understanding of trauma that renders historical and modern perspectives relevant and beneficial for conceptualizing violence and health matters (Frazier et al., 2022).

KEY TERMS FROM THIS CHAPTER

- Skeletal trauma
- Perimortem trauma
- Blunt force trauma
- Projectile trauma
- Healing response
- Taphonomy
- Cut marks
- Interpersonal violence
- Trauma timing
- Antemortem injury
- Postmortem damage
- Sharp force trauma
- Fracture patterns
- Bone remodeling
- Paleopathology
- Stress fractures
- Accidental injury
- Microscopic analysis

CRITICAL THINKING QUESTIONS

1. **Which of the following best describes a perimortem injury?**
   a. Occurs after death and shows no healing
   b. Occurs after death and shows signs of healing
   c. Occurs at or near the time of death and lacks healing
   d. Occurs long before death and fully heals
2. **A greenstick fracture is most commonly observed in:**
   a. Elderly individuals
   b. Subadults
   c. Athletes
   d. Decomposed remains
3. **What distinguishes postmortem fractures from perimortem fractures?**
   a. Color and texture of the fracture edges
   b. Presence of hematoma
   c. Degree of bone remodeling
   d. Location on the skeleton
4. **Blunt force trauma is best characterized by:**
   a. Clean, sharp linear incisions
   b. Radiating and concentric fractures
   c. Thermal alterations
   d. Projectile penetration
5. **A depressed fracture in the skull is typically caused by:**
   a. Gunshot wounds
   b. Low-velocity blunt force trauma
   c. Sharp force injury
   d. Thermal exposure

Short Answer Questions

1. What are the key differences between blunt force trauma and sharp force trauma on bones? Provide one example of each.
2. How can forensic anthropologists determine whether a fracture occurred before or after death?
3. Describe the typical features of a gunshot wound in the skull, including entry and exit wounds.
4. What is the significance of fracture healing in trauma analysis? How can the stage of healing inform the time since injury?
5. Explain how thermal trauma affects bone and how it can be differentiated from other forms of trauma.

Answers to Critical Thinking Questions

1. (c); 2. (b); 3. (a); 4. (b); 5. (b)

REFERENCES

1. Adamić, A., Petaros, A., & Šlaus, M. (2015). Bioarcheology–A discipline that encompasses the past, present and future of mankind. https://core.ac.uk/download/33279524.pdf (accessed on 21st July 2025).
2. Anderson, C. (2017). *The Bioarcheology of Inequality During the Middle Bronze Age in Central Anatolia*. https://digitalscholarship.unlv.edu/cgi/viewcontent.cgi?article=3938&context=thesesdissertations (accessed on 21st July 2025).
3. Apoh, W., & Lamptey, P. S. N. O. (2020). The restitution debate and return of human remains: Implications for bioarcheological research and cultural ethics in Africa. https://core.ac.uk/download/478450776.pdf (accessed on 21st July 2025).
4. Assis, S., Santos, A., & Keenleyside, A. (2016). Paleohistology and the study of human remains: past, present and future approaches. *Revista Argentina De Antropología Biológica*, *18*(2). https://doi.org/10.17139/raab.2016.0018.02.02Baier, W., Burnett, B., Harrison, N. P., Hunt, T., et al. (2017). Novel application of three-dimensional technologies in a case of dismemberment. https://core.ac.uk/download/74227383.pdf (accessed on 21st July 2025).
5. Bass, W. M., Brothwell, D. R., Buikstra, J. E., Dieppe, P., Felson, D., Gagnon, C. M., Gagnon, C. M., et al. (2019). Evaluating elbow osteoarthritis within the prehistoric Tiwanaku state using generalized estimating equations (GEE). https://core.ac.uk/download/323311271.pdf (accessed on 21st July 2025).
6. Botta, F. N., & Seldes, V. (2014). Violence indicators in Quebrada de Humahuaca, Jujuy, Argentina: The Regional Development Period from a regional perspective. https://core.ac.uk/download/159288092.pdf (accessed on 21st July 2025).
7. Buikstra, J. E., Byers, S. N., Cheverko, C. M., Field, A., Gunz, P., London, M. R., London, M. R., et al. (2018). A statistical method for reassociating human tali and calcanei from a commingled context. https://core.ac.uk/download/153531718.pdf (accessed on 21st July 2025).
8. Carew, R. M., French, J., Morgan, R. M., Rando, C., et al. (2023). Exploring public perceptions of creating and using 3D printed human remains. https://core.ac.uk/download/564421283.pdf (accessed on 21st July 2025).
9. Christie, S. M. (2023). *Deconstructing Decapitation in Late Roman Gloucestershire and Oxfordshire, UK*. https://core.ac.uk/download/589986599.pdf (accessed on 21st July 2025).
10. Domett, K. (2014). Bioarcheology in Southeast Asia and the Pacific: Newsletter. https://core.ac.uk/download/303766613.pdf (accessed on 21st July 2025).
11. Fibiger, L., Moreno-Ibáñez, M. Á., & Saladié, P. (2023). Unraveling Neolithic sharp-blunt cranial trauma: Experimental approach through synthetic analogues. https://core.ac.uk/download/553368387.pdf (accessed on 21st July 2025).
12. Frazier, E. M. (2022). Combating frailty: Application of a modified skeletal frailty index in modern military and civilian populations. https://core.ac.uk/download/534817570.pdf (accessed on 21st July 2025).
13. Graham, L. (2014). A bioarcheological comparison of oral health at three postbellum African American cemeteries in coastal and central Georgia. https://core.ac.uk/download/71425430.pdf (accessed on 21st July 2025).

14. Hitchens, G. E., Needham, A., Spikins, P., Tilley, L., et al. (2018). Calculated or caring? Neanderthal healthcare in social context. https://core.ac.uk/download/146487591.pdf (accessed on 21st July 2025).

15. Lewis, M. (2017). Fetal paleopathology: An impossible discipline? https://core.ac.uk/download/42153730.pdf (accessed on 21st July 2025).

16. Lockau, L. (2012). Bioarcheological analysis of trauma in a skeletal sample from Smith's Knoll Historic Cemetery. https://core.ac.uk/download/639162311.pdf (accessed on 21st July 2025).

17. Meier-Augenstein, W., Rai, N., & Sehrawat, J. S. (2020). Identification of Ajnala skeletal remains using multiple forensic anthropological methods and techniques: A bioarcheological report. https://core.ac.uk/download/326520745.pdf (accessed on 21st July 2025).

18. Morrone, A. (2020). *Balso Suteikimas Mažiesiems: Baltijos Šalių Vaikų Bioarcheologija*. https://core.ac.uk/download/401879905.pdf (accessed on 21st July 2025).

19. N/A. (2022). *Recent Advances in Forensic Anthropological Methods and Research*. https://core.ac.uk/download/543578187.pdf (accessed on 21st July 2025).

20. Ornot, D. E. (2024). *Assessment of Forensic and Clinical Criteria of Orbital Blowout Fractures for Use in Bioarcheological Analysis*. https://core.ac.uk/download/645913001.pdf (accessed on 21st July 2025).

21. Simon, A. (2020). The accuracy of age estimation using transition analysis in the Hamann-Todd Collection. https://core.ac.uk/download/323061960.pdf (accessed on 21st July 2025).

22. Tegtmeyer, C. E. (2017). *Violence in the Canyons: The Human Cost of Raiding and Warfare in Northeastern Arizona (AD 300–~1300)*. https://digitalscholarship.unlv.edu/cgi/viewcontent.cgi?article=4178&context=thesesdissertations (accessed on 21st July 2025).

23. Vega Dulanto, M. del C. (2016). *A History of Violence: 3000 Years of Interpersonal and Intergroup Conflicts from the Initial to the Early Colonial Periods in the Peruvian Central Coast. A Bioarcheological Perspective*. https://core.ac.uk/download/61690164.pdf (accessed on 21st July 2025).

TAPHONOMY AND POSTMORTEM CHANGE

5

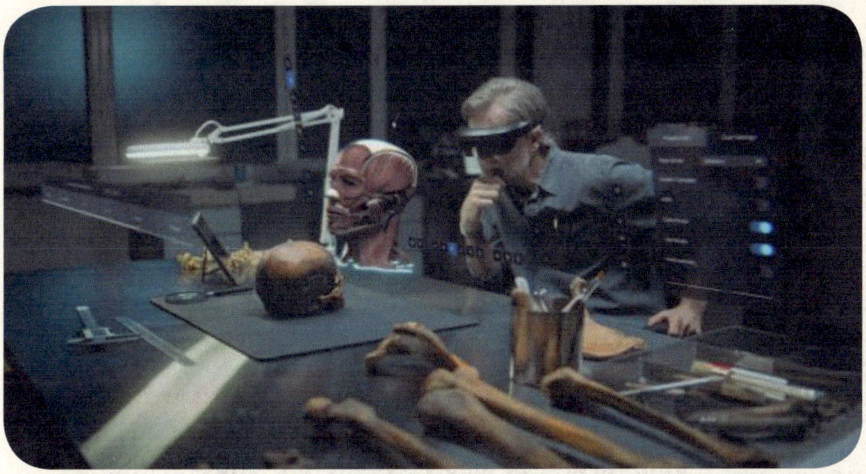

LEARNING OBJECTIVES

After studying this chapter, you will be able to:

1. Describe the historical background of taphonomy
2. Understand the process of decomposition
3. Explain the biotic and abiotic factors
4. Know taphonomic analysis techniques
5. Evaluate forensic applications of taphonomy
6. Learn about ethical considerations in taphonomic research

Introduction

Understanding the mechanisms of taphonomy and postmortem alteration is crucial in anthropology and forensic science. Taphonomy describes how organisms fossilize and decay, involving biological, chemical, and environmental factors that influence decomposition rates. In determining the postmortem interval (PMI), several factors are considered, including temperature, humidity, and the activity of microorganisms, insects, and scavengers. This complex interaction calls for a careful investigation of the causes of deterioration, as these factors are typically not included in current models. As scientists develop a conceptual framework that accounts for these interdependencies, they can gain a clearer understanding of PMI, which could enhance forensic practice and techniques (Cieśla et al., 2023). Another central aspect of decomposition is the release of volatile organic compounds (VOCs), which have also been in the spotlight for their potential as valuable forensic tools. The odorant compounds undergo change with time and are influenced by environmental conditions, associated microorganisms, and the decompositional stage. The specific odor released during decay has also been used for training detector dogs, underscoring its relevance in crime scene investigations. However, the variation in research on VOCs and decomposition requires an organized approach to studying these compounds. Through the convergence of past research on VOCs, scientists can enhance detection methods and maximize the use of these odors in forensic investigations (Cieśla et al., 2023). Moreover, the complexity of the decomposition process requires multidisciplinary research. As more research reveals the complex interactions between biological and environmental variables in taphonomy, there must be a unified structure. Current PMI models generally do not incorporate new data and are thus limited in their contribution to forensic use. By encouraging an adaptive cycle of study with experimentation, modeling, and testing, scientists can evade such confinement and reduce uncertainty in PMI estimation. This not only enhances theoretical understanding but also improves day-to-day applications, hence advancing the efficacy of forensic science and its practice in criminal investigations (Dawson et al., 2023).

Definition of Taphonomy

Taphonomy is the term that emerges as a crucial branch of the study of fossilization and decay processes, particularly for representing the complex interactions that occur with organic remains after death. Utilized initially by Russian scientist Ivan Efremov in the 1940s, the term encompasses the many factors that determine how organisms are represented in the geologic record. The factors range from biological agents such as bacteria to ecological processes, chemical environments, and physical forces that modify remains over time. By analyzing how these elements interact, taphonomy seeks to gain insights into the conditions of fossilization and the effects these processes have on our understanding of ancient life. Both paleobiologists and forensic scientists are interested in this broad view because it makes sense out of the life cycles of living organisms from the moment they die to how they come to be buried in blankets of sediment. Studying the taphonomic function of postmortem modifications reveals that climatic conditions have a significant effect on decomposition. Post-mortem interval (PMI) is the period after death that largely determines how biological tissues break down. Certain environmental factors, such as temperature, humidity, and exposure to bacteria, regulate the rate and nature of decay. For instance, research has shown that human tissue decomposition can vary significantly geographically and ecologically. Toward this end, such studies in some regions, e.g., southeastern Pennsylvania and the Delaware River Valley, emphasize the need for region-specific approaches toward PMI estimation.

These investigations not only reaffirm the significance of local forensic examination standards but also increase the understanding of how taphonomic processes can vary geographically, as attested by Guerra et al. (2014). The integration of taphonomic theory with fossilization and forensic science invokes a multifaceted view of past and present biological processes. Notably, the preservation quality of remains is regulated by many factors after death, so that behavioral, formational, intravolumetric, and post-formational sources of variation need to be addressed. For instance, fossil footprints reflect behavior, but their quality could be significantly influenced by how they formed, unknowingly complicating the morphological interpretations. Researchers advocate a subtle approach to assessing the preservation of such biological remains, calling for clarity in distinguishing among causal effects. In questioning these in a taphonomic context, researchers can acquire a more precise understanding of both fossilization processes and the central implications they hold in piecing together life histories—crucial to both paleontology and forensic science, based on Falkingham et al. (2017) (Figure 5.1).

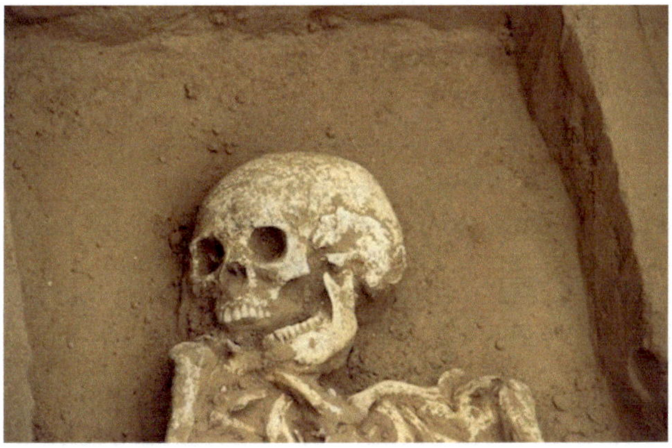

Figure 5.1. The concept of taphonomy.

Source: https://study.com/cimages/multimages/16/sias_ancient_grave_excavation_of_elite_burial_with_excellent_teeth_20146782173861357428762.jpg.

Importance of Studying Postmortem Changes

Studying postmortem changes is vital to understanding decomposition processes, which significantly contribute to our knowledge base in anthropology, forensic science, and archaeology. Postmortem changes constitute a series of biological, chemical, and environmental changes that occur in a dead body. Through the analysis of these changes, scientists are able to find timelines for decomposition that are vital in forensic research to calculate the time of death. Furthermore, these analyses can give valuable information about conditions of rot in comparison with environmental influences such as temperature, moisture, and microbial growth. This data not only contributes to our knowledge of human decomposition but also aids police in solving crimes by providing critical data for evidence collection and analysis, serving as justification for in-depth studies of postmortem processes. A critical aspect of postmortem change research is reflection on isotopic variation in human remains, particularly in forensic anthropology . Research has established that hair isotopic ratios can provide information on a person's diet and geographic displacements throughout life, but these are not guaranteed to be stable upon death. For instance, research at the Anthropology Research Facility determined that carbon and nitrogen isotopes in hair are stable with time, whereas hydrogen, oxygen, and strontium are affected by environmental circumstances. Understanding of these isotopic differences is crucial to both anthropologists and forensic scientists because they improve forensibility of dietary and geographic histories from hair analysis. Thus, scientific studies of postmortem changes are a vital element in guaranteeing that forensic analyses yield meaningful and accurate results that can hold water in court proceedings, as evidenced by the findings in Saul et al. (2017). Moreover, the emerging discipline of forensic archaeology underscores the value of incorporating archaeological techniques into forensic analyses. Much of the literature, however, has been written with professionals who have extensive experience in these fields in mind, making it disadvantageous for law enforcement personnel with limited access to archaeological methods. The importance of understanding postmortem changes becomes even more relevant as such techniques are adapted and made accessible to a broader audience, enabling effective teamwork on forensic scenes. This has implications for the need for comprehensive manuals that merge archaeological techniques into applicable practice by experts outside archaeology and forensic anthropology. Such resources can significantly enhance their understanding of taphonomic principles and further facilitate the investigation process, complementing the significance of studying postmortem changes in forensic cases as presented in Garcia et al. (2024) (Figure 5.2).

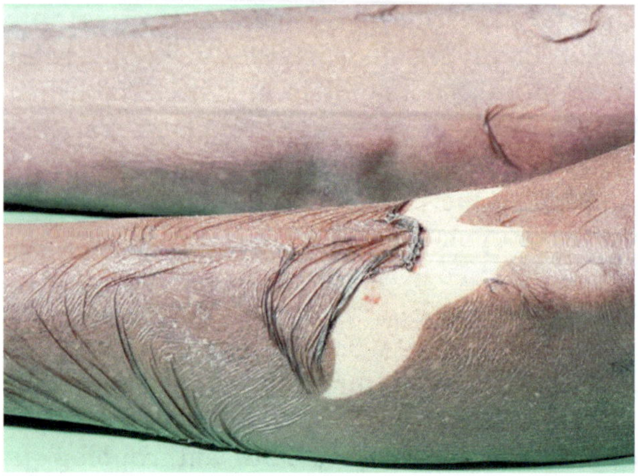

Figure 5.2. Studying postmortem changes.

Source: https://media.springernature.com/lw685/springer-static/image/chp%3A10.1007%2F978-1-61779-058-4_8/MediaObjects/978-1-61779-058-4_8_Fig33_HTML.jpg.

5.1. Historical Background of Taphonomy

Learning Outcome

1. Origins of the term "taphonomy"
2. Key figures in taphonomic research
3. Evolution of taphonomic studies over time

The discipline of taphonomy, which includes the processes that act upon organisms from the moment of death to their discovery, has developed exceedingly over its history. Initially proposed in the mid-20th century, the term encompassed a wide range of biological, chemical, and physical variables that influence fossilization. Comprehension of the complex mechanisms of decay and what happens to them afterward requires the synthesis of a wide range of disciplines, such as geology, biology, and anthropology. By understanding bone structure and chemical changes under varying environments, scientists began to see how pre-burial and post-burial modifications affected the fossil record. Specifically, Alcalá Martínez et al. (2002) noted that several conditions, both pre- and post-burial, can alter the bone structure and composition, emphasizing complexity in detecting these modifications and their role in paleontology. The course of taphonomy in the past has marked major advances in understanding the roles that specific environments play in dictating the fate of remains. Taphonomic research has progressed from mere recording of fossil finds to the study of their origins and environments during decomposition. For instance, the science of fossil remains typically identifies structural abnormalities that indicate the presence of specific taphonomic agents, thereby enabling the reconstruction of past conditions. The study of processes such as the opisthotonic posture demonstrates the need for an integrated understanding of postmortem processes. It raises questions about the processes underlying the formation of skeletal attitudes at fossilization. Referring to Reisdorf et al. (2018), the investigation of fossils in the Solnhofen Archipelago highlights the diversity of depositional environments, which makes universal statements about taphonomic conditions in paleontological settings problematic and further supports the need for targeted studies to interpret the fossil record properly. The combination of ecological and chemical processes engaged in taphonomy also calls for consideration of historical contexts and sedimentary settings. Some researchers in the field have developed models to study bone preservation that consider microbial activity, sedimentation rates, and physical burial dynamics. These models are crucial for explaining how these factors drive diagenetic processes that enhance or hinder fossilization. A continental paleoenvironmental study, as reported by Alcalá Martínez et al. (2002), indicates that transformation can be initiated by a number of agents that affect bones and influence their ultimate chemical composition and physical condition. A better understanding of these processes allows taphonomists to infer the life, death, and eventual fossilization of organisms, leading to improved interpretations of the fossil record and the environments they inhabited.

5.1.1. Origins of the Term "Taphonomy"

The term taphonomy was coined from the Greek words taphos, meaning burial, and nomos, meaning laws or processes that relate to a specified phenomenon. Initially used in paleontological literature, taphonomy was meant to elucidate the processes associated with the fossilization and decomposition of organic matter upon death. By studying the physical, chemical, and biological processes involved, scientists realized how these conditions had affected skeletal remains over the years. The evolution of this term and its application reflect a significant shift in the practice of archaeology, underscoring the value of context in interpreting human remains and their relationship with mortuary rituals, as defined in studies on funerary taphonomy, which integrate contextual and state-associated data on remains (Knüsel et al., 2016). This contextual data allows researchers to reconstruct historical post-death behaviors, opening windows onto cultures that would otherwise be inaccessible. The multidisciplinary nature of taphonomy has expanded its relevance, extending well beyond its original paleontological context and combining anthropology, archaeology, and forensic science. As the discipline advanced, scientists have increasingly become aware of numerous variables that influence post-death alterations, including environmental contexts and biological processes. These variables not only build the state of the skeletal body but also provide valuable information on the conditions of death and burial rites. For instance, the study of cut marks on bones is capable of unveiling butchery methods as well as trade relations. The advancement of technology, such as scanning electron microscopy (SEM), has enhanced the precision and consistency of these analyses, enabled increasingly subtle interpretation of evidence, and opened the door to future studies (Pollio et al., 2009). The broader applications of Taphonomy demonstrate its core significance for explaining ancient and contemporary human behavior with respect to death and group practice. Over the last few decades, taphonomic studies have extended far beyond their original scope, especially in osteoarchaeology and bioarcheology. With an emphasis on taphonomic processes affecting skeletal collections, researchers are revealing the intricacies underlying human depositional processes—mapping the ways in which cultural activities shape the dead. For example, funerary taphonomy analysis employs different methodologies to investigate human remains and reveal information about the traditions and values of societies related to death (Knüsel et al., 2016). Growing interest in the intersection of culture and taphonomic processes underscores that physical remains following death are not mere artifacts but rather essential sources of information regarding the lives of individuals and communities. Thus, the evolution and history of taphonomy are profound in their implications, as they place our understanding of postmortem change within a continuing dialogue among environmental, biological, and cultural processes (Figure 5.3).

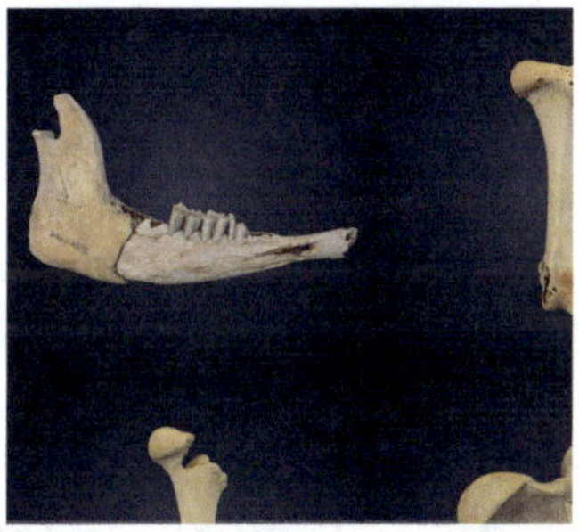

Figure 5.3. Origins of the term "taphonomy."

Source: https://external-content.duckduckgo.com/iu/?u=https%3A%2F%2Fwww.si.edu%2Fsites%2Fdefault%2Ffiles%2Fedan%2FOCIO3D%2Fobjectgroup%2Ftaphonomy_thumb.png&f=1&nofb=1&ipt=05263ee18aa19b62aa51cd9c12c85980341cbff81d7864392dbf2f564a301287.

5.1.2. Key Figures in Taphonomic Research

Taphonomy has produced some of its most influential figures, who have guided the field by adopting an interdisciplinary approach. Some of these key players include researchers like William R. Belche, who have operated across archaeological settings with emphasis on the clinical analysis of skeletons. The value of interdisciplinary cooperation is illustrated in projects by researchers like Sophia Perdikaris, whose research on Barbuda Island has highlighted the complexity of site operations and rescue excavations. Perdikaris group not only excavated sites but also used osteobiographical analyses to shed light on the biological profiles and histories of the people depicted in the skeletal evidence. This approach emphasizes the need for global models of archaeology, combining field observation and theoretical models to understand the processes that act on postmortem changes across diverse environments. Moreover, the impact of modern warfare on burial has led to widespread taphonomic research with an emphasis on mass graves and the consequences of human rights violations. The rise in mass graves in instances of genocide and war has come with it the need for investigation into how heavy machinery involved in burials alters the skeletal remains. This is revealed in research that focuses on the impact of heavy machinery like bulldozers and dump trucks during exhume, where documenting postmortem breakage and fragmentation of bones becomes extremely vital. A study on this aspect not only highlights the physical transformation of remains but is also important evidence in documenting atrocities linked to war crimes and genocide. By carefully observing these processes, researchers can gain insight into the intricate dynamics between taphonomic variables and the socio-political settings that give rise to mass burial situations. In addition, laboratory experiments have enhanced understanding of taphonomic processes by replicating natural conditions. Experimental work on the effects of artifacts, such as backhoes, on the disturbance of remains provides a controlled method for systematically evaluating postmortem alterations. For instance, one such study carried out at Boston University's Outdoor Research Facility investigated the taphonomic impacts of backhoe disturbance on juvenile Sus scrofa remains and recorded varied forms of fractures and patterns due to mechanical interference. Not only do these experimental techniques validate findings from the field, but they also provide essential data on the role of external forces during secondary burial processes. Finally, their research, exemplified by quantitative empirical studies and innovative methodologies, continues to illuminate the taphonomic nuances and how it may be used in understanding both past and present postmortem alterations.

5.1.3. Evolution of Taphonomic Studies Over Time

The evolution of taphonomic studies has been marked by a move from descriptive fossil remnant analysis towards an improved understanding of the processes controlling postmortem alterations. Previous taphonomic research primarily focused on fossil assemblage searches and the explanation of paleoecological context. However, the progression towards fine-grained research on the processes of decay, as exemplified by studies on the opisthotonic posture of non-avian theropods such as Compsognathus longipes and Juravenator starki, underscores the importance of integrating anatomical, ecological, and environmental perspectives into taphonomy. Scientists have begun to redefine traditional explanations, suggesting that certain specific physical postures preserved in the fossil record are not the result of pre-burial processes but rather postmortem expressions driven by resistance to decay and environmental conditions during burial (Reisdorf et al., 2018). This observation follows in the wake of the evolving view that recognition of taphonomic processes entails embracing a multidimensional approach that addresses heterogeneous decay dynamics with time. With progressing taphonomic studies, there was stunning interdisciplinarity among paleontology, archaeology, and forensic science. The use of bone surface modifications (BSMs) in forensic science demonstrated how postmortem change knowledge could be applied in criminal investigations. With the ability to identify a range of modifications caused by various agents, from environmental conditions to scavengers, investigators were now able to reconstruct the perimortem and postmortem intervals with greater precision. The discovery that BSMs can yield significant data on burial conditions and chemical interactions with the environment redirected taphonomic research away from observation and towards the detection of cause-and-effect relationships. This innovation emphasizes rigorous methodologies and invites multidisciplinary collaboration, as advocated by advocates seeking to enhance interanalyst concurrence through objective definitions and rigorous testing of BSM identifications in forensic contexts (Egeland et al., 2020). Furthermore, the evolution of taphonomic science has been mainly influenced by technological improvements, allowing increasingly sophisticated examinations of decay processes and fossilization. Digital imagery, multivariate predictive modeling, and advances in analytical techniques have transformed the approach to taphonomic problems in the hands of scientists, providing valuable tools with which to explore the intricate interaction between organic matter and depositional environments. Thus, modern taphonomic science is constantly in flux, underscoring the necessity of both empirical and theoretical frameworks for understanding the complexity of postmortem change. The recognition of varied depositional environments, such as those in the Solnhofen Archipelago, illustrates the need for context-dependent analysis that takes local conditions and sedimentation regimes into account (Reisdorf et al., 2018). The ongoing advancement of taphonomic techniques reflects the field's commitment to elucidating the dynamic processes that shape our understanding of death and decay in both the archaeological and forensic contexts (Figure 5.4).

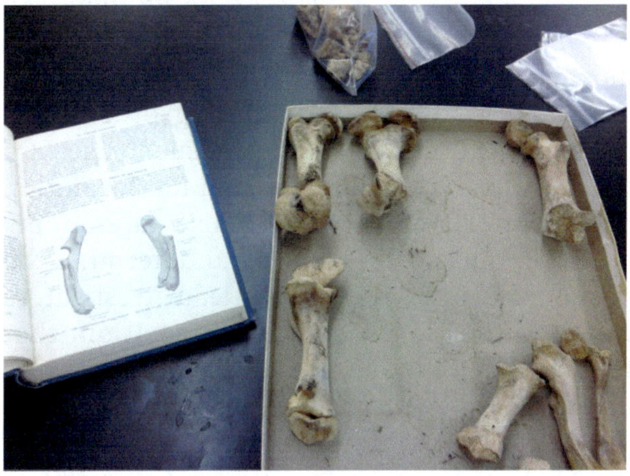

Figure 5.4. The evolution of taphonomic studies.

Source: https://bonebroke.org/wp-content/uploads/2014/02/img_20140210_172444.jpg.

Test Your Knowledge

1. What is taphonomy, and how did the concept develop historically?
2. Who were the key contributors to the early development of taphonomic studies?

5.2. The Process of Decomposition

Learning Outcome

1. Stages of decomposition
2. Factors influencing decomposition rates
3. Role of environmental conditions

The process of decomposition is a complex series of biological and environmental interactions that ultimately leads to the breakdown of organic matter upon death. Decomposition could be influenced by numerous factors, including environmental conditions, availability of scavengers, and way of body disposal. Decomposition typically begins hours post-mortem, initiated by microbial activity, setting the stage for the ongoing rotting process. As the bacteria break down body tissues, gases are trapped, leading to bloating and the formation of characteristic odors. Forensic taphonomy relies on these early changes to determine the postmortem interval (PMI) and lead investigators through the course of decomposition that follows." As a case in point, there has been an investigation to record the role location has in decomposition, with temperature and humidity levels at various sites resulting in varying outcomes. One significant aspect of investigating decomposition is the identification of varying rates with burial depth, as in studies of mass graves. In a pair of burial mass experiments with rabbit corpses, rates of decomposition varied radically by burial position. Shallow carcasses decomposed faster than deeper carcasses, with the inference that environmental factors like soil density and temperature in the burial complex have a role to play. The reported variations, with an internal carcass temperature range of approximately 1°C between shallow and deep, emphasize the significance of these factors in models of decomposition formulated by forensic practitioners. The studies have far-reaching implications beyond mere curiosity; they enhance the accuracy of forensic investigations where time since death is a significant factor. With further study of variables influencing decomposition, forensic science can more effectively improve approaches to calculating PMI more accurately and more efficiently. Photographic proof has established itself as an innovative method in forensic taphonomy, particularly for determining the decomposition of remains. Researchers have begun examining the efficacy of digital photographs during decomposition, noting that scoring mechanisms contribute to accuracy. For example, the study found that while one scoring system yielded drastic inconsistencies between photographic and real-time measurements, another method showed greater correlation with real decomposition. This finding illustrates the potential of photographs in forensic examination, especially when physical remains are unavailable. By improving photographic measurements, forensic investigators can reconstruct the death process more accurately. As the field continues to evolve, further study of photographic technique will be critical to further build the foundations of forensic taphonomy and enhance the validity of assessments of postmortem change (Figure 5.5).

Decomposition - Definition, Types, Process, Advantages

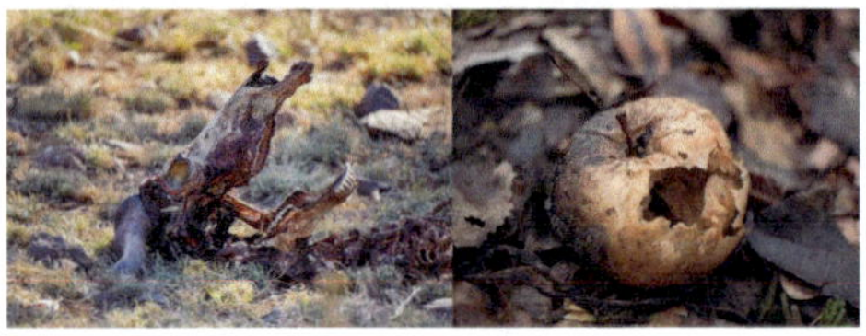

Figure 5.5. The process of decomposition.

Source: https://external-content.duckduckgo.com/iu/?u=https%3A%2F%2Fbiologynotesonline.com%2Fwp-content%2Fuploads%2F2024%2F11%2FDecomposition-Definition-Types-Process-Advantages-1024x576.jpg&f=1&nofb=1&ipt=0feddcd7c1b9476427676e3ab9e1bdc117352eb50e6c30d8cc75bf21c31f7d3f.

5.2.1. Stages of Decomposition

The decomposition stages are a vital area of study in taphonomy, and they provide insight into the process by which a body is altered postmortem. The decompositional process is typically divided into a series of stages, including fresh, bloat, active decay, advanced decay, and dry remains. Each stage is characterized by specific physiological and environmental factors that influence the decomposition rate. The enzymatic degradation process begins immediately after death during the fresh stage, triggering cellular death and the onset of autolysis. As the body progresses into the bloat stage, accumulation of gases produced by microbial breakdown results in distension, which is externally visible. Forensic investigators should be cognizant of these stages because they can help establish time of death, particularly regarding external environmental influences on the rate of decomposition. As decomposition progresses, the active decay stage manifests, marked by intense tissue breakdown and increased scavenger activity. This stage is significant in taphonomic studies as it yields valuable information regarding the interactions between the ecology surrounding the remains and the remains themselves. Various conditions, including temperature, moisture, and the presence of insects may influence the rate at which a body decomposes in this stage. For instance, in warmer climates, the process can occur more quickly, so forensic experts should ensure they perform their calculations for postmortem intervals with that in mind. It has been determined that procedures such as photography analysis can assist in objectively documenting the active decay process, enabling more accurate estimations and comparative analyses of decomposition across different environments, thereby enhancing the reliability of forensic conclusions (Carter et al., 2018). Rapid decay leads to significant loss of mass as water and organic material continue to be lost. In this case, bared skeletal remains can begin to appear, giving rise to greater examination of the forensic origin of the body. Of note, subsequent research has examined new ways to quantify the post-burial interval (PBI) by determining decomposition fluid conductivities under burial conditions (Cassella et al., 2010). By studying the conductivity of fluids from rotting remains, researchers can yield timelines that assist forensic investigations in human and animal burial cases. The ability to convert decay measurement into correlatable data, such as accumulated degree days, enhances the accuracy of forensic assessments and underscores the value of interdisciplinary approaches to taphonomic investigations. Generally, a good understanding of the stages of decomposition is essential to achieving justice in forensic science (Figure 5.6).

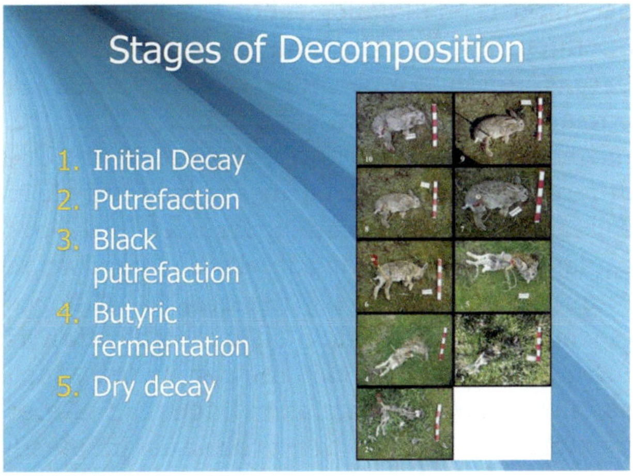

Figure 5.6. The stages of decomposition.

Source: https://external-content.duckduckgo.com/iu/?u=https%3A%2F%2Fimage2.slideserve.com%2F4141721%2Fstages-of-decomposition-l.jpg&f=1&nofb=1&ipt=a87d066110df5dac26763796d9383319b9361c61df9c6f15a282d45503d042e9.

5.2.2. Factors Influencing Decomposition Rates

Decomposition is influenced by numerous environmental and biological factors that determine the rate at which the body decomposes after death. A notable factor is the location of the remains relative to the substrate, as it determines the conditions that influence microbial activity. For instance, research in mass graves has indicated that carcasses buried to shallower depths will decompose at considerably higher rates than those buried deeper in the substrate. Specifically, studies reported significant differences in decomposition rates across burial positions, suggesting that both temperature and oxygen availability can vary substantially with depth and grave closure (Adlam et al., 2014). This finding emphasizes the importance of the burial context as a controlling factor in decay processes, implicating the localized environment in the taphonomic process.

Furthermore, temperature is pivotal in the decomposition of biological tissues via its effect on microbial activity and enzymatic action. Carcass body temperature is determined by burial depth and environmental exposure. In mass graves, a noticeable temperature difference was observed in shallow and deep carcasses, with higher temperatures in deeper carcasses corroborating lower decomposition rates (Adlam et al., 2014). Besides, the influence of ambient temperature on decomposition is further enhanced by climatic parameters, such as humidity and rainfall, which can either facilitate or hinder the processes involved. It is necessary to appreciate the dynamics of temperature in combination with other environmental factors so as to make the correct interpretations of decay patterns, which in turn can facilitate forensic analysis and paleontologic reconstruction. The matrix composition and structure of the immediate surroundings also control decomposition rates. For instance, various soil types may differ in parameters such as pH and oxygenation, influencing microbial activity and decay resistance. The results pertaining to the burial environment of several species, including those belonging to Solnhofen Archipelago, demonstrate how certain depositional environments may form special conditions that have a profound impact on taphonomic results. Analyses further show that sedimentation rates and the presence of certain minerals may affect preservation, facilitating or inhibiting processes like adipocere formation, which can arrest decay temporarily. Recognizing the complexity of such interactions is essential to constructing an integrated model for explaining decomposition paths and their implications for taphonomic analysis.

5.2.3. Role of Environmental Conditions

The role of the environment in taphonomy, particularly in postmortem change, is relevant to examine in terms of how varying factors influence the decay process. Temperature, water content, soil type, and even microbial presence are significant factors that contribute to the rate and manner of decay. For instance, warmer temperatures will accelerate decay, whereas wet conditions will augment the effects of microbial activity. Interactions between these environmental factors are often portrayed through experiments on decomposition rates in laboratory-controlled environments, with depth of burial and substrate type controlled.

These experiments highlight that real differences in these conditions can have a considerable effect on the timing of decomposition, thereby affecting forensic examination and analysis of remains found in various environments. Examining differential patterns of decay can inform about the environmental context within a grave. Research with mass graves, for example, demonstrates how grave location affects decomposition rates. Shallow bodies decompose quickly than deeper-buried bodies, with huge temperature differences between these horizons. And the atmospheric environment also gets its turn, affecting the occurrence and activity of decay agents such as insects and microbes. The studies at varied burial depths reveal that the compactness of the mass and the substrate in which the mass is interred, among other factors, plays a crucial role in decomposition processes and periods. Hence, awareness of these patterns would enhance investigative methods, particularly in cases involving clandestine burials, where conditions are often unpredictable and beyond control. The application of environmental data in post-burial interval (PBI) estimation is increasingly important in forensic science.

Existing innovations in geoscientific methods, such as measuring the conductivity of decomposition fluids within buried remains, have demonstrated robust correlations with environmental factors. From observations on conductivity comparisons from controlled burial scenarios, soil types and moisture levels significantly influence the properties of decomposition fluids, enabling more accurate time-since-burial estimates. The ability to use accumulated degree days (ADD) and soil moisture to refine PBI estimates underscores the need for a multidimensional method of testing taphonomic scenarios. Also, sustained research on these techniques is imperative to improve resting estimates of human and animal remains and fully understand environmental conditions for proper forensic interpretation (Cassella et al., 2010; Adlam et al., 2014) (Figure 5.7).

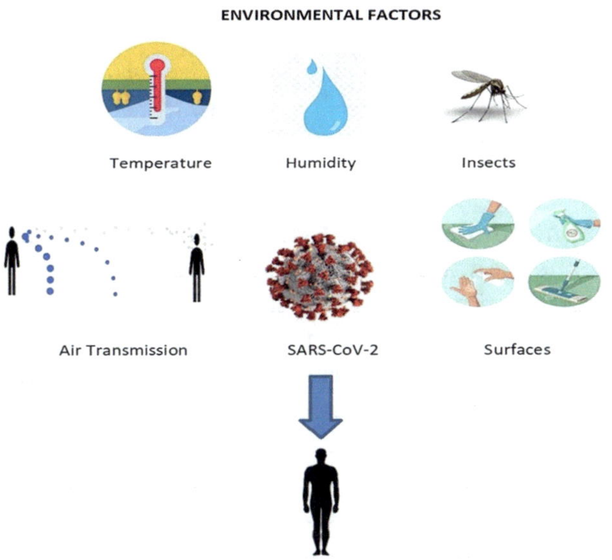

Figure 5.7. The role of environmental conditions in taphonomy.

Source: https://media.springernature.com/lw1200/springer-static/image/art%3A10.1007%2Fs10311-022-01418-9/MediaObjects/10311_2022_1418_Fig1_HTML.png.

Test Your Knowledge

1. What are the main stages involved in the process of decomposition?
2. How do environmental factors influence the rate and pattern of decomposition?

5.3. Biotic and Abiotic Factors

Learning Outcome

1. Influence of microorganisms on decomposition;
2. Effects of scavengers on remains;
3. Impact of climate and soil composition.

Taphonomic investigations have a strong connection with abiotic and biotic factors, both playing important roles in the decomposition process. The abiotic factors include factors such as temperature, humidity, pH of the ground, and nutrient concentration, all jointly influencing the rate as well as the process of body decomposition. Research at the University of Tennessee's Anthropology Research Facility has determined that variations in these abiotic properties are directly proportional to the intensity of decomposition at any location. For instance, soil samples from major areas with high decomposition that showed significant variations in physicochemical properties compared to control samples. This temporal variation in abiotic properties is a significant indicator of the decay stage and can be used by forensic scientists to obtain pertinent information about postmortem intervals, thereby making manifest the complex relationship between environmental conditions and decay processes observed in prior studies (Damann et al., 2010). Besides abiotic components, biotic entities such as microorganisms, insects, and scavengers also contribute significantly to the decomposition of cadavers. The structure of microbial communities in soil may change significantly with organic matter decomposition, indicating a clear response to biotic and abiotic cues. Specifically, studies show increased activity of certain groups of bacteria, e.g., chemoorganotrophic and sulfate-reducing bacteria, in soil samples from locations under severe decomposition pressure. This shift in microbial diversity not only points to the greater availability of nutrients from decomposition but also elucidates the role these organisms play in nutrient cycling and the breakdown of complex organic material. These findings tend to substantiate the interaction between microbial processes and abiotic conditions and lend credence to the realization of their applicability to forensic taphonomy (Damann et al., 2010). The synthesis of both abiotic and biotic perspectives accounts for the complex ecosystem that emerges during decomposition, attesting to the utility of interdisciplinarity in forensic science. Soil ecological studies, as exemplified by experiments involving burial of organic matter in controlled environments, demonstrate the ways in which microbial ecosystems emerge through shifting carbon sources and environmental conditions. Research has identified statistically significant alterations in soil pH and biodiversity when nutrients associated with cadavers come into contact with the soil community, reflecting a direct impact of decomposing material on microbial and soil health. Such findings are invaluable for improving estimates of the postmortem interval and for detecting clandestine graves. Finally, integration of biotic and abiotic information in taphonomic research presents a potential pathway for deciphering and applying ecological interactions in forensic analysis (Figure 5.8).

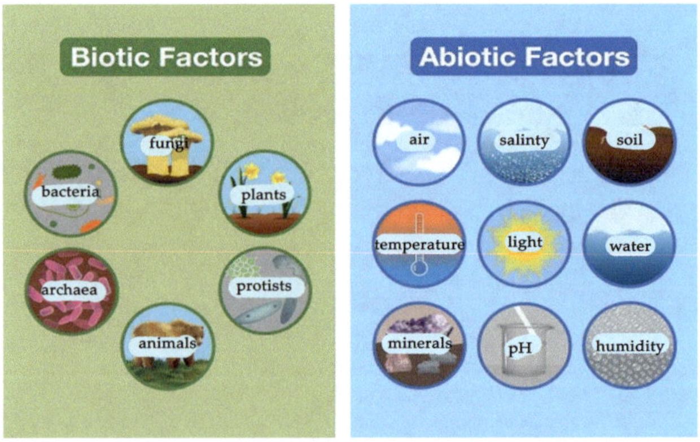

Figure 5.8. Biotic and abiotic factors.

Source: https://cdn.britannica.com/82/199682-004-BDDF7230.jpg.

5.3.1. Influence of Microorganisms on Decomposition

Microorganisms' intricate role in decomposition is at the core of taphonomic research, playing a pivotal role in the decomposition of post-mortem organic matter. These microbes, including fungi and bacteria, utilize cadaveric tissue as a source of nutrition and accelerate decomposition via biochemical degradation. Microbial populations can impact the rate of decay, nutrient release into the environment, and overall soil health in the region around decaying organisms. This association is particularly significant from a forensic context, as microbial dynamics are used to estimate time since death and identify remains. Thus, scientists have turned their attention to ecogenomic approaches to investigate cadaver-soil microbiome associations, elucidating the complex relationship between decomposing bodies and their given ecosystem (Olakanye et al., 2015). Microbial community changes under decomposition shed valuable light on the ecological succession that occurs in decomposing organic material. In experimental settings, e.g., sealed microcosms, it has been reported that the addition of cadaveric substances can provoke profound changes in soil microbial diversity. For instance, pig cadaver experiments show statistically significant changes in soil parameters, such as pH and microbial population dynamics, demonstrating the dynamic role of microorganisms in breaking down cadaveric material. Changes in community richness and diversity are most pronounced in the top layer of the immediate vicinity around the remains, with measures of biodiversity exhibiting dramatic increases over time. This is a testament to the profound effect that decomposition has not only on the body itself but also on microbial communities within and interacting with the soil matrix (Ager et al., 2014). The effects of microbial activity far outweigh mere decomposition, often leading to forensic investigation in clandestine burials (Houck et al., 2014). A detailed understanding of microbial dynamics can potentially improve the accuracy of time-of-death estimates and the environmental circumstances under which human remains are discovered. Researchers have indicated that varying soil depths have varying degrees of microbial activity, and cadaveric addition leads to increased and varied microbial communities. This implies that taphonomic changes during decomposition have significant ecological effects, including nutrient cycling and soil health. Besides, information from cadaverous decomposition research is applied to inform the development of predictive models for forensic settings, making it imperative to integrate microbial ecology into broader taphonomic schemes (Ager et al., 2014; Olakanye et al., 2015).

5.3.2. Effects of Scavengers on Remains

Scavengers are at the center of the process of decay in the sense that they affect the observable changes to remains after death. The interaction between scavengers and remains is influenced by factors such as scavenger type, environmental conditions, and the state of the remains. For instance, vertebrate scavengers, such as birds and rodents, exhibit specific scavenging behavior. Literature indicates that birds, including the buzzard (*Buteo buteo*) and carrion crow (*Corvus corone*), exhibit varying scavenging behavior, taking into account variations in seasons and the decomposition process. These differences significantly affect the quantities and types of tissue ingested, posing challenges to forensic examiners. The findings highlight the need for a sophisticated understanding of these activities, particularly across different regions of the globe, as they tend to have a major effect on the integrity and interpretability of human remains for forensic examiners (Amendt et al., 2014). Moreover, the role of scavengers not only involves surface modification but also involves vertical stratification of remains. Studies, such as the observation of scavenging activity in raccoons, show that some scavengers are involved in defleshing actions that make soft tissue susceptible, while the bones remain intact. Through studies of scavenging events, scientists have come to know specific scavenging behaviors, including nocturnal foraging and social scavenging among collectives. Interestingly, both activities appear to be influenced by food and mating seasons, thus emphasizing the environmental pressure responsiveness of scavengers.

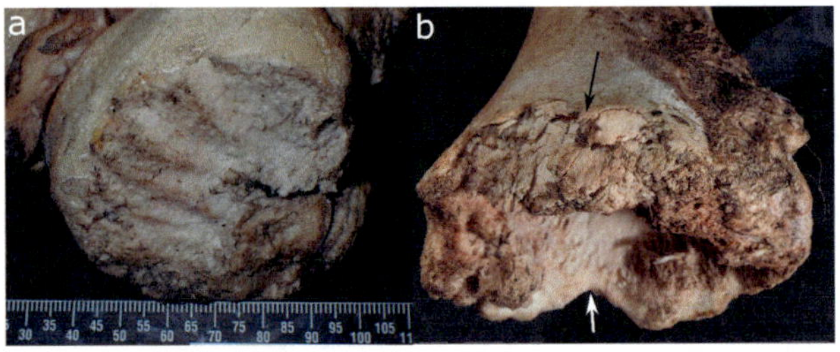

Figure 5.9. Effects of scavengers on remains.

Source: https://www.mdpi.com/biology/biology-11-00601/article_deploy/html/images/biology-11-00601-g004.png.

The cumulative effect on remains thus depends not only on the species of scavenger used but also on ecological parameters that vary seasonally, making it extremely critical that forensic examiners take these dynamics into account (Hannigan et al., 2015). The taphonomic significance of scavenger activity on remains extends to the broader field of taphonomy, necessitating multidisciplinary approaches to assess the extent of modification caused by such animals. An understanding of how different scavengers interact with human cadavers can be crucial in providing valuable information for forensic case investigation, in particular, the reconstruction of postmortem intervals and appreciation of the circumstances of death. This data is essential for forensic analysts tasked with putting pieces together from tampered remains. As scavenging activity is non-uniform, but regional, forensic professionals need to include local research in their analytical systems. In addition, technological advances, e.g., motion-detection cameras, have further enhanced scavenger surveillance, enabling more accurate predictions of the breakdown of remains and improving the overall accuracy of field forensic examination for taphonomy (Amendt et al., 2011; Hannigan et al., 2015) (Figure 5.9).

5.3.3. Impact of Climate and Soil Composition

Understanding the influence of climate and soil structure on taphonomic processes is critical to understanding postmortem change. Temperature variation, humidity, and levels of rainfall significantly influence decomposition rates and hence the preservation of remains. For instance, in hot climates, microbial activity accelerates, leading to rapid degradation. Conversely, low temperatures may slow these processes, leading to preservation. Soil characteristics, such as pH, water content, and nutrient levels, further interact with climatic variables to create the degradation setting. These work together to create a decisive framework that not only controls decomposition rate but also the particular pathways through which remains break down, ultimately influencing forensic examination and the validity of postmortem interval predictions. Empirical work in recent years underscores the necessity of integrating climate and soil analysis with forensic taphonomy. For example, decomposition studies of pig carcasses across different settings demonstrate that some soils are more prone to stimulate or inhibit decomposition depending on their composition. Variation in organic matter content, drainage capacity, and microbial communities is all contributing to the taphonomic environment. These findings emphasize the need for adaptive approaches that account for regional environmental settings. The potential to predict decomposition processes based on climate and soil analysis is important for increasing the credibility of forensic findings, particularly when optical recording techniques such as photography are used in the examination of remains (Carter et al., 2018). Furthermore, the interaction between intrinsic and extrinsic forces during decomposition highlights the complexity of taphonomic investigations. Although external factors such as climate and soil composition are central, internal biological processes also regulate decay. Studies have begun to reveal the importance of postmortem metabolomics in elucidating how remains behave within their contexts (Hoeland et al., 2021). The metabolic signatures emitted by decomposing organic material can affect the surrounding soil, thereby shaping a dynamic process between the remains and their burial environment. Effective taphonomic research thus must not only highlight postmortem transformation evident on the surface but also consider deeper biochemical reactions in various substrates. Having this multi-dimensional consideration allows forensic professionals to understand better the forces acting during decomposition, and hence enhances forensic assessments' credibility (Figure 5.10).

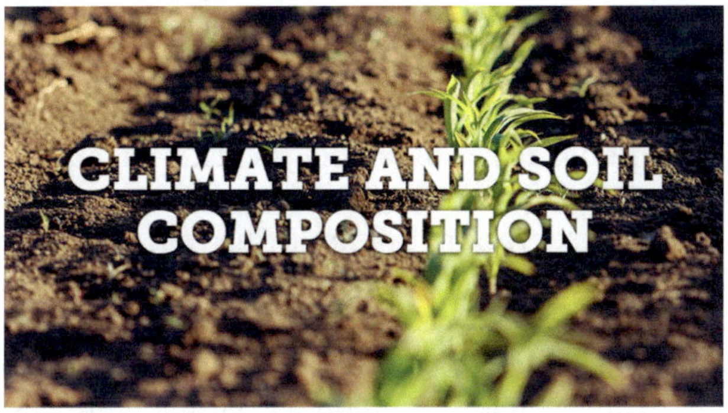

Figure 5.10. The impact of climate and soil composition on taphonomic processes.

Source: https://learn.weatherstem.com/modules/learn/lessons/85/screenshot-og.jpg.

Test Your Knowledge

1. What are biotic and abiotic factors, and how do they differ in affecting decomposition or preservation?
2. How do biotic and abiotic factors influence the condition of skeletal remains?

5.4. Taphonomic Analysis Techniques

Learning Outcome

1. Methods for studying skeletal remains
2. Use of chemical analysis in taphonomy
3. Role of imaging technologies in taphonomic research

Techniques of taphonomic analysis are significant for understanding the processes of decay and fossilization that organisms undergo after death. These involve a range of scientific disciplines, including sedimentology, chemistry, and biology, that together constitute a wide overall framework for research on postmortem change. Using a range of approaches, from examination of bone histology and chemical composition to biological interactions, researchers can reconstruct the environmental conditions at the time an organism perished. Not only do these analyses clarify the order of decomposition, but they also provide insight into specific taphonomic pathways that result in exceptional preservation, which is vital to untangling the fossil record. For instance, determining various levels of decay can demonstrate the differential resistance of soft tissues and record how environmental conditions or rapid burial may slow the decomposition. In addition, taphonomic analysis methods are applicable to the exploration of depositional environments that influence fossil preservation. Using sophisticated imaging tools like scanning electron microscopy (SEM) and energy-dispersive X-ray spectroscopy (EDAX), scientists can study the microstructure of fossils in minute detail. For instance, they have been used to explain Lagerstätten preservation patterns under which some conditions lead to exceptional fossil assemblages. The Sirius Passet Lagerstätte is a case in point; the exceptional taphonomic pathways discovered there differ from standard models such as Burgess Shale Type (BST) preservation. By employing these analytical techniques, a clearer picture of the ecological and environmental factors in fossilization is achieved, advancing our overall understanding of ancient ecosystems and their processes, as indicated by the outcomes analyzed in Chapters 3 and 4 of Strang et al. (2017). Understanding the ramifications of taphonomic analysis methods is equally important when reevaluating existing hypotheses on fossil posture and preservation. As an example, the opisthotonic posture hypothesis was tested with these methods, and it was demonstrated that some bone positions habitually attributed to pre-mortem conditions might indeed be the result of post-mortem muscle spasms and subsequent fossilization processes. This reinterpretation of bone positioning indicates the need for rapid burial and special microenvironmental conditions in order to preserve such features, as discussed by Reisdorf et al. (2018). In addition, these updated explanations stress that taphonomic processes are complex and that a single viewpoint can fall short of accounting for the intricate interplay of environmental factors involved. Therefore, using multiple taphonomic analysis methods is paramount for developing an integrated knowledge base on postmortem changes and their implications for both paleontology and broader biological principles (Figure 5.11).

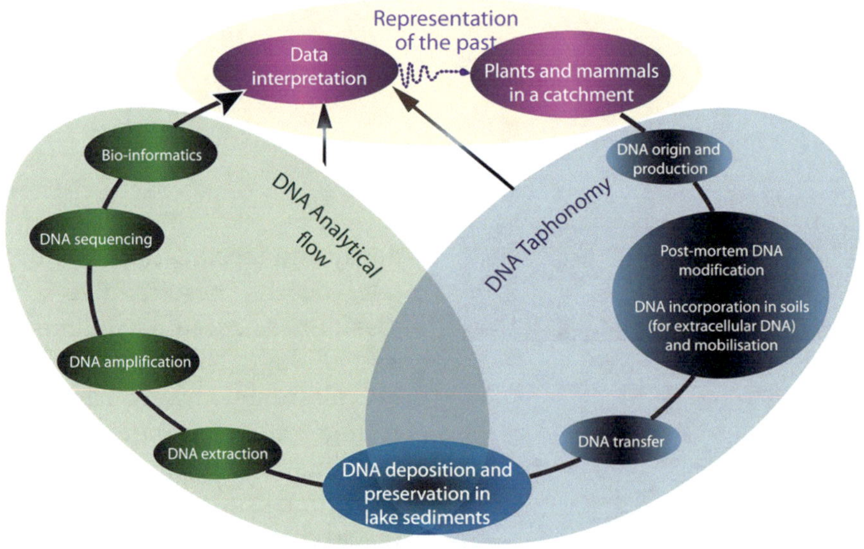

Figure 5.11. Taphonomic analysis techniques.

Source: https://www.researchgate.net/publication/336413491/figure/fig4/AS:959537716662283@1605783027438/Flow-chart-of-taphonomic-and-analytical-processes-likely-to-affect-reconstructions-of-the.png.

5.4.1. Methods for Studying Skeletal Remains

The analysis of skeletal remains employs several methods that further enhance our understanding on taphonomy and postmortem processes. One significant method is the observation of weathering effects on bone stability, which has been applied in studies of white-tailed deer long bones. The study in this case aimed to establish the relationship between environmental exposure duration and the pressure required to fracture these bones. By successive recordation of weathering processes over a nine-month period, the scientists provided insight into how bone morphology and strength can be altered by environmental conditions, allowing the reconstruction of postmortem interval and discrimination between perimortem and postmortem breakage patterns. This method highlights the important interaction between environmental exposures and skeletal deformation, illustrating the broader implications for forensic archaeology and anthropology to correctly analyze skeletal remains (LaCroix et al., 2013). Another method critical to skeletal remains analysis is anthropological and taphonomic analysis of commingled human bones, such as those excavated from the Farneto rock shelter located in northern Italy. The research addresses difficulties posed by the commingled and disarticulated state of human remains with caution, focusing particularly on radiocarbon dating to establish the time context of the human remains. Furthermore, the anthropological analysis offers comprehensive biological profiles of the individuals while investigating the impact of postmortem processes, including deliberate body alteration such as cleaning and dismemberment. Such intense scrutiny enables researchers to draw conclusions about funeral practices, thereby augmenting knowledge of death-related cultural practices in Eneolithic and Neolithic cultures. Lastly, the methodology emphasizes contextual and biological evaluations of human remains (Belcastro et al., 2023). A third crucial method applied in the analysis of the skeletal remains is the application of the biochemical analysis, which can elucidate information about the diet, health, and life of the individual. Bone collagen isotopic analysis, for instance, can trace dietary variations by revealing the diet of an individual through specific foods and origins. Similarly, trace element analysis may indicate exposure to multiple environmental conditions or dietary deficiencies throughout a lifetime. Combining these biochemistries with standard morphological analysis can assist scientists in constructing a fuller history of bony remains, adding texture to the tale of individuals' and populations' history. These methods not only provide taphonomic interpretations but also offer subtle insights into how all the factors affect the preservation and alteration of skeletons over time.

5.4.2. Use of Chemical Analysis in Taphonomy

The role of chemical analysis in taphonomy offers great improvements in interpreting postmortem changes and aiding forensic analyses. Using techniques such as soil water conductivity measurements in clandestine graves, researchers can estimate victims' post-burial interval (PBI) and likely post-mortem interval (PMI). These estimates are key to assisting law enforcement agencies in preparing timelines that sufficiently connect or rule out suspects in crimes. Notably, studies have revealed that conductivity in burial fluids increases enormously shortly after burial, providing the potential for a quantifiable means of further refining the understanding of rates of decomposition in varying soils and environments. This ability to transform post-burial days into accumulated degree days (ADDs) permits more accuracy in comparative examination between differing case studies, thereby enriching the forensic framework constructed by previous scholarship (Cassella et al., 2010). In addition to soil analysis, the integration of chemical analysis in entomology also shows highly promising implications for taphonomy. Forensic entomology focuses on the behavior of insects in decomposing cadavers, using their well-organized patterns of colonization and responses to volatile organic compounds (VOCs) emitted during decomposition. Current advances in analytical chemistry, such as gas chromatography-mass spectrometry (GC-MS), enable detailed examination of these VOCs, aiding in defining the decomposition process. Death's stench, a complex blend of more than a hundred VOCs, evolves sequentially, with some compounds being uniquely attractive to necrophagous insects.

The specific identification of such semiochemicals has the potential to enhance the accuracy of entomological estimates of post-mortem interval and thereby solidify the role of chemical analysis in forensic science (Dekeirsschieter et al., 2012). Additionally, chemical analysis is more than just decomposition analysis, offering potential avenues for legal investigation. Through the definition of chemical signatures present with decay, forensic entomologists can obtain information on the environmental parameters influencing the rate of decomposition and the presence of particular species.

For example, examining the interaction between VOCs produced by cadavers and the insect population may elucidate factors influencing the behavioral responses of sarcosaprophagous insects during decomposition. Such studies can improve ecological dynamics within taphonomy, yielding robust evidence that can strengthen forensic conclusions. The emphasis on a multidisciplinary approach, such as combining chemical analysis with other forensic sciences, improves the accuracy and reliability of investigative methods, which is necessary in order for justice to be established in a courtroom setting (Cassella et al., 2010; Dekeirsschieter et al., 2012).

5.4.3. Role of Imaging Technologies in Taphonomic Research

The integration of imaging technologies in taphonomic research has significantly transformed forensic experts' analysis of postmortem changes in human remains. Magnetic resonance imaging (MRI) and computed tomography (CT) are now indispensable for imaging skeletal anatomy without invasive procedures. These non-destructive methods not only preserve the integrity of the remains but also allow researchers to investigate complex questions regarding patterns of decay and artifact placement. For instance, CT imaging allows for close examination of bone architecture that can reveal the extent of postmortem trauma or the effect of environmental conditions on decay and thereby provide important information regarding the timing and cause of death.

Furthermore, novel imaging devices have enabled the intensification of commingled human remains analysis, a common taphonomic issue. An example of such an approach is mesh-to-mesh value comparison (MVC), employing three-dimensional digital models to make bones comparable, and how imaging aids individualization. Studies demonstrate that the MVC method performs with high specificity and sensitivity to correctly pair-match individual skeletal elements, thereby increasing identification for forensic anthropologists handling mixed remains (Frelat et al., 2016). It is such a paradigm shift in the field that it creates the potential to improve the quality of forensic studies through better imaging techniques. Additionally, the ongoing development of newer imaging modalities is invaluable for expanding forensic science applications in practice.

The Journal of Forensic Radiology and Imaging has highlighted the expansion of image-based modalities, illustrating the significance of active and passive surface-scanning technologies and three-dimensional printing (Carew et al., 2019). This transition to cutting-edge imaging technologies makes it easier to generate systematic case studies that emphasize their significance in capturing the complex nature of taphonomic processes. As forensic scientists increasingly depend on such technologies, the integration of imaging and taphonomy will continue to enhance our understanding of postmortem change and ultimately improve the methods employed in forensic examinations (Figure 5.12).

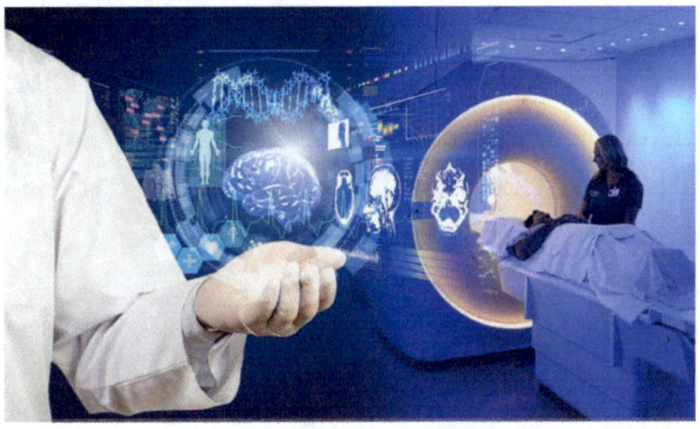

Figure 5.12. The integration of imaging technologies within taphonomic research.

Source: https://external-content.duckduckgo.com/iu/?u=https%3A%2F%2Fadmissionxpert.in%2Fwp-content%2Fuploads%2F2020%2F09%2FMedical-Imaging-min.jpg&f=1&nofb=1&ipt=6619f8e5f92bf829517f7946cd236d2eaa177e05259cece4437e592c37aa289f.

Test Your Knowledge

1. What techniques are used in taphonomic analysis to study post-mortem changes in remains?
2. How does taphonomic analysis help distinguish natural processes from human or animal activity?

5.5. Forensic Applications of Taphonomy

Learning Outcome

1. Importance in criminal investigations
2. Case studies illustrating taphonomic principles
3. Challenges faced in forensic taphonomy

The field of forensic taphonomy provides critical information on the stages of decomposition, which is crucial for estimating postmortem intervals and aiding criminal investigations. By examining how various environmental conditions affect decay processes, forensic scientists can make significant determinations about the conditions of death. A good example is the impact that soil texture and water content have on the rate of decomposition. Studies have shown that one can accurately determine the post-burial interval (PBI) for clandestine graves by measuring the conductivity of decomposition fluids in burial environments. Higher conductivity levels, which are discovered to dominate a period of time, may supply information to law enforcement officers about the timeline of a death, linking probable suspects with the crime and assisting law enforcers in solving homicides (Cassella et al., 2010). The incorporation of taphonomic concepts enables forensic pathologists to present scientifically sound evidence in court, thereby enhancing the probative value of their findings. In addition to outdoor environments, taphonomic forensic applications also include varied indoor environments, each with its own array of problems and data on the processes of decomposition. Decomposition studies in different indoor environments name temperature and humidity as essential variables influencing rates of decay. Cadaver model tests using piglets in various environments, for example, demonstrate that corpses decomposing in water experience higher rates of decay than those in arid environments. However, the studies show that relying solely on decomposition scales is statistically inadequate for postmortem interval estimates. This deficiency necessitates that numerous scientific analyses are included, thereby making conclusions from decomposition assessments sufficient for legal use (Santos et al., 2019).

Forensic examiners, therefore, need to embrace a multi-dimensional approach combining taphonomic understanding with other methodologies to make them more credible. The principal contribution of forensic taphonomy is its ability to inform on the complex relationships between the environment and biological remains, thereby yielding more accurate time since death estimates. In examining decay patterns and the conditions that affect decomposition, the forensic taphonomy can separate between natural death, homicide, or even postmortem manipulation. In addition, taphonomic science is developing, with particular emphasis on quantitative methods for estimating decay rates through statistical modeling, yielding results. The application of accumulated degree days (ADDs) has been found to allow one to compare more satisfactorily across varied soils and environments and enhance the accuracy in postmortem interval estimation (Cassella et al., 2010). Such methodological advancements underscore the significance of taphonomy in forensic science, underscoring the need for interdisciplinary teams to improve investigative outcomes and, ultimately, achieve justice (Figure 5.13).

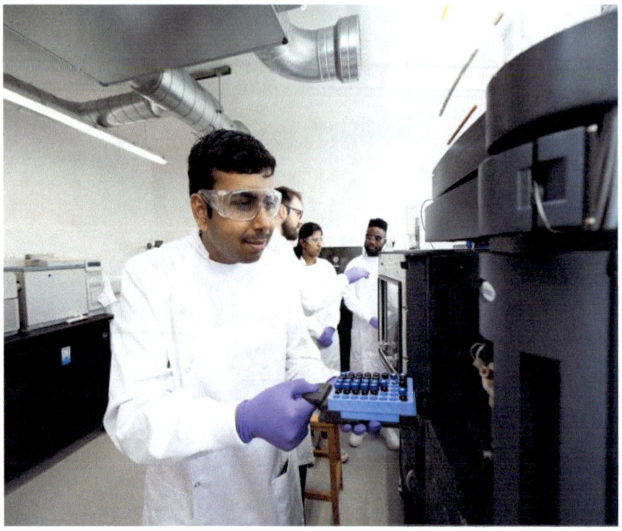

Figure 5.13. The field of forensic taphonomy provides critical insights into the stages of decomposition.

Source: https://external-content.duckduckgo.com/iu/?u=https%3A%2F%2Fwww.uclan.ac.uk%2Fimage-library%2Ffacilities%2Fforensic-taphonomy-lab-2.xe04b9ba2.jpg%3Ff%3Dwebp%26q%3D75%26w%3D740&f=1&nofb=1&ipt=b42927c9dd84bf217424a5003e5e76b8f3270fc572f4c1ade02f1cb568b2a7bd.

5.5.1. Importance in Criminal Investigations

The significance of taphonomy in criminal investigations cannot be overstressed, particularly in the estimation of the postmortem interval (PMI). It is critical that precise PMI estimates are used to create timelines and, potentially, identify suspects in murder cases. Determining PMI requires a firm understanding of how decomposition occurs under varying environmental conditions, making taphonomic studies central to forensic science. New developments in photographic taphonomic analysis have underscored the importance of sound scoring techniques in determining decomposition. For instance, research indicates that applying certain scoring methods to photographic records can yield more accurate results than previous approaches. By using high-quality photographic documentation, investigators can gather critical information even when it is not possible to observe the remains directly, thereby enhancing the quality of the overall forensic inquiry and resulting in more accurate conclusions regarding the time of death and the circumstances of the case (Carter et al., 2018). In addition to refining the accuracy of PMI estimates, taphonomy is crucial for gaining insight into the broader context of the crime scene. Patterns of decomposition in human remains can convey information about the context of a death, including possible postmortem movements of the body. This multimodal insight is particularly valuable in complex cases where the context of a death is not immediately apparent. By employing diverse techniques, such as soil chemistry, mite analysis, and analysis of micro-Eukaryotes, forensic experts can construct a more detailed investigation narrative of the decomposition process. Not only do these analyses aid in estimating post-mortem interval, but they also aid in identifying whether a body has been transported post-mortem, thereby enhancing the investigatory narrative and informing law enforcement responses (Perez et al., 2018). In addition, combining different taphonomic techniques enhances the validity of results, supporting the integrity of evidence in a legal setting. Forensic analysis that utilizes interdisciplinary methods is capable of yielding more credible conclusions, facilitating an easier time for the police to resolve inconsistencies and issues that can be encountered during a case. The potential for high inter-observer reproducibility in photo analyses is a classic example of how technologically advanced data can be used to make taphonomic investigations more consistent. As illustrated by recent research, judicious selection of scoring systems and analytical methods can enhance transparency in forensic investigations. These advances in taphonomic methods ultimately render criminal investigations more efficient and assist the broader judicial process, in which scientifically based evidence has a considerable influence on the pursuit of justice (Carter et al., 2018) (Figure 5.14).

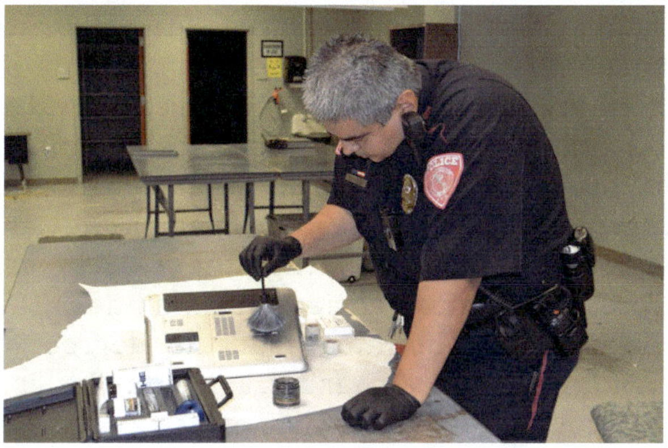

Figure 5.14. Importance in criminal investigations.

Source: https://external- co ntent.duckduckgo.com/iu/?u=http%3A%2F%2 Fww w.ta mi u.edu%2Fadmi n is%2Fpolice% 2Fima ges% 2F3.1.JPG &f=1&no fb=1&i p t=f285 f2c4c8bf275d6a 957 00 e49bdc4fb5b5 b04056ecf201ba63bb1a71989c42a.

5.5.2. Case Studies Illustrating Taphonomic Principles

Research into case studies that illustrate taphonomic principles provides valuable insights into postmortem biological activity and the factors controlling the preservation of organic matter. An excellent example is provided by the early Cambrian North Greenland Sirius Passet Lagerstätte, renowned for its remarkable fossil preservation. Studies reveal a characteristic mat-dominated, tissue-specific taphonomic route that contrasts with the commonly accepted Burgess Shale Type (BST) preservation. Using a suite of advanced analytical techniques, such as SEM and elemental mapping, researchers have been able to determine key aspects of this site's depositional setting, thereby providing insight into the overall implications for Cambrian ecosystems. The results emphasize the importance of taphonomic pathways in deciphering how exceptional preservation can mold our understanding of ancient biota and provide a window into the intricacies of early life (Strang et al., 2017). In another enlightening example, work on glaciomarine and estuarine sediments has revealed profound patterns of shell preservation among different bivalve and gastropod species. This study examined 5065 samples and revealed the dominance of infaunal suspension feeders in high-latitude environments, reflecting the ecological processes of these ancient communities. The research demonstrated that the degree of shell disarticulation and fragmentation can be accounted for by environmental processes such as sea ice scouring and sedimentation rate. Interestingly, the Hiatella and Astarte shells of the genus exhibited different preservation potential, indicating differences in the energy regimes and sediment facies from which they were sampled.

These findings highlight how taphonomic parameters can influence the fossil record and argue that interpreting the paleontological record in depositional contexts is crucial (Cai et al.). Overall, these case studies highlight the complexity of taphonomic processes and products. The Sirius Passet Lagerstätte demonstrates the exceptional ability to preserve under particular ecological conditions, yet the taphonomic control of bivalve assemblages in glaciomarine sediments illustrates preservation determinism based on environmental parameters. Understanding these principles of taphonomy is more than mere taxonomy of fossils; it inspires further research into the interactions between organisms and the environment over geological time scales. By closely examining these examples, one can appreciate the intricate interplay between postmortem modification and the environmental forces driving the fossilization process, ultimately contributing to our understanding of life on Earth in the past.

5.5.3. Challenges Faced in Forensic Taphonomy

Forensic taphonomy encompasses a set of challenges that affect how accurate and trustworthy postmortem analyses are. These are compounded by the need to examine a range of environmental factors influencing decomposition rates, such as temperature, water, and scavenging. The complexity arises when forensic experts need to factor in how these external factors interact and affect the decomposition process. The progress of digital imaging has allowed for improved recording of the decomposition stages, but little has been done regarding the effectiveness of photographic examination versus live observations. As noted, the scoring system employed can make a significant difference in outcomes, raising questions about the reproducibility and standardization of forensic taphonomic studies (Carter et al., 2018). The use of sound methodologies is of cardinal importance for advancing the discipline and providing credible postmortem interval estimates. Moreover, the impact of scavengers on human remains poses a significant impediment to forensic taphonomy and, most times, leaves postmortem interval (PMI) estimates inconsistent. Although numerous scoring systems have been proposed to quantify decomposition, few address the important role of scavenger activity, especially during the early stages of decay. Experiments have shown that scavengers such as raccoons and canids expedite processes such as skeletonization and mummification, making the application of standard PMI estimation challenging (Smith et al., 2015). This supervision puts the validity of current forensic investigations at risk, as such systems do not incorporate the consequences of animal contact with remains. There is thus a necessity for a more complex understanding of the interaction of decomposition variables and scavenging behavior. Finally, the challenge of interdisciplinary work in forensic taphonomy makes the reliability of investigations problematic. Forensic taphonomists must work with entomologists, ecologists, and other professionals to gain an integrated understanding of decomposition processes.

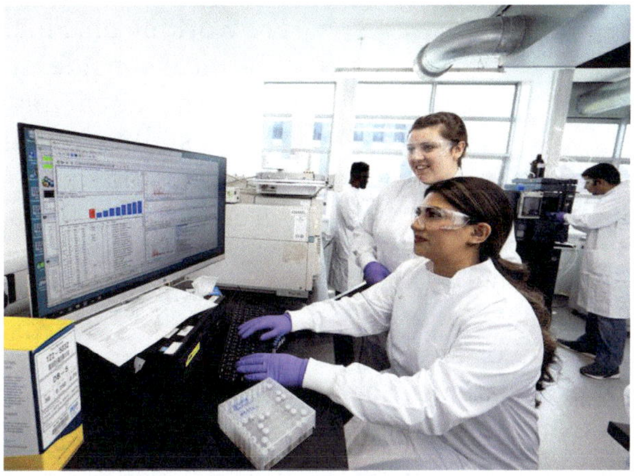

Figure 5.15. Challenges faced in forensic taphonomy.

Source: https://external-content.d uckduckgo.com/iu/?u=https%3A%2F%2Fw ww.uclan.ac.uk%2Fimage-library%2Ffa cilities%2Fforensic-taphonomy-lab.x611ce287.jpg%3Ff%3Dwebp%26q%3D75%26w%3D740&f=1&nofb=1&ipt=7e 626b9ca8c0b27744d403568 4e1d1cf9f9a5ec21ca7f6c5fda6d4dc768fa323.

This variety of scientific input, however, generates methodological conflict because procedures and terminologies differ between disciplines. Such a divergence in diversity hinders communication and application of results, usually resulting in uneven conclusions and methodologies in forensic investigations. The need for standardized protocols across these fields is key to overcoming these challenges and ensuring greater accuracy in interpreting taphonomic evidence (Smith et al., 2015). As the landscape of forensic science continues to evolve, promoting interdisciplinary collaboration will be key to advancing knowledge and addressing the complexities inherent in forensic taphonomy (Figure 5.15).

Test Your Knowledge

1. What are the main techniques used in taphonomic analysis to examine post-mortem changes?
2. How do taphonomic analysis techniques help interpret the burial environment and post-depositional processes?

5.6. Ethical Considerations in Taphonomic Research

Learning Outcome

1. Respect for human remains
2. Cultural sensitivities in taphonomic studies
3. Legal implications of taphonomic research

Ethics in the science of taphonomy are of paramount concern, particularly when employing human cadavers and animal proxies in experiments. The use of house pigs as model cadavers has been the topic of ongoing controversy regarding the appropriateness of employing non-human subjects in the study of decomposition. While pigs provide a realistic and viable substitute for understanding postmortem changes—a mirror of their anatomical and physiological makeup compared to that of human beings—this practice tests the ethical grounds for using animals. Hall et al. (2019) further state that the utilization of pig cadavers, which have now become part of forensic science, demands a stringent ethics procedure that maintains respect and humane treatment towards life. Therefore, scientists need to walk very carefully on the razor-sharp knife of dividing the frontiers of scientific knowledge and upholding ethical standards in their methodological strategies. Moreover, ethical concerns in taphonomy are not limited to managing cadavers but also encompass the total control of skeletal remains exposed during archaeodigging. The Island of Barbuda case is a classic example of the challenges researchers face when working with human skeletal materials altered by environmental factors or development programs. Excavations at sites such as Seaview and Indian Town Trail have uncovered human remains over threats posed by erosion and commercial development. Researchers involved in such excavations are obligated to conduct the work sensitively and respectfully towards the dead and the societies, as set forth by Klemm et al. (2024). This involves practicing moral excavation methods, being transparent with nearby communities, and maintaining that excavation methods adhere to values of respect for the human and archaeological heritage they are working on. Finally, the broader implications of ethical considerations in taphonomic science raise the need for reiterative debate on the responsibility of scientists. Ethical principles need to advance with improvements in forensic methods to ensure that they not only address current scientific challenges but also maintain the dignity of human remains and sensitivity towards Aboriginal communities. The intersection of law, ethics, and science in taphonomy calls for ongoing education and collaboration between professionals to seek optimal practices that honor these values. It is the researcher's responsibility to remain constantly aware of their ethical responsibilities, particularly because the impact of research extends beyond the academy to affect the communities of origin of the remains directly. It is this ethical seriousness that will ultimately enrich the field, leading to responsible and meaningful contributions to our understanding of postmortem change.

5.6.1. Respect for Human Remains

The concept of respect for human remains is core to the fields of archaeology and forensics, and taphonomy and postmortem change in particular. This respect is expressed by handling human remains ethically, being respectful of the cultural, religious, and historical significance of the dead. Through the observation of burial practices and postmortem changes, practitioners have a greater appreciation not only of the biological process of decay but also of the social narratives surrounding death. For instance, the study of mass graves resulting from genocide or war crimes, such as those that have been documented in Bosnia and Herzegovina and Rwanda, necessitates strong respect for the identity and history of the victims. Intervention by heavy machinery and subsequent disarticulation of remains, as in a study on the taphonomy of juvenile pig remains, is representative of the exigent ethical considerations that must be followed when excavating and analyzing human remains (Gilligan et al., 2018). The key to maintaining respect for human remains is to address the societal implications as well as the possible trauma caused to the descendants and communities that have an association with the deceased. Analysis of human remains, particularly in the context of mass graves, requires sensitivity and a conscious effort to weigh the scientific questions against the tales of the people behind the data. The researchers must present their findings with the understanding that behind every fragment of bone lies the memory of an individual or a group of individuals whose experience deserves commemoration. Through approaches centered on the dignity of the dead, such as the meticulous mapping and documentation of remains, archaeologists can preserve the dignity owed to deceased individuals who were interred in their time under austere conditions. The effect of machinery on remains sets the broader conversation of ethical excavations and the significance of representing victims with respect (Gilligan et al., 2018). Further, taphonomic process analysis provides data on ancient burial behavior that encourage respect for human bodies by fostering appreciation for death customs and beliefs. As an example, the study of Iron Age British burial traditions demonstrates diversified mortuary practices and suggests that societies possess a level of sophistication in treating the dead. The application of microscopic taphonomic analysis has enabled a more detailed understanding of changes in and positions of remains, focusing on varied cultural responses to death. This precise attention is a respect to the deceased as it allows them to speak through the remnants of their existence, informing us about past exhumation and burial practices. The intersection of taphonomy and respect for the dead establishes the necessary balance between scientific inquiry and cultural preservation, highlighting the paramount imperative to maintain respect throughout the inquiry (Figure 5.16).

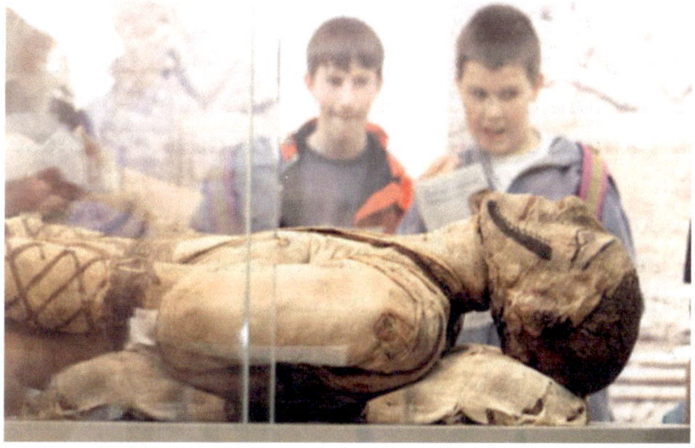

Figure 5.16. The concept of respect for human remains.

Source: https://i.guim.co.uk/img/static/sys-images/Guardian/Pix/pictures/2010/10/25/1288002054029/mummy-in-case-006.jpg?width=465&dpr=1&s=none&crop=none.

5.6.2. Cultural Sensitivities in Taphonomic Studies

Cultural sensitivities play a very significant role in taphonomic studies, especially when dealing with mass graves and the corpses of individuals of multicultural descent. Postmortem alteration needs to be analyzed not just by scientists, but also about the cultural and ethical implications of handling human remains. In the majority of cases, such as the excavation of mass graves for human rights violations, cultural concerns become paramount. Researchers must walk a narrow line between scientific inquiry and respect for the victims and their nation. This sensitivity can impact the methodology employed and interpretation of findings so that the dead are afforded dignity at all times during the investigative process (Hayes et al.,

2023). Moreover, taphonomic studies frequently overlap with legal and ethical frameworks that vary across cultures. Researchers ought to appreciate that sociocultural context can influence how the remains are treated and interpreted. For example, burial practices can vary widely across cultures, and therefore the rates of decomposition and formation of taphonomic signatures on the local environment are affected. It is essential to understand these cultural nuances to apply appropriate evidence-recovery methodologies and determine whether a study's results can be applied to impacted communities. The inclusion of culturally appropriate practices not only makes a study more valid but also fosters maximum trust between researchers and communities, paving the way for fruitful collaboration in forensic and archaeological studies (Soltani et al., 2021). The ethical implications of taphonomic research are more than the direct research itself, necessitating a broader consideration of the social impact of such work. With each excavation and analysis of human remains, an embodied history of injustice accompanies it, most clearly in areas that have been contested or colonized. Academics are tasked with ensuring that the lessons derived from their research contribute to healing and knowledge rather than to further marginalization of affected communities. This involves ongoing interaction with cultural leaders and stakeholders to ensure the stories generated from the research are authentic to the deceased's accounts. By engaging with these cultural susceptibilities, taphonomic studies can move beyond their scientific bounds and meaningfully contribute to broader societal debates on identity, memory, and justice in the face of trauma (Hayes et al., 2023).

5.6.3. Legal Implications of Taphonomic Research

The legal implications of taphonomic studies are multifaceted and intersect with forensic science, criminal law, and ethical concerns regarding the handling of human remains. Taphonomy, the examination of postmortem processes acting on corpses, can be extremely important in legal cases, especially homicides or suspicious fatalities. Determining the postmortem interval, or the time elapsed since death, depends largely on understanding how environmental factors affect decomposition. These data not only assist police forces in shortening timelines but also serve as clinching evidence in court trials, exposing the potential culpability of suspects or demonstrating innocence. However, the utilization of taphonomic data within a courtroom environment poses significant challenges to scientific precision and reliability and reaffirms the importance of strict protocols and peer-reviewed procedures in forensic taphonomy.

Additionally, the handling of remains in taphonomic research, especially those of deceased individuals, raises serious ethical and legal issues. Whether it is legal to study human remains is essentially a matter of jurisdiction, with the laws about burial and respecting the dead commonly dictating this. For instance, exposure of corpses to environmental elements, in scavenging studies, can have ramifications according to law where it exists regarding the treatment of human corpses. Given that vertebrate scavengers can significantly remold remains, as in other similar studies, it is critical that forensic scientists and researchers adhere to ethical protocols that protect the dignity of the dead while advancing science (Amendt et al., 2014). This synthesis of legality and ethics encapsulates the basis of responsible taphonomic research. Additionally, the implications of taphonomic study findings carry over into public attitudes toward crime and justice and influence public policy and societal norms regarding death investigations. Taphonomic processes are informative not only for illuminating forensic procedures, but also for enhancing public awareness regarding the intricacies of decomposition and the factors governing the preservation of remains through time. For instance, public officials and law enforcers need to be aware of how environmental conditions may influence the gathering of evidence and the prosecution. The finer details of taphonomy, e.g., specific modes of decay and forensic significance, can inform legal systems, hence leading to legislative reform based on the most current scientific understanding. Hence, policymakers, scientists, and legal scholars must work more closely together to ensure the processes uncovered by taphonomic research are adequately covered by the law, enabling better and more equitable use of investigations (Reisdorf et al., 2018).

Test Your Knowledge

1. Why are ethical considerations important when conducting taphonomic research on human remains?
2. What ethical guidelines should be followed during the collection and analysis of taphonomic evidence?

SUMMARY

Postmortem change and taphonomy are research that provide crucial information on the processes underlying the preservation or decay of organic remains after death. By investigating various habitats and environments, researchers illuminate how temperature, salinity, and biological processes influence both the initial state and the ultimate fate of carcasses. Not only does this interaction contribute to the reconstruction of ancient ecosystems, but it also contributes to our understanding of modern ecological processes. Research on the habits of giant lung-breathing sea tetrapods, as evidenced by ichthyosaurs, supports revisiting earlier assumptions about carcass buoyancy and decay. Research diverges from earlier hypotheses, positioning taphonomic investigations at the center of understanding the enigmatic phase shift between life and fossilization (Benecke et al., 2018). In addition, the use of state-of-the-art analytical methods, such as cathodoluminescence and elemental mapping, significantly enhances understanding of exceptional preservation conditions within single sites, such as the Sirius Passet Lagerstätte. With these analytical techniques, scientists can create an integrated story around single fossils, revealing their subtle taphonomic history and the processes that led to their preservation. By comparing across various taphonomic modes, researchers can uncover trends on larger scales of ecological and geological processes from geochronologically and geographically heterogeneous settings, particularly during the Cambrian Explosion. A diversified approach opens the way for fresh dialogue on biota preservation and has far-reaching implications for paleobiology, demanding a more in-depth exploration of the lifecycles of ancient and contemporary species (Strang et al., 2017). Finally, taphonomic research has implications beyond scholarship, touching on conservational practice and body recovery in aquatic environments. Knowledge of the processes that determine what happens to decaying organisms guides measures for safeguarding modern marine ecosystems and resolving problems in recovering bodies from the ocean. Moreover, as new technologies and higher levels of analytical science evolve, the ability to uncover complex taphonomic histories grows exponentially. This ongoing improvement in technique not only further enhances an appreciation of the fossil record but also emphasizes the interconnectedness of life, death, and preservation in the natural world. Taphonomy is thus a transcendent research area that informs many disciplines and acts as a connecting link between paleontology, ecology, and conservation biology.

Taphonomy and postmortem transformation research examines processes acting on organic remains after death and provides significant insights into decomposition patterns. An interesting fact is how burial conditions can affect the rate of decomposition. It has been discovered that where carcasses are situated in mass graves significantly affects their rate of decomposition. For example, carcasses resting in shallow graves decompose faster than those buried deeper, and the internal carcass temperature also varies according to position in the grave. This indicates that extrinsic factors, such as the availability of oxygen and substrate contact, also play important roles in determining the decomposition rate, illustrating the complex nature of taphonomic processes and the need for ongoing investigation of the interactions among these variables (Adlam et al., 2014). The other key component of taphonomy is postmortem interval (PMI) estimation, which supports forensic recovery by providing a chronology of death. Current research focuses more on what is now termed a subtler appreciation of the potential for intrinsic (personal biological factors) and extrinsic (environmental factors) factors to influence rates of decomposition. For example, research from the Great Plains ecosystem shows that regional climatic factors and scavengers can significantly alter decomposition. New literature in vertebrate scavengers illustrates their importance in decomposing soft tissue and possibly biasing PMI estimates. Such an observation may prompt the inclusion of these biotic factors in existing predictive models, underscoring the need for a broader understanding of the taphonomic environment and its implications for forensic science (Alexander et al., 2024). Furthermore, the need for region-specific models of PMI estimation has been emphasized in existing taphonomic research. This includes efforts to constrain predictive algorithms with parameters that account for variation in decomposition across geographic locations and environmental conditions. For example, the proposed extension factor (Ef) calculated on localized data can refine PMI estimations. By employing a cubic polynomial regression on total degree days and corresponding total body scores, new functions for PMI estimation are established that are based on both the upper and lower limits of predicted decay. This blending of qualitative assessments enables a better sense of how patterns of decomposition can be predicted to change over time, ultimately offering greater reliability to forensic practice and the attainment of justice in court proceedings (Alexander et al., 2024).

KEY TERMS FROM THIS CHAPTER

- Adipocere Formation
- Burial Environment
- Decomposition
- Disarticulation
- Mummification
- Postmortem Breakage
- Postmortem Interval (PMI)
- Rodent Gnawing
- Root Etching
- Skeletonization
- Soil Staining
- Sun Bleaching
- Surface Modification
- Taphonomy
- Water Transport
- Weathering

CRITICAL THINKING QUESTIONS

1. **What is the primary focus of taphonomy in forensic anthropology?**
   a. Determining ancestry from skeletal remains
   b. Studying disease in ancient populations
   c. Understanding the processes that affect a body after death
   d. Estimating stature from bones
2. **Which of the following is a biotic factor influencing postmortem change?**
   a. Sunlight exposure
   b. Soil acidity
   c. Root etching
   d. Carnivore scavenging
3. **The postmortem interval (PMI) refers to:**
   a. The time between trauma and death
   b. The time between death and burial
   c. The time between death and discovery of the remains
   d. The time between death and bone mineralization
4. **A key indicator of scavenger activity on bones is:**
   a. Eburnation
   b. Chop marks
   c. Spiral fractures
   d. Punctures and scoring

Short Answer Questions

1. Define taphonomy in the context of forensic anthropology and bioarcheology.
2. What is the significance of understanding postmortem interval (PMI) in forensic investigations?
3. Explain how scavenger activity can alter human remains.
4. Describe two postmortem changes that can be confused with perimortem trauma. How can they be distinguished?
5. Explain the difference between postmortem staining and heat-induced color changes in bones.

Answers to Critical Thinking Questions

1. (c); 2. (d); 3. c); 4. (d); 5. (d)

REFERENCES

1. Santos, J. A. (2019). Decomposition of pig carcasses at varying room temperature. *Themis Research Journal of Justice Studies and Forensic Science*, *7*(1). https://doi.org/10.31979/themis.2019.0703Adlam, A., Arnold, B., Bachmann, C., Baraybar, J. P., Burns, K. R., Carter, D. O., et al. (2014). A preliminary examination of differential decomposition patterns in mass graves. https://core.ac.uk/download/1441337.pdf (accessed on 21st July 2025).
2. Ager, A. O. O., Bandeira, B., Barry, T., Bull, I. D., Campobasso, C. P., Carter, D. O., et al. (2014). Changes to soil bacterial profiles as a result of *Sus scrofa domesticus* decomposition. https://core.ac.uk/download/153371381.pdf (accessed on 21st July 2025).
3. Alcalá Martínez, L., Andrews, P., Fernández Jalvo, Y., Fernández López, S., et al. (2002). Morphological taphonomic transformations of fossil bones in continental environments, and repercussions of their chemical composition. https://core.ac.uk/download/19725679.pdf (accessed on 21st July 2025).
4. Alexander, J. L. (2024). Scavenging as an accelerant in the postmortem interval estimate: Refining quantitative regressions for decomposition analyses in Southeast Nebraska. https://core.ac.uk/download/636660809.pdf (accessed on 21st July 2025).
5. Amendt, J., Asamura, H., Baker, A. M., Bass, W. M., Byard, R. W., Campobasso, C. P., Coard, N. J., et al. (2014). An experimental study of vertebrate scavenging behavior in a Northwest European woodland context. https://core.ac.uk/download/42143110.pdf (accessed on 21st July 2025).
6. Belcastro, M. G., Benazzi, S., Lenzi, F., Mariotti, V., et al. (2023). On the traces of lost identities: Chronological, anthropological and taphonomic analyses of the Late Neolithic/Early Eneolithic fragmented and commingled human remains from the Farneto rock shelter (Bologna, northern Italy). https://core.ac.uk/download/564348487.pdf (accessed on 21st July 2025).
7. Benecke, M., Bux, R., Fornaro, P., Klug, A., et al. (2018). Float, explode or sink: Postmortem fate of lung-breathing marine vertebrates. https://core.ac.uk/download/159156116.pdf (accessed on 21st July 2025).
8. Booth, T. J., & Madgwick, R. (2016). New evidence for diverse secondary burial practices in Iron Age Britain: A histological case study. https://core.ac.uk/download/42531553.pdf (accessed on 21st July 2025).
9. Cai, S. (2025). Paleoenvironmental interpretation of late glacial and post-glacial fossil marine molluscs, Eureka Sound, Canadian Arctic Archipelago. https://core.ac.uk/download/226137190.pdf (accessed on 21st July 2025).
10. Carew, R. M., & Errickson, D. (2019). Imaging in forensic science: Five years on. https://core.ac.uk/download/188365686.pdf (accessed on 21st July 2025).
11. Carter, D. O., Morgan, R. M., Rando, C., Ribéreau-Gayon, A., et al. (2018). The suitability of visual taphonomic methods for digital photographs: An experimental approach with pig carcasses in a tropical climate. https://core.ac.uk/download/144582757.pdf (accessed on 21st July 2025).
12. Cassella, J. P., Jervis, J. R., & Pringle, J. K. (2010). Preliminary soil water conductivity analysis to date clandestine burials of homicide victims. https://core.ac.uk/download/28874724.pdf (accessed on 21st July 2025).

13. Cieśla, J., Skrobisz, J., Niciński, B., Kloc, M., Mazur, K., Pałasz, A., Javan, G. T., et al. (2023). The smell of death: State-of-the-art and future research directions. *Frontiers in Microbiology, 14*. https://doi.org/10.3389/fmicb.2023.1260869 (accessed on 21st July 2025).
14. Damann, F. E. (2010). Human decomposition ecology at the University of Tennessee Anthropology Research Facility. https://core.ac.uk/download/268764702.pdf (accessed on 21st July 2025).
15. Dawson, B. M., Ueland, M., Carter, D. O., McIntyre, D., & Barton, P. S. (2023). Bridging the gap between decomposition theory and forensic research on postmortem interval. *International Journal of Legal Medicine, 138*, 509–518. https://doi.org/10.1007/s00414-023-03060-8 (accessed on 21st July 2025).
16. Dekeirsschieter, J., Frederickx, C., Haubruge, E., & Lognay, G., et al. (2012). Comment les insectes communiquent-ils au sein de l' «écosystème-cadavre»? L'écologie chimique des insectes nécrophages et nécrophiles. http://orbi.ulg.ac.be/bitstream/2268/124146/1/Dekeirsschieter-etal-2012-FE.pdf (accessed on 21st July 2025).
17. Egeland, C. P. (2020). Cruel traces: Bone surface modifications and their relevance to forensic science. https://core.ac.uk/download/489534638.pdf (accessed on 21st July 2025).
18. Falkingham, P. L., & Gatesy, S. M. (2017). Neither bones nor feet: Track morphological variation and "preservation quality." https://core.ac.uk/download/82964465.pdf (accessed on 21st July 2025).
19. Frelat, M., Halazonetis, D., Karell, M. A., Kranioti, E. F., et al. (2016). A novel method for pair-matching using three-dimensional digital models of bone: Mesh-to-mesh value comparison. https://core.ac.uk/download/305118311.pdf (accessed on 21st July 2025).
20. Garcia, J. R. (2024). *A Manual on The Planning and Integration of Archaeological Methods into Outdoor Forensic Search Investigations*. https://core.ac.uk/download/610528751.pdf (accessed on 21st July 2025).
21. Gilligan, J. (2018). An experimental clandestine grave: Analysis of postmortem fractures and remains distribution of an intentional backhoe reinterment. https://open.bu.edu/bitstream/2144/33000/5/Gilligan_bu_0017N_14090.pdf (accessed on 21st July 2025).
22. Guerra, S. C. (2014). Qualifying and quantifying the rate of decomposition in the Delaware River Valley region. https://core.ac.uk/download/76395174.pdf (accessed on 21st July 2025).
23. Hall, M. J. R., Matuszewski, S., Moreau, G., Schoenly, K., et al. (2019). Pigs' vs people: The use of pigs as analogues for humans in forensic entomology and taphonomy research. https://core.ac.uk/download/334608154.pdf (accessed on 21st July 2025).
24. Hannigan, A. (2015). A descriptive study of forensic implications of raccoon scavenging in Maine. https://core.ac.uk/download/217052491.pdf (accessed on 21st July 2025).
25. Hayes, H. (2023). Locating the missing: A critical examination of the taphonomic alterations and the archaeological and forensic techniques that can be used to identify them during the search for mass graves. https://core.ac.uk/download/567876279.pdf (accessed on 21st July 2025).
26. Hoeland, K. M. (2021). Investigating the potential of postmortem metabolomics in mammalian decomposition studies in outdoor settings. https://core.ac.uk/download/524887815.pdf (accessed on 21st July 2025).

27. Klemm, M. M. (2024). *The Osteobiography of Human Remains from The Seaview and Indian Town Trail Archaeological Sites*. https://core.ac.uk/download/610528749.pdf (accessed on 21st July 2025).

28. Knüsel, C. J., & Robb, J. (2016). Funerary taphonomy: An overview of goals and methods. https://core.ac.uk/download/77413943.pdf (accessed on 21st July 2025).

29. LaCroix, M. N. (2013). A study of the impact of weathering upon the minimal force required to fracture bone. https://open.bu.edu/bitstream/2144/12140/6/LaCroix_Marcelle_2013_nosig_nocv.pdf (accessed on 21st July 2025).

30. Olakanye, A. O., Bandeira, B., Barry, T., Bergmann, G. T., Bull, I. D., Campobasso, C. P., Carter, D. O., et al. (2015). Shifts in soil biodiversity—A forensic comparison between *Sus scrofa domesticus* and vegetation decomposition. https://core.ac.uk/download/153371389.pdf (accessed on 21st July 2025).

31. Perez, A. E., Anderson, B., Lindahl, B. D., Sharanowski, B. J., O'Connor, B. M., Berney, C., et al. (2018). Comparative analysis of bones, mites, soil chemistry, nematodes and soil micro-eukaryotes from a suspected homicide to estimate the post-mortem interval. https://core.ac.uk/download/145628179.pdf (accessed on 21st July 2025).

32. Pollio, C. J. (2009). Cut mark analysis of protohistoric bison remains from EfPm-27 utilizing the scanning electron microscope. https://core.ac.uk/download/226137630.pdf (accessed on 21st July 2025).

33. Reisdorf, A., & Wuttke, M. (2018). Re-evaluating Moodie's opisthotonos-posture hypothesis in fossil vertebrates. Part I: Reptiles—the taphonomy of the bipedal dinosaurs *Compsognathus longipes* and *Juravenator starki* from the Solnhofen Archipelago (Jurassic, Germany). https://core.ac.uk/download/159149524.pdf (accessed on 21st July 2025).

34. Saul, T. B. (2017). An exploration of the effects of taphonomy on isotope ratios of human hair. https://core.ac.uk/download/268796633.pdf (accessed on 21st July 2025).

35. Smith, J. K. (2015). Raccoon scavenging and the taphonomic effects on early human decomposition and PMI estimation. https://core.ac.uk/download/268808456.pdf (accessed on 21st July 2025).

36. Soltani, S. K. (2021). Antemortem health indicators and burial status: A study of the Tepe Hasanlu Bronze–Seleuco-Parthian period burials, Iran. https://core.ac.uk/download/388588340.pdf (accessed on 21st July 2025).

37. Strang, K. M. (2017). Aspects of the taphonomy of the Cambrian Explosion in North Greenland. https://core.ac.uk/download/141198887.pdf (accessed on 21st July 2025).

FORENSIC OSTEOLOGY AND IDENTIFICATION

6

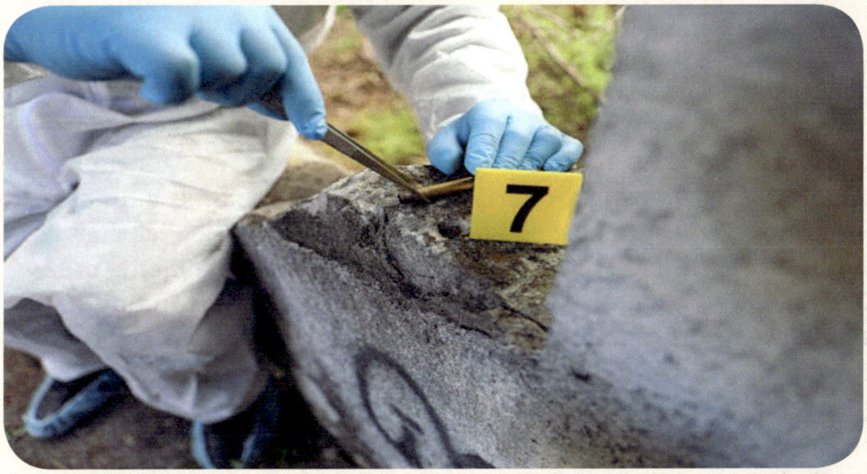

LEARNING OBJECTIVES

After studying this chapter, you will be able to:

1. Discuss the historical background
2. Explain the role of osteologists
3. Understand techniques in forensic osteology
4. Know determining age, sex, and ancestry
5. Discuss the trauma analysis
6. Identify case studies that play a pivotal role in the field of forensic osteology

Introduction

Forensic osteology, being a professional field of anthropology, is a valuable resource in identification and criminal justice. Forensic osteology specifically examines remains using macroscopic and microscopic techniques to reconstruct the biological profiles of unidentified individuals. As osteologists investigate the intricacies of bone morphology, they are not merely recording physical attributes; rather, they are unlocking narratives about age, sex, lineage, and, in some cases, the life experiences of the deceased. The integration of osteological methods with forensic anthropology has, in large part, enhanced the ability to ascertain significant information regarding death conditions, particularly within settings commonly crowded with legal and human rights dynamics. These analyses emphasize the worth of forensic osteology not merely as a scientific discipline but also as a significant tool for social justice, as attested by its application in countless cases and cases in court (Bosnar et al., 2010). The evolution of forensic osteology in the 21st century is evidence of its continued relevance and vibrancy. As new methods and technologies become available, professionals use them to continue enhancing the accuracy and effectiveness of identification and analysis. High-level radiographic imaging, for instance, and three-dimensional reconstruction continue to redefine the landscape of forensic science, enabling the analysis of the skeleton more precisely and revealingly than ever before. In addition, forensic representatives increasingly engage with archaeologists and physicians to blend multidisciplinary expertise that not only enables identification but also provides a better understanding of ancient and sociocultural environments. This enhanced collaboration helps to reinforce the adaptive nature of forensic osteology, showcasing its ability to meet new challenges confronting the field, with an emphasis on mass casualties and human rights abuses (Bosnar et al., 2010). Furthermore, forensic osteological technique is not just used for identification purposes but is also crucial in ascertaining the conditions of human remains, as exemplified by high-profile cases like Amelia Earhart. The excavations for her potential skeletal remains illustrate the complexity involved in osteological testing and the necessity of strict, scientific procedure. Despite differing interpretations of evidence, as seen in differing evaluations of her recovered remains, professional criticism underscores the importance of honest and authoritative forensic processes. These instances do not so much draw attention to the intricacies of bone identification as underscore the ethical responsibility of forensic professionals who operate to provide closure to family members and justice to judicial systems. Through a comprehensive study of osteology, the field will be in a position to develop further, contributing significantly to uncovering truths used by both the legal system and societal narratives.

Definition of Forensic Osteology

Forensic osteology is a specialized field of anthropology that focuses on the examination and identification of human remains composed of bone within a legal context. It plays a key role in the recovery, analysis, and interpretation of bone remains found at crime scenes, sites of disaster, or mass graves. The science borrows from archaeological practice with biological anthropology, allowing forensic osteologists not only to identify dead individuals but also to reveal valuable information on how they died. This interdisciplinary approach is required because the bones may yield valuable data such as age, sex, ancestry, and even specific pathologies or trauma incurred prior to death. Forensic osteology is basically a link between the law and the sciences, providing evidence that may be absolutely vital in criminal investigations and cases. The dynamic nature of forensic osteology is attested by the fact that it is required to keep pace with developments in analytical techniques and technologies. Today's forensic osteologists have utilized a variety of tools, ranging from imaging techniques to genetic testing, which facilitate a greater understanding of human remains. For instance, advanced non-invasive methods such as CT scans and advanced 3D modeling can be used to image and analyze skeletal details that might not be readily apparent during physical examinations. Furthermore, the necessity of considering factors such as the environment and context in which the remains were found makes it more complicated, as decomposition and preservation can vary significantly. This highlights the importance of forensic osteologists maintaining a multidisciplinary frame of mind, incorporating biological and contextual considerations to enable proper identification and the reconstruction of life history from bones. Forensic osteology education and training are also important to address the increasing complications of cases being worked on in this specialty. As noted in various studies, remote learning techniques have been modified to facilitate the teaching of human osteology more effectively, especially in the context of the current pandemic. Students must be taught both practical and theoretical components of the subject to study effectively, developing proficiency in areas such as identification of bones and age determination (Gamble et al., 2024). The importance of practical experience cannot be overstated; it is essential for attaining competency in the subject of study. Moreover, given that forensic cases often yield incomplete remains, osteologists ought to know techniques to assess incomplete bones appropriately. Such elementary knowledge equips practitioners to contribute meaningfully to forensic inquiry and improves the overall integrity of the legal process in which their contribution is applied (Figure 6.1).

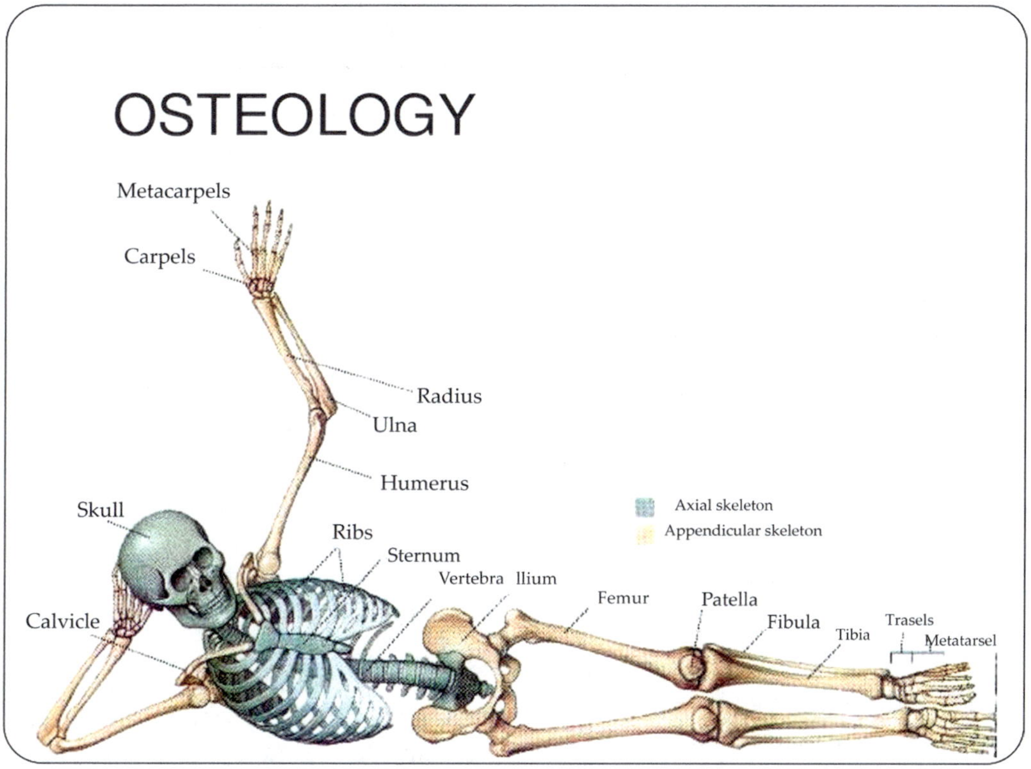

Figure 6.1. Forensic osteology.

Source: https://external-content.duckduckgo.com/iu/?u=https%3A%2F%2Fimage.slidesharecdn.com%2Fforensicosteology-190518074252%2F95%2Fforensic-osteology-2-1024.jpg%3Fcb%3D1558165625&f=1&nofb=1&ipt=b0e66255c9a6f7271f72db0053432c7432c35d8c4723cc83ab6fbdd9ec210891.

Importance in Criminal Investigations

The use of forensic osteology in criminal investigations plays a pivotal role in identifying human remains, particularly when other methods are not adequate. If a body is decomposed or severely decomposed, forensic anthropologists analyze skeletal remains to obtain vital information, such as age, sex, ancestry, and stature. This information is crucial for restricting potential matches in missing persons cases and provides police with excellent leads. Furthermore, the application of morphological characteristics of bone is used to determine the cause of death or reconstruct the circumstances of one's death, thereby contributing to the investigative narrative and informing future action by criminal justice agencies. Exhumation procedures, as a term used in forensic anthropology, serve a significant function in the criminal investigation process by allowing for the legally regulated recovery of buried remains. Exhumations are frequently central in the majority of cases when new evidence is produced, or initial investigations yield inconclusive leads. For instance, the Ribeirão Preto Medical School-University of São Paulo's Medico-Legal Centre demonstrates that exhumations continue forensic processes for humanitarian and investigative purposes.

This approach not only aligns with legal regulations but also fulfills forensic professionals' ethical duty to seek justice for victims, ensuring that overlooked cases receive further inquiry—a necessity in the realm of cold cases and missing persons involving institutional violence or historical injustices (Arrabaça Francisco et al., 2017). The historical context of exhumation is highlighted by the role it plays in handling politically sensitive cases, such as those resulting from Brazil's civil-military dictatorship, 1964–1985.

Through conducting detailed investigations into such deaths, forensic osteology goes beyond the usual crime-solving to encompass broader societal needs for truth and healing. The alliance of social justice and forensic science finds support in the analysis of skeletal material to identify patterns of human rights abuses and violence. In this manner, the utilization of forensic osteology does not just confine itself to legal recourse; it resonates with the political and cultural life of society to achieve closure for families and accountability for past atrocities. As demonstrated through some case studies, the minutiae work of forensic anthropologists demonstrates the relevance of this science in today's criminal investigations (da Silva et al., 2017) (Figure 6.2).

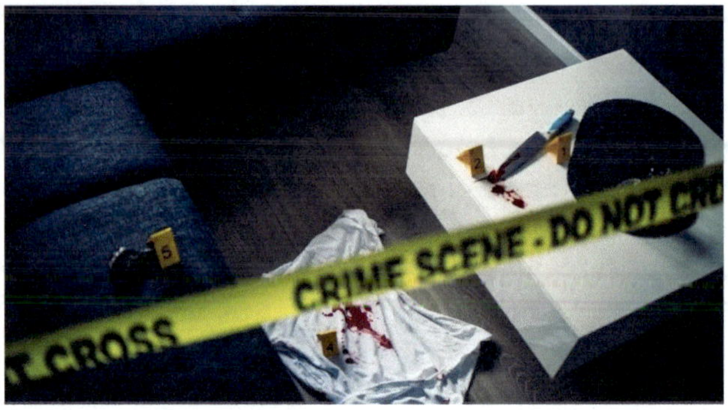

Figure 6.2. The integration of forensic osteology in criminal investigations.

Source: https://www.theaftercare.com/wp-content/uploads/2022/01/blood-analysis.jpg.

6.1. Historical Background

Learning Outcome

1. Origins of forensic osteology
2. Key developments in the field
3. Notable cases that shaped forensic practices

Forensic osteology, as a branch of science, has undergone dramatic evolution over the centuries, fueled by scientific advancements and the experience of landmark cases that have shaped its practice. The historical backdrop of this science begins during the early 20th century, when scientific methods of analyzing human remains began to emerge simultaneously with increasing numbers of criminal investigations. Pioneering practitioners focused on skeletal analysis of remains to identify individuals, which is now a standard forensic procedure. With techniques refined, anthropology and archaeology crossed over into disciplines like morphological analysis and DNA extraction, which allowed forensic experts to glean data from even the most battered remains. These developments underscore the importance of context in interpreting skeletal evidence, as modern forensic osteology continues to look to past precedent for inspiration in its practices and approaches. One of the most high-profile historical instances, with a strong impact on forensic osteology, is that of the disappearance of Amelia Earhart in 1937. Although a plethora of theories have been put forth regarding her disappearance, some of them in particular have suggested the potential identification of remains found that are associated with her case. In 1940, British officials analyzed fragmentary skeletal remains found on Gardner Island and, from it, decided that these belonged to a muscular, middle-aged male. The initial investigation was seminal to the discipline, marking both the potential and limitations of osteological analysis. Later evaluations in 1998 sought to reinterpret results using advanced cranial analysis software, speculating that the remains were indeed Earhart's, illustrating how assumptions from the historical record can profoundly shape forensic conclusions. However, as methodology and technology have advanced, a close examination of each study reveals that stronger conclusions show the same associations as the original British study, further reinforcing the challenge of constructing identity from skeletal remains, especially given the limitations of the data (Cross et al., 2015). Matters also arise when analyzing cremated remains, presenting particular challenges to forensic osteologists wishing to glean information about historical populations. The cremation process is distinguished by its worldwide history and decisively influences the conservation and examination of skeletal human remains. In studies of East Lithuania as a case region from the 3rd to the 12th centuries, researchers noted significant differences between cremated and buried samples, particularly in the number of subadult groups. The study identified macroscopic-analysis-inherent biases in the analysis of cremated human remains that run the risk of underestimating infant and early child mortality rates since they are difficult to establish in cremated remains. The biases are not only distorting demographic data but also complicating the interpretation of earlier social structures and health implications among population groups. The historico-complex nature of cremation supports the need for context-specific approaches in forensic osteology to minimize bias and maximize interpretative accuracy (Kurila et al., 2015).

6.1.1. Origins of Forensic Osteology

Forensic osteology traces its origins to an overlap of anthropology, archaeology, and the need for scientific precision in the courts. As a branch of forensic science, forensic osteology primarily focuses on the excavation and analysis of human remains to create biological profiles, aid identification, and support the pursuit of justice in unexplained deaths or crimes. Historical influences are evident in early physical anthropology methods, in which bones were measured and categorized, laying the groundwork for present methods. By the turn of the 19th century, developments in the field of human osteology started to standardize the practice of work in legal contexts, leading to the use of skeletal analysis not just for identification purposes but also for gaining an insight into several aspects of a deceased person's life and the conditions of his death. An important step in the development of forensic osteology was the systematic investigation of commingled remains, especially within archaeological conditions. Notably, an in-depth examination of Minnesota's Acacia Park Cemetery skeletal remains demonstrates such application. In this context, researchers compared skeletal fragments to reconstruct demographic profiles, estimate health status, and evaluate activity patterns among those buried over a broad temporal range. By applying standardized techniques to ascertain age, sex, height, and ancestry, the study demonstrated how forensic osteology extends beyond identification, providing deep insight into the past and cultural histories of the dead. Such precise examination highlights the importance of forensic osteology in the past and present, revealing the intricate relationship between bone remains and human existence and ultimately enhancing our knowledge of community history. Furthermore, the use of histological techniques is a significant part of the evolution of forensic osteology, enhancing the discipline's ability to distinguish between human and non human bones, especially in cases involving charred remains. A feasibility study that evaluated the histological characteristics of charred as well as non-charred cranial bones provided a decision tree analysis that pinpointed differentiating features that facilitate forensic identification. This revolutionary strategy not only provides us with a final key for identification but also guarantees 100% accuracy in discriminating human remains under unfavorable conditions. Therefore, the focus on histology highlights how forensic osteology continually develops and adapts, bringing new technologies and methods into legal investigation procedures. The dedication to its continued improvement positions forensic osteology at the forefront as a valuable resource for the identification and understanding of skeletal remains in legal and social contexts, ultimately opening avenues for future development in the field (Figure 6.3).

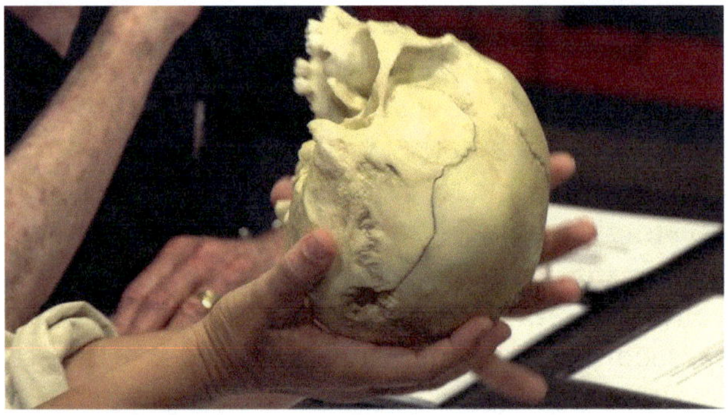

Figure 6.3. The origins of forensic osteology.

Source: https://i.ytimg.com/vi/eU3TqdZHLbg/hq720.jpg?sqp=-oaymwE7CK4FEIIDSFryq4qpAy0IARUAAAAAGAElAADIQj0AgKJD8AEB-AH-CYAC0AWKAgwIABABGGUgTyg8MA8=&rs=AOn4CLCFSXM0UuO3TG8kd7gy2cV13cZ7zA.

6.1.2. Key Developments in the Field

The development of forensic osteology has been largely marked by advances in methodology that have contributed to the accuracy of biological profiling. Forensic osteology, a branch of forensic anthropology, employs a broad range of techniques to determine key features such as age, sex, ancestry, and stature from skeletal remains. According to the literature, the application of digital tools such as 3D imaging and computer-aided design has revolutionized forensic anthropologists' analysis and interpretation of skeletal data. They support a more refined sensitivity to bone morphology, thereby strengthening the accuracy of identifications and reconstructions of biological profiles. Improvements in osteological methods do not simply improve the accuracy of existing methods but also increase the chances of forensic applications. This development reflects how modern technology and traditional osteological knowledge come together to advance identification and enhance the accuracy of forensic analysis (Bryson et al., 2016). In addition to methodological creativity, forensic osteology has been driven by interdisciplinary approaches that draw on knowledge from a broad spectrum of research. The integration of osteology with genetics, archaeology, and even bioinformatics enables forensic professionals to recover comprehensive details about the deceased's life and the manner of death. Such collaboration has enhanced DNA extraction and analysis from skeletal remains, adding to identification procedures. Forensic osteologists are increasingly involved in humanitarian efforts through their skills to combat human rights violations and unidentified human bodies in mass casualty events. This wide-ranging approach not only optimizes the discipline's academic value but also optimizes its social relevance, further solidifying forensic osteology's position as a core element in the overall scheme of forensic science and legal justice (Bosnar et al., 2010). Continuous development of teaching models in forensic osteology has also played a key role in developing the subject. Institutions are increasingly recognizing the merit of pedagogical reforms, such as the use of digital badge systems that award students badges for mastery of specific skills in osteology and forensic anthropology. These types of systems encourage student engagement by bridging theory and practice applications in real-world contexts. The University of Derby case studies demonstrate the effective use of badges as a mechanism for enhancing students' learning outcomes and demonstrating competence in key areas of osteology (Bryson et al., 2016). These pedagogical practices not only enrich academic life but also prepare prospective professionals to address the evolving demands of forensic science, building a new generation of experts adept at managing the complexities of identification in forensic contexts (Bosnar et al., 2010).

6.1.3. Notable Cases That Shaped Forensic Practices

Forensic practice has vastly improved via high-profile cases that have emphasized the importance of osteological analysis in forensic investigation. A prime example was the application of non-destructive taxonomic identification, whereby scientists demonstrated that it could be used to identify skeletal remains via a microscope from fragmentary bones sampled from varying taxa. Non-destructive identification enabled species identification without destructive histological methods. This new approach led to a very high correctness of 96.2% for identifying human bones, with a high 7.9% of non-human bones as human. These findings have significant forensic applications, particularly in instances where only small bones remain for analysis. By establishing reliable methods in forensic osteology, this case ultimately contributed to the standardization of practices within the field and enhanced the overall reliability of forensic evidence itself (O\u27Brien et al., 2019). Another significant advancement emerged from the examination of skeletal remains for sex estimation using osteological methods. Historically, the pelvis has been regarded as the most accurate indicator of biological sex; however, when only long bones were available, identification proved challenging. Because of this limitation, research has focused on the metric size of long bones and has used discriminant analysis to assess predictive validity. The analysis, using a large sample, produced consistent classification results ranging between 70% and 90%. Such methods are important to test, particularly given their ability to make accurate sex estimations without the need for population-specific collections.

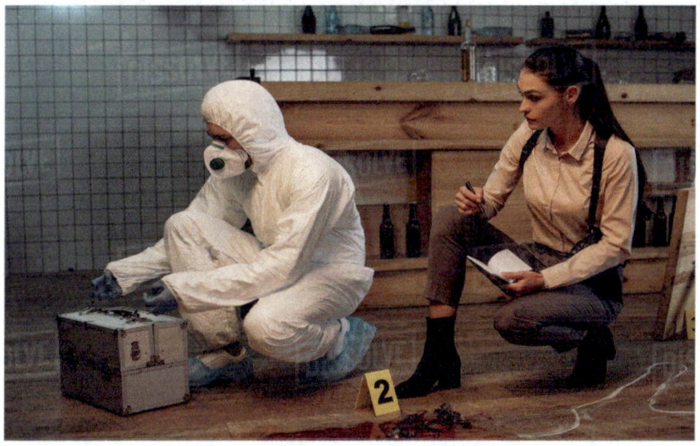

Figure 6.4. The development of forensic practices.

Source: https://external-content.duckduckgo.com/iu/?u=https%3A%2F%2Fcdn8.dissolve.com%2Fp%2FD2115_167_162%2FD2115_167_162_1200.jpg&f=1&nofb=1&ipt=0ec8d444dcc37d553154193fb3d2d587607f39e3d4ac45f18066dd86ce6c475c.

The development of such methods provides a basis for cases in which traditional biological profiling is compromised, thereby broadening the scope of forensic osteological analysis in human remains identification (Sanchez et al., 2025). Besides these advancements, even high-profile forensic osteology cases have outlined the crucial intersection of morphological and non-destructive approaches to further identification. The integration of new technologies with traditional osteological practices has revolutionized the discipline, enabling forensic practitioners to extract valuable information from even the most disarticulated skeletons. These established techniques not only improve forensic identification yields but also address ethical concerns regarding the preservation of skeletal remains in criminal cases. As the field of work continues to develop and improve, findings from such cases will inevitably influence future applications, making forensic osteology a focal aspect of human identification investigations. By bridging the gap between historical methodologies and modern technological applications, forensic practices continue to demonstrate their significance in the criminal justice system, solidifying osteologists' role as vital contributors to forensic science overall (O\u27Brien et al., 2019; Sanchez et al., 2025) (Figure 6.4).

Test Your Knowledge

1. How did forensic osteology develop as a scientific discipline over time?
2. Who were the key pioneers in the historical development of forensic osteology and what were their contributions?

6.2. The Role of Osteologists

Learning Outcome

1. Responsibilities of forensic osteologists
2. Collaboration with law enforcement
3. Importance of expert testimony in court

In forensic osteology, osteologists play a crucial role in identifying and examining human skeletal remains. Their involvement is not only pivotal in determining the age, sex, and ancestry of unidentified bones but also in establishing the cause and manner of death.

Through various methods, such as osteometric analysis, osteologists can provide vital information that helps law enforcement crack cold cases or ongoing investigations. It is particularly useful in mass catastrophes, where there is a need for rapid identification of victims to achieve closure and justice. Besides, osteologists must keep pace with technologies that enhance their ability to analyze bone remains, thereby establishing more accurate post-mortem intervals and trauma, thereby validating their role in forensic and anthropological analysis. Osteology is perhaps the most interdisciplinary of all fields, bridging anthropology, archaeology, and forensic science. Osteologists generally need to collaborate with forensic pathologists, law enforcement officials, and anthropologists to provide a comprehensive understanding of skeletal evidence. Their findings may provide insight into the historical context of remains, offering invaluable information on the person's life and living conditions. Further, as with more recent training courses such as the use of plastic model skeletons in distance education, pedagogy in human osteology is adapting to new needs, focusing on haptic learning experience for instruction (Gamble et al., 2024). This interconnection creates a well-rounded expertise among osteologists, enabling them to make practical contributions to forensic analysis and rendering them indispensable to the criminal justice system. Moreover, the activity of osteologists extends the immediate realm of forensic identification; it also includes ethical sensitivity and decolonizing the field. As highlighted by available debate, the most pressing need is to transcend the abuse and misuse of Indigenous people in anthropological studies (Hill et al., 2020). Osteologists must address such ethical issues, recognizing their work's cultural sensitivities and maintaining themselves within the realm of social justice. Such persistent discussion of the issues involved in their work reconfigures osteologists' role toward an inclusive, reflective practice in forensic anthropology. Therefore, in their efforts to provide scientifically sound analyses, osteologists also have to be champions of open practices that honor the history and identities of the populations they study, enriching their multifaceted role within both forensic and anthropological contexts.

6.2.1. Responsibilities of Forensic Osteologists

The responsibilities of forensic osteologists encompass a wide range of tasks, including the identification of skeletal remains and the interpretation of skeletal trauma. One of their primary duties is to analyze and document the condition of bones, typically determining the cause of death, post-mortem interval, and any potential pathological conditions. Forensic osteologists meticulously investigate the morphology and condition of bones to ascertain individual characteristics, such as age, sex, ancestry, and stature, and therefore, a critical amount of information is used to identify victims. Moreover, their profession extends to the examination of patterns of trauma that may be suggestive of homicide or accidents; hence, their expertise is crucial in criminal investigations. Findings derived from such experts not only assist the police but are also of fundamental significance in court, where their depositions can have a considerable impact on court decisions. Apart from the physical inspection of remains, forensic osteologists must also work with other forensic experts, which assist in the overall conclusion of cases. Interdisciplinarity is important because integrating various forms of forensic evidence makes conclusions more robust. Working with forensic anthropologists, crime scene examiners, and radiologists allows osteologists to build an overall picture of skeletal remains that they investigate. For example, the addition of radiographic imaging techniques can help estimate chronological age based on skeletal characteristics that cannot be seen with the naked eye. Awareness of the union of these disciplines is important to forensic osteologists, as it informs their approaches and enhances the quality of evidence in investigations and in court. As the literature has highlighted, training programs must address gaps in training so that practitioners gain the necessary knowledge and skills to enable practical interdisciplinary work (Fish et al., 2004). Forensic osteologists are also required to remain current with the new advances in forensic science and technological hardware that will aid their practice. For instance, technological advances in radiographic techniques have revolutionized age estimation methods, which play a crucial role in identifying remains, particularly when other techniques are inconclusive. New findings have illustrated the utility of radiographic examination in assessing skeletal features that reflect changes in body form throughout life, such as the development of epiphyseal scars that persist into adulthood (Schmeling et al., 2016). To carry out their responsibilities, forensic osteologists must continually build their expertise through ongoing learning and professional refreshers. Such passion for continuous learning not only strengthens their individual skills but also promotes the growth of forensic osteology as a discipline. By embracing new procedures and techniques, forensic osteologists make sure they can provide the reliable and accurate analysis required in the criminal justice system (Figure 6.5).

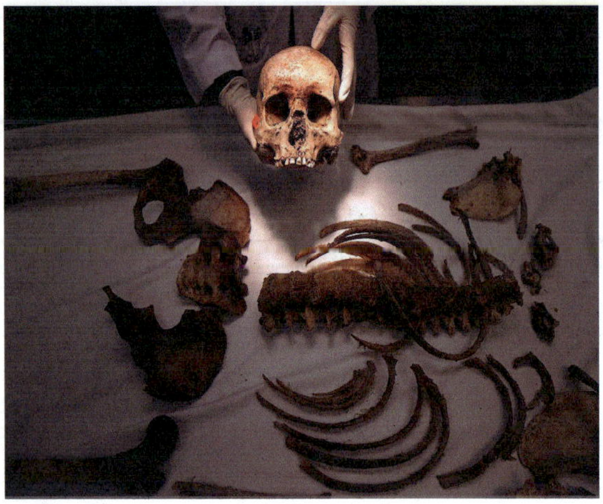

Figure 6.5. The responsibilities of forensic osteologists.

Source: https://www.thoughtco.com/thmb/9Zekgu7JKFgYudG8xVceed9XEFQ=/1500x0/filters:no_upscale():max_bytes(150000):strip_icc()/forensicanthropologist-5c771363c9e77c0001e98db3.jpg.

6.2.2. Collaboration with Law Enforcement

A successful partnership between forensic osteologists and the police is critical to the successful outcome of cases relating to skeletal remains. Such a partnership provides a holistic approach to crime scene investigation, especially in establishing the identity of unidentified remains and determining how a death occurred. Law enforcement professionals typically provide valuable context within the case, such as previous reports and neighborhood information, that may inform forensic analysis. These collaborations are typically established through formal training programs and workshops intended to meet at the interface of forensic science and investigative processes. Moreover, as indicated in recent surveys, investigative practitioners have given significant value in exchanging knowledge to enhance field practices. Taken together, these efforts reinforce the indispensable role of forensic osteology in the investigation of crime and emphasize the need for ongoing collaboration to maximize recovery of human remains (Klein et al., 2014). The establishment of human decomposition laboratories, such as the University of Tennessee's Anthropological Research Facility, represents a paradigm for collaborative forensic osteological and law enforcement investigations. These centers provide controlled environments in which scientists can study the effects of decomposition on human remains and thus better observe taphonomic change across various environments. Police forces can use their findings to refine investigative protocols as well as training programs.

The understanding developed not only enhances academic understanding but also offers practical applications in real-world situations, resulting in improved evidence collection and analysis at crime scenes. All these are required to enhance an atmosphere that allows both law enforcement and forensic science to develop and ultimately impact judicial outcomes (Fish et al., 2004). Along with this finding, the discovery of key skills needed in crime scene investigation identifies the immediate need for multidisciplinary collaboration in forensic science education. An examination of current graduate-level forensic science programs revealed curricular gaps that do not adequately prepare students for the challenges of forensic investigations. With the addition of experiential knowledge gained through collaborative work with police, training can better prepare new practitioners to function competently in advanced crime scenes. This progressive alignment of academic training with current research needs is critical to creating an effective workforce capable of conducting scientific and procedural aspects of forensic activities. As professional societies aim to formulate standard curricula, frequent collaboration with law enforcement will ensure that educational products remain relevant and useful in addressing the emerging challenges in forensic osteology and identification (Klein et al., 2014).

6.2.3. Importance of Expert Testimony in Court

In the court process, the provision of expert testimony is an important component in establishing facts and guiding juries through complex evidence. In under identification and forensic osteology, expert witnesses provide critical analysis of the skeleton, providing information pertinent to cases involving unidentified human remains. In line with research on the reliability of biological profiles derived from forensic anthropology reports, the specificity and uniqueness of expert testimony are crucial to ensuring reliable results in court. The validity of such evidence directly affects the judicial process because juries are likely to use knowledge provided by experts to make informed decisions regarding the guilt or innocence of defendants.

The presence of heavily validated expert evidence thus ensures that high standards of evidence are upheld in securing justice, particularly in cases based on forensic anthropology. With advancing forensic methods, the importance of statistical confirmation in expert evidence is all the more clear. The study's findings reveal that while the biological profile is highly accurate in determining sex and ancestry, certain differences should be used with caution if presented in court. For example, when ancestry estimates were correct in 99% of cases, issues encountered—especially with the Hispanic category—highlight the need for expert witnesses to be able to describe the nuances and limitations of their work effectively. Such variation not only enhances the credibility of expert testimony but also educates juries on the inherent complexity of forensic science. Therefore, professionals working in the field must specifically ascertain the findings of their analysis so that the court will comprehend the very high significance of these findings in identifying people and making case decisions, particularly where significant variations are involved in the creation of victims' bio-profiles. Additionally, the establishment of specialized research laboratories for human decomposition, such as Human Taphonomy Facilities and Green River Human Decay Laboratories, reflects the ongoing evolution of forensic sciences and the consequent need for informed expert testimony. Such laboratories support comprehensive studies of decomposition, which can provide insights into significant factors accountable for forensic identification.

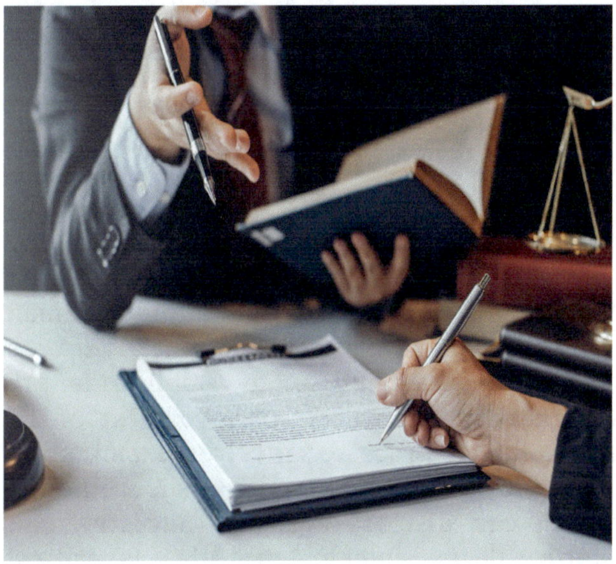

Figure 6.6. Importance of expert testimony in court.

Source: https://external-content.duckduckgo.com/iu/?u=https%3A%2F%2Flitiligroup.com%2Fwp-content%2Fuploads%2F2023%2F09%2Fshutterstock_1476113657.jpg&f=1&nofb=1&ipt=6d867014c5a2727a4803d3403cb4644dacd3efa8c19a4803aebf0e8d47646a14.

As forensic scientists become increasingly

involved in investigating the implications of decomposition processes, the demand for well-founded expert testimony grows, especially in grappling with the legal ramifications of what is found. In addition, as in the literature review of HTF development, the debate over their necessity underscores the complexity of delivering expert information in a legal setting. Through rigorous academic training, experts are prepared to appear in courtrooms where their evidence must bridge the gap between research and application, eventually leading to the closure of cold cases and solidifying the paramount significance of expert testimony in seeking justice (Figure 6.6).

Test Your Knowledge

1. What are the primary responsibilities of osteologists in research and forensic investigations?
2. How do osteologists contribute to the identification and interpretation of skeletal remains?

6.3. Techniques in Forensic Osteology

Learning Outcome

1. Methods of skeletal analysis
2. Use of technology in identification
3. Challenges in analyzing remains

Forensic osteology, the examination of human skeletal remains in forensic application, uses many techniques in order to establish identity and ascertain how death occurred. One of the fundamental processes involves examination of bone morphology and measurements, which can disclose age, sex, ancestry, and stature. This biological profiling is critical for identification, especially when deformed remains are encountered. The foot has been particularly identified as a precious asset in forensic identification, with its unique characteristics serving to reduce the number of possible individuals in missing persons' databases. Although so precious, there remains a considerable lack of literature on the contribution of the foot to forensic identification, underscoring the need for further research in this area (Barrett et al., 2014). The thorough study of such anatomical regions fortifies the forensic specialist's ability to provide reliable conclusions when only incomplete remains are available. In addition to morphology-based approaches, forensic osteology also integrates high-tech technology-based techniques such as imaging and DNA testing. Radiographic techniques such as X-ray and CT scans allow for non-destructive analyses of bone anatomy, which not only identify pathologies but also disclose features that can be used to identify. Besides, DNA profiling and extraction from bone remains have revolutionized forensic identification, particularly in cases of degraded remains where conventional visual examination may be unreliable. The deployment of such advanced techniques is evidence of the progression of forensic science, demonstrating how interdisciplinarity has significantly enhanced the precision of identification. Evidence shows that, through the convergence of traditional morphological techniques and modern scientific discoveries, the likelihood of successful identification even in unfavorable circumstances is enhanced (Studebaker-Reed et al., 2018). Such integration between methodologies is at the heart of forensic osteology. Training and experience are key determinants of the effectiveness of forensic osteology methodologies. Research shows substantial increases in the rate of recovery of evidence when individuals are formally trained in methods of skeletal recovery, with a focus on experiential learning (Studebaker-Reed et al., 2018). For practicing investigators involved in forensic investigations, understanding the aspects of skeletal recovery and identification is vital, as this knowledge directly affects whether their investigations are successful. Involvement of senior team members can assist junior researchers, ensuring that significant evidence is not overlooked. Additionally, new technologies and methods in the field require ongoing training for forensic professionals. With advances in forensic osteology, dedication to practice and learning will be key to maximizing overall efficiency in identifying human remains, thereby improving justice.

6.3.1. Methods of Skeletal Analysis

The analysis of skeletal remains is the basis for forensic osteology, and it performs critical functions in the identification of human beings and the estimation of demographic parameters. Methods of skeletal analysis encompass a range of techniques that assess skeletal attributes such as age, sex, ancestry, and stature. All of these attributes contribute a different element to the construction of a biological profile that helps forensic examiners to narrow potential identities. For example, pelvic morphology is usually employed to determine sex based on its dimorphic nature. Conversely, cranial measurements can provide strong evidence regarding ancestry. The creation of these profiles becomes important, especially in situations where fragments of human bones are recovered, a demonstration of how skeletal analysis can be used to identify individuals even when there are severe decomposition issues. These methods allow forensic specialists to make logical decisions based on skeletal integrity and morphological information to identify the probable victims in forensic investigations (Barrett et al., 2014). Moreover, retrieval of skeletons is complicated with fractured bones typically spread across crime scenes or natural surroundings. Research established the critical need for standardized techniques in evidence recovery to improve identification. A study that compared multivariate evidence recovery efforts found degrees of success to depend on searcher training and ability. Civilian volunteers conducted line searches through professionally trained forensic anthropologists and showed the critical role experience and specialized training have in successfully recovering human skeletal remains.

Understanding these distinctions is crucial to developing effective training protocols for law enforcement and recovery staff, thereby enhancing their ability to accurately identify remains through improved search methods (Studebaker-Reed et al., 2018). Increased knowledge of these factors leads to greater success in forensic examinations. Finally, avenues for future investigation and innovation in skeletal analysis methods are needed in order to advance forensic osteology. There is a lack of literature for the full analysis of certain skeletal components, such as the foot, which can significantly contribute to forensic identification. Research highlights the significance of the foot in human identification, particularly its distinguishing features, which are not well researched (Barrett et al., 2014). By closing these knowledge gaps, future research may once again ensure the validity and applicability of skeletal analysis in forensic anthropology, ultimately leading to higher identification rates in complex cases. Additionally, the integration of accessible technologies, such as 3D imaging and printing, could completely transform the way skeletal remains are compared and analyzed, paving the way for more precise forensic applications. The advancement of skeletal analysis methods will definitely continue to be a significant aspect of forensic investigations (Figure 6.7).

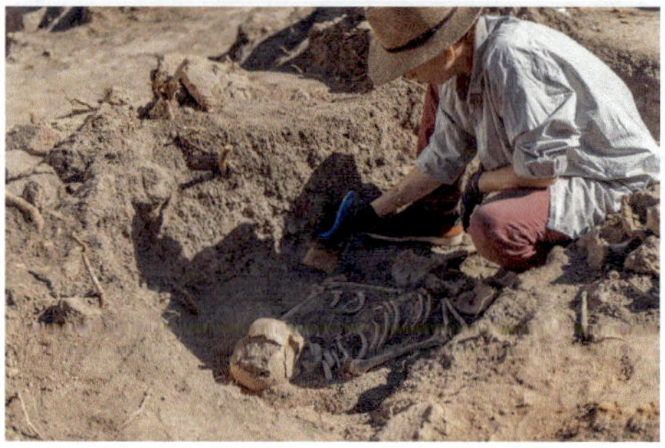

Figure 6.7. Methods of skeletal analysis.

Source: https://external-content.duckduckgo.com/iu/?u=https%3A%2F%2Fimperialacademy.org.uk%2Fwp-content%2Fuploads%2F2021%2F04%2FForensic-Anthropology-Skeletal-Analysis.jpg&f=1&nofb=1&ipt=ba9d62205991922f8ab71638e7245cc35a2605bdf23f6134a76c97562b74b2cd.

6.3.2. Use of Technology in Identification

Progressive technology has extensively altered the protocols of forensic identification, notably in forensic osteology. The use of DNA analysis has enabled forensic scientists to recover genetic material from skeletal remains, providing a more reliable means of identification. Emerging studies illustrate the application of emerging technologies such as peptide nucleic acid (PNA)-based DNA sequencing to identify age-related mutations in bone samples. This is an approach that not only improves the estimation accuracy of age but also enables validation of identity through genetic markers, thereby complementing standard osteological analysis. Therefore, the use of modern technology in forensic identification is a critical advancement that can improve the credibility of evidence in both new and old cases (Brandstätter et al., 2008). Also, the combination of diverse forensic sciences demonstrates how technology can be employed to develop integrated identification methods. A case had shown that the collaboration between anthropology, odontology, facial reconstruction, and genetics was instrumental in identifying a motorcycle accident victim whose body was nearly skeletonized. With intensive analysis, investigators were able to establish the age, sex, and perimortem trauma of the victims, thereby creating a complete profile. Worth highlighting, DNA analysis further confirmed the finding, having identified genetic material against that of the victim's family. Multidisciplinary in its approach, this strategy underscores the value of using diverse technological means to streamline and reinforce identification efforts—virtually reducing the list of potential candidates and optimizing resource allocation for law enforcement agencies (Eliopoulos et al., 2025). Accompanying these innovations are computer models and three-dimensional imaging that have further transformed forensic identification procedures. With the of skeletons, forensic anthropologists can create more realistic visual images of individuals from their skeletons. In addition to helping with public identification procedures, such technology also facilitates the reintegration of missing individuals into their social units. With evolving forensic methods, the potential for even more accurate identification is even greater. The integration of osteology and technology clearly illustrates how these tools can be brought together for the overall goal of forensic science, ultimately delivering more effective case resolutions for cases involving unidentified remains. This ongoing blending of technology is a testament to the field's commitment to constantly be better for the sake of justice and truth.

6.3.3. Challenges in Analyzing Remains

Skeletal analysis poses significant challenges that can complicate forensic osteologists' operations. One of the primary challenges is the commingling of remains, which can occur in a scenario where a grave is disturbed or a mass grave is excavated. For example, while conducting a study of a mixed sample from Minnesota's Acacia Park Cemetery, scholars were faced with the challenge of collecting the minimum number of individuals that are in a complication of a cluster of bones. It was a challenge that required keen metric and visual inspection to differentiate and enumerate each individual, finally revealing at least 25 distinct bones.

These demands require not only advanced osteological techniques but also extensive background information on ancient contexts, since burial practices themselves and how they change over time can pose additional difficulties for analysis. Distinguishing between human remains and nonhuman skeletal material is another significant problem and involves particularly great difficulties in contexts where both are prevalent. This issue is commonly faced by forensic anthropologists working in medical examiner's offices, where animal and human bones may coexist. An interesting study conducted in Kenosha County revealed that about 74% of the bones recovered were nonhuman, predominantly those of white-tailed deer and domestic pigs. Such overlapping demands require extensive training in osteological distinction and identification, since misidentification may lead to incorrect inferences about the remains being analyzed. Effective forensic analysis relies heavily on the accuracy of these judgments, so the challenge of distinction is not theoretical but practical, with concrete implications for justice and identification processes. Furthermore, the environment in which the remains were found can significantly affect their analysis and interpretation. As in the case of the Acacia Park Cemetery skeletal remains, understanding the demographic and cultural context of individuals is crucial. The cemetery held significance for European settlers and the Dakota people alike, underscoring the need to incorporate socio-cultural aspects into osteological analysis. Historical records of the remains can inform investigators about the deceased's health patterns and lifestyle behaviors, but these are typically obscured by the physical degradation of the remains over time. Therefore, forensic osteologists must contend not merely with problems in the biological examination of remains but also with retelling the narratives that such remains can tell us about the past, thereby compounding the problem of forensic identification (Figure 6.8).

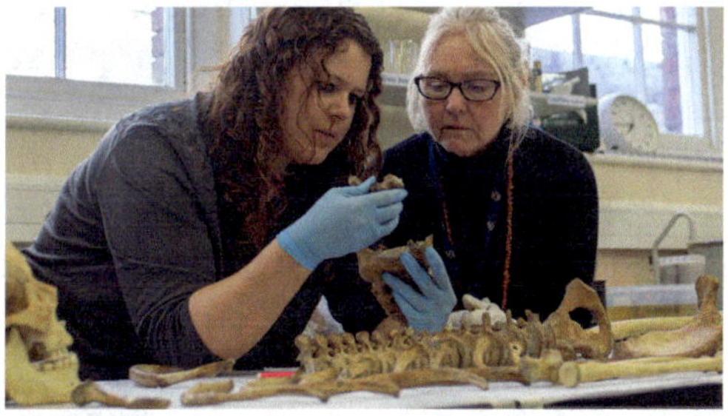

Figure 6.8. The analysis of skeletal remains poses significant challenges.

Source: https://external-content.duckduckgo.com/iu/?u=https%3A%2F%2Fmaryrose.org%2Fwp-content%2Fuploads%2F2024%2F03%2Fhuman-remains-examine.jpg&f=1&nofb=1&ipt=b4a4eada6bed4472e6285be5d04e7e21f5afec0f996e284385ea917302f9740f.

Test Your Knowledge

1. What techniques are commonly used in forensic osteology to analyze skeletal remains?
2. How do osteological techniques assist in determining age, sex, and ancestry of skeletal remains?

6.4. Determining Age, Sex, and Ancestry

Learning Outcome

1. Techniques for estimating age from bones
2. Methods for determining biological sex
3. Ancestry estimation through skeletal features

In forensic osteology, determining age, sex, and ancestry from skeletal remains is essential to the identification process. Careful evaluation of these biological factors can often significantly narrow the range of possible matches for unidentified individuals. This multidimensional evaluation includes comparisons of bone morphological features, which can vary significantly across age groups, sexes, and ancestral populations. Dental attrition, epiphyseal fusion, and cranial development characteristics are typically used to estimate age, while pelvic and cranial measurements play an important role in determining sex. Specific skeletal characteristics associated with various ancestral populations also play a vital role in reconstructing the biological profile of the deceased, thereby supporting the identification process as a whole. Furthermore, improvements in forensic methods have reinforced the credibility and validity of these findings. With further development in forensic science, it has embraced the latest technologies, such as DNA analysis and three-dimensional imaging, which enable forensic scientists to extract more in-depth information from remains. These technologies have been shown to be capable of validating or enhancing age, sex, and ancestry determinations on empirical grounds, thereby overcoming the limitations of traditional morphometric analyses. Of particular interest, however, are situations in which challenges arise, such as when the remains are degraded or fragmented, thus complicating the identification process. In this case, investigative experts should be cognizant of the impact on forensic evidence, particularly in high-profile cases with media and public interest, as exemplified by reports of unidentified remains in various incidents in North America (Barrett et al., 2014). The complexities of forensic osteology extend beyond mere physical observation to include moral factors in cases of historical significance or general interest. The fame surrounding Amelia Earhart's disappearance is a haunting case in point; attempts at identifying potential remains attributed to her demonstrate the delicate distinction between scientific interest and popular opinion. A 1940 examination had concluded the skeletal remains were those of a middle-aged, stocky male, but subsequent examinations in 1998 put forth other conclusions hypothesizing feminine traits that could equate to Earhart (Cross et al., 2015). This is against the notion and controversy of calculating age, sex, and ancestry in forensic examination, echoing the need to think cautiously about results and to encourage collaborative discourse among multidisciplinary teams to draw informed conclusions. Consequently, ongoing investigation and methodological advancement will increasingly enhance the fidelity of identifications in forensic osteology.

6.4.1. Techniques for Estimating Age from Bones

Age estimation from bones is a core component of forensic osteology, applied to yield the biological profiles required for identification. Various methodologies have evolved, each playing a different tune to accuracy and practicability. Among these methods, dental development anatomy is a good technique, especially at the adolescent and juvenile levels. Teeth develop in a stable order and can provide an estimate of age within a year or two. Moreover, the analysis of epiphyseal fusion in long bones is particularly useful: growth plates fuse at known ages, and anthropologists can determine levels of maturity and infer age ranges. The techniques, while effective, may require additional analyses to complement them due to variation caused by nutrition, health, etc., highlighting the value of a multifaceted approach in forensic identification. Histological techniques have also emerged as a forefront approach in bone age estimation, particularly in adults. Histomorphometry, a quantitative examination of bone tissue microstructure, provides informative data on bone density and bone remodeling rates. Using this technique, forensic experts can measure osteon morphology quantitatively, thereby revealing a person's age at the time of death. This method counteracts biases inherent in examiner subjectivity by relying on measurable factors that can be compared across populations. Specifically, the method has been effective in analyzing numerous skeletal components, such as the femur and clavicle.

Though the latter has not been extensively investigated, it offers distinguishing features that could improve forensic use, thereby making it a target of current research into osteology and identification (Inthasan et al., 2017). Lastly, the harmonization of age-estimation methods underscores the importance of an integrated approach in forensic osteology. While traditional methods that rely on macroscopic features are rich sources of information, histological assessments enhance understanding of skeletal development and lifespan. The dynamics of human biological growth call for an integrated approach that accounts for demographic variations. Techniques must not be taken individually; they must instead inform and complement one another to increase the precision of age estimates. As forensic practitioners confront increasingly challenging cases, e.g., fragmentary or deteriorated remains, the ongoing refinement of these techniques will be critical for shaping forensic science and for correctly identifying humans (Barrett et al., 2014) (Figure 6.9).

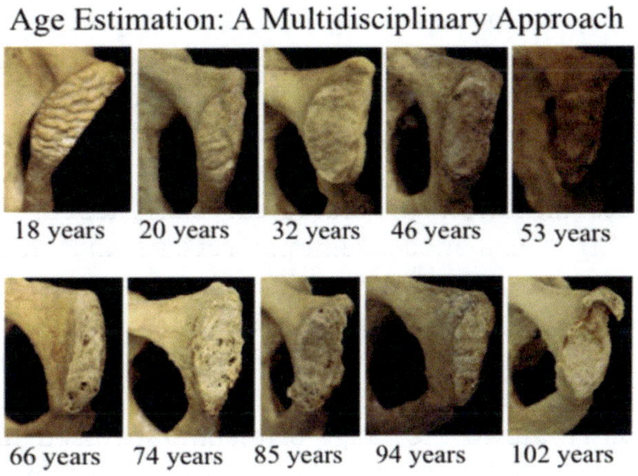

Figure 6.9. Techniques for estimating age from bones.

Source: https://ars.els-cdn.com/content/image/3-s2.0-B9780128144916000054-f05-01-9780128144916.jpg.

6.4.2. Methods for Determining Biological Sex

Determination of biological sex from bones is among the most important aspects of forensic osteology. Various bone structures provide important information for sex determination, but two are of particular interest: the pelvis and the skull. The pelvis, since it is structurally adapted for childbirth, exhibits strong sexual dimorphism; males have typically a narrower pelvis inlet and a greater sciatic notch, while females exhibit wider structures to facilitate childbirth. However, the skull is also characterized by distinct features, including brow ridge, mastoid process, and mandible shape strength, that are usually variable and associated with biological sex. Such osteological attributes are applied by forensic anthropologists in establishing a plausible biological profile, which plays a crucial role in linking cases in forensic casework (Bosnar et al., 2010). While sex determination centers on the skull and pelvis, the mandible has not yet been pushed to its maximum in this respect. Recent studies have explored morphological and metrical methods for assessing sexual dimorphism in the mandible, which is especially important in cases where other skeletal parts are unavailable. Bimental breadth and corpus thickness have emerged as significant parameters in sexual determination of biological sex. Research using these measurements reveals that the mandible can generate discriminant function equations that enable sex identification with an accuracy of up to 77.3%. The research reveals that mandibular measurements can contribute to the range of techniques used to determine biological sex and thus provide a valuable tool for forensic anthropology in cases involving poorly preserved skeletons (Borrini et al., 2017). It is the application of over one skeletal indicator to determine biological sex that gives forensic evaluations more strength. With the incorporation of a combination of old methods with new ones, such as geometric morphometrics and advanced statistical tests, forensic anthropologists can gather more precision when making sex estimations. The multi-level approach can overcome the variation observed in human skeletal remains, thereby improving identification outcomes. Besides this, methodological refinement, for instance, in terms of fresh discriminant functions and indices from different samples of populations, is a necessity. Not only does it enhance biological sex determination, but it also offers methods to further precision in forensic analysis toward ultimately realizing justice in court cases (Bosnar et al., 2010).

6.4.3. Ancestry Estimation Through Skeletal Features

Ancestry estimation based on skeletal traits is an essential aspect of forensic osteology, as it is a significant part of the human remains identification process. Based on assessments of certain morphological traits of bones, forensic experts can infer an individual's geographical and ancestral origins. The process becomes particularly complex when dealing with fragmented remains, a common scenario in forensic investigations. As noted in the literature, practical interpretation of skeletal characteristics is often hampered by the fact that crime scene or other evidence recovered is usually fragmentary, and therefore advanced approaches are needed for accurate ancestry estimation. Therefore, not only is the determination of skeletal characteristics a scientific endeavor, but it also bleeds into cultural elements that pertain to personal identity and forensic conclusions in the law (Barrett et al., 2014). When determining ancestry from skeletal characteristics, markers such as cranial characteristics, dental morphology, and postcranial measurements are thoroughly examined. All these markers play an important role in estimating demographic estimates.

For instance, cranial shapes and sizes can be related to particular population groups, allowing forensic anthropologists to make reasonable estimates of an individual's ancestry. Also, techniques such as geometric morphometrics are used to quantify variation in skeletal features, enabling researchers to achieve higher accuracy in ancestry estimation. This method has extensive applications, particularly in forensic use, where accurate identification can benefit legal proceedings, the general population, and health outcomes across various populations (Winter et al., 2016). The use of advanced forensic techniques to calculate ancestry has revolutionized the traditional process, thereby enhancing the accuracy of demographic reconstructions.

In particular, the analysis of mixed remains, as demonstrated through the investigation of skeletal samples from the Acacia Park Cemetery, shows the step-by-step approach required for successful estimation of ancestry and other biological profiles. By applying established osteological standards, researchers can analyze diverse skeletal remains to reconstruct demographic profiles based on variables such as health condition and activity patterns. Such a close inspection not only aids in forensic identification but also contributes to anthropological knowledge of the patterns of populations through time. As such, ancestry prediction based on skeletal features is a valuable contribution to forensic osteology, enhancing knowledge of human diversity and the fascination surrounding identity in a forensic context (Winter et al., 2016) (Figure 6.10).

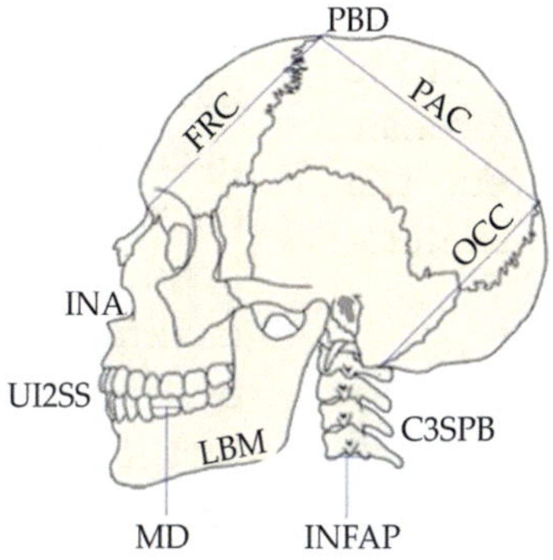

Figure 6.10. Ancestry estimation through skeletal features.

Source: https://wires.onlinelibrary.wiley.com/cms/asset/9143d663-477e-4e82-8479-a5da4ebf4427/wfs21369-toc-0001-m.jpg.

Test Your Knowledge

1. What skeletal features are used to determine age, sex, and ancestry in forensic osteology?
2. How do methods for estimating age, sex, and ancestry differ between subadult and adult skeletal remains?

6.5. Trauma Analysis

Learning Outcome

1. Identifying perimortem versus postmortem injuries
2. Types of trauma commonly analyzed
3. Implications of trauma findings in investigations

In forensic osteology, the examination of trauma is of critical significance in identifying the circumstances of death of a skeletal individual. Trauma can be broadly divided into perimortem and postmortem injuries, both providing diverse information regarding the timing and nature of the incident. Perimortem fractures will often have characteristic features that indicate the circumstances under which they were sustained. Researchers have come to recognize features such as layered breakage and crushed margins that are associated with injuries sustained at or near the time of death. They are important as they can be utilized to differentiate between violent interaction-caused injuries and those caused by forces of the environment after death, thus helping forensic scientists develop a clearer account of events leading up to death. Also, understanding the decomposition process adds vital context to forensic analysis of trauma. Mass grave analysis provides information on how rates of decomposition are influenced by several variables, thus making the presence of observable trauma on skeletal remains determinable. Research into carcass decomposition patterns at various burial depths indicated significant differences by position, with more deeply buried carcasses exhibiting higher decomposition levels. This understanding underlines the importance of conditions of the environment and burial practices in forensic osteology because they directly affect the preservation or destruction of the skeletal markers for trauma.

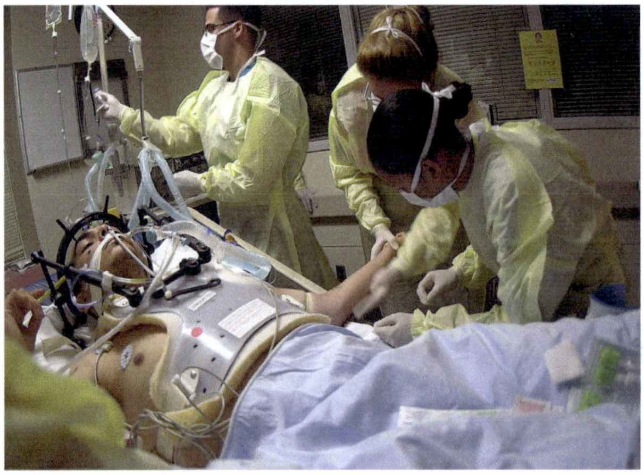

Figure 6.11. The trauma analysis is critical for establishing the circumstances surrounding a skeletal individuals death.

Source: https://upload.wikimedia.org/wikipedia/commons/thumb/a/aa/US_Navy_040723-N-8977L-008_Navy_Hospital_Corpsmen_and_Medical_Officers_assess_the_treatment_and_prognosis_of_a_patient_with_a_gunshot_wound.jpg/960px-US_Navy_040723-N-8977L-008_Navy_Hospital_Corpsmen_and_Medical_Officers_assess_the_treatment_and_prognosis_of_a_patient_with_a_gunshot_wound.jpg.

The integration of decomposition analysis with the assessment of trauma is of paramount importance in reaching a proper understanding of the skeletal remains, thus aiding legal investigations by providing forensic experts with information regarding the probable time and nature of injury caused. Besides these, establishing the timing of an injury remains a challenging aspect of forensic anthropology. The typical perimortem fracture features can serve as the significant markers in assessing the trauma context. Wave lines and resultant flake defects have been found to be possible perimortem condition indicators that allow forensic analysts to infer biomechanical forces involved in injury. These indications not only facilitate discrimination among various types of fractures but also allow one to explore further the physical dynamics of trauma. As research continues, the inclusion of more detailed analyses of these characteristics will enhance understanding of skeletal remains in forensic cases, ultimately leading to more conclusive findings in criminal investigations and to the identification of trauma in intra vitam conditions, in line with conclusions reached in the field of forensic osteology and identification (Figure 6.11).

6.5.1. Identifying Perimortem Versus Postmortem Injuries

Identification of perimortem vs. postmortem injuries is crucial in the science of forensic osteology to understand the circumstances under which death has happened. Perimortem injuries refer to those that occur around the time of death and are typically associated with physiological phenomena at that moment, whereas postmortem injuries are those that occur after death. In contrast, postmortem injuries occur after the subject's biological processes have ceased. Assessing these types of injury involves a critical analysis of the break patterns, as some characteristics may indicate the time of injury. For example, fractures that exhibit layered break, bone scales, and crushed edges typically indicate perimortem conditions. Comparative research between fresh and dry bone injuries shows that these markers inherently point back to the biomechanics and trauma suffered at the moment of life, thus assisting forensic practitioners in creating more accurate timelines relative to the injuries that the deceased had sustained (Dalmases et al., 2017). When looking at cranial traumas suffered in human remains from the past, it becomes more essential to establish whether injuries are perimortem or postmortem. Current studies analyzing cranial trauma from specific archaeological sites validate the high incidence of perimortem trauma, hence interpersonal violence.

The study of 84 adult crania revealed that there was a high incidence of perimortem injuries, and the occurrence varied by sex. For instance, male subjects presented with trauma in greater frequency than females, revealing societal interactions that may have contributed to the high occurrence of such trauma. This information is crucial in reconstituting the life context and social culture of former communities, eventually completing our understanding of human interactions and violence in the past (Bedić et al., 2021). Furthermore, the importance of identifying perimortem and postmortem wounds extends to law enforcement situations, where the validity of remains is assessed for criminal investigations. Accurate differentiation can significantly contribute to homicide investigations by validating the nature of the injury and its relation to cause of death.

Forensic anthropologists employ precise protocols and tests to determine skeletal injury timing, and their opinions carry greater legal significance. Because aspects of perimortem injuries not just show the level of physical force but also the victim's state when they died, they may become key evidence in court cases. Therefore, the intersection of forensic science and anthropological studies provides an empathetic interpretation of osteological research, which assists forensic scientists in making comprehensive narratives around human death and trauma (Dalmases et al., 2017) (Figure 6.12).

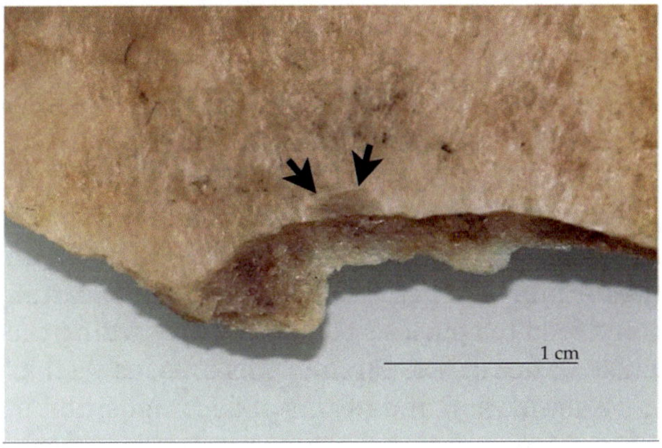

Figure 6.12. Identifying perimortem versus postmortem injuries.

Source: https://media.springernature.com/lw1200/springer-static/image/art%3A10.1007%2Fs00414-020-02356-3/MediaObjects/414_2020_2356_Fig4_HTML.jpg.

6.5.2. Types of Trauma Commonly Analyzed

In forensic osteology, various types of trauma are analyzed to shed light on the circumstances in which the skeletal remains existed. Such traumas are all generally categorized as perimortem and postmortem injuries, which have specific characteristics that may prove beneficial to forensic examiners when investigating. Perimortem trauma is caused close to death, and as such, the individual ought to have still been alive upon the injury, and as would be expected, manifests itself as fractures that show features like layered fracture and crushed margins.

The features explain the biomechanics of the trauma and are employed to ascertain the time and cause of death. Understanding of these fractures is not just important for identification but also for reconstruction of the events leading to an individual's death, heightening the situational analysis skill of the forensic anthropologists. Postmortem trauma, however, is trauma inflicted after death, commonly by the forces of the environment, animals, or man. This form of trauma does not have the same well-defined features as perimortem trauma and is harder to assess. Brittle, dry fractures, which remain intact under some environmental conditions, are among the common features of postmortem changes. Forensic analysts must develop a good sense of discrimination between these injuries because incorrect identification could lead to spurious conclusions regarding the cause of death. Research in this area, as well as the examination of patterns of decomposition in mass graves, has clarified how various factors can influence the appearance of postmortem trauma and provide valuable information regarding the circumstances under which skeletal remains are deposited (Adlam et al., 2014).

The determination of trauma types in forensic science can be significantly enhanced through quantitative research methods, whereby forensic scientists can extractively study findings and offer patterns. Research has cited some features that are associated with perimortem fractures, such as wave lines and related flake defects, which are not only markers of the type of trauma but also the severity of the force that resulted in it.

By correlating such distinct patterns with specific circumstances, forensic anthropologists can gain a clearer understanding of the mechanisms and, perhaps, the intent behind inflicting the trauma (Dalmases et al., 2017). The determination of trauma thus remains a core aspect of forensic osteology, providing significant data that serves to assist legal identification processes as well as feeding into broader investigative discourses of violent crime or unintentional death (Figure 6.13).

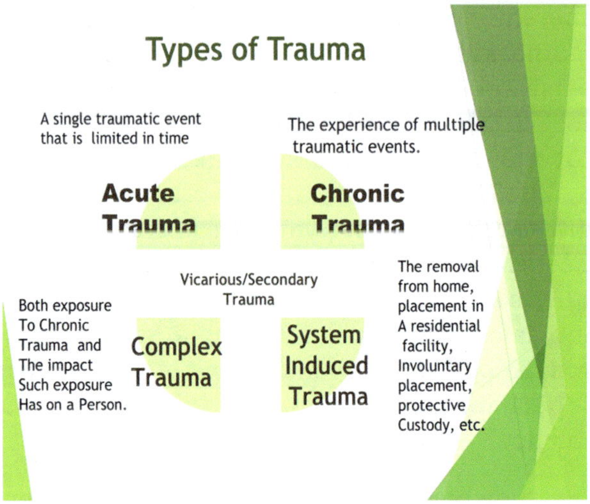

Figure 6.13. Types of trauma commonly analyzed.

Source: https://external-content.duckduckgo.com/iu/?u=https%3A%2F%2Fimage4.slideserve.com%2F8780773%2Ftypes-of-trauma-l.jpg&f=1&nofb=1&ipt=098e0e8c45e2cc8cb484691c45cb2a31d396057d8fb3ca0159ed4601eae98b4b.

6.5.3. Implications of Trauma Findings in Investigations

The examination of trauma findings in forensic osteology plays a critical role in investigations, particularly in the identification of remains and determining the circumstances of death. By analyzing skeletal injuries, forensic experts can differentiate between ante-mortem, peri-mortem, and post-mortem traumas, which significantly impacts the interpretation of findings. This nuanced understanding helps establish timelines and causes of death, providing insight into the events leading up to and following the individual's demise. Moreover, trauma analysis can offer vital information regarding the manner of death, whether it be due to accident, homicide, or other causes. This information is not solely of interest to the forensic community; it also holds implications for legal proceedings, as accurate trauma assessment can influence judicial outcomes and the provision of justice for victims and their families. Additionally, trauma findings can reveal patterns of violence that may suggest broader social issues, such as domestic abuse or systemic violence within communities. Forensic osteologists are not just examining individual cases but, through thorough documentation of trauma types and frequencies, can contribute to larger datasets that inform public health responses and policymaking. Through research, it has been demonstrated that conditions such as compactness within burial contexts can influence decomposition rates and, consequently, the visibility of trauma on remains. The implications of understanding such environmental factors extend to the interpretation of trauma, as outlined by research into mass graves, which reveals that specific trauma patterns may be obscured or accentuated depending on burial methods and conditions (Adlam et al., 2014). This body of knowledge can guide future investigations, providing a framework for understanding trauma in different contexts. Moreover, the examination of skeletal remains can extend beyond traumatic injuries to inform about the lived experiences of individuals, including maternal and fetal health. The study of fetal paleopathology, for instance, demonstrates the potential of skeletal analysis to provide stratified insights into the lives of mothers and infants, shedding light on past societal structures and health outcomes. Such research also underscores the complexities of trauma analysis as it relates to the social and health dynamics of historical populations (Lewis et al., 2017). The integration of trauma findings into broader historical and social narratives enhances the interpretative value of forensic osteology, allowing investigators not solely to solve cases but to contribute to a more nuanced understanding of human life and societal health trends across time. Consequently, trauma findings in forensic investigations do not exist in isolation; they are integral to a holistic comprehension of history and the multidimensional impacts of trauma on individuals and communities alike.

Test Your Knowledge

1. What are the key methods used to analyze skeletal trauma in forensic and archaeological contexts?
2. How can trauma analysis distinguish between ante-mortem, peri-mortem, and post-mortem injuries?

6.6. Case Studies

Learning Outcome

1. Famous forensic osteology cases
2. Lessons learned from these cases
3. Impact on the field and future investigations

Case studies are at the heart of forensic osteology, serving as digital representations of digital complexity in human identification remains. They provide a detailed illustration of forensic practitioners' techniques and variations in recovery methods based on the skill level of the searchers. For instance, a study that compared evidence recovery conducted by scientists with varying levels of experience nicely showed that learning significantly enhances the recovery success rates. By contrasting civilian volunteers with first responders and forensic anthropology students, researchers could not only test the effectiveness of different searching strategies but also highlight the importance of specialized training programs in optimizing the recovery of forensic data (Studebaker-Reed et al., 2018). These studies underscore the central importance of case studies in refining identification methods and debunking recovery process mythologies. Moreover, case studies highlight the specific recovery and identification challenges posed by fragmented remains, which tend to elude simplistic approaches. For instance, recent incidents where severed lower limbs and feet were washed up on the coastlines have underscored the challenges facing forensic practitioners in the process of identifying these remains. Media reporting of such a case increases public curiosity but also identifies significant gaps in the hitherto literature on anatomical human identification problems, particularly concerning the foot (Barrett et al., 2014). By studying such specific cases, case studies not only contribute to the knowledge base necessary for forensic science but also necessitate further focused research in fields that are yet underrepresented. The interconnectedness of these problems is characteristic of how case studies drive the creation of forensic osteological procedures. Finally, case studies in forensic osteology extend beyond descriptive use; they directly influence the creation of policy and procedures within the field. By documenting a single case in depth, professionals can compare forensic outcomes and develop best practices that can be applied to all future investigations. This feedback mechanism ensures continuous improvement in human remains recovery and identification methods, especially in the presence of emerging forensic technologies. Synthesizing information from incongruent case experiences enhances coordination among forensic professionals and fosters interdisciplinary measures that integrate anatomical science, law enforcement practices, and public health concerns. Therefore, the application of case studies in forensic osteology can never be overstressed, because not only do they enhance scholarship but also bridge the gap between theory and practice for forensic identification (Figure 6.14).

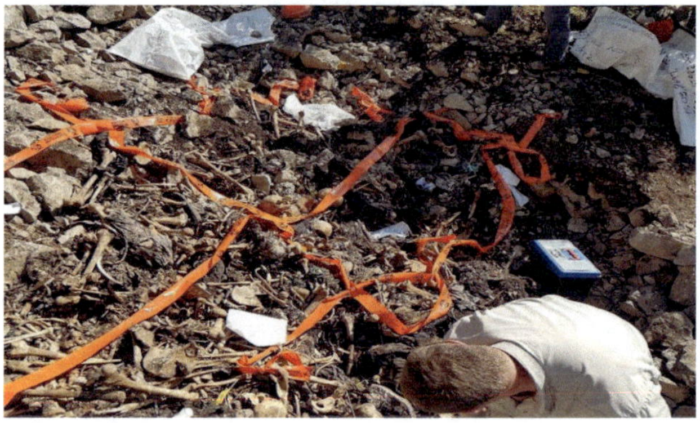

Figure 6.14. Case studies play a pivotal role in the field of forensic osteology.

Source: https://cdn-wordpress-info.futurelearn.com/info/wp-content/uploads/48836409886_970af20cb9_c-768x577.jpg.

6.6.1. Famous Forensic Osteology Cases

The connection between forensic osteology and criminal cases runs deep, as attested by numerous celebrity cases that illuminate the science's critical role in interpreting skeletal remains. One case was the exhumation of human skeletons from a mass grave in Southern Estonia, where anthropological analysis played a key role in determining the biological sex and age at death of the victims buried there. Scientists used conventional aging and sexing methods and demonstrated the usefulness of forensic osteology by comparing the findings with the historical records of the deceased. This case shows how sound methodology in forensic investigation can reveal information about historical events while demonstrating the utility of skeletal remains in establishing identity and acquiring knowledge of past social hierarchies (Allmäe et al., 2015). A stronger example of forensic osteology is the Vigilante serial killer case, where the study of bone remains played a key role in solving the case. In this instance, forensic osteologists used high-tech imaging techniques to analyze the skeletal features of the victims. These processes not only verified the identities of the victims but also played a significant role in reconstructing the sequence of events in the crimes. By analyzing factors such as the stage of bone growth and trauma, forensic scientists provided investigators with persuasive evidence that informed the direction of the investigation and directly helped apprehend the perpetrator. This shows how forensic osteology can be applied both as a diagnostic tool and as narrative media, telling, in the language of story, that already inheres within bones (Ahmed et al., 2017). Forensic osteology's application goes beyond individual cases to contribute to a' larger understanding of human remains within both the past and the present. Worthy of mention is the contribution of osteology to the detection of mass disasters in the modern era, with forensic practitioners making strides in analyzing remains from war and natural disasters. This not only helps identify victims but also provides closure to affected communities and families touched by the disasters. Forensic osteologists apply a combination of historical understanding and modern techniques, such as 3D reconstruction, to bring light to commonly disorganized situations. With the power of skeletal examination, forensic specialists uphold the integrity of the deceased while facilitating the meticulous process of identification and accountability after tragedies (Allmäe et al., 2015).

6.6.2. Lessons Learned From These Cases

In examining forensic osteology and the identification of remains, several valuable lessons can be drawn from analyses of various cases. Most significant among these is the need for careful, precise differentiation between skeletal remains of human or nonhuman origin, as highlighted by the occurrence of nonhuman bone accumulation in forensic cases. For example, the Office of the Chief Medical Examiner of Kenosha County identified that a high proportion of skeletal remains were not human, emphasizing the need for special training in this regard. Accurate identification can significantly influence investigative results and the ensuing legal procedures. Hence, integrating inclusive training courses that focus on common nonhuman taxa such as white-tailed deer and domesticated animals has the potential to augment the ability of forensic anthropologists to perform timely and sound assessments of remains in diverse conditions (Fourshee et al., 2022). Information from Disaster Victim Identification (DVI) missions also enhances forensic osteology and observes the absolutely indispensable essence of interdisciplinarity. Forensic anthropologists are now well known for their functions in DVI, where they apply their expertise to improve the identification process in mass disasters significantly. What has been learned from recent DVI experiences indicates that the work of forensic anthropologists goes beyond identification; they play a significant role in implementing systematic processes that include the use of various forensic procedures, such as imaging and tissue sampling, to support DNA analysis.

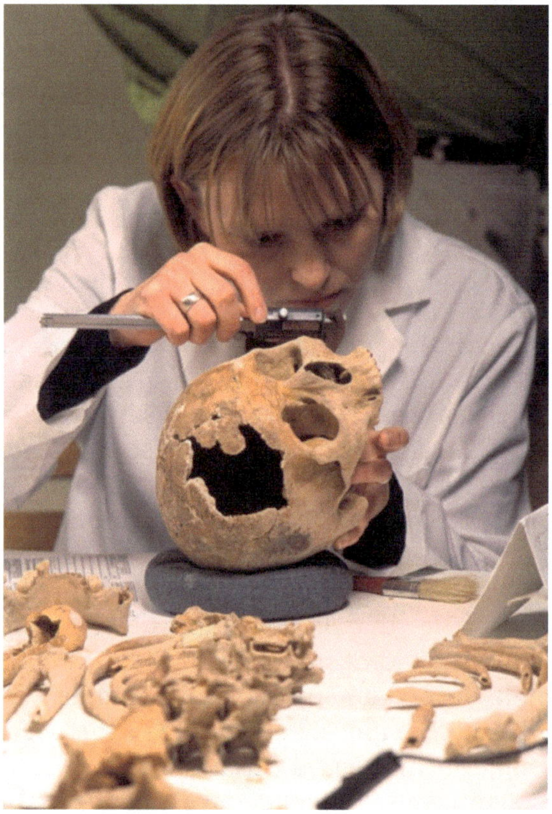

Figure 6.15. In examining forensic osteology and the identification of remains.

Source: https://wp.stu.ca/forensicscience/wp-content/uploads/sites/22/2015/04/Forensic-Anthropology-forensic-anthropology-6380688-1200-1783-689x1024.jpg.

Given the above complexities, it is apparent that multidisciplinary cooperation among forensic specialists is of utmost significance for fruitful case management and identification procedures in such perilous disaster scenarios (Acharya J et al., 2018). In addition, the cases highlight the ethical measures and the psychological preparedness required in forensic anthropological practice. Since practitioners are exposed to emotionally charged scenarios, particularly in relief operations during disasters, the matter of self-care and resilience should be highlighted enough. Without sacrificing scientific rigor, compassion ensures that concerns of both the remains under study and their families are addressed with respect and sensitivity. This holistic perspective is intended to remind forensic anthropologists of their important social role in addressing not only the scientific aspects of identification but also the emotional weight their work will carry. Consequently, the lessons from these experiences highlight the importance of establishing and maintaining strict training protocols alongside a sensitive practice style in forensic osteology and identification (Figure 6.15).

6.6.3. Impact on the Field and Future Investigations

The discipline of forensic osteology has witnessed significant advancements, particularly through the use of new methods that enhance the accuracy and confidence of identification. The use of antemortem and postmortem radiographs has traditionally been set against a backdrop of sparse antemortem records. However, recent studies show that using more readily accessible radiographic data, such as panoramic dental radiographs, can address this deficiency. These images provide excellent visualization of the maxillary sinus region, enabling forensic anthropologists to leverage advanced analyses to make identifications. According to research findings, geometric morphometric and visual analyses of maxillary sinus shape yield promising results for positive identification and have the potential to revolutionize methodologies in the field (Collins et al., 2014). These are valuable because they have the direct potential to aid in the resolution of unidentified remains, ultimately fulfilling the interests of justice and society. The implications of such developments extend beyond immediate uses in identification, influencing the future direction of forensic science and inter-disciplinary collaborations. Institutions committed to reconciling the various disciplines, such as ToScA North America, have a key role in facilitating the evolution of forensic methodologies. Through facilitating synergy between multi-modal imaging techniques, earth sciences, and biological sciences, they pave the way for an integrated methodology for forensic osteology (Ahmed et al., 2017). This convergence is essential to solving the problems surrounding human remains because it not only raises the methodological level of forensic investigation but also broadens the pool of knowledge available to researchers and practitioners. Through this academic institution's evolution, it will drive further innovations that enhance investigative efficiency, further solidifying forensic osteology's role as an anchoring pillar of medicolegal processes. In addition, as forensic osteology continues to advance, it can potentially influence educational models and training programs in the field. Shifting new techniques and modes of analysis to students and professionals alike is highly important for developing capable professionals who can address the challenges of modern forensic testing. Educational outreach programs, along with hands-on research experience, will ensure that the next generation of forensic anthropologists is well equipped with the requisite skills and expertise to utilize the latest technologies effectively. Furthermore, ongoing collaborative research activities that utilize the latest imaging and analysis tools will not only render existing practices more sophisticated but also instill an ethos of ongoing learning and adaptation. Finally, the forward momentum in forensic osteology can further enhance overall investigative capabilities, with a significant impact on current and future methods in pursuit of identification and justice.

Test Your Knowledge

1. Who are some key figures that have played a pivotal role in the development of forensic osteology?
2. What contributions have these pioneers made to the methods and applications of forensic osteology?

SUMMARY

Forensic osteology plays a dominant role in human remains identification, bridging the gap between archaeology and forensic science. Through detailed study of skeletal remains, forensic osteologists can unlock valuable information vital to legal inquiries and archaeological research. The importance of human osteology enables these professionals to ascertain data such as age, sex, ancestry, and, in certain instances, even trauma, which is invaluable to law enforcement agencies as it helps in closing missing persons or homicide cases. The integration of recent technologies, such as three-dimensional scanning, has further enhanced the accuracy of these examinations, enabling better identification and placing forensic and archaeological contexts in greater value. Furthermore, the Amelia Earhart case illustrates the complexities and challenges of forensic identification. Although initial investigations suggested that the skeletal remains found on Nikumaroro belonged to Earhart, subsequent examinations challenged such findings. The re-examination of the evidence based on modern methods indicates the need for continual questioning of forensic science. Reliance on early findings alone, without concern for changes in methodology, would lead to incorrect conclusions; thereforethe necessity of finding , the necessity of finding an equilibrium that involves both established knowledge and new analytical methods. As forensic osteology continues to evolve, it is essential to identify the high standards that make up the science to ensure that all findings are aligned with the bigger picture in the science. Briefly, forensic osteology is where science, law, and history come together to give a unique lens through which human identity can be rebuilt and understood. The incorporation of biometric processes alongside sophisticated analytical technology enables more reliable identification, which can be of inestimable value to both criminal investigations and historical research. The multidisciplinary nature of forensic osteology not only enriches the field but also promotes interaction among numerous disciplines, from anthropology to computer science. With the field's development, the use of new technologies will be imperative for advancing methodologies and enhancing the quality of identifications in forensic cases. Ultimately, by adhering to high scientific standards themselves, forensic osteologists ensure that their conclusions are as much as possible not only correct but also ethical, enhancing faith in an evolving science that comes perilously close to human identity and recognition at its very essence.

Forensic osteology is particularly significant for human remains identification, especially when standard identification methods are hindered by deterioration or loss of identifying details. Examination of the skeletal remains allows forensic experts not just to establish the biological profile of the victim, such as age, sex, ancestry, and height, but also to ascertain the conditions under which death occurred, for instance, disease or trauma. Growing research highlights the importance of understanding decomposition patterns, as they may play a fundamental role in the preservation and recovery of skeletal material. For instance, studies contrasted mass graves' decomposition rates. They identified that interment depth and position of the remains within a grave can have a considerable impact on how well the remains will be preserved at exhumation (Adlam et al., 2014). Evidence like these underscores how important it is for forensic scientists to be well-versed in decomposition science so that they can adequately interpret evidence for investigative purposes and for use in the legal system (Adlam et al., 2014). The identification of remains can also be dependent on more sophisticated techniques, particularly where past cases are involved, for instance, the case of Amelia Earhart's disappearance. Forensic examination in this instance raises questions about the credibility of osteological inferences from incomplete remains. The differing assessments between the British officials' early reports and the new cranial analysis computer program illustrate the complexities of skeletal identification. Even though the historical context and previous research provide a treasure trove of information, they also indicate potential for misinterpretation with developments in forensic science and altered methods. This case highlights the importance of developing a robust, evidence-based system of forensic identification to prevent false conclusions based on incomplete or misidentified skeletal remains (Cross et al., 2015). Furthermore, the uses of forensic osteology go beyond individual identification to broader issues, including legal culpability, humanitarian work, and mass fatality situations. The addition of various scientific methodologies, from isotopic studies and DNA typing to anthropology and paleodemography, enhances the potential not only to identify victims but to reconstruct individuals' life courses and populations' social life. An understanding of how sociocultural problems interact with osteological evidence is vital in cases involving mass graves or archaeological excavations. As forensic science advances, so must the paradigms employed to decipher such evidence, underscoring the interdisciplinary nature of the job. Lastly, the evolution of forensic osteology is a constant interaction between scientific inquiry and ethical questions, focused on delivering justice to people and adding to the broader historical record.

KEY TERMS FROM THIS CHAPTER

- Age Estimation
- Ancestry Estimation
- Ante mortem Records
- Biological Profile
- Comparative Radiography
- Craniofacial Reconstruction
- Craniofacial Superimposition
- DNA Analysis
- Forensic Osteology
- Individualizing Features
- Isotope Analysis
- Metric Analysis
- Non-metric Traits
- Pathological Markers
- Positive Identification
- Sex Estimation

CRITICAL THINKING QUESTIONS

1. **Forensic osteology primarily involves:**
   a. The study of ancient human artifacts
   b. The diagnosis of genetic disorders in living people
   c. The analysis of human bones to aid in identification and cause of death
   d. The excavation of archaeological sites
2. **Which of the following bones is most commonly used to estimate sex in skeletal remains?**
   a. Femur
   b. Skull
   c. Tibia
   d. Radius
3. **The pelvis is considered the most reliable skeletal element for determining:**
   a. Age
   b. Stature
   c. Sex
   d. Ancestry
4. **Cranial sutures can provide information about:**
   a. Biological sex
   b. Trauma history
   c. Age at death
   d. Stature
5. **Which bone is most often used to estimate stature in forensic anthropology?**
   a. Humerus
   b. Clavicle
   c. Femur
   d. Scapula

Short Answer Questions

1. What is the biological profile in forensic osteology, and what key components does it include?
2. How can cranial features assist in estimating ancestry in skeletal remains?
3. Explain how the femur can be used to estimate stature.
4. How are dental records used in the identification of skeletal remains?
5. Describe two skeletal markers that can indicate antemortem trauma.

Answers to Critical Thinking Questions

1. (c); 2. (b); 3. (c); 4. (c); 5. (c)

REFERENCES

1. De Boer, H. H., Blau, S., Delabarde, T., & Hackman, L. (2018). The role of forensic anthropology in disaster victim identification (DVI): recent developments and future prospects. *Forensic Sciences Research*, *4*(4), 303–315. https://doi.org/10.1080/20961790.2018.1480460Adlam, T., Arnold, J., Arnold, M., Bachmann, B., Baraybar, J. P., Burns, K. R., Carter, R. F., et al. (2014). A preliminary examination of differential decomposition patterns in mass graves. https://core.ac.uk/download/1441337.pdf (accessed on 21st July 2025).
2. Ahmed, F., & Maisano, J. A. (2017). *ToScA North America (6–8 June 2017, The University of Texas, Austin, TX) Program*. https://core.ac.uk/download/211334283.pdf (accessed on 21st July 2025).
3. Allmäe, R., & Limbo-Simovart, J. (2015). Conventional ageing and sexing methods based on teeth and dry bone morphology in the person's identification (victims of Red Terror in 1946). https://core.ac.uk/download/43658427.pdf (accessed on 21st July 2025).
4. Anderson, M., Davy-Jow, S., Lorenz, K., et al. (2012). Roman portraiture and biometric identification. https://core.ac.uk/download/42505482.pdf (accessed on 21st July 2025).
5. Arrabaça, F., Raffaela, C., Castro Pinheiro, M. E., da Silva, R., et al. (2017). Procedural and political aspects of forensic exhumation in Brazil. https://core.ac.uk/download/80693793.pdf (accessed on 21st July 2025).
6. Arregui Dalmases, C., Galtés Vicente, I., Malgosa, A., et al. (2017). New insights in the analysis of blunt force trauma in human bones. Preliminary results. https://core.ac.uk/download/132528495.pdf (accessed on 21st July 2025).
7. Barrett, H., Bidmos, M. A., Bidmos, M. A., Bidmos, M. A., Bilge, Y., British Broadcasting Corporation (BBC), British Broadcasting Corporation (BBC), et al. (2014). The foot in forensic human identification–A review. https://core.ac.uk/download/30660095.pdf (accessed on 21st July 2025).
8. Bedić, Ž. (2021). Evidence of interpersonal violence at two sites of the Bijelo Brdo culture in eastern Croatia. https://core.ac.uk/download/482001871.pdf (accessed on 21st July 2025).
9. Borrini, M., Cole, C., Eliopoulos, C., et al. (2017). An anthropometric method for sex determination from the mandible: Test on British Medieval skeletal collections. https://core.ac.uk/download/131226347.pdf (accessed on 21st July 2025).
10. Bosnar, A., Petaros, A., & Čengija, M. (2010). When osteology is put into practice: Forensic anthropology. https://core.ac.uk/download/14420112.pdf (accessed on 21st July 2025).
11. Brandstätter, A., Brandstätter, A., Chomyn, A., Cormio, A., Schmitt, A., Kadenbach, B., Ludes, B., et al. (2008). Detection of the A189G mtDNA heteroplasmic mutation in relation to age in modern and ancient bones. https://core.ac.uk/download/50543720.pdf (accessed on 21st July 2025).
12. Bryson, D., Hadi, M., & Petronzi, D. (2016). Developing badge eco-systems to support engagement in class-based and online learning. https://core.ac.uk/download/77059939.pdf (accessed on 21st July 2025).
13. Cassella, J., Rogers, C., & Williams, A. (2025). Does the UK need a Human Taphonomy Facility? https://core.ac.uk/download/186333008.pdf (accessed on 21st July 2025).

14. Collins, K. M. (2014). Visual and geometric analysis of maxillary sinus region variability for identification of unknown decedents. https://core.ac.uk/download/267571339.pdf (accessed on 21st July 2025).

15. Crawley, M., Forbes, G., Mulhern, D. M., Nelson, R., & Stout, S. (2016). Decision tree analysis as a supplementary tool to enhance histomorphological differentiation when distinguishing human from non-human cranial bone in both burnt and unburnt states: A feasibility study. https://core.ac.uk/download/42137084.pdf (accessed on 21st July 2025).

16. Cross, P. J., & Wright, R. (2015). The Nikumaroro bones identification controversy: First-hand examination versus evaluation by proxy–Amelia Earhart found or still missing? https://core.ac.uk/download/76945212.pdf (accessed on 21st July 2025).

17. da Silva, R., Evison, M., Francisco, R., et al. (2017). Forensic investigation, truth and trust in the context of transitional justice in Brazil. https://core.ac.uk/download/80693795.pdf (accessed on 21st July 2025).

18. Eliopoulos, C., Falsetti, C., Mitsea, A. G., et al. (2025). Multidisciplinary approach to the forensic identification of a late discovery victim of a motorcycle accident. https://core.ac.uk/download/42477548.pdf (accessed on 21st July 2025).

19. Fish, J. T. (2004). *The Evidence Does Not Lie: A Forensic Investigation Program to Bridge the Gaps Between Crime Scene Investigation and Forensic Science.* https://core.ac.uk/download/268768091.pdf (accessed on 21st July 2025).

20. Fourshee, J. L. (2022). Differentiating human from nonhuman bone: Insights from a medical examiner's collection, Kenosha, Wisconsin. https://core.ac.uk/download/554010999.pdf (accessed on 21st July 2025).

21. Gamble, J. A., & Gilmour, R. J. (2024). Bones at home: Supporting haptic learning and universal design beyond the biological anthropology laboratory. https://core.ac.uk/download/644028705.pdf (accessed on 21st July 2025).

22. Hill, E. (2020). A review of the mandible. https://core.ac.uk/download/323028614.pdf (accessed on 21st July 2025).

23. Inthasan, C., & Mahakkanukrauh, P. (2017). Age estimation from clavicle by histomorphometry method: A review. https://core.ac.uk/download/159613125.pdf (accessed on 21st July 2025).

24. Klein, N. S. (2014). *A Comparative Study of Human Decomposition Research Facilities in The United States: The Role of Body Farms in Forensic Applications.* https://core.ac.uk/download/217403349.pdf (accessed on 21st July 2025).

25. Kurila, L. (2015). Cremation as limitation? A paleogeographic inquiry into the accuracy of macroscopic analysis of cremated human remains based on an East Lithuanian sample. https://core.ac.uk/download/43658404.pdf (accessed on 21st July 2025).

26. Lewis, M. (2017). Fetal paleopathology: An impossible discipline? https://core.ac.uk/download/42153730.pdf (accessed on 21st July 2025).

27. O'Brien, H. N. (2019). Human vs. non-human bone: A non-destructive histological method. https://core.ac.uk/download/267596207.pdf (accessed on 21st July 2025).

28. Sanchez, R. P. (2025). Establishing metric methods to identify variation in human biological sex using the upper and lower.

29. Schmeling, A., Schmeling, A., Schmeling, A., Schmeling, A., Schmeling, A., Lewis, A. B., Davies, C., et al. (2016). The persistence of epiphyseal scars in the distal radius in adult individuals. https://core.ac.uk/download/30664060.pdf (accessed on 21st July 2025).
30. Studebaker-Reed, M. S. E. (2018). The impact of training and experience on the recovery of evidence in outdoor forensic scenes: Implications for human remains recovery. https://open.bu.edu/bitstream/2144/31280/5/StudebakerReed_bu_0017N_13567.pdf (accessed on 21st July 2025).
31. Winter, R. M. (2016). Analysis of a commingled skeletal sample from Acacia Park Memorial Cemetery. https://core.ac.uk/download/230810544.pdf (accessed on 21st July 2025).

BIOARCHEOLOGY OF IDENTITY AND SOCIAL LIFE

7

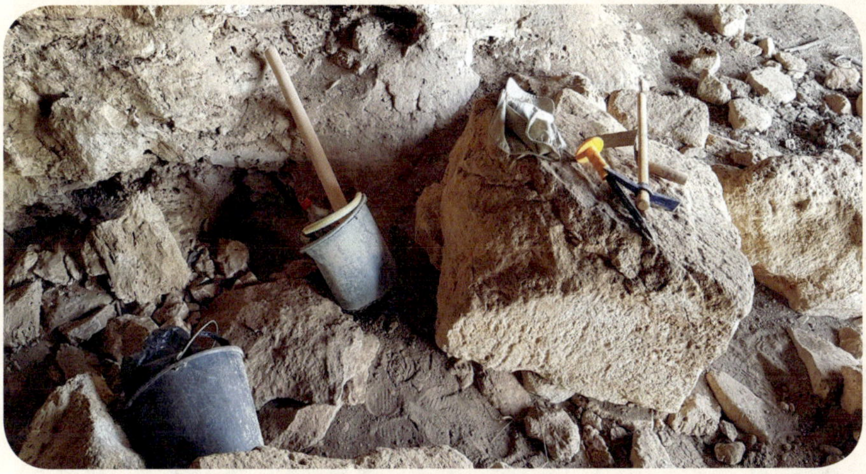

Introduction

The field of bioarcheology is a critical intersection of the social and biological facets of identity, providing a rich dividend of information about communities in the past and their multifaceted social structures. By examining human remains and bioarcheologists associated cultural material, bioarcheologists can infer individuals' lived experiences and sketch the roles they played within communities. The concept of "community" has shifted dramatically throughout the centuries, acquiring many different meanings responsive to changing social theory. A profound understanding of these changes is required, for it precedes a nuanced examination of how identity is formed and lived in life and death. As constructed, research into a "bioarcheology of community" can facilitate a more profound understanding of identity as a social construction that reflects its context, such that the tension between belonging and exclusion is articulated in the archaeological record (Kakaliouras et al., 2017). In recent years, bioarcheology has focused primarily on children, a minor minority in archaeology, and it has things

LEARNING OBJECTIVES

After studying this chapter, you will be able to:

1. Discuss the historical context of bioarcheology
2. Explain the theoretical frameworks
3. Understand bioarcheological methods
4. Identify case studies in bioarcheology
5. Identify construction in ancient societies
6. Focus on contemporary implications of bioarcheology

to say about central aspects of society and identity formation. Physical health, gender, and age disparities in childhood can clarify broader social stratifications and prejudices against different groups. For instance, the mortuary analysis reveals how children were perceived and treated within their respective societies, providing an indication of parental treatment and societal ranking. Researchers can tell volumes concerning society organization and identity formation procedures through patterns in mortality, health, and burial treatments with intense study. These studies are significant because they help fill knowledge gaps regarding childhood experiences and their contribution to shaping wider social identities within the past narrative (Davis et al., 2024). Bioarcheology of identity and social life, therefore, not only adds to our current understanding of the past but also poses significant questions regarding how identities were created, performed, and negotiated in varying contexts. The multifaceted nature of identity—intersecting with bioarcheological factors such as age, gender, and group status—tests bioarcheological inquiry with both problems and possibilities. By examining the treatment of people and groups alive and dead, researchers can unearth historical norms and beliefs that framed human relationships. This process offers a greater understanding of social dynamics, provoking us to reexamine contemporary notions of identity in light of earlier practice. Lastly, by combining biological data with sociocultural knowledge, bioarcheology offers a robust framework for interpreting how identity and social existence intersect throughout human history (Kakaliouras et al., 2017).

Definition of Bioarcheology

Bioarcheology is an interdisciplinary interface between the biological and cultural aspects of human life, which offers profound insight into identity and social existence in archaeological contexts. Defined as the study of human bone remains in their cultural and environmental setting, bioarcheology uses a variety of methods such as osteological analysis, paleopathology, and isotopic analysis to reconstruct previous populations' lives. By studying skeletal indicators of nutrition, health, and physical activity, it is possible for researchers to determine the influence of social structures and cultural practices on individuals' well-being and lifespan. Thus, bioarchaeology brings to light that light not just social membership and cultural display negotiate identity, but also biological experience through a response to numerous stressors over time, and thus offers an interesting critique of how biology and culture intersect in order to imbue meaning into human experience. At the center of bioarcheology's questions are the study of skeletal remains as coded histories of the dead, with implications for wider changes in society as well as personal experiences. The study of burial practices, burial orientation, and grave goods adds further depth to understanding identity construction, showing how cultural beliefs and social structures have shaped the treatment of the deceased. In the majority of contexts, such as the Mochica of the Lambayeque Valley in Peru, scholars have discovered complex interactions between indigenous cultural practices and colonialism, with a focus on adaptation and resilience during times of significant social change. The area's bioarcheology reveals not just that biological stress intensified after colonial contact but also that there was massive cultural hybridization that ensued as a reaction, reflecting on the dynamic nature of social life and identity in the presence of colonization (Klaus et al., 2008). New technologies in bioarcheological practice, such as isotopic analysis and 3D scanning, have also enabled more personal knowledge of ancient populations. Through isotope analysis of diet, migration, and health, scientists can reconstruct the physical lives of past people and complement this with 3D imaging of skeletal deformities and pathologies that mark lifestyle and social status. This multidisciplinary approach enables bioarcheologists to study issues of identity, for example, how gender, age, and work contributed to social positioning and biological existence. Thus, the definition of bioarchaeology is not confined to bones only; it involves a complete understanding of the individuals who lived before in different landscapes and societies, which would help better understand how identity and social life are entangled in human history (Becker et al., 2019) (Figure 7.1).

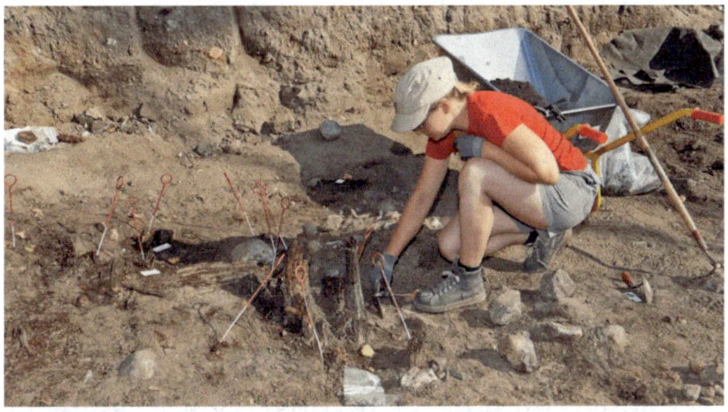

Figure 7.1. The domain of bioarcheology.

Source: https://anthroholic.com/wp-content/uploads/2023/02/Bioarcheology-Anthroholic.webp.

Importance of Studying Identity and Social Life Through Bioarcheology

The examination of identity and social life through bioarcheology produces unique viewpoints regarding how prehistoric populations lived, behaved, and socially organized themselves. By analyzing human remains, scientists cannot only detect biological processes but also identify cultural practices that shape identity. Bioarcheology provides the material link to ancient societies because it defines the ways in which people responded to one another and their environments. Such analyses incorporate a variety of factors, such as health indicators, eating habits, and death rites, all of which are important for reconstructing social organization. The addition of genetic information also provides more insight into identity and offers a more complete picture of kinship and community dynamics. Defined in current studies, focusing on bone diseases such as osteoarthritis and biomechanical stress can reveal the physical impact of social activities on health, expressing the intricate interaction between identity, social life, and biology in previous environments (Becker et al., 2019). To better enhance our comprehension of identity and social interactions, bioarcheology applies advanced techniques, particularly in geographic information systems (GIS) and spatial analysis. These technological advances allow researchers to approach burial sites, excavation yields, and artifact distributions with meticulous precision. For instance, as in the Tell Abraq example, GIS use not only connects fragmentary remains to geographic locations but also allows the incorporation of hand-written archaeological reports into a coherent digital format. This approach brings richness and complexity to bioarcheological interpretation, providing essential insight into mortuary patterns and societal organization. The complexity revealed through spatial analyses contributes to the reconstruction of social hierarchies and cultural rituals, and it adds rich context to the interpretation of past community interaction. The geospatial linkage of GIS with bioarcheological data transforms our understanding of identity and social organization by exposing underlying patterns that would otherwise remain invisible (Calleja et al., 2016). Secondarily, the inquiry of identity and social life through bioarcheology raises the multidisciplinary tone of the study, closing the gap between biological, cultural, and historical research. The integration of osteologists, archaeologists, and anthropologists becomes essential to construct a holistic approach toward comprehending human pasts. This framework of integration enables a more refined explanation of how people and communities negotiated their social worlds. For instance, through research into how osteological conditions relate to lifestyle habits and environmental factors, scholars can more critically evaluate the role of cultural behaviors in bodily health and vice versa. These interdisciplinary approaches not merely enhance the discipline of bioarchaeology but also promote broader debate regarding questions of identity and social inequality in the present day. As fresh research continues to challenge methodological horizons, the significance of exploring identity and social life through bioarcheology remains key to unearthing the richness of human experience through the centuries.

7.1. Historical Context of Bioarcheology

Learning Outcome

1. Development of bioarcheology as a field
2. Key figures and milestones in bioarcheological research
3. Evolution of methodologies in bioarcheology

The historical development of bioarcheology attests to a key evolution in human remains' comprehension and their relation to identity and social organizations. Bioarcheology emerged during the late 19th and early 20th centuries, with its early years spent on the physical aspects of the skeletal remains, primarily through anatomical and osteological examinations. The initial practitioners would attempt to reconstruct population profiles solely from skeletal features, often overlooking the cultural associations inherent in burial rites. However, as scholars came to appreciate the limitations of the method, the field began to adopt techniques from anthropology, archaeology, and history that enabled a more holistic interpretation of burial contexts and the social identities they represented. The transition from an exclusively biological perspective to one that embraces death studies' more interdisciplinary approach has led to research on how physical remains can reveal ancient cultures and their practices. The addition of mortuary archaeology has been enormously influential in bioarcheology, where it centers upon burial practice and material culture associated with death. Mortuary archaeology extends beyond the analysis of the skeletal record to encompass the broader cultural perceptions of death. Mortuary archaeology draws on a variety of disciplines, combining biological data with archaeological strategies to interpret funerary environments, grave offerings, and the spatial organization of burial places in relation to their topographies. By analyzing how these aspects shaped the social identity of the dead, bioarcheologists can recover narratives on social ranking, community position, and cultural behavior. This bioarcheological context increases our understanding of how people were perceived within their social groups, thereby enhancing our understanding of identity construction in premodern societies. Bioarcheology is informed by a broad background of past history research methods that traverse the biological and cultural divide. With advances in the discipline, contemporary bioarcheology emphasizes sound methods that facilitate such bioarcheological contexts. Scientists are now adopting holistic approaches in evaluating conditions such as osteoarthritis and other skeletal transformations, discovering their relevance to the day-to-day lives and social interactions of ancient humans (Becker et al., 2019). Moreover, the need to develop standardized methods and procedures for research on ancient human remains has been highlighted to ensure reliability and consistency in research findings. The interdisciplinary collaboration among experts, including osteologists, paleopathologists, and cultural anthropologists, signals a shift toward a more refined understanding of how human skeletal evidence illuminates social dynamics and identities in archaeological assemblages (Meyers et al., 2014). In the process, past bioarcheological history continues to shape current studies, leading to more profound understanding of the complexities of human life and identity in the past.

7.1.1. Development of Bioarcheology as a Field

The rise of a key transformation of human social life and identity knowledge, in which it is studied through the examination of bones and associated mortuary practices. Osteology, originally founded, bioarchaeology has expanded its foundations through interdisciplinary approaches as it now encompasses mortuary archaeology, cultural anthropology, and social history.

This multidisciplinary framework allows scholars to investigate not only the biology of bones but also the cultural and social implications of death and burial. The area of study's emphasis on understanding individual identities—age, sex, status, and health—has led archaeologists to rethink funerary contexts as complex representations of past societies' beliefs and social systems, augmenting evidence of the necessity to include multiple methodologies in bioarcheological analysis (Meyers et al., 2014). In parallel with the advancement of methodologies in bioarcheology, social dynamics among ancient populations also received greater focus. Scientists use techniques such as stable isotope analysis, DNA extraction, and trauma analysis to provide information on diet, health, migration, and inter-personal violence. For instance, studies in certain places, such as Quebrada de Humahuaca in Argentina, reveal patterns of inter-personal violence that can provide insights into social tensions and conflicts at the community level (Botta et al., 2014). These findings expand the identity narrative beyond simple labels to rich knowledge of individuals navigating complex social worlds. Such a focus on individual history allows for a more nuanced understanding of collective identities, accounting for the way individual reactions to trauma and resilience shape the norms and relations of societies over time. The development of bioarcheology has promoted a critical dialogue between the past and present, facilitating a more comprehensive understanding of the human condition. By linking biological data with death-related cultural practices, researchers can investigate how early individuals established their identity in relation to death, kinship, and group membership. Mortuary archaeology, as a valuable subsidiary, takes this further by examining burial artifacts and spatial structure and thereby placing biological information within context. This way, this integrated approach not only tells us how people lived and died but also how they were commemorated and remembered, and, thereby, about wider social values and constructions of identity and social integration. Accordingly, bioarcheology is a crucial mode of understanding the intersection of social life and identity and provides depth in our knowledge of humanity's plural pasts (Meyers et al., 2014) (Figure 7.2).

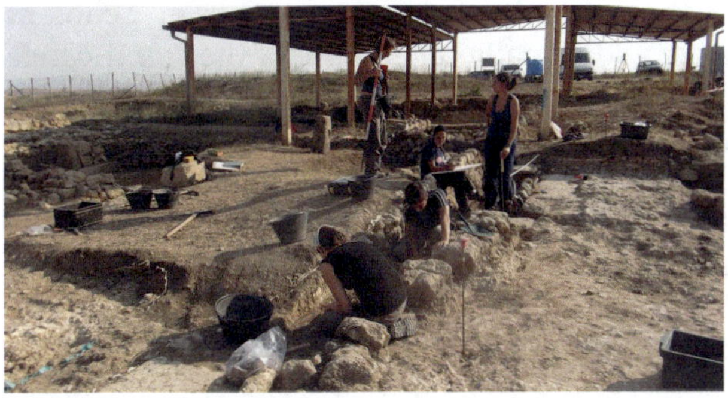

Figure 7.2. Development of bioarcheology as a field.

Source: https://external-content.duckduckgo.com/iu/?u=https%3A%2F%2Fwww.magd.cam.ac.uk%2Fsites%2Fdefault%2Ffiles%2Fstyles%2F1302x600%2Fpublic%2F2024-06%2Ftarquinia_excavation_image_credit_tarquinia_project_1300.jpg%3Fitok%3DWOJJkYhq&f=1&nof b=1&ipt=55f8e6da9a007b2e84eecc9dd93e1bc36de964f4f051bae6b246d4c5b937a9e2.

7.1.2. Key Figures and Milestones in Bioarcheological Research

Bioarcheology has been shaped considerably by the contributions of several key figures whose innovative research approaches have expanded our understanding of human identity and social living from the study of skeletons. At the top of the list is Dr. Douglas W. Owsley, whose diverse research on human skeletons from various archaeological sites has elucidated social organization, health, and identity among ancient societies. Owsley's integration of the bioarcheological techniques, such as stable isotope analysis, has enabled the reconstruction of the diet and migration of ancient populations, which is important for the determination of people's identities. The emphasis on the boundary between the biological and the cultural and the construction of laboratory protocols is a watershed moment in bioarcheology, as it has encouraged a more nuanced understanding of how identity and social life were interwoven in past communities. Apart from Owsley, scholars have additionally taken note of the significance of children in bioarcheology so that they may learn more about social dynamics and the construction of identity. The establishment of the archaeology of children as a distinct subdiscipline underscores the necessity of investigating the experience of childhood and material culture as a representation of social hierarchies and identity. As analyzed in recent scholarship, theory-driven frameworks that emphasize childhood allow one to examine how children engage with their communities and worlds and to uncover larger societal expectations and norms. These new approaches, for example, phenomenological explanations of children's lives in terms of spatiality, have helped locate their position within family configurations and larger social networks, thereby providing a rich tapestry of information about identity formation at critical moments in life (Lillehammer et al., 2025). Bioarchaeological breakthroughs have also been marked by collaborative research involving advanced scientific techniques to pinpoint the impacts of systemic stress among groups, particularly in oppressive contexts. For instance, recent comparisons of enamel microdefects known as Wilson bands in colonial Peruvian skeletal material have provided astounding insight into the stress to which native populations were subjected under Spanish domination. The frequency of these markers of stress highlights the struggles encountered during early developmental crises and contributes to narratives of resilience and adaptation under social and environmental stress. These outcomes demonstrate the significant role played by bioarcheology in analyzing identity not just from a physiological standpoint, but also from social and cultural angles, enhancing our understanding of past human circumstances and social structure (Garland et al., 2014).

7.1.3. Evolution of Methodologies in Bioarcheology

Methodological development in bioarcheology reflects a shift toward more interdisciplinarity within practices to allow for more advanced interpretations of past societies and individual identities. Early bioarcheological work was predominantly focused on osteological analysis and mortuary practices, and these provided the initial foundation for fundamental knowledge of demographic reconstruction and health. However, as the field developed, researchers began to introduce methods from social theory, archaeology, and genetics. This combination has deepened understanding of community dynamics, prompting researchers to consider the role that social life and identity play in forming archaeological knowledge. Through the emphasis on the dynamic interaction between biological information and social constructs, contemporary bioarcheology seeks to create a more nuanced picture of past human experience with an emphasis on the diversity of identities that existed among past populations, thereby facilitating richer interpretation of the material in the archaeological record. Furthermore, the application of advanced methods such as isotopic analysis reflects technological advances that have come to redefine bioarcheological analysis. For example, isotopic analysis, as applied in the research on isolated skulls found at the Elizabeth site, has provided evidence on diet and movement among ancient populations. The method provides the most important information on social organization by detailing the complexities of identity shaped by environment and lifestyle. The isotopic results, which provided evidence of both genetic homogeneity and extensive individual variation in the skulls, confirm that, even though the community appeared cohesive, there were various identities and experiences.

Thus, bioarcheological approaches have embraced a holistic context in which the biological evidence is employed to support broader social narratives, which show how identity is negotiated within communities and supports our own understanding of social life in the past. In addition to the synthesis of various scientific approaches, methodological advancement in bioarchaeology also entails critical reevaluation of community concepts inspired by social theory. Scholars have begun to reassess the very concept of "community," taking into account its complexity and implications for interpreting the archaeological record. This reevaluation has much in common with the aims laid out in recent studies that seek to disentangle the social fabric of the early populations through examining their interconnectedness. According to recent analyses, social theory-driven bioarcheologists aim to illuminate the daily lives of individuals within their societies, including their class, gender, and ethnic divisions. Through the promotion of debate regarding the various aspects of community, particularly with respect to identity and sociality, bioarcheology goes on to evolve techniques that not only record the past but attribute it contextual relevance, ultimately broadening our understanding of human history and social processes (Jones et al., 2015; Kakaliouras et al., 2017) (Figure 7.3).

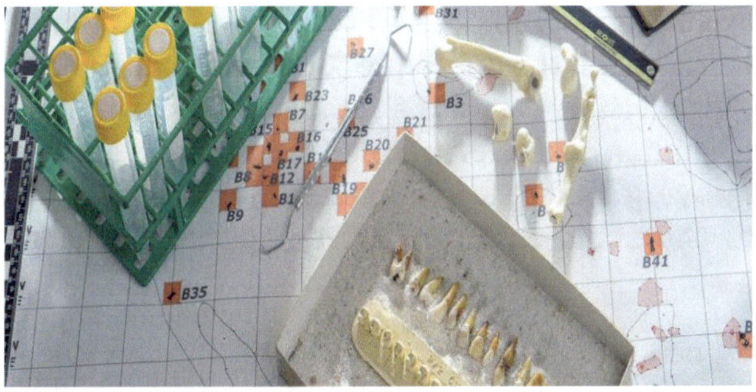

Figure 7.3. The evolution of methodologies in bioarcheology.

Source: https://external-content.duckduckgo.com/iu/?u=https%3A%2F%2Fshesc.asu.edu%2Fsites%2Fdefault%2Ffiles%2Fbioarcheology-hero.jpg&f=1&nofb=1&ipt=75aed92dd9a158de6060c38433b875ab48d037557a23f9a47d5d70fba65dbdad.

Test Your Knowledge

1. How did bioarchaeology emerge as a discipline, and what historical developments contributed to its formation?
2. Who were the key figures in the early development of bioarchaeology, and what were their contributions?

7.2. Theoretical Frameworks

Learning Outcome

1. Social identity theory in bioarcheology
2. Intersectionality and its relevance to bioarcheological studies
3. The role of material culture in understanding identity

The integration of theoretical approaches in bioarcheology is a vital framework for understanding the complex dynamics of identity and social living. Traditional academic regimes have a tendency to perpetuate a separation between social theory and scientific analysis, excluding the full possibility of cross-disciplinary work within the discipline (Gowland et al., 2020). This division impedes a complete understanding of human behavior in relation to bone remains by overlooking the contextual subtleties inherent to the socio-cultural environments of ancient populations. With these divisions dismantled, researchers can perform more sensitive analyses that incorporate both biological and sociocultural facets, thereby augmenting our understanding of identity construction and societal dynamics in ancient times. Highlighting a biocultural perspective permits the bioarchaeologist to link skeletal remains with their corresponding social meanings. Through the utilization of frameworks like Tilley's four-stage "bioarcheology of care" approach, scientists are able to extract evidence of caregiving activities from human skeletons (Ouellette et al., 2014). This systematic practice enables scholars to examine which health, illness, and social roles intersect profoundly, laying bare the profound connections among people and communities. Such questions not only enrich our understanding of identity but also prompt a broader consideration of how practice constructs caregiving and shapes social structures, compelling us to reshape our assumptions about the biological and the social.

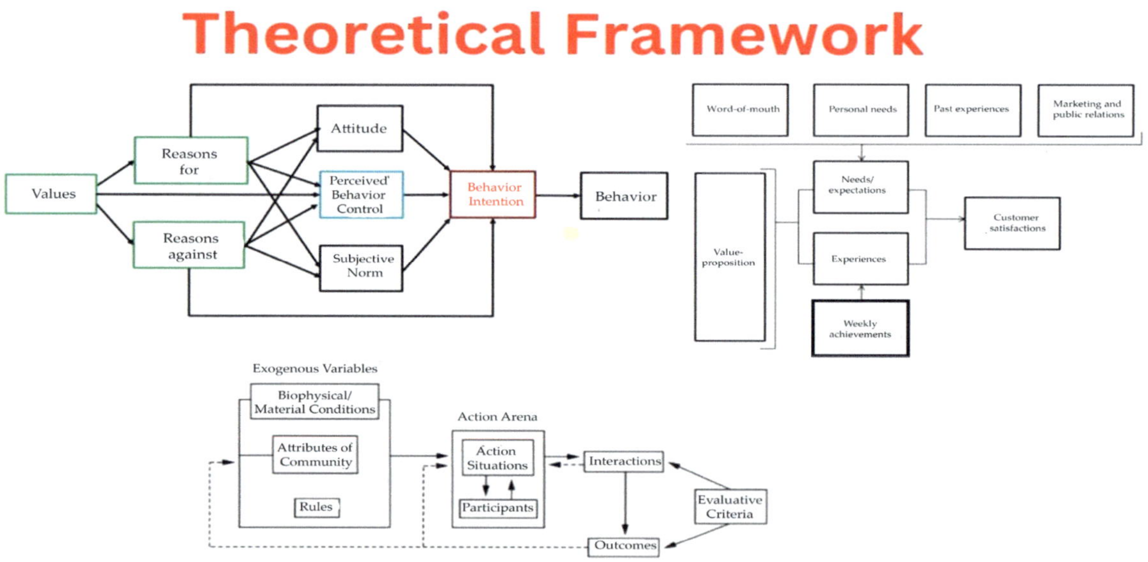

Figure 7.4. The integration of theoretical frameworks in bioarcheology.

Source: https://external-content.duckduckgo.com/iu/?u=https%3A%2F%2Fresearchmethod.net%2Fwp-content%2Fuploads%2F2023%2F04%2FTheoretical_Framework-1140x641.jpg&f=1&nofb=1&ipt=9623eb4fe0daa53fd140a44ee0006877121f28d2a1a36ef4da0925f8cd5180fe.

The blending of diverse theoretical traditions encourages a broader exploration of identity and social life in bioarcheology. The complementarity of biological analysis and social theory deepens explanations of human remains while allowing for more critical examination of identity formation across time and space. Blending these approaches challenges scholars to examine how environmental, cultural, and individual factors intersect to shape identity (Gowland et al., 2020). As interdisciplinary works increase, the field of bioarcheology can benefit from introducing social theories that account for the complexities of human existence. This revolution will ultimately enrich our understanding of the complex relationships among identity, care, and social life over time (Figure 7.4).

7.2.1. Social Identity Theory in Bioarcheology

The use of social identity theory in bioarcheology offers a more nuanced platform for researchers to understand better the complex dynamic between identity formation and bioarcheological evidence. Based on this theory, individuals identify with specific social groups, and it plays a very crucial role in forming their behavior, perception, and interactions. Bioarcheological analysis of skeletons and burial rituals reveals the biological past of ancient populations but also traces the social structures and identities that characterized such groups. It is particularly pertinent when explaining how external pressures, such as colonial contact, affected indigenous identities and social solidarity. For instance, bioarcheological evidence for burial practices can trace alterations in identity formation after European colonization and highlight the construction and reconstruction of social identity through history, as demonstrated in studies on the Colonial Mochica of Peru (Klaus et al., 2008). Social identity theory also allows us to ask questions about ethnogenesis—how new social identities are formed—through bioarcheological evidence. The ethnogenesis process is especially relevant within contexts of social disruption, including the contact between Native Americans and Europeans. For the Colonial Mochica, researchers have recorded a hybridization of identities that occurred in the aftermath of colonial disruptions. This syncretism of pre-Hispanic and Catholic burial rites, as practiced, is a testament to a shift in social identity and not to an essential collapse in culture. Instead of responding to external pressure, the Mochica negotiated their identity in advance by employing both biological resistance and new forms of cultural representation as survival strategies. These findings emphasize the importance of integrating social identity theory in bioarcheology because it accounts for the malleability of identity in the face of historical conflict, providing a better sense of human resilience and cultural persistence (Klaus et al., 2008). Second, applying social identity theory allows bioarcheologists to assess the broader social ramifications of disease and health in ancient populations. The intersection of identity and health is critical for understanding individuals' lived experiences in the past, as social stratification often influenced access to resources and overall well-being. Investigations into skeletal remains reveal telltale signs of stress, illness, and nutritional deficiencies, which can be intricately tied to social identity affiliations. For example, examining demographic patterns in skeletal populations can reveal how identities influenced reproductive experiences and health outcomes. Methodologically, adopting holistic strategies that couple social identity theory with quality osteological analysis, as mentioned with respect to recent developments in bioarcheological methods, increases the depth of our understanding of the interplay between social and biological forces in shaping human experience. Thus, infusion of social identity theory into bioarcheology allows for greater understanding of the richness of identity and social life through history (Figure 7.5).

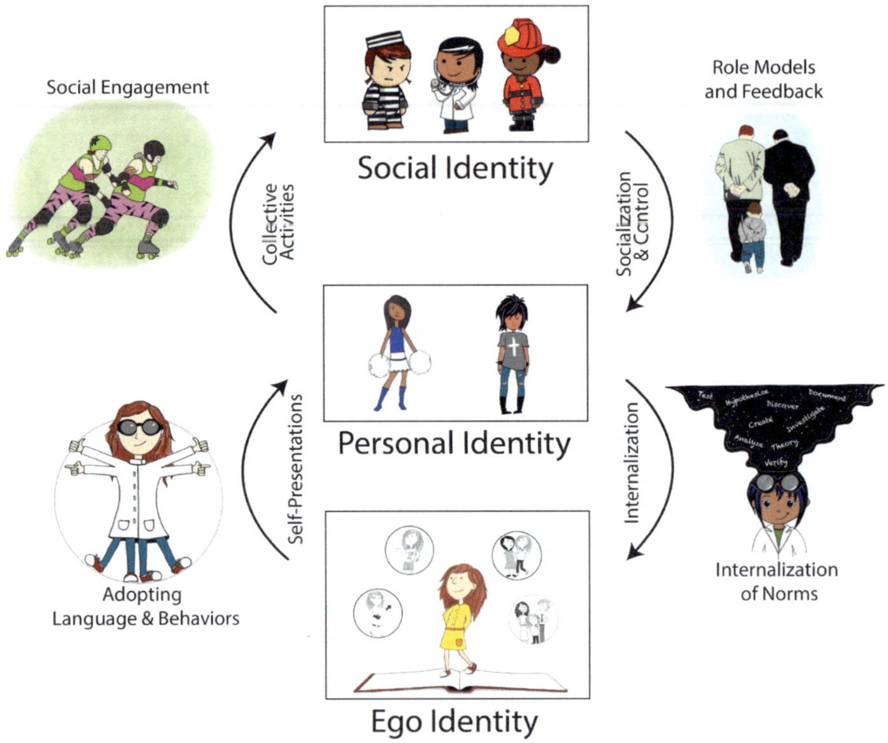

Figure 7.5. The integration of social identity theory within the field of bioarcheology.

Source: https://external-content.duckduckgo.com/iu/?u=https%3A%2F%2Fimages.squarespace-cdn.com%2Fcontent%2Fv1%2F55b7e5afe4b0d5f73e652870%2F1541983330167-P7DEVV97EQ7XCIO9BMYB%2F7_SIFT(graphic)%2Bcopy.jpg&f=1&nofb=1&ipt=3a4126025654a877670835b89eb0b9384fea6abea2b5302bd838643c5661e619.

7.2.2. Intersectionality and its Relevance to Bioarcheological Studies

Intersectionality is yet another critical framework in bioarcheological research, which significantly enhances our understanding of identity and social relationships among past groups. This approach recognizes that social categories, including race, class, gender, and health, intersect and form specific experiences and identities. By applying this intersectional approach, bioarcheologists can evaluate the influence of such compound identities on the health consequences, community participation, and social functioning of past populations. This approach helps researchers transcend reductionist analysis of human remains and address the socio-political and environmental forces that structure the experiences of individuals and groups. Therefore, intersectionality not only provides more nuance in the analysis of populations in the past but also more relevance for the applicability of bioarcheological findings to contemporary arguments about social justice and health disparity. Incorporating intersectionality within bioarcheology allows for scholars to analyze disease and health inequality patterns through the lens of social determinants. For instance, the syndemic approach brought into bioarcheology enables an appreciation of how interlinked disease affects various populations in different ways, emphasizing that health becomes unseparable from social context. With examples of diseases like tuberculosis and vitamin D deficiency in the 18th and 19th centuries, authors have demonstrated how effectively this intersectional methodology will work by demonstrating how socioeconomic status and environmental factors indeed contributed to health conditions, and that the morbidity burden was not only borne by everyone. This methodology enriches our historical understanding of health and also emphasizes the urgent present-day relevance of these inequalities in public health discourse, most significantly by addressing the system inequalities that persist (Gowland et al., 2022). Furthermore, intersectionality complicates earlier dichotomies in bioarcheological debate, most significantly a binary way of dealing with sex and gender. Current texts advocate a more encompassing model that shatters these dichotomies, recognizing the interconnectedness of social and biological constructs.

Using feminist and queer theory, bioarcheologists can approach the complexity of identity without imposing austere categorical distinctions on the past. This shift not only widens the range of methodological approaches to the study of human skeletal remains but also invites renewed discussion of constructed and performed identities in mortuary settings. Ongoing criticism of binary models permits deeper analysis of lived experiences and social positions, emphasizing respect for diversity in responding to the complexity of human existence (Hämäläinen et al., 2020).

7.2.3. The Role of Material Culture in Understanding Identity

Material culture is a significant lens that researchers utilize to understand human identity and social life, particularly in the bioarcheological realm. The artifacts, tools, and death rituals found at an archaeological site offer valuable insights into the cultural norms, values, and societal structures of past individuals. These materials provide physical traces of how individuals lived their identities in a specific cultural context. Grave goods, for instance, reflect the social status or gender roles present in society, and this suggests how identity was enacted and constructed through materiality. An analysis of these artifacts permits a more nuanced understanding of the dynamics of identity formation due to the fact that, although they symbolize individual characteristics, they also indicate the broader cultural stories that ruled over communal experiences and social engagement in historic settings. In examining the dynamic between material culture and identity, mortuary archaeology is an exceptionally fruitful research field. By looking at burial practices, the scholar can discover how individuals dealt with the crossroads of collective and individual identity.

The presence of specific objects in burial contexts typically indicates the deceased's social status, beliefs, and affiliations within their society. For example, the transition from orthodox to hybrid burial practices in postcontact societies, such as the Colonial Mochica, exemplifies how identity is transformed as a result of outside influence and social pressure. As proposed in more recent bioarcheological research, such alterations reflect not only personal behavior changes but also societal changes overall, thus reinforcing the importance of material culture as a means of understanding identity in both past and present contexts (Klaus et al., 2008). Furthermore, new methods applied in mortuary archaeology and related fields also illustrate the dynamic interaction between material culture and identity.

Techniques used to investigate burial grounds—like spatial organization and the presence of ecofacts—allow for a holistic study of how societies handled death and respected their dead (Meyers et al., 2014). Tracing changes in burial practices over time allows scholars to better understand how identity is negotiated, constructed, and reconstructed across diverse cultural environments. This interdisciplinary emphasis on mortality both reveals the material practices of identity and invites critical debate across disciplines, raising our consciousness about how individuals engage with past and present identities created through both social and environmental conditions. This addition of material culture to identity analysis is crucial to developing a more expansive and nuanced understanding of human social life (Figure 7.6).

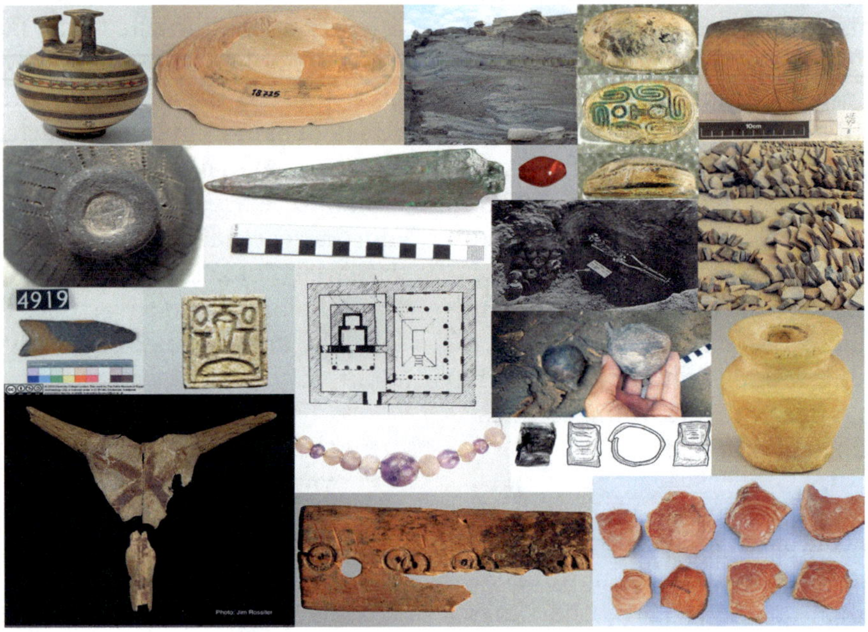

Figure 7.6. The role of material culture in understanding identity.

Source: https://external-content.duckduckgo.com/iu/?u=https%3A%2F%2Fwww.oeaw.ac.at%2Ffileadmin%2FInstitute%2FOREA%2FEvents%2F2019%2FDocumentingMaterialCulture%2FDocumentingMaterialCulture.jpg&f=1&nofb=1&ipt=5dc38dd5012eb0bbf9f6805e105244ba9ff92841682e236cdad9619cf17937a1.

Test Your Knowledge

1. What are the main theoretical frameworks used in bioarchaeology to study identity and social life?
2. How do these frameworks help interpret the social roles, status, and cultural practices of past populations?

7.3. Bioarchaeological Methods

Learning Outcome

1. Osteological analysis and its significance
2. Isotopic analysis for dietary and mobility insights
3. Bioarchaeological fieldwork techniques

It is through bioarchaeological methods that we have a lot to understand about the exploration of identity and social life in skeletal remains. bioarcheologists use different methods to detect patterns of health, nutrition, and social structure in ancient populations. The analysis of skeletal trauma, for instance, informs us about the violence and interpersonal dynamics in a population. Case studies, such as the Quebrada de Humahuaca, provide us with examples of how bioarchaeological information generates evidence that demonstrates high levels of interpersonal violence, and research shows that such trauma was ubiquitous in both male and female individuals and across all ages. The results of these analyses contribute to the understanding of conflict within society and the daily lives of citizens, and significantly enhance the interpretation of the complexity of identity in ancient societies (Botta et al., 2014). Bioarcheological methods further extend to researching diet and eating habits and their social identity implications. By employing dental analysis, researchers can make nutritional inferences and health conditions through the analysis of oral pathological conditions. For example, comparisons of two contemporaneous Inka sites, Salapunku and Sacsayhuaman, indicate differing patterns of dental wear and tooth loss in the probable, differently functioning populations of the sites. The differences in dental pathology reflect not only differing diets but also differing subsistence strategies in keeping with the more general social and economic functions of each site. Therefore, by using methods of bioarcheology, researchers can reconstruct the subtle lifestyles of ancient people, ultimately making it possible for a richer comprehension of their social identities (Orrand et al., 2020). Besides a physical check-up, quantitative analysis allows an enrichment of the bioarcheological research.

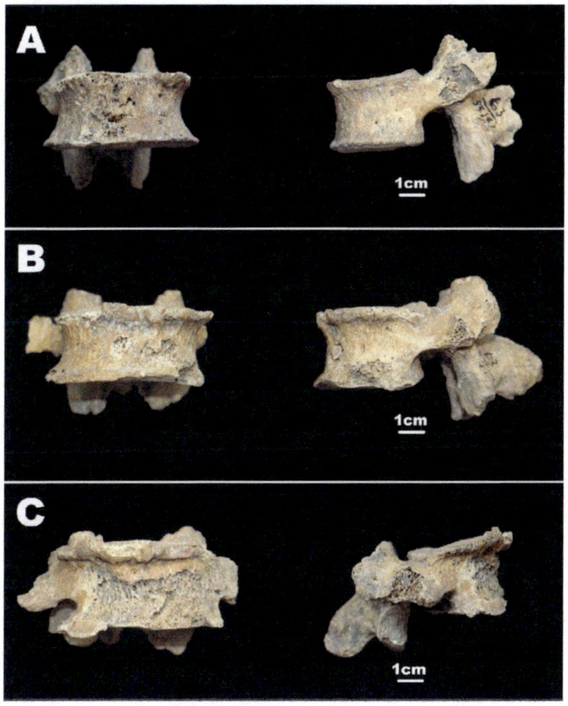

Figure 7.7. The exploration of identity and social life through bioarcheological methods.

Source: https://external-content.duckduckgo.com/iu/?u=https%3A%2F%2Fwww.researchgate.net%2Fpublication%2F367965884%2Ffigure%2Ffig1%2FAS%3A11431281117095922%401675375864419%2FIntervertebral-disc-disease-grades-based-on-the-Bioarchaeological-Intervertebral-Disc.png&f=1&nofb=1&ipt=6dc31c61299f311f1c41aa5874fb54398b7588d97d547a42abbba9fac461506e.

Statistical methods may be used to investigate trauma frequencies and health states within any demographic characteristic, such as sex and age, and provide a general picture of community health and social organization. Comparative analysis of skeletal trauma in a sequence of sites, such as is available with the evidence from Quebrada de Humahuaca, offers the potential for inter-site comparison and the demonstration of geographic and social differences. By such intensive approaches, bioarcheologists provide an evidence-based perspective of identity, emphasizing how common social experience sheds light on individual narratives across historical populations. In the long run, such approaches determine nuanced layers of identity formation and social existence, indicating the importance of interdisciplinary research across the discipline of bioarcheology (Figure 7.7).

7.3.1. Osteological Analysis and Its Significance

Osteological analysis is a key aspect of bioarcheology, particularly in the determination of where identity and social life intersected in prehistoric populations. Osteological analysis, by examining skeletal remains, allows scientists to discover patterns of health, stress, and social organization, as well as to clarify the daily lives of prehistoric individuals. The osteological signs of stress, such as enamel hypoplasia and additional signs of malnutrition or illness, provide critical insight into how social identities—gender, age, and social status—influenced people's biological health. In struggling with the complexity of these markers, scientists have circumvented traditional configurations, emphasizing that identity is realized through socio-cultural environments rather than solely biological factors. This method is consistent with the purposes of bioarcheological inquiry, seeking to unlock the stories hidden in the human skeleton and thus bridge the gap between the biological information and the constructed meanings of identity (Casserly et al., 2022). In children's contexts, osteological analysis yields revelations of depth regarding how social structures framed the lives and deaths of children in past societies. As highlighted in recent studies, the study of children's skeletal remains can inform the demographic and health implications of social identity. Bioarchaeological analysis of mortuary treatment, age, and health provides insight into the status and roles assigned to children in their populations. For instance, contrasts in funeral rites combined with stress markers in skeletons can illustrate different social statuses that children were assigned to based on gender or family background. Such findings not only enhance our understanding of infants and child mortality but also extend our understanding of identity construction and social stratification within the ancient world, informing us that even the most minor society members were integrated into multifaceted social systems (Davis et al., 2024). Also, osteology has the potential to redefine accounts of past populations by integrating biocultural accounts for both the social and biological roles of identity. Through the use of techniques such as proteomic analysis in conjunction with traditional skeletal analysis, bioarchaeologists can offer information on previously neglected themes of social differentiation, such as status and gender, among children in different cultural environments. For example, skeletal analysis of individuals discovered in Byzantine cemeteries has identified differential treatment in mortuary practices by age and sex, illuminating the intricate interrelationship between identity and death in these societies. Thus, osteological analysis is not just a method for researching health but also for examining the intimate connections between identity, social life, and cultural practices in the past (Casserly et al., 2022; Davis et al., 2024).

7.3.2. Isotopic Analysis for Dietary and Mobility Insights

Isotopic analysis of carbon and nitrogen is a fundamental technique in bioarcheology that provides unprecedented insight into past diets and mobility. By analyzing stable isotopes in human and animal collagen, researchers can reconstruct sources of food plants and animals consumed and even specific geographical origins of individuals. This methodological approach allows for an interdisciplinary appreciation of how environmental circumstances, subsistence strategies, and social identity interacted in building the lives of ancient societies. For instance, isotopic variation is capable of recording dietary change in response to environmental or socioeconomic variables, and researchers are thus able to map dietary adaptation in the context of overall cultural transformation in a society, revealing important dimensions of their social life and identity. Isotopic analysis findings, such as those conducted in the Avondale Burial Place, reveal the importance of mobility in societal dynamics. Stable isotope analysis of dental remains in this research indicated restricted mobility among community members, suggesting that people lived and died close to their birthplaces. Restricted mobility has implications for social organization and family relations within the community. By integrating isotopic data with cooperative osteological and mortuary analysis, scientists can construct a more nuanced model of early-life diets that shaped social networks and cultural identities, illuminating how the community managed the complexities of social life during the post-Civil War era. Such insights are fed directly into the broader discourse on identity formation and continuity amid historical upheaval.

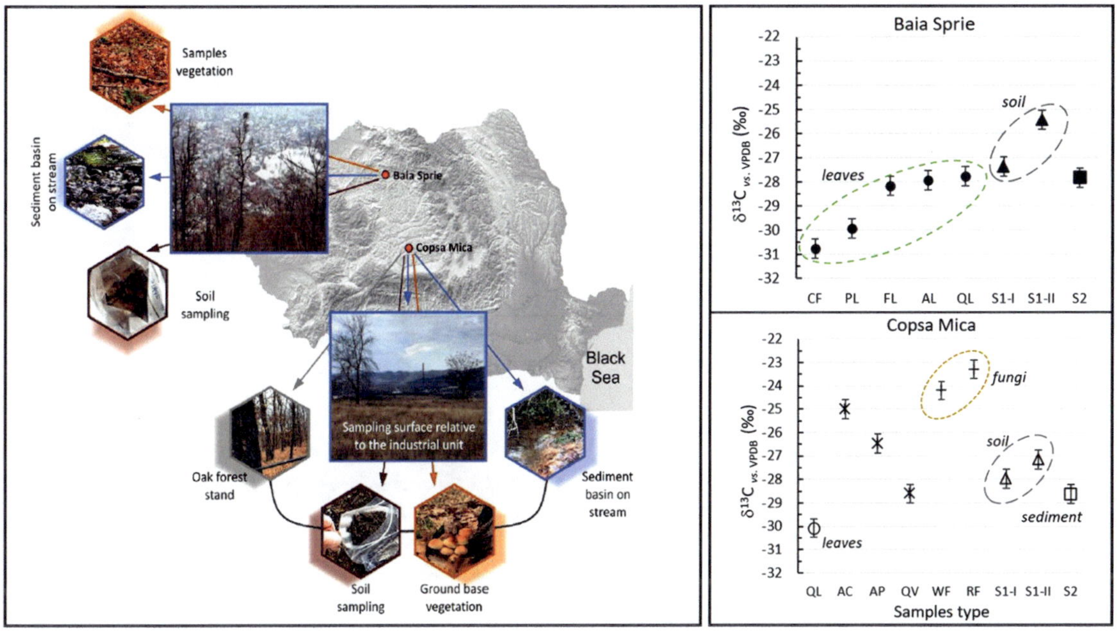

Figure 7.8. Isotopic analysis, particularly of carbon and nitrogen.

Source: https://external-content.duckduckgo.com/iu/?u=https%3A%2F%2Fwww.notulaebotanicae.ro%2Fpublic%2Fjournals%2F2%2Farticle_12138_cover_en_US.jpg&f=1&nofb=1&ipt=9d13bf89b524f196a051df9e014a790190b216ffd89cc39270c2f4f261139b01.

Moreover, isotopic analysis transcends dietary reconstruction, opening a window to past human-environmental relations. The methodological advances mentioned in recent literature, such as collaborative studies funded by various academic and research institutions (Bogaard et al., 2017), underscore the significance of multiscalar analysis in unmasking patterns of mobility and subsistence. This technique not only deepens our understanding of past populations but also augments genealogical analysis, providing a foundation for the contextualization of past testimonies. For communities such as Avondale Cemetery, isotopic analysis can reveal demographic patterns and social affiliation, thereby filling gaps in historical records and contributing to a better understanding of their identities. As the field evolves, these approaches will continue to retell social life stories in bioarcheology, emphasizing the intricate interplay among diet, mobility, and group identity (Figure 7.8).

7.3.3. Bioarchaeological Fieldwork Techniques

The bioarcheological fieldwork process lies at the heart of understanding the intricate interplay among social life and identity as expressed in mortuary practices. Using a range of excavating techniques and meticulous recording procedures, it is possible for bioarcheologists to ultimately retrieve not just skeletal deposits but also burial ritual-related artifacts, spatial contexts, and ceremonial practices. Mortuary archaeology, which is a subdivision of bioarcheology, is more than an examination of the skeletal remains because it crosses disciplines that include anthropology, art history, and sociology, among others, and thus facilitates a full breakdown of how individuals engaged with death and remembrance in their cultures.

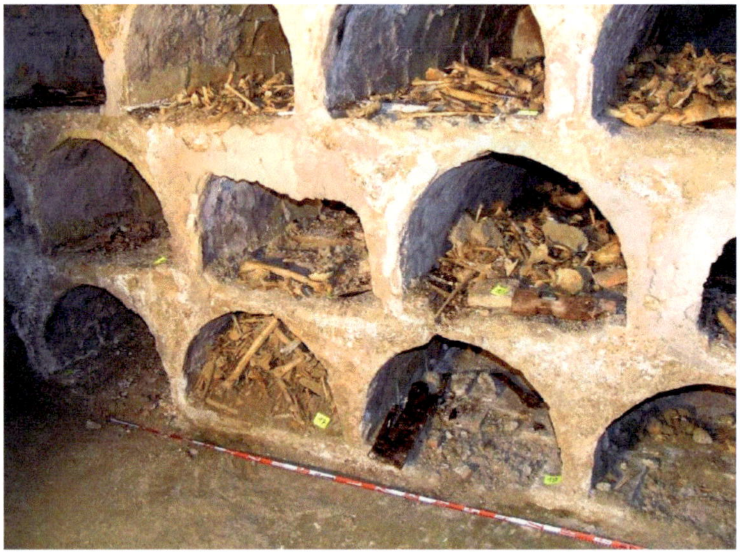

Figure 7.9. The process of bioarcheological fieldwork.

Source: https://external-content.duckduckgo.com/iu/?u=http%3A%2F%2Farchaeology.institute%2Fimg%2F053-5g-funerary-crypt-bioarcheology-fieldschool.jpg&f=1&nofb=1&ipt=8d6b28005f24958fc510b70c88ba459d5c0dc215083a67b557f7f5844cab0a48.

This integrative approach enhances our understanding of social norms and individual identity regarding death, and of how mortuary practice reflects broader cultural constructs and social hierarchies (Meyers et al., 2014). As well as normal excavation techniques, bioarcheological fieldwork now includes advanced scientific techniques such as isotopic analysis and DNA testing. These technologies not only provide information about individual health and diet but also explain patterns of migration, kinship, and social organization in ancient populations. By analyzing the skeletal remains of adults and children, researchers can crack stories about community adaptation and resilience in the face of environmental adversity. A focused research interest in non-adult skeletal remains, for instance, can reveal important information about the survival strategies and well-being of societies, speaking to the voiceless in society within the social hierarchy. In line with this, knowledge of these remains allows for a deeper appreciation of childhood and family forms in historical contexts, including insight into a better grasp of social vulnerability and support networks in communities (Morrone et al., 2020). Ethics is a core component of bioarcheological fieldwork, where human remains and cultural materials should be treated with respect. Engagement with descendant populations is crucial because it fosters communication and partnership in research design and interpretation, ensuring that identity and social life studies are conducted respectfully within the historical narrative. Synthesizing these ethical frameworks enriches the research's findings through culturally sensitive interpretations of social structure and burial practices. Further, using collaborative paradigms provides a rich appreciation of how social status, age, and gender influenced individuals' contributions to their communities, thereby enabling a grasp of identity formation as such. This multi-layered perspective is essential for fully addressing the socio-cultural dimensions of mortality and memory within the broader bioarcheological context (Meyers et al., 2014) (Figure 7.9).

Test Your Knowledge

1. What are the common bioarchaeological methods used to analyze human skeletal remains?
2. How do bioarchaeological methods help reconstruct the health, lifestyle, and demographic patterns of past populations?

7.4. Case Studies in Bioarcheology

Learning Outcome

1. Analysis of burial practices and their implications for social identity
2. Examination of health and disease patterns in past populations
3. Insights from specific archaeological sites and their findings

The domain of bioarcheology intersects archaeology, anthropology, and biology in providing valuable information regarding the identity and social structure of past populations. The most essential characteristic of the field is the examination of skeletons to acquire knowledge of how socio-cultural conditions have impacted biological reactions over time. The research method employed in such analyses involves careful observation of osteological conditions, such as osteoarthritis and entheses. According to the research of scholars such as Ortner (2011, 2012) and Verano (1997), researchers strive to precisely determine such conditions to elucidate the pathogenesis of skeletal changes in historically significant populations. In such analyses, demographic variables such as age and sex are necessary, as they dictate individual experience and responses to biomechanical stress and, by extension, the understanding of identity in social life, as noted in Becker et al. (2019). Case studies from Argentina's Quebrada de Humahuaca are similarly reflective of the dynamics of violence, identity, and health in bioarcheological contexts. Research in this discipline has produced evidence of interpersonal violence in the form of a quantitative analysis of skulls between locations. Cranial trauma surveys—antemortem and perimortem fractures—have revealed that both women and men were subjected to violence equally, unlike expected gendered patterns of exposure to trauma. Significantly, the presence of such injuries differed by location, with specific sites recording an observed higher rate of trauma as well as trophy skulls.

These findings not only shed light on the physical effects of social conflict but also provide invaluable insights into the cultural traditions of such ancient societies, deepening our understanding of identity construction in times of sociopolitical unrest, as supported by research by Botta et al. (2014). The integration of osteological evidence with broader cultural discourses further encourages the appreciation of how social identities were constructed and shaped over time. For instance, the study of variation patterns in trauma can enable researchers to reconstruct social organization, conflict, and community resilience among past populations. By combining skeletal data with archaeological and ethnographic data, bioarcheologists can generate comprehensive narratives of the ways that several social groups lived their lives and responded to one another and to their environmental contexts. Such an interdisciplinary approach is crucial to untangling multi-stranded identities created by both biological and sociocultural processes. The imperative of employing stringent methodological frameworks, according to Becker et al. (2019), ensures that the data collected are credible and can truly contribute to the debate of the bioarchaeology of identity and social life. These integrative practices not only encourage scholarly debate but also enhance appreciation of legacies left by past societies (Figure 7.10).

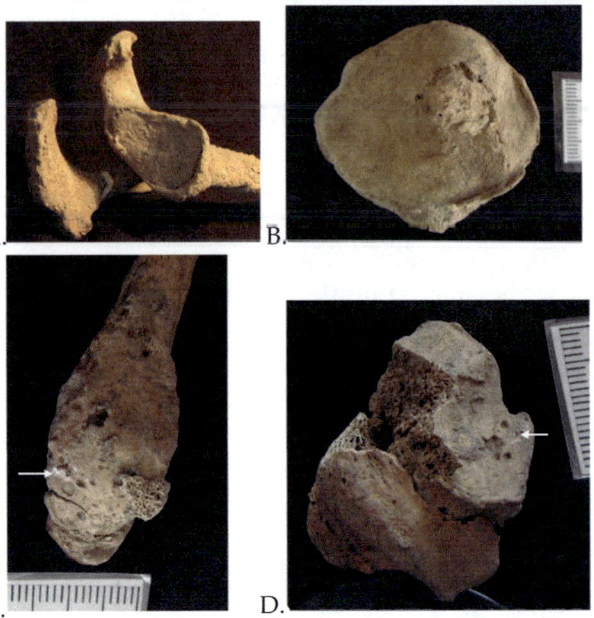

Figure 7.10. The field of bioarcheology intersects the disciplines of anthropology.

Source: https://ars.els-cdn.com/content/image/1-s2.0-S2352409X16302589-gr5.jpg.

7.4.1. Analysis of Burial Practices and Their Implications for Social Identity

Burial practices are a significant reflection of social identity, resonating with the religious, cultural, and socio-economic contexts of ancient communities. Archaeological evidence suggests that mortuary ritual can distinguish among social strata and markers of identity, such as class, ethnicity, and gender. The burial style, whether in elaborate offerings over the grave or in a simpler form, in any society presupposes a lot about the status of the dead and their clan affiliations. Therefore, for example, the aristocracy may be buried at visible sites with luxury items, revealing their higher status and the importance of ancestor worship in perpetuating lineage and power. These rites honor not just the deceased but also serve to support existing social hierarchies within the group and indicate an intersection between identity and mortality, as the burial of the dead becomes an act of social organization and group memory. Bioarcheological analysis of burial rites enables a greater understanding of complex, multifaceted identities that people held in life and potential legacies. Cardiovascular and skeletal analysis, combined with isotopic analysis, provide fundamental information about dietary practices and geographic mobility that specify an individual's social network and identity. In a study of 52 Maya individuals, isotopic ratios could differentiate local and migrant individuals to illustrate how burial context can convey an individual's role in political and economic systems (Cormier et al., 2018). The osteobiographies that combine personal stories challenging homogenized perceptions of ancient populations, demonstrating that even within shared cultural practices such as burial, various identities remained preserved and celebrated. Complexity highlights how individualized life narratives add to a richer understanding of societal identity and cohesion. Contrariwise, child morbidity studies demonstrate that burial practices might also represent societal inequalities, providing insight into the lives of peripheral groups. Research indicates that urban and rural burial plots exhibit distinct health patterns and the placement of remains of youth, thereby illuminating social grading in Roman England (Adams et al., 2017). For instance, higher infant mortality and some poverty-related pathologies were common in rural cemeteries, meaning that these children's living conditions were poorer and the availability of resources was lower than in urban areas. These discoveries raise fundamental questions about how mortuary structures influence life paths, especially for marginalized populations. By converging bioarcheological and sociocultural understanding, one is able to measure how death rituals move beyond individual markers to symbolize broader stories about resources, health, and social identity and therefore create a more advanced understanding of ancient societies and their complexities.

7.4.2. Examination of Health and Disease Patterns in Past Populations

The examination of patterns of health and disease in ancient populations provides crucial information regarding the lived experiences, environmental challenges, and socio-organization of ancient societies. Through the examination of the skeletal remains, bioarcheologists can determine traces of chronic conditions such as osteoarthritis and other pathologies that point to underlying socio-economic contexts and life decisions. Standard techniques that are employed include examination of osteological changes and biomechanical stresses that inform on the manner in which individuals accommodate to their physical environment and social requirements. As explained in the current literature, examining such health markers entails a small-data paradigm that is responsive to how pathology needs to be correctly labeled and framed. Understandings of these skeleton expressions allow researchers to build histories of the well-being and health of populations over time, not just their biological adaptation but also social resilience within an environment of adversity (Becker et al., 2019). In addition, examination of postcontact health patterns among indigenous populations, particularly in regions such as the Central Andes, allows for complex interactions between colonization and regional health dynamics. After European contact, evidence indicates a radical shift in health patterns, characterized by increased morbidity and the introduction of new diseases that severely affected indigenous societies. Bioarchaeological evidence would capture that while populations experienced an increase in biological stress through avenues such as poor nutrition and increased traumatic injury, they also engaged in cultural adaptation to these changes. The case of the Colonial Mochica in Lambayeque Valley illustrates this duality; rather than yielding completely to colonial disruption, these cultures exhibited resilience through individual adaptation, integrating traditional practices with innovative influences from European customs. This change not only suggests health changes but also a deeper narrative of identity emergence under colonial coercion (Klaus et al., 2008). Speculating about ancient communities' health and disease patterns, and particularly viewing them through the lens of bioarcheology, contributes to increased understanding of identity and social life in such societies. Health is also a significant indicator of social stratification, resource availability, and quality of life. Variability in the skeletal manifestations across different demographic groups reveals variations within societal institutions, with dissimilarities pointing potentially to class, occupation, or access to food. Secondly, these bioarcheological findings tell us about identity since health inequality often intersects with cultural practices and societal conventions. Through the integration of skeletal data with broader cultural interpretations, scientists can construct a more nuanced account of the balance between health, identity, and social interaction within ancient communities, upon which rests an understanding of how history influences contemporary social life (Becker et al., 2019) (Figure 7.11).

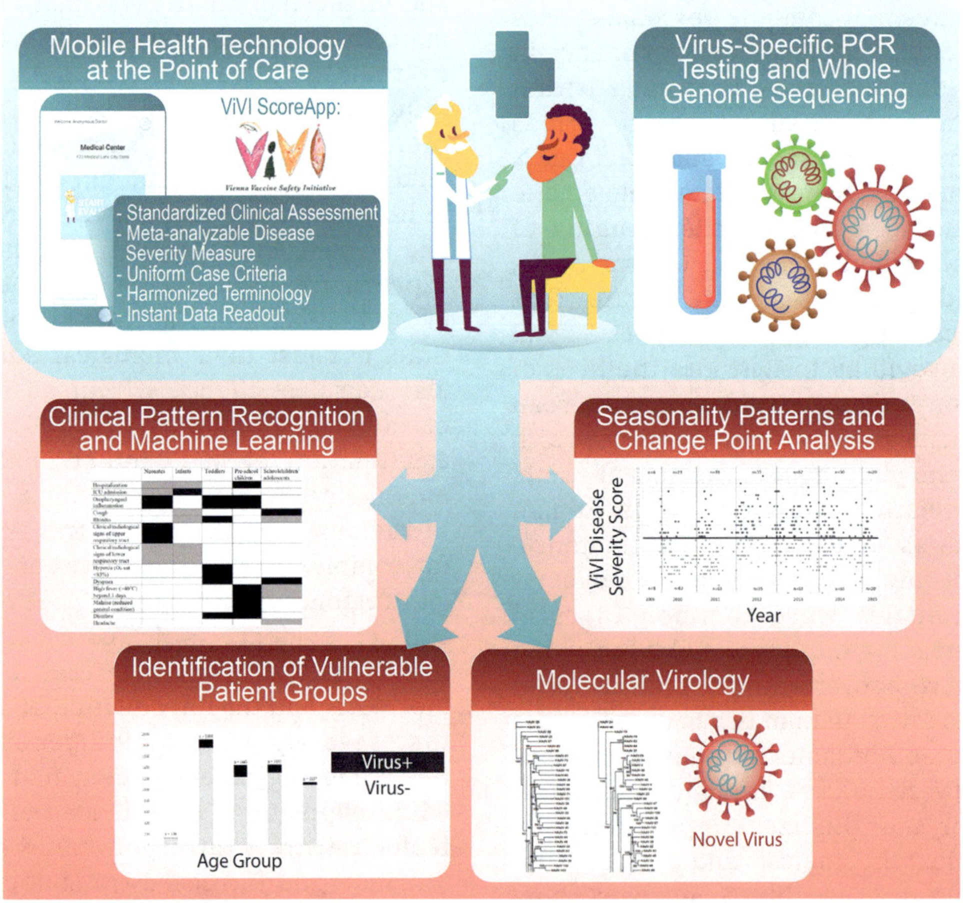

Figure 7.11. Examination of health and disease patterns in past populations.

Source: https://ars.els-cdn.com/content/image/1-s2.0-S2589004222005466-fx1_lrg.jpg.

7.4.3. Insights From Specific Archaeological Sites and Their Findings

Uncovering bioarcheological remains from significant archaeological sites has presented profound information on the social existence and identity of prehistoric populations. For instance, studies of Andean skeletons provide significant information on lifestyle, health, and social status. They have emphasized conditions such as osteoarthritis and entheses, showing how biomechanical stressors reflect the labor and locomotor patterns of these prehistoric populations. Through the alignment of methodological advances in osteological studies with the cultural identities of these societies, scholars have begun untangling the complicated interrelations among biological information and social behavior, underlining a rich understanding of life in the Andes. The emphasis on "small data" techniques allows researchers to study carefully detailed skeletal remains that are well preserved, enabling a detailed examination of the pathogenesis of the conditions and their effects on identity and status within the communities they served (Becker et al., 2019).

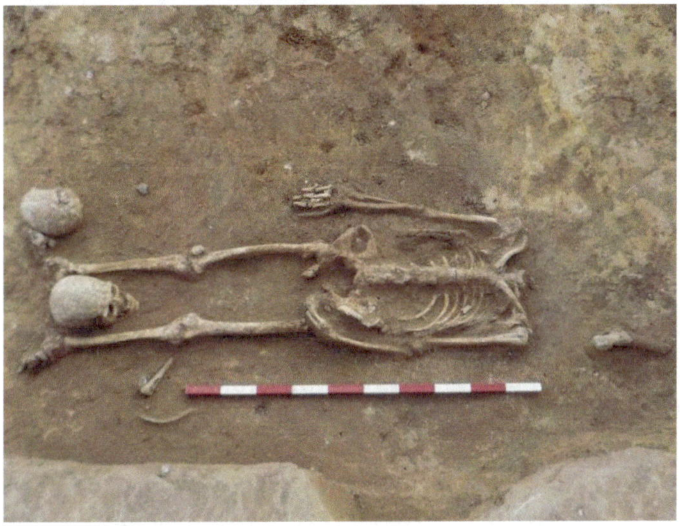

Figure 7.12. The exploration of bioarcheological findings.

Source: https://external-content.duckduckgo.com/iu/?u=https%3A%2F%2Fcdn.nexusnewsfeed.com%2Fimages%2F2019%2F11%2FArc1-1577507383439.jpg%3Fw%3D992%26h%3D744&f=1&nofb=1&ipt=fe230040b506d23fcca39aa65e9a2bab22c428901629c0431170050660bcd011.

Besides the data obtained from adults' remains, bioarcheological research on children also yields valuable insights into social identity and life experience in ancient societies. An analysis of a Byzantine cemetery at Syedra in Türkiye illustrates how the mortuary treatment of children may serve as an indicator of power relations and identity-formation processes within larger social structures. Through a combination of bioarcheological and proteomic studies, researchers have returned patterns for infant/child mortality, health, and status. Notably, evidence indicated female domination of the sample of burials, or gendered differences in treatment, which were likely to continue into life. The study of space in relation to mortuary practice also points to the interconnected nature of societal values, identity, and the perceived value of individuals by sex and age, thereby increasing our knowledge of social hierarchies during the Late Antique period in Anatolia (Davis et al., 2024). Furthermore, the combination of bioarcheology and interdisciplinary methods has enlightened us about the most essential aspects of both social life and identity in ancient societies. By combining proteomic analysis with traditional osteological techniques, researchers can explore more intricate social stories that help understand identity. The exploration of spatial placement in burials, as at the Syedra site, sheds light on how human beings were laid to rest according to social status and community organizational patterns, hinting at a sophisticated approach to understanding identity. Such collaborative approaches not only enrich our accounts of treatment and mortality in life but also lead to a richer engagement with how such phenomena influence present knowledge of person and social worth. In doing so, these archaeological findings advance discussion of identity and social structure, which remains relevant to contemporary readings of the human condition (Becker et al., 2019; Davis et al., 2024) (Figure 7.12).

Test Your Knowledge

1. How are case studies used in bioarchaeology to understand past human populations?
2. What insights can individual skeletal case studies provide about health, diet, and social life in ancient communities?

7.5. Identity Construction in Ancient Societies

Learning Outcome

1. Gender roles and identity in bioarcheological contexts
2. Ethnicity and cultural identity as reflected in skeletal remains
3. Social stratification and its bioarcheological indicators

The intricate tapestry of identity construction in ancient societies can be approached from the vantage point of bioarcheology, which sheds light on how social identities were constructed and perpetuated. Among the central tenets of this research is the examination of burial and skeletal remains, which reveal broader socio-economic formations and cultural narratives. By examining osteological evidence such as labor-related trauma, degenerative joint disease, and physiological responses to work, researchers can identify patterns that reveal individuals' daily experiences within their particular societies. This approach is congruent with approaches supported by researchers who focus on categories like osteoarthritis and entheseal alteration and require adequate description and observation of the aforementioned conditions in a bid to assess social dynamics (Becker et al., 2019). Thus, bioarcheological analysis is an important step through which physical evidence can be connected to the socio-political and economic constructions of identity within ancient societies. Furthermore, identity construction in ancient societies must consider the socio-economic stratification that shaped individual roles. Examining burial contexts, particularly how individuals were treated according to their estimated social class, offers tremendous insight into the identities they constructed based on occupation and status. Through an experimental look at societies' mortuary rituals, bioarcheologists discover how identity was inextricably connected to occupation, social status, and even ethnicity. For instance, research on pre-Hispanic coastal Peru's labor organization shows a complex dynamic between elite and commoner identities and suggests that popular narratives of oppression may have oversimplified the realities of labor organization (Muno et al., 2018). Thus, bioarcheological strategies for interpreting death and identity make complex not just our accounts of the individual but also larger narratives of class relations in past societies. In addition, the multifaceted nature of identity construction in ancient societies underscores the impact of biology and environment on identity formation in the past. Climatic factors, resource availability, and labor requirements had straightforward impacts on the physical health and social role of the individuals within their communities. Bioarchaeological analyses involving detailed observation of enthesial changes and other skeletal indicators reveal that these biological reactions are not isolated from social contexts but rather reflect communal practices and identities. The definition of identity and physicality—physicality, how labor and social status configured the body's health—highlights the fluidity of social interaction and the creation of identity. This process questions the usual dichotomous understanding that personalizes individuals as purely elite or laborers and concludes that identity in ancient societies was a performance defined by social, environmental, and biological variables embedded within the day-to-day experience (Becker et al., 2019).

7.5.1. Gender Roles and Identity in Bioarchaeological Contexts

The examination of gender identity and roles by bioarcheology uncovers a rich and complicated weave of social relationships that go beyond simplistic duality. As researchers increasingly acknowledge the shortcomings of classical categorical models, bioarcheology takes an insistent and multifaceted view of the interaction among sex, gender, and identity. By addressing and drawing upon a variety of theoretical schools of thought, especially those based on poststructuralist, feminist, and queer theory, scientists are demystifying the entanglements of gender construction. This analytical shift challenges the normative assumptions embedded in archaeological data, enabling more nuanced insights into the social identities individuals held throughout their lifetimes. In response, the discipline of bioarcheology is shifting to take on intersectionality, creating a broader context through which to explore how identities were constructed, performed, and reproduced across various cultural landscapes (Fausto-Sterling et al., 2016). Children, as a crucial focus in bioarcheological studies, provide a critical insight into the evolution of gender identities and social identity. Studies of children's mortuary treatment demonstrate how social organization dictated their lives and deaths and reveal identities that are otherwise forgotten in broader archaeological narratives. For instance, burial analysis can inform us about how children's experiences were determinative of social status, genotypic sex, and age in past societies. A perfect example is the cemetery of Syedra, Türkiye, which is Byzantine. Analysis of skeletal groups revealed differential patterns of treatment by gender and social rank. Such findings underscore the interplay of childhood and gender, exploring how these dimensions of identity were navigated and represented in the social landscape of the past (Davis et al., 2024). As bioarcheologists pursue these multiple layers of identity more intensely, an understanding emerges that transcends easy biological determinism. The application of interdisciplinary methods, such as proteomic analysis in conjunction with skeletal analysis, enhances our comprehension of gendered experience over time. Such rich data not only contributes to the growth of the discipline of bioarcheology but also illustrates a heightened concern towards recognizing the multiplicity of identities living in earlier social structures. By critically analyzing gender, status, and spatial relations, scholars are better able to deconstruct obsolete perceptions of identity. The ongoing desire to know about how gender roles were negotiated, constructed, and performed in premodern societies justifies the importance of bioarcheology in illuminating the social lives of ancient individuals and populations (Fausto-Sterling et al., 2016) (Figure 7.13).

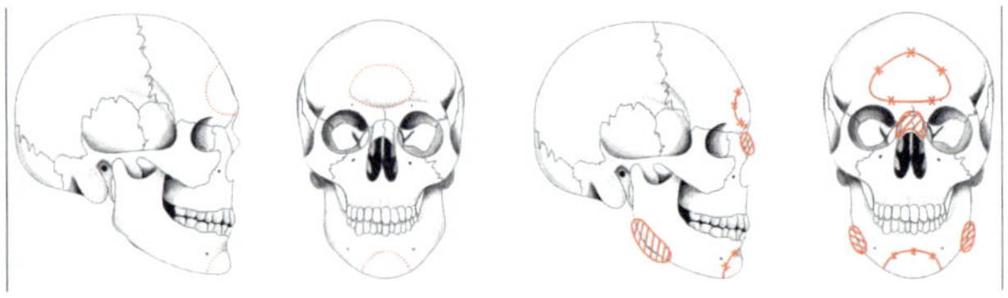

Figure 7.13. The exploration of gender roles and identity through bioarcheology reveals a complex tapestry of social dynamics that transcends simplistic binaries.

Source: https://pub.mdpi-res.com/humans/humans-04-00011/article_deploy/html/images/humans-04-00011-g001.png?1718698201.

7.5.2. Ethnicity and Cultural Identity as Reflected in Skeletal Remains

Skeletal remains provide a single vantage point from which to study cultural identity and ethnicity in ancient societies. Skeletal morphology, patterns of health, and burial ritual are often indicative of the complex interaction between culture and biology in shaping identity.

For instance, variation in skeletal traits can be employed to indicate geographic origins and migration patterns, and frequencies of particular disease processes may clarify social contacts and lifestyle activities related to ethnicity. Moreover, funeral rites, such as body orientation or grave offerings, are also rich in cultural significance that can determine the assumptions and values of the community. From these remains, bioarcheologists are informed about how individuals in a society constructed their identities and verify material entanglement between the social life and the body in ancient communities (Kakaliouras et al., 2017). In bioarcheological identity, there is the need to consider the broader socio-cultural context that regulates people's lives. It is not so much biology that determines ethnicity; instead, it is embedded in the fabric of community as a product of social relations, politics, and environment. Skeletal analysis, therefore, needs to unravel the dynamics of identity through an integrated approach bringing together both biological data and contextual socio-cultural data. For instance, by comparing demographic data with skeletal analysis, scientists can gain a deeper understanding of how past notions of identity might differ from those in the present.

This holistic approach helps appreciate the multifaceted realities of ethnicity and cultural identity, and how societal constructs change over time and influence how one interprets past populations (New et al., 2021). Moreover, some case studies illustrate the challenges and potentialities of using ethnicity and identity to extrapolate skeletal remains. For example, forensic identification of casualties in the 1943 Battle of Tarawa illustrates the issues when historical demographics are matched against more recent identity knowledge. The skeletal evidence does not correspond as easily with historical racial classifications, leading to interpretative biases. By applying a biosocial model that encompasses biological analysis, genetic data, and material culture, researchers can more accurately depict the identities of individuals and their populations. By an integrative approach, it underscores the necessity of bioarcheologists to constantly revise and expand their methodologies as the definitions of identity change, significantly affecting the narrative of human history (Kakaliouras et al., 2017).

7.5.3. Social Stratification and Its Bioarchaeological Indicators

Social stratification examined with bioarcheological markers presents a multifaceted approach to the study of ancient societies, particularly the relation of people to labor and social identity. The skeletal remains yield information concerning the experiences of people of different social levels. For instance, variations in trauma, osteoarthritis, and morphology of the attachment sites of muscles are bioarcheological markers that define the quality and amount of physical labor individuals have performed. In a study of the Late Intermediate Period of coastal Peru, these skeletal indicators are used to disprove assumptions that commoners were seriously overworked and oppressed compared to elites. Through the application of activity and health measures, the bioarcheological debate has the potential to reconfigure laborers and elites' relations in a way that is more in keeping with social reality than classical Marxist theory posits they are to do so, an aspect paramount to understanding the social dynamics of such past epochs (Muno et al., 2018). Dental pathology and oral health are also significant determinants of social stratification, indicating diet and socio-economic status in prehistoric societies. A comparative analysis of dental remains from sites within the Inka heartland, specifically Salapunku and Saqsahuaman, reveals significant contrasts in oral health and indicators of stress by socio-economic status. The higher rates of antemortem tooth loss and edentulism at Saqsahuaman point to dietary habits and spheres of physical demand distinct from those at Salapunku, which was an administrative center. This difference points to how bioarcheological analyses can illuminate the complexities of social identities based on economic positions within the Inka state context that relied on diverse servant populations for control. The dramatic disparity in dental health among these populations encapsulates key aspects of daily life and labor that inform our understanding of social stratification and hierarchies (Orrand et al., 2020). In addition, the effect of these bioarcheological indicators is not only to offer health figures but to revisit identity among past societies. By integrating skeletal evidence with cultural practices and burial context, researchers can construct narratives that capture individuals' positions within society. By analyzing funerary treatment alongside physical markers, researchers gain a sensitive appreciation for how identity was negotiated and performed during life and death. As bioarcheology research continues to uncover, the interaction dynamics of labor, health, and identity make hierarchies overly simplistic assumptions too rigid and instead show the dynamic nature of social stratification. An emic approach that considers a variety of indicators provides a deeper understanding of the social hierarchies that governed ancient communities, thereby enriching debate around identity in both modern and ancient communities (Muno et al., 2018).

Test Your Knowledge

1. What materials and techniques were commonly used in construction by ancient societies?
2. How did construction practices reflect the social, economic, and cultural aspects of ancient communities?

7.6. Contemporary Implications of Bioarcheology

Learning Outcome

1. Relevance of bioarcheological findings to modern social issues
2. Ethical considerations in bioarcheological research
3. The impact of bioarcheology on public understanding of history

The contemporary relevance of bioarcheology extends beyond mere archaeological interpretation and influences broader discussions in human adaptation and human conduct to environmental change. With increasing climate change, most state agencies maintain a causal link between such environmental changes and outbreaks of violence and assert that human beings have a tendency to resort to aggression automatically when faced with ecological stressors. This is answered, however, by bioarcheologists using historical evidence, which indicates that human communities have adapted mainly to climatic fluctuation through peaceful adaptation, utilizing social structures to confront hardship.

This well-balanced perspective highlights human agency, suggesting that social responses are less an outcome of inherent violence and more a matter of widespread cultural praxis. According to this, therefore, as the contemporary world crises keep unfolding, a revisit of past transitions using bioarcheological methods can provide important insight into today's policy-making disputes, which translates into more informed policy on environmental matters (DOCKS at Appalachian State University et al., 2017). The bioarcheological contribution to the study of social dynamics is complemented by how it approaches the study of caregiving practices as a way of achieving valuable insights into identity formation and social relationships across human history. Through biocultural approaches, researchers can bridge the gap between biology and the sociocultural environments that made up the life of an individual. This perspective is particularly applicable in considering caregiving behavior, not only reflects individual relationships but also overall societal values upon which they are predicated. Tilley's model of a "bioarcheology of care" presents a template for using skeletal remains to identify caregiving practice across cultures. By incorporating social theory into bioarcheological inquiry, researchers can reveal the intricacies of how communities and individuals care for each other, claiming caregiving as essential to what is fundamental to social life and identity (Ouellette et al., 2014).

Adding bioarcheology to the fray of contemporary debate allows a specific perspective from which to approach pressing issues that concern the world, such as public health and environmental sustainability. The emphasis upon the reconstruction of ancient social patterns and identities also fosters a greater appreciation for human interconnectedness, and from which the present can gain valuable lessons for contemporary problems, such as climate change and disparity. Through the dissemination of bioarchaeological information through modern channels of outreach, such as online media, researchers can facilitate greater public awareness of these lessons.

These efforts have the potential to connect community practice and academic scholarship, with a conversation about how earlier trends of flexibility can inform current practices. Lastly, the uses of bioarchaeology extend far beyond skeletal collection; they entail a careful examination of identity, hardness, and community facing ongoing transformations in society (DOCKS at Appalachian State University 2017 et al., 2017; Ouellette et al., 2014) (Figure 7.14).

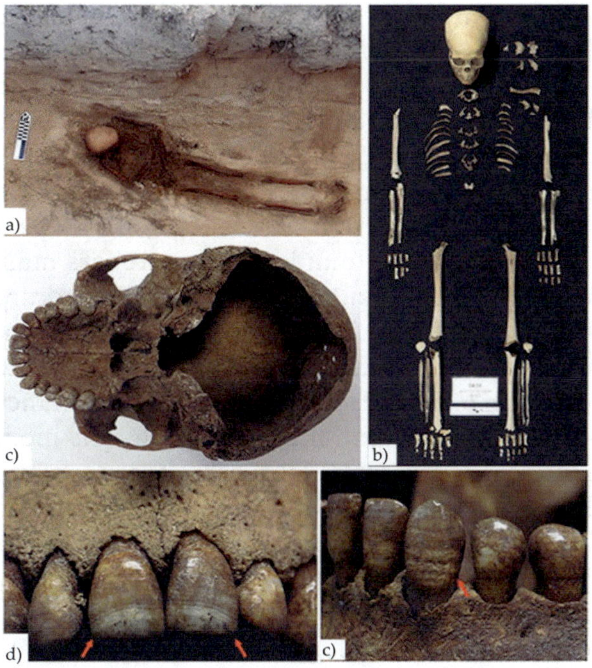

Figure 7.14. The contemporary implications of bioarcheology.

Source: https://www.tandfonline.com/cms/asset/a50a53be-cd9c-4470-aaee-75db2eb8e1b6/raaa_a_2403796_f0002_c.jpg.

7.6.1. Relevance of Bioarcheological Findings to Modern Social Issues

Bioarcheology is more than skeletal analysis; it is a lens by which modern societal issues can be examined. In this context, evidence with respect to osteoarthritis and other skeletal diseases is employed as an example of the manner in which bioarcheological research can inform us about past human life and modern social realities. For instance, investigating the prevalence of osteoarthritis among prehistoric populations reveals aspects of lifestyle, such as labor intensity and social stratification. By employing scientific studies to evaluate bone changes in terms of occupational strains, researchers can make comparisons with current work-related health. This convergence brings to the forefront a broader context for physical welfare and health, allowing for an informed consideration of the impact of socio-economic contexts on human wellness in the past and present, as embodied in the comprehensive treatment of osteoarthritis offered by Becker et al. (2019). Beyond issues of health, bioarcheology brings significant illumination to caregiving and social support systems. Analysis of burial and skeletal markers for care may reveal insights into how previous societies structured social networks and caregiving responsibilities. Through the use of Tilley's (2012) bioarcheology of care model, researchers are able to analyze and interpret caregiving behavior within the skeleton and contribute to a greater understanding of past support systems. It is beneficial in contemporary discussions around the worth of social support for vulnerable populations, such as the elderly or handicapped.

This capacity to make use of biocultural knowledge assists scholars in positioning ancient practices in juxtaposition with current caregiving practices to highlight the worth of social bonding and accountability across time. These findings support the efficacy of interdisciplinary approaches to resolving modern social issues, as noted in Ouellette et al. (2014). Further, the use of bioarcheological evidence is relevant to identity and social dynamics among ancient people's debates. Through examination of the intersection between biological identity and cultural practice, bioarcheologists are able to contribute to modern debates regarding race, ethnicity, and identity politics. Revealing identities through skeletal analysis can capture the wealth and depth of past social identities that find echoes in contemporary protests for representation and justice. As contemporary society is grappling with the implications and meanings of identity constructs, the bioarcheological focus on reconstructing the ways that identities were created and controlled through social hierarchies provides a temporal depth for contemporary arguments. Addressing these issues from a bioarcheological approach allows for more comprehensive investigation of how identity has always been tied to social convention, health, and interactions within communities, and therefore offers valuable insights into contemporary social problems.

7.6.2. Ethical Considerations in Bioarchaeological Research

Within bioarcheology, ethical concerns come forward most prominently, particularly regarding the treatment and interpretation of human remains. As researchers investigate the socialities and lives of the dead in the past, they strive to balance scholarly research with commemoration and remembrance of the deceased. There are ethical issues that arise when determining how to approach burial assemblages, especially when they might be spiritually or culturally significant to descendant groups. It is necessary to identify such cultural contexts because, as well as being a measure of respect for the memory of people interred, it also promotes mutually beneficial relationships between bioarcheologists and extant communities. These, in turn, can lead to more nuanced appreciations of prehistoric social forms and identities and thereby further enrichen the bioarcheological record while simultaneously maintaining ethical integrity within the research processes. Furthermore, the utilization of advanced scientific techniques in bioarcheology, i.e., paleopathology, raises other ethical concerns which should be tackled by researchers. The relatively recent science investigates earlier health and disease through an interface of disciplines, from archaeology and anthropology to the biochemical sciences. While such interdisciplinary approaches have the potential to yield more nuanced insights into the lives and struggles of ancient societies, they also entail a critical examination of the ethical considerations involved in their use. Scholars will be faced with having to address not just contributing to knowledge but potentially the ramifications of their discovery, particularly with regard to issues of representation and health disparities' historical contexts. This requirement of careful ethical evaluation makes the maintenance of informed consent, respect, and the welfare of the studied populations and their living descendants equally important. The ethical discourse of bioarcheological research has to be dynamic and responsive to the evolving social order. The entwining of past and present is profound, and researchers must be attentive to its implications in contemporary societal settings. Engaging with descendant communities and incorporating their voices into research proposals can significantly enhance ethical practices and make study designs more inclusive. This way, researchers can ensure their work makes positive contributions to discussions of identity, memory, and social life. Through the encouragement of interdisciplinary collaboration and respectful treatment of human remains, bioarcheology is well positioned to illuminate the complicated texture of human lives further while being attuned to ethical considerations that honor the past, its people, and their legacies, as highlighted in mortuary archaeology's richness (Meyers et al., 2014) and the obligations that underlie paleopathological inquiry (Grauer et al., 2022).

7.6.3. The Impact of Bioarcheology on Public Understanding of History

Bioarcheology provides a necessary intersection between the natural sciences and the humanities that profoundly influences the wider public's conceptualization of history. By examining human skeletal remains, bioarcheologists are able to reconstruct different aspects of individuals' lives in the past, including health, diets, and social structure. This scientific inquiry provides a tangible link to the past, transforming intangible historical narratives into physical stories that move people today. As , they examine conditions such as osteoarthritis and indicators of skeletal stress, revealing how individuals adapted their worlds and social requirements. This forensic practice not only increases popular understanding for history but also facilitates broader discussion of identity, community, and what it is to be human, showing the subtlety of ancient cultures in a way more conventional historical approaches risk losing (Becker et al., 2019). Furthermore, bioarcheology expands the horizon of history study through its incorporation of perspectives from various fields, thereby expanding our collective knowledge of humanity's past. The field intersects with mortuary archaeology and material culture research by investigating how burial practice, artifacts, and ritual provide insight into cultural perceptions of death and person (Meyers et al., 2014). By examining the burial of the dead across cultures, bioarcheology reveals the relationships between religious customs, social norms, and geography. With this multi-disciplinary inquiry, the public is made more able to comprehend the nuances of death and life in the past, fostering greater sensitivity to how societies change over time and what they leave behind. Therefore, the integration of bioarcheological evidence in public discourse encourages a more inclusive history, where many different voices and histories are acknowledged and honored. Finally, the role of bioarcheology in public understanding is reinforced by its application in pedagogical and heritage environments. Public monuments and museums increasingly incorporate bioarcheological research to explain things more in an interactive way to the public. By presenting skeletal remains alongside anecdotes about individuals' lives, institutions can effectively bridge the gap between scientific analysis and public engagement. These kinds of presentations make it possible to critically examine identity, community relationships, and the connection between past and contemporary social values. Moreover, collaborative research programs with emphasis on community participation foster inclusive discourses of heritage and identity, demonstrating the utility of bioarcheology in constructing an integrated understanding of history pertinent to contemporary issues of social justice and cultural identity (Meyers et al., 2014).

Test Your Knowledge

1. How does bioarchaeology inform our understanding of modern human health and disease patterns?
2. In what ways can bioarchaeological research influence contemporary social, ethical, and public health discussions?

SUMMARY

Bioarcheology offers a sophisticated understanding of the analysis of identity and social life using the study of human remains. This discipline goes beyond traditional archaeological methods by integrating biological data with cultural contexts, enabling the interpretation of past societies with a more advanced methodology. Through novel technologies, such as Geographic Information Systems (GIS), scientists can clarify their analyses and reveal social interaction patterns, caregiving regimes, and community organization. The application of such technologies, as in the case of the Bronze Age burial at Tell Abraq, demonstrates the possibility of accurate spatial analyses that provide a deeper understanding of mortuary practices and social organization and, ultimately, of the broader social identities of persons and groups within ancient contexts (Calleja et al., 2016). Furthermore, the interdisciplinary method of bioarcheology provides significant insight into the way in which human biology meets with sociocultural dynamics. Adopting a biocultural approach, as highlighted through recent scholarship on caregiving within skeletal analysis, researchers can reveal complex patterns of behavior to illuminate identity. This new method facilitates an increasingly integrated presentation of human experience, marrying biological properties with social histories. As suggested by Tilley's four-stage bioarcheology of care approach, the field can shed light on how systems of care and support existed in previous societies, thus advancing our understanding of the determinants shaping social identity and cohesion (Ouellette et al., 2014). In summary, bioarcheology of identity and social life not only informs us more on ancient society but also raises relevant questions on modern social constructs. Through continued use of methodologies that place material remains within sociocultural practice, academics can advance deeper debates about identity, community, and care in past and contemporary contexts. The ongoing growth of this field, bolstered by developments in technology and theory, has the potential to continue revealing further intricacies around the human condition and values contained within past cultures. Therefore, bioarcheology remains a core component of anthropological inquiry, integrating biological information and cultural knowledge, ensuring that the stories of our ancestors remain truthfully stored and interpreted in their entirety.

The analysis of the bioarcheological aspects of identity and social life reveals vital information regarding the health and living standards of people in Roman England, which points out the contrasts between urban and rural populations. In a classic work on child morbidity, the authors conducted a close examination of the health indicators at various sites. They concluded that rural children had higher rates of certain illnesses compared to urban children. The accounts presented drastic pathologies associated with poverty, and it was deduced that farming activities in the Roman period extensively shaped the health of low socio-economic groups. This research challenges the assumption that urban locations like Poundbury Camp reflect experiences of Romano-British childhood, thereby revealing the need for a more refined appreciation of health inequalities by social stratification (Adams et al., 2017). Another significant area of the bioarcheological research entails the examination of race as a biological anthropology phenomenon. The most recent expert questionnaires have shown a consensus that race is not primarily a biological classification but rather a social one; as a result, an analysis of how these ideas affect investigation and public discourse is in order. Most anthropologists advance a system of classification by geographical regions rather than reciting the discredited race classifications, and the demand for responsible discussion on these sensitive issues follows. The survey findings stress both the ethical costs of talking about race and the sense of stifling critical discourse. By debating these matters, bioarcheologists can position themselves within the broader debate around race, thus contributing to a more socially aware understanding of identity and diversity throughout the past (Adams et al., 2021). Additionally, the implications of these findings extend far beyond academic circles; they emphasize the crucial relevance of bioarcheology in shaping contemporary understandings of identity and social relations. Public engagement is key as scholars move forward to address the legacies of colonialism and racism within anthropology. The rhetoric demands a rethinking of pedagogy around race and ancestry, one that calls for standardized curricula that engage these topics in depth. The call for further consideration of the moral and ethical aspects of anthropological practice aims to minimize the risk of misappropriation by ideologically driven organizations. This way, bioarchaeology not only provides a window into past societies but also serves as a place to consider current social organizations and foster a greater integration of understanding of identity and heritage (Adams et al., 2021).

KEY TERMS FROM THIS CHAPTER

- Activity Markers
- Bioarcheology
- Biocultural Approach
- Burial Treatment
- Community Structure
- Cranial Modification
- Dental Modification
- Dietary Reconstruction
- Funerary Context
- Grave Goods
- Health Inequality
- Isotopic Analysis
- Mobility Patterns
- Mortuary Practices
- Social Identity
- Status Differentiation

CRITICAL THINKING QUESTIONS

1. **What does the "bioarcheology of identity" primarily focus on?**
   a. The chemical composition of bones
   b. Cultural and social meanings derived from human remains
   c. Taxonomic classification of ancient hominins
   d. Preservation techniques in archaeological sites
2. **Which of the following can be used to infer occupational stress in skeletal remains?**
   a. Porotic hyperostosis
   b. Harris lines
   c. Enthesopathies (muscle attachment changes)
   d. Dental wear
3. **Isotopic analysis of bones and teeth can provide information about:**
   a. Ancestry and biological sex
   b. Mobility and diet
   c. Trauma and disease
   d. Age at death
4. **Artificial cranial modification is often interpreted as evidence of:**
   a. Nutritional deficiency
   b. Chronic infection
   c. Cultural identity or group affiliation
   d. Trauma from interpersonal violence
5. **Which of the following is not typically considered a marker of identity in bioarcheology?**
   a. Dental modification
   b. Grave goods
   c. Mitochondrial DNA
   d. Burial orientation

Short Answer Questions

1. What is meant by the term "bioarcheology of identity," and how does it differ from traditional osteological analysis?
2. How can burial context and grave goods contribute to interpretations of social identity in the past?
3. Explain how skeletal markers can provide evidence of occupation or labor in ancient societies.
4. What are some of the challenges in interpreting gender from skeletal remains in bioarcheological contexts?
5. How can isotopic analysis inform our understanding of past diet and migration, and what does this reveal about identity?

Answers to Critical Thinking Questions

1. (b); 2. (c); 3. (b); 4. (c); 5. (c)

REFERENCES

1. Adams, D. M., & Pilloud, M. A. (2021). Perceptions of race and ancestry in teaching, research, and public engagement in biological anthropology. *Human Biology*, *93*(1), 9. https://doi.org/10.13110/humanbiology.93.1.01Adams, M., Allen, L. H., Armelagos, G. J., Baker, B. J., Brickley, M., Brickley, M. B., Britton, K., et al. (2017). Poundbury Camp in context–A new perspective on the lives of children from urban and rural Roman England. https://core.ac.uk/download/59989550.pdf (accessed on 21st July 2025).
2. Becker, S. K. (2019). Osteoarthritis, entheses, and long bone cross-sectional geometry in the Andes: Usage, history, and future directions. https://core.ac.uk/download/323311202.pdf (accessed on 21st July 2025).
3. Bogaard, A., Kjellström, A., Linderholm, A., Onsten-Molander, A., Rand, A., Lamb, A. L., Ingvarsson, A., et al. (2017). Integrating isotopes and documentary evidence: Dietary patterns in a late medieval and early modern mining community, Sweden. https://core.ac.uk/download/131023965.pdf (accessed on 21st July 2025).
4. Botta, F. N., & Seldes, V. (2014). Violence indicators in Quebrada de Humahuaca, Jujuy, Argentina: The Regional Development Period from a regional perspective. https://core.ac.uk/download/159288092.pdf (accessed on 21st July 2025).
5. Calleja, M. (2016). Commingled tombs and ArcGIS: Analyzing the mortuary context and taphonomy at Bronze Age Tell Abraq. http://digitalscholarship.unlv.edu/cgi/viewcontent.cgi?article=3649&context=thesesdissertations (accessed on 21st July 2025).
6. Casserly, A. M. (2022). Assessing stress biomarkers as embodied identity in Kentucky's Green River Archaic. https://core.ac.uk/download/541431151.pdf (accessed on 21st July 2025).
7. Cormier, A. A. (2018). Maya Oste biographies of the Holmul region, Guatemala: Curating life histories through bioarcheology and stable isotope analysis. https://core.ac.uk/download/215940331.pdf (accessed on 21st July 2025).
8. Davis, M. R. (2024). Social identity and personhood at an early Byzantine cemetery: Late antique child burials at Syedra, Türkiye. https://core.ac.uk/download/639328724.pdf (accessed on 21st July 2025).
9. Fausto-Sterling, A., Jagose, A., Oakley, A., Zihlman, A., Jordan, A. M., Alberti, B., Alberti, B., et al. (2016). Introduction to "Binary Binds": Deconstructing sex and gender dichotomies in archaeological practice. https://core.ac.uk/download/153514013.pdf (accessed on 21st July 2025).
10. Garland, C. J. (2014). Biocultural consequences of Spanish contact in the Lambayeque Valley region of northern Peru: Internal enamel micro-defects as indicators of early life stress. https://core.ac.uk/download/71425135.pdf (accessed on 21st July 2025).
11. Gowland, R. L., & Perry, M. A. (2022). Compounding vulnerabilities: Syndemics and the social determinants of disease in the past. https://core.ac.uk/download/578086411.pdf (accessed on 21st July 2025).
12. Gowland, R., & Kacki, S. (2020). Theoretical approaches to bioarcheology: The view from across the pond. https://core.ac.uk/download/578142155.pdf (accessed on 21st July 2025).
13. Grauer, A. (2022). Introduction. https://core.ac.uk/download/614446076.pdf (accessed on 21st July 2025).

14. Hämäläinen, R. (2020). Gender matters: Material-cultural theory of sex-gender in mortuary archaeology. https://core.ac.uk/download/328853618.pdf (accessed on 21st July 2025).
15. Jones, D. (2015). Bioarcheological analysis of isolated crania from the Elizabeth site in the Lower Illinois River Valley. https://core.ac.uk/download/71427328.pdf (accessed on 21st July 2025).
16. Kakaliouras, A. M. (2017). 2 Theory for a bioarcheology of community: Potentials, practices, and pitfalls. https://core.ac.uk/download/337304564.pdf (accessed on 21st July 2025).
17. Klaus, H. (2008). Bioarcheology of life and death in colonial South America: Systemic stress, adaptation, and ethnogenesis in the Lambayeque Valley, Peru AD 900–1750. https://core.ac.uk/download/159583890.pdf (accessed on 21st July 2025).
18. Lillehammer, G. (2025). *Archaeology of Children*. https://core.ac.uk/download/pdf/38828355.pdf (accessed on 21st July 2025).
19. Meyers, K., & Williams, H. (2014). Blog bodies: Mortuary archaeology and blogging. https://core.ac.uk/download/20250427.pdf (accessed on 21st July 2025).
20. Morrone, A. (2020). Balso suteikimas mažiesiems: Baltijos šalių vaikų bioarcheologija. https://core.ac.uk/download/401879905.pdf (accessed on 21st July 2025).
21. Muno, S. K. (2018). Labor and social identity in ancient Peru: A bioarcheological perspective. https://core.ac.uk/download/213558269.pdf (accessed on 21st July 2025).
22. New, B. T., Taylor, R. J., & Tegtmeyer, C. E. (2021). Navigating identity: The intersection of social and biological identity from the WWII Battle of Tarawa. https://core.ac.uk/download/480389530.pdf (accessed on 21st July 2025).
23. Orrand, M. (2020). Oral health in the Inka heartland during the Late Horizon: A tale of two sites. https://core.ac.uk/download/344771103.pdf (accessed on 21st July 2025).
24. Ouellette, L. (2014). The bioarcheology of care. https://core.ac.uk/download/61661236.pdf (accessed on 21st July 2025).
25. Parnell, E. K. (2017). Bioarcheology and climate change in the public realm. https://core.ac.uk/download/345084797.pdf (accessed on 21st July 2025).
26. Vanderpool, E. (2011). Bioarcheological investigations of community and identity at the Avondale Burial Place (McArthur Cemetery), Bibb County, Georgia. https://core.ac.uk/download/71421738.pdf (accessed on 21st July 2025).

DENTAL ANTHROPOLOGY AND CRANIOFACIAL ANALYSIS

8

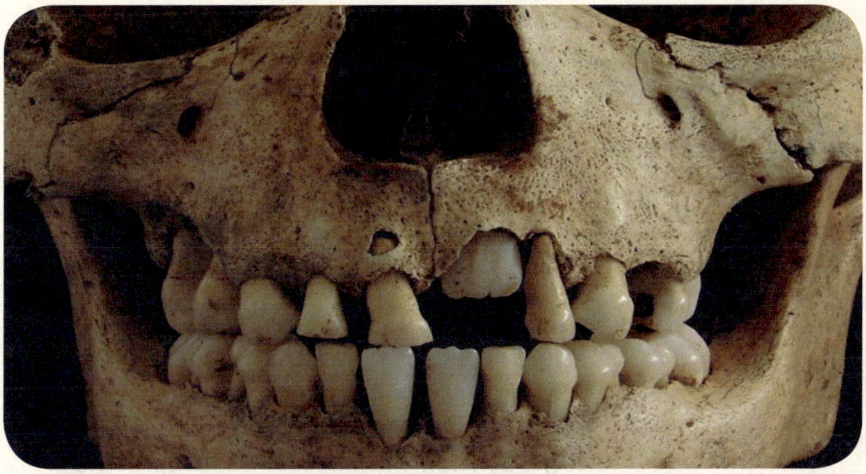

LEARNING OBJECTIVES

After studying this chapter, you will be able to:

1. Describe the historical background of dental anthropology
2. Discuss the role of teeth in anthropology
3. Focus on craniofacial anatomy
4. Describe the methodologies in craniofacial analysis
5. Know applications of dental anthropology
6. Identify ethical considerations in dental anthropology

Introduction

The science of dental anthropology and craniofacial analysis offers a profound understanding of the evolutionary, behavioral, and health-related features of human beings and their ancestors. The interdisciplinary field of study encompasses ideas from anthropology, biology, and medicine and offers a unified framework for researchers to study differences in dental morphology and craniofacial structures across populations. By studying such differences, scientists can find out about dietary adaptations, social trends, and environmental influences that have shaped human evolution over millennia. Further, the correlation of craniodental traits with other variables generates hypotheses about the adaptive significance of specific morphological and thus talk about human evolutionary lineages and potential future adaptations becomes feasible. Therefore, dental morphology is a valuable tool for reconstructing extinct and extant species' diets and habits, and it provides context for interpretations in the fossil record. The dental characters, such as occlusal surface shape, inform us a lot about an organism's mode of feeding and ecological niche. For instance, it has been hypothesized in studies that the interaction between dietary and dental variation could be complex, given what research on the variation in occlusal surfaces among primates has revealed. Elliptical Fourier Functional Analysis and multivariate analysis were utilized in this work to identify unexpected trends in dental adaptation and dentition. Consequently, examination of these correlations provides additional insight into how dental characteristics may have evolved in response to environmental pressures and dietary needs, adding to the controversy within dental anthropology (O\u27Neill et al., 2016). Further still, no stress can be put on the importance of robust methodologies to craniofacial analysis, particularly in terms of issues of accuracy and risks of traditional imaging techniques. To address these issues, new approaches, such as high-definition webcams, have proven effective alternatives for capturing facial images and identifying soft tissue landmarks. These low-tech methods underscore the importance of accuracy in facial analysis and have enabled the identification of reliable landmarks in facial images. Results show that certain landmarks are more consistent when measured by a single examiner, highlighting the need to adopt standard practices and to explore avenues for improving current methodologies used in craniofacial research. This shift towards using less intricate and less accurate methods opens new avenues for future research in dental anthropology and craniofacial analysis, thereby extending the field's contribution to human biodiversity and evolution (Payne et al., 2013).

Definition of Dental Anthropology

The discipline of dental anthropology is a branch of biological anthropology that examines the relationship between dental structures and human biological variation. Dental anthropology encompasses the examination of teeth and jaws to interpret varied aspects of human adaptation, evolution, and health. Using dental morphology, experts can infer dietary habits, genetic relationships, and population social behaviors. This is a continuation of the dental applications in the real world, where dental variation can shed light on historical population movements and contacts. Dental anthropology, hence, becomes a vital means through which one can understand not only the physiological significance of dental characteristics but also their cultural as well as evolutionary significance. In addition, dental anthropology supports craniofacial analysis in establishing a model for understanding the coordination of dental structure with cranial shape. Using tools such as geometric morphometrics, researchers can identify correlations between mandibular shape and muscle mass, thereby gaining a broader understanding of functional adaptation.

As shown in studies using imaging technology, coordination between dental morphology and craniofacial structures is key to reconstructing evolutionary trajectories. For example, the correlation between mandibular form and the cross-sectional areas of masticatory muscles indicates how functional needs can shape anatomical structures over time (Bresin et al., 2018). These findings continue to validate the importance of dental anthropology in understanding the complexity of craniofacial growth. In addition, advances in diagnostic methods have enhanced dental anthropology's ability to provide valid information on facial morphology. The availability of low-cost imaging techniques, such as high-definition webcam photography, enables standardized facial image capture, thereby enabling landmark identification for further analysis. Studies have shown that certain facial landmarks, once correctly identified, can be used to obtain key data for quantitative analysis of craniofacial relationships (Payne et al., 2013). This increased precision helps anthropologists uncover unique patterns of variation, integrating dental health into the broader anthropological context and establishing dental anthropology as a fundamental component of research into human biology and cultural evolution (Figure 8.1).

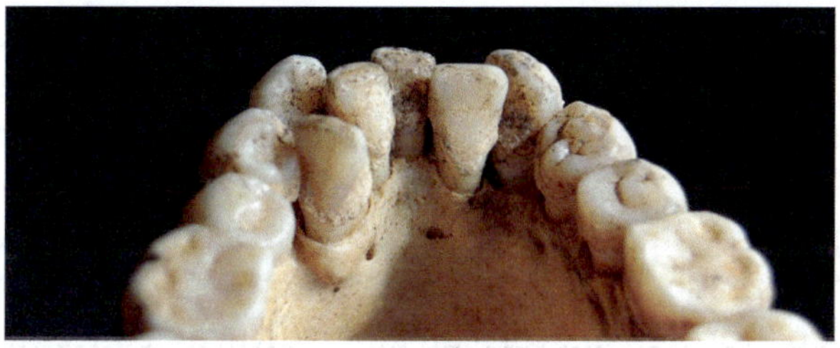

Figure 8.1. The field of dental anthropology.

Source: https://images.squarespace-cdn.com/content/v1/552ade7fe4b0ee740debb251/1497387337744-JJPAXVZNTNRL59C7OE6E/Banner9.jpg?format=1500w.

Importance of Craniofacial Analysis

Craniofacial analysis has an important role in interpreting the evolutionary course of various species, particularly in the field of dental anthropology. By studying craniofacial forms, researchers can infer dietary adaptations that drove morphological evolution over time. The relationship between dental form and ecological niches is highlighted by studies that measure how occlusal surface shapes vary among non-hominin primates and hominins. These studies show that dental form and size can be utilized as markers of phylogenetic relationships as well as of ecological habits and thus enhance our understanding of how craniofacial features are shaped by pressures from the environment. This morphological data not only aids in reconstructing the lifestyles of extinct species but also provides a comparative framework for assessing contemporary populations and their adaptive features, establishing craniofacial analysis as a cornerstone of anthropological research (O\u27Neill et al., 2016). Moreover, integrating genetic factors into craniofacial analysis reveals another layer of complexity in understanding morphological variation within a species. Research has also established that an individual's craniofacial traits are influenced not only by environmental factors but also by genetic factors. For instance, inbred strains of mice research indicates the way genetic interaction can contribute significantly to the establishment of craniofacial morphology, and this demonstrates that the expression of some traits can be affected by the interaction of multiple genetic factors. Specifically, research on Sprouty gene mutant models has demonstrated that variation in craniofacial shape can be attributed to both genotype and genetic background. The findings confirm the necessity of accounting for genetic variation when assessing craniofacial characteristics, as this may reveal the complexity of physical attributes across populations, underscoring the significance of craniofacial analysis within the broader context of dental anthropology (Hallgrímsson et al., 2017). The uses of craniofacial analysis extend beyond evolutionary biology and genetic interaction because they also interpenetrate with modern clinical practice. An understanding of craniofacial variation can inform dental and medical practitioners about congenital deformities and appropriate interventions for correction. Accurate mapping of craniofacial morphology can assist in surgical planning, prosthetic design, and orthodontic intervention, thereby improving patient outcomes. Also, as clinicians and anthropologists collaborate, they create opportunities for more integrated models of healthcare that consider both the biological and social factors. This interdisciplinarity underscores the value of craniofacial analysis not only as a research tool but also as a practical tool for the management of craniofacial problems in contemporary populations. All in all, the significance of craniofacial analysis goes beyond its historical origins, as it is now a fundamental pillar for the description of intricate biological processes in dental anthropology and beyond (Figure 8.2).

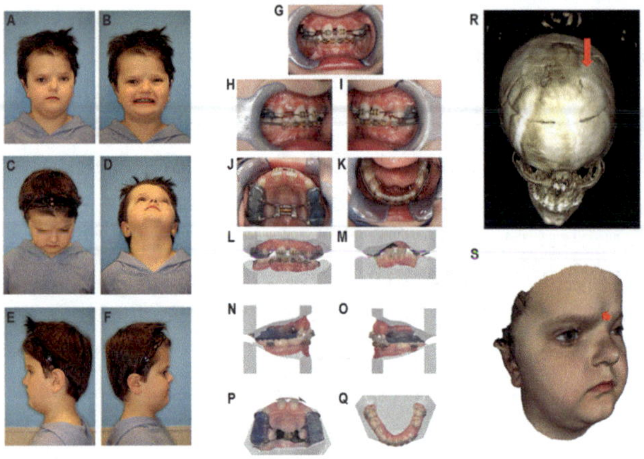

Figure 8.2. Craniofacial analysis serves a pivotal role in understanding the evolutionary trajectories of various species.

Source: https://external-content.duckduckgo.com/iu/?u=https%3A%2F%2Fwww.mdpi.com%2Fjdb%2Fjdb-09-00039%2Farticle_deploy%2Fhtml%2Fimages%2Fjdb-09-00039-g002-550.jpg&f=1&nofb=1&ipt=82d9d19dfbef4485be1751af31230887d30dd537fef835e11ce049a176fe0084.

8.1. Historical Background of Dental Anthropology

Learning Outcome

1. Early Studies and Discoveries
2. Key Figures in the Field
3. Evolution of Research Methods

The origins of dental anthropology are traceable to the point where archaeology merged with dental science, and anthropologists began examining skeletal remains to deduce ancient populations' dietary and health trends. This field grew significantly in the late 19th and early 20th centuries as scholars sought to understand population variation at the biological level through dental features. Dental anthropologists have previously focused on dental morphology to examine evolutionary relationships and migration patterns. As research progressed, it became necessary to add cultural and environmental factors in consideration. This rising awareness spurred a more advanced conceptualization of how lifestyle, diet, and inheritance interact to shape craniofacial development, thereby marking a shift from descriptive studies to a more mature interpretative model that incorporates historical and cultural contexts, further enhancing our appreciation of human dental diversity across different locales and populations. Throughout the 20th century, science was transformed by the inclusion of modern methodologies and technologies. Metric analysis, radiographic imaging, and computer modeling were introduced, facilitating precise measurements of craniofacial structures and enabling researchers to study the intricate interrelationships between dental structures and anthropological measurements. Comparative studies at the international level became feasible with these developments, shedding light on the variability of craniofacial structures in some populations. One of the best examples is the focus on Central and South American native populations, in which recent studies identify characteristic craniofacial patterns resulting from historical events and migration. Understanding this morphological variation not only enriches our anthropological knowledge but also is relevant to contemporary oral health strategies aimed at specific demographic needs, underscoring the ongoing importance of dental anthropology in addressing health disparities among multicultural populations (Hubbe et al., 2024). In addition, the contemporary context of dental anthropology increasingly emphasizes interdisciplinary collaborations that merge anthropological, dental, and public health knowledge. This convergence is particularly observed in addressing pressing oral health issues prevalent in certain regions. For instance, societies in Central and South America are confronted with extensive prevalence of dental caries and inadequate access to healthcare centers (Fornai et al., 2024). Thus, researchers are advocating for an integrative approach that combines anthropological data on traditional food practices and habits with dental science to develop successful public health interventions. These collaborative efforts not only advance our understanding of the craniomandibular system and its pathologies but also promote community engagement, in that research is not merely culturally responsive but ethically conducted. This paradigm clearly demonstrates that dental anthropology is not a scientific field in isolation but an integral subject with sheer health and wellness ramifications for populations globally (Figure 8.3).

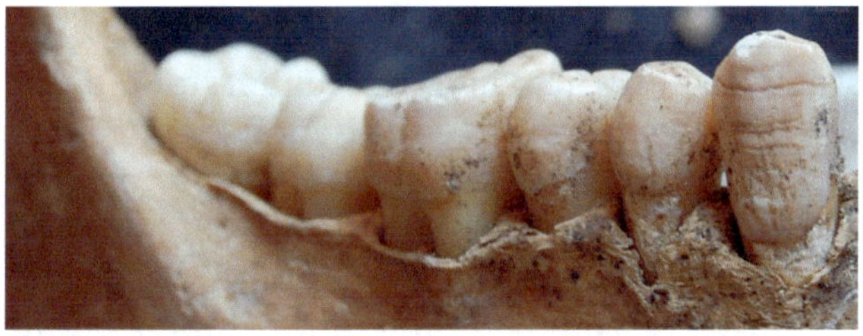

Figure 8.3. The foundation of dental anthropology can be traced back to the intersection of archaeology and dental science.

Source: https://external-content.duckduckgo.com/iu/?u=https%3A%2F%2Fimages.squarespace-cdn.com%2Fcontent%2Fv1%2F552ade7fe4b0ee740debb251%2F1497387176870-NMKF7RFQ5YR0EJEOV2CY%2FBanner1.jpg&f=1&nofb=1&ipt=d97b484c1fb83c38a0ee34e1602fa65c1c7a8bc474e42f3c7131d6bc7f71f406.

8.1.1. Early Studies and Discoveries

Research in dental anthropology has established basic principles for the study of human evolution and diversity. Dental remains were used in early research to make inferences about population migration, health, and the social organization of prehistoric societies. Considerable progress has been made through such techniques as craniometry, the examination of skull morphology to acquire information on craniofacial variation across different human groups. By applying statistical techniques, scientists have established patterns of dental trait distribution correlated with geographic and environmental factors. These techniques have illuminated not just the physical adaptations of populations but also their migratory and cultural heritage. The results gained through these initial attempts serve to underscore the merit of dental anthropology in building integrated profiles of prehistoric man, from diet to social group, laying the groundwork for subsequent research in the field. Beyond immediate population analysis, initial results in non-human dental morphometry are significant for understanding overall evolutionary processes. Research on the franciscana dolphin has revealed that suture closure patterns in the skull differ among species, highlighting the intricacies of adaptations during evolution (Cappozzo et al., 2015). The results of such research provide insights for human craniofacial investigation, indicating that differences in dental and cranial forms can be indicative of functional and evolutionary histories. In addition, exploring these morphological differences enhances our understanding of anatomical development in extant and extinct species. As such, initial studies on this front have given us a lush tapestry of details, placing the importance of dental features within the larger context of evolutionary biology and ecological adaptation. studies. However, pioneering investigations have brought to the forefront its important contribution to explaining the peopling of areas, particularly the Americas. Greenberg, Turner, and Zegura's early work, which proposed models of migration based on dental traits, emphasized its role in anthropological history (Duncan et al., 2013). Through research on dental morphology in Paleoindians, researchers identified unique similarities and differences that they attributed to geographic dispersal and environmental adaptation. This is an indication that while genetics plays a significant role in giving insights into lineage and variation, dental anthropology alone captures the dynamic history of interaction between cultural practices, diet, and health. By combining these findings with new genetic research, scholars can build a clearer picture of the complex patterns of human settlement and migration in the New World.

8.1.2. Key Figures in the Field

Several key scholars within the disciplines of dental anthropology and craniofacial research have assisted in advancing the knowledge and the process of science. Deserving of mention among so long a roll of pioneers is Dr. C. Loring Brace, who has made his career in the study of the evolutionary meaning of dental morphology for ecological and cultural adaptation. Having worked extensively with skeletal samples from an enormous range of populations, Brace has made significant observations on the use of dental characteristics as markers for both genetic heritage and functional adaptation. His works emphasize the importance of integrating anthropological principles with dental analysis to shed light on the intricate dynamics between phenotype and environment, thereby harmoniously bridging the gap between biological anthropology and dental sciences. Dr. Susan H. E. Smith is another pivotal figure who has made significant contributions to the forensic use of craniofacial analysis. Her investigation into craniofacial superimposition as a tool for identifying remains when standard methods are ineffective has the potential to transform forensic science. Although it has a century-old history, the use of craniofacial superimposition usually does not have standardized criteria for its practitioners. In a recent collaborative research effort with practitioners from 16 institutions, Smith campaigned for the establishment of objective, clear criteria for skull-face analysis and for closing existing loopholes in methodological standards (Abramov et al., 2025). This research not only enhances the reliability of forensic identifications but also underscores the importance of interdisciplinarity in advancing dental anthropology. Furthermore, researchers like Dr. Anna M. P. Fischer have expanded the understanding of the adaptive value of dental morphology in herbivorous mammals and have therefore provided information that can be applied to hominins. Using model animals such as rabbits, Fischer's study describes how variations in the mechanical properties of food during chewing influence jaw adaptation and chewing patterns. The results outline contrasting perspectives of common assumptions of relationships among food toughness, jaw-loading patterns, and chewing investment, and that diets with inferior nutritive value require longer processing to ensure maximum extraction of nutrients (Fling et al., 2015). This study not only expands our understanding of the adaptive significance of dental morphology but also provides a compelling framework for investigating the interface between dietary behavior and evolutionary biology in the human condition through dental anthropology and craniofacial analysis.

8.1.3. Evolution of Research Methods

The evolution of research methods in dental anthropology and craniofacial analysis has progressed from traditional observation techniques to more sophisticated, technology-driven approaches. Early anthropological studies were mainly based on comparative dental morphology and cranial measurements, often with poor-quality measurement instruments such as calipers and rough sketches. While these initial studies offered rudimentary data on human variation and evolution, they were stamped with human bias and subjective interpretation. As the field matured, researchers became increasingly sensitive to the value of formalized quantitative analysis. Techniques such as geometric morphometrics have evolved, allowing precise measurements of dental and craniofacial shape variation to provide a clearer picture of evolutionary relationships and functional adaptations in extant and extinct species. In the last few years, the integration of advanced imaging technologies with computational methods has further revolutionized techniques in dental anthropology. Techniques such as 3D surface scanning and digital photogrammetry enable accurate, non-destructive records of craniofacial morphology. This technology has been particularly groundbreaking, as it enables researchers to obtain more detailed information than before, further enhancing the accuracy of morphological analysis. For instance, the analysis of tooth occlusal surface profiles using methods such as Elliptical Fourier Analysis has illuminated dietary adaptations and their influence on morphological variation within species. The use of such quantitative approaches not only deepens our understanding of dental variation but also refines the empirical basis for understanding the evolutionary mechanism controlling craniofacial growth, thereby giving credibility to dental anthropology research in general (O\\\\u27Neill et al., 2016). Additionally, the incorporation of genetic analysis in the study of craniofacial is a significant leap in the comprehension of interactions between genetics and morphology. Current studies investigating the connections between genetic mutations and craniofacial features demonstrate the value of multi-disciplinary studies. For example, efforts to establish correlations between FGFR1 gene mutations and some craniofacial measurements show how genetic factors contribute to the determination of human facial morphology (Kalra et al., 2015). Despite some unsubstantiated findings in such genetic correlations, the marriage of molecular techniques with traditional morphological assessment is a real testament to an integrated approach towards the study of human evolution. Such research evolution testifies to the field's dynamic nature, opening new frontiers and enabling anthropologists to explore complex correlations among genetics, environment, and morphology, adding depth to knowledge of human diversity and its evolutionary history (Figure 8.4).

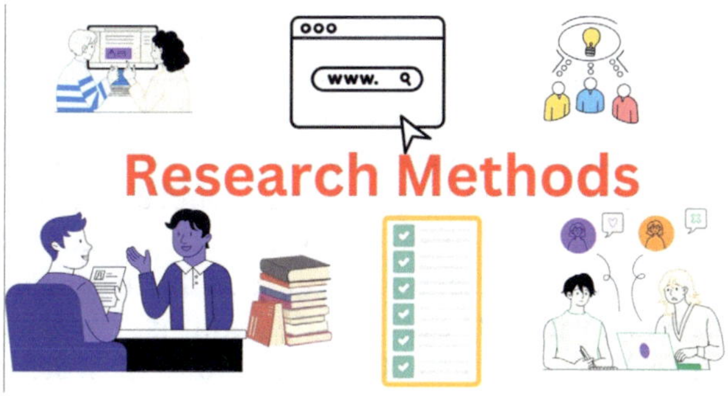

Figure 8.4. Evolution of research methods.

Source: https://media.licdn.com/dms/image/v2/D4D12AQHrsTBad5drvw/article-cover_image-shrink_720_1280/article-cover_image-shrink_720_1280/0/1687518877198?e=2147483647&v=beta&t=PssWpRdrem36OQ_1PJhD8ada2Y-1zmM2ONqUa7NIY00.

Test Your Knowledge

1. How did dental anthropology develop as a scientific discipline over time?
2. Who were the key figures in the historical development of dental anthropology, and what were their contributions?

8.2. The Role of Teeth in Anthropology

Learning Outcome

1. Teeth as Indicators of Diet
2. Teeth and Genetic Heritage
3. Dental Pathologies and Their Implications

When exploring human evolution, the role of teeth in anthropology extends beyond function; they are vital indicators of diet, signs of environmental adaptation, and markers of evolutionary relationships between species. Dental morphology, including tooth shape and size, provides much information. For instance, differences in occlusal surfaces of teeth can shed light on dietary patterns and ecological niches of extinct and living species. This association is apparent among primates, where dietary adaptations vary as do differences in premolars and molars. These dental attributes hold secrets to how the earliest hominins, such as Paranthropus robustus, adapted to their world, suggesting a complex interaction between diet, environment, and evolutionary pressures, which can be critically assessed by observing variations in tooth size and shape among species, as determined in similar work (O'27Neill et al., 2016). Anthropological scientific analysis of tooth shape not only reveals dietary habits but also reveals phylogenetic similarities among various species. Scientists use techniques such as Elliptical Fourier Functional Analysis to quantify occlusal surface contours, allowing intra- and interspecific variation at a sophisticated level. Variational analysis can provide insights into the evolutionary paths of related species and their adaptive strategies in new environments. For example, discoveries that larger teeth in certain species are linked to specific dietary requirements underscore the significance of teeth as functional adaptations. In addition, such an analysis can shed light on ecological pressures behind dental attributes and therefore contribute to a better understanding of how anatomical attributes, in this case teeth, reflect overall evolutionary trends (O\27Neill et al., 2016). Additionally, the relevance of mastication and its implications for dental morphology contribute further understanding to human and primate evolution. Model-organism research, including the use of the rabbit, demonstrates how mechanical properties of the diet affect masticatory behaviors and, ultimately, tooth wear and shape. The study indicates that determinants such as food stiffness are prime predictors of jaw loading during mastication, suggesting that the quality of the food consumed has immediate ramifications for dental adaptations. Contrary to common assumptions, hardness and dental structure have a complex relationship, underscoring the need to eat more resistant foods to meet nutritional needs, thereby affecting chewing frequency and duration. These findings lend credence to the argument that teeth are not just biological structures but are also deeply implicated in behavioral and dietary practices, enabling anthropologists to decode the complex interrelationships between diet, landscape, and evolutionary change (Figure 8.5).

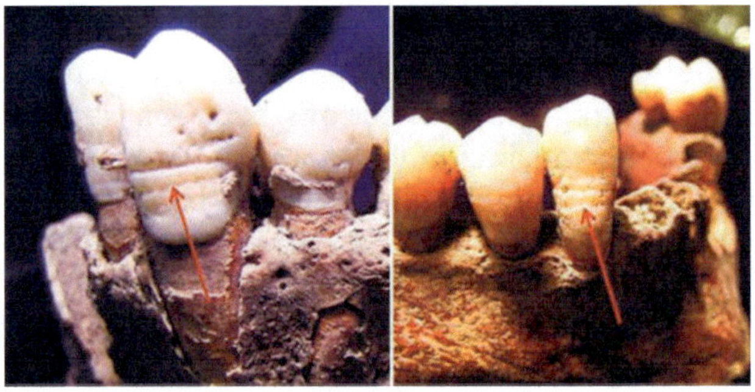

Figure 8.5. The role of teeth in anthropology extends beyond mere functionality.

Source: https://media.springernature.com/lw685/springer-static/image/chp%3A10.1007%2F978-3-319-51726-1_138-2/MediaObjects/184254_0_En_138-2_Fig4_HTML.jpg.

8.2.1. Teeth as Indicators of Diet

Dental morphology vs. dietary practice has been a focus of interest in dental anthropology and much has been discovered about the dietary adaptations of extinct organisms. Teeth are not just mastication tools; they are also influenced by organisms' eating habits. Studies have found that the shapes of teeth's occlusal surfaces can tell us much about an organism's diet and ways of feeding. For example, the range of shapes on the occlusal surface of hominins and non-hominin primates can reveal particular dietary preferences, as certain shapes are linked to specific types of food. Morphological examination is important to realizing how ancient species lived in relation to their environments. It can be observed that these modifications of the teeth are not random; they show the relation between an organism's ecological niche and its evolutionary history and explain how diet is the causation of dental shape and function in the animal world (O\\&u27;Neill et al., 2016). The fossilized teeth can also provide further insight into earlier human subsistence modes and behavior. By inspecting dental remains from varying archaeological contexts, researchers can identify dietary patterns corresponding to environmental and cultural changes. The analysis of teeth from the site of Tepe Hissar is a good example that provides significant data on dietary change during large-scale socio-cultural reorganizations. These changes affected subsistence economies and, in turn, the general health of the population. The dynamic interdependence of cooking methods, the use of teeth as tools, and changing dietary sources reveals how dental anthropology can provide an integrated view of the complexity of ancient diets (Afshar et al., 2014). Moreover, dental health indicators may also reflect larger socio-economic patterns within a community. The research conducted at Tepe Hissar indicates that, while there was no mass population replacement, there were significant changes in diet and oral health. The evidence demonstrated that subsistence strategy and changes in way of life were closely associated with fluctuations in dental disease across different phases. Understanding these aspects allows anthropologists to attribute the condition of health of populations to economic and socio-cultural determinants. To this extent, teeth are not only biological artifacts but also cultural markers that chart the evolution of human societies against environmental stresses and dietary changes (Afshar et al., 2014) (Figure 8.6).

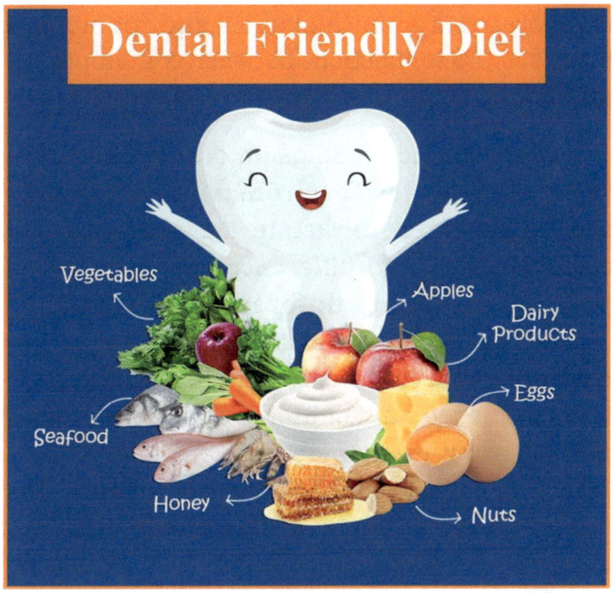

Figure 8.6. The relationship between dental morphology and dietary practices.

Source: https://www.magizhchidental.in/wp-content/uploads/2024/04/395953d1-4e11-44e8-8e42-ac6f5fcae90a.jpeg.

8.2.2. Teeth and Genetic Heritage

Teeth provide insights into genetic heritage, particularly in dental anthropology. Teeth are not just functional to chewing and speech; they are a robust repository of genetic information, divulging the ancestry and developmental history of an individual. Varying dental features, such as tooth size, shape, and structure, are suggestive of inheritance patterns and population affinities.

For instance, the presence of particular dental anomalies, e.g., developmental pathologies, is indicative of the health and environmental status to which individuals were exposed during development. Studies of such morphological features enlighten us about how specific traits have been passed down through generations, a physical link to evolutionary forces and genetic disparities among populations. When researching the genetic past through dental characteristics, researchers tend to use comparative analyses of contemporary and fossilized specimens. The comparative approach enables anthropologists to determine connections between contemporary populations and their extinct relatives.

For example, findings on orangutan dental health reveal how environmental influences can be observed to dictate the prevalence of certain flaws, with differences noted between populations from different environments. These findings have indicated that genetics and environmental context are not distinguishable in their influence on dental morphology. In terms of evaluating developmental defects and their frequencies, anthropologists can deduce the quality of the habitat and nutritional offerings available to particular species, thus providing a comparative insight into the relationship between genetics and environment in the development of teeth, as indicated in the case of both living and extinct primates (Nater et al., 2016).

Furthermore, the integration of advanced imaging techniques, such as micro-CT scans, plays an important role in dental anthropology by providing precise images of internal dental structures. Scientists can study dental morphology more accurately using these methods, thereby elucidating genetic tendencies and developmental patterns that influence craniofacial features. The dental traits of the different species examined reveal adaptations created by evolution and indicate how crucial teeth are as indicators of genetic origin. As researchers continue to explore the relationship between teeth and genetic inheritance, dental anthropology is revealed as a key tool for reconstructing the intricate pasts of human evolutionary histories and for understanding the genetic diversity observed among present-day populations (Cucchi et al., 2015).

8.2.3. Dental Pathologies and Their Implications

Research on dental pathologies using dental anthropology provides significant insight into the well-being and lifestyle of ancient individuals. Dental diseases, such as caries and periodontal disease, are not only indicators of individual health but also more widespread social and environmental conditions. In areas like Central and South America, where professional health care is limited, caries frequency indicates issues in public health and socioeconomics. There needs to be an interdisciplinary collaboration between dental health professionals and anthropologists in this regard, enabling a deeper understanding of how oral diseases relate to eating patterns, cultural behaviors, and healthcare accessibility within a given population.

By combining findings from various disciplines, researchers can develop effective programs to address these pathologies and to improve public health programs and policies more broadly (Fornai et al., 2024). In addition, developmental dental pathologies are significant for interpreting primate health on evolutionary time scales. Such defects, as those observed in orangutans, provide insight into the relationship between developmental conditions and dental health. Variation in the prevalence of enamel defects among orangutans across environments indicates a link between oral health patterns and environmental stressors. In populations facing hardships such as overpopulation or starvation, these pathologies will be exacerbated. Such findings have broader implications, as they allow scientists to infer the quality of environments and adaptive strategies in existing and extinct primate populations, ultimately enhancing our understanding of evolutionary processes and species resilience (Nater et al., 2016). Moreover, the treatment of dental pathologies goes beyond academic concern; it has implications for contemporary health policy and intervention. Effective response strategies to oral disease must consider social determinants of oral health, such as education, access to care, and oral health-related cultural beliefs. Field surveys and epidemiological research may help identify risk groups and formulate interventions tailored to their specific needs. With enhanced awareness and facilitation of preventive practices within populations, such as education on dietary and hygiene practices, stakeholders can contribute more significantly to reducing the prevalence of dental pathologies. Such efforts will not only foster well-being at the individual level but will also contribute towards enhancing the health of populations at large, facilitating the essential interface of dental anthropology with public health (Fornai et al., 2024) (Figure 8.7).

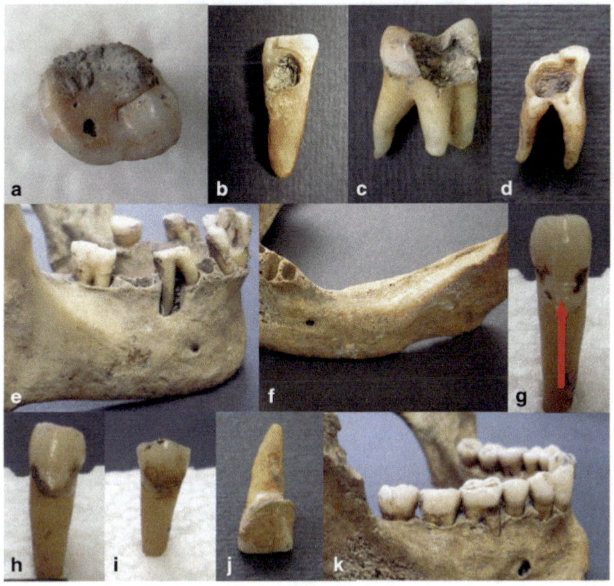

Figure 8.7. The exploration of dental pathologies within the framework of dental anthropology.

Source: https://www.researchgate.net/profile/Alessandra-Varalli/publication/322087498/figure/fig1/AS:962369878499335@1606458267151/Examples-of-dental-pathologies-in-Ballabio-remains-a-d-Different-severity-of-caries-in.gif.

Test Your Knowledge

1. What information can teeth provide about diet, health, and lifestyle in anthropological studies?
2. How are teeth used to determine age, sex, and ancestry in human populations?

8.3. Craniofacial Anatomy

Learning Outcome

1. Basic Structure of the Human Skull
2. Variations in Craniofacial Features
3. Significance of Craniofacial Measurements

Craniofacial anatomy provides a basic foundation for understanding human morphological variation and its implications in dental anthropology and forensic science. The extremely intricate skull formation, composed of various bones and sutures, not only protects the brain but also serves as a support system vital to the structures of the face. The zygomaticotemporal suture, for instance, exemplifies the intricate relationship between skeletal form and functional adaptability. As explained, this suture facilitates dynamic interaction between the zygomatic and temporal bones, allowing movement with preserved structural stability. These points highlight the importance of precise anatomical data for anthropological studies, as variations in craniofacial morphology can significantly contribute to evolutionary biology and clinical applications in dentistry. Beyond mere structural examination, analysis of craniofacial features is highly significant for human identification, particularly when other methods are unsuccessful. The correlation of skulls with facial images, a sharpening method in forensic anthropology, reflects the intricate relationship between cranial configurations and their surface appearances. The relationship is discussed in the context of recent studies comparing manual and computerized craniofacial superimposition techniques that enhance the accuracy of human identification. As indicated, some facial photo characteristics, particularly profile and three-quarter views, are more effective for confirmation tasks. In consequence, knowledge of craniofacial anatomy is indispensable for developing methodologies that optimize the efficiency of identification procedures, particularly in the context of disaster victim identification, where standard information may not be available. The evolutionary relevance of craniofacial anatomy extends to a broader context, underscoring how adaptations have shaped human population dynamics.

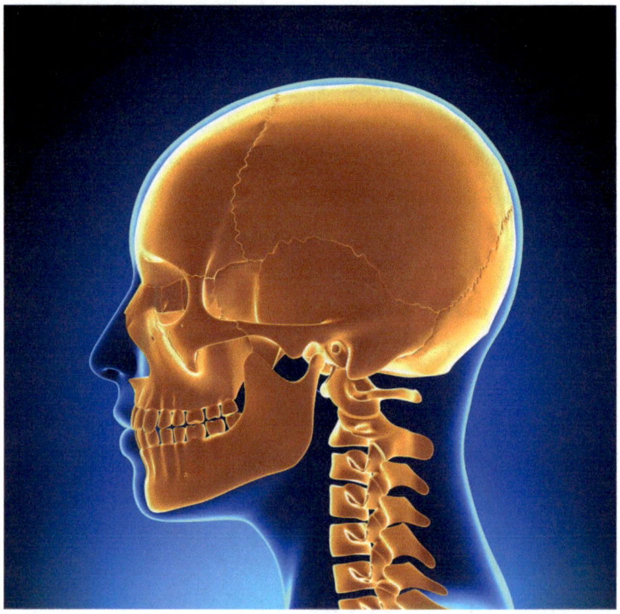

Figure 8.8. Craniofacial anatomy serves as a crucial foundation for understanding human morphological variation.

Source: https://craniofacialteamtexas.com/wp-content/uploads/2015/06/craniofacial-anatomy.jpg.

Characteristics such as dental occlusion, jaw morphology, and zygomatic arch morphology all exhibit not only individual differences but also responses to pressures over time. A greater understanding of these responses can yield useful insights into dietary habits, social behaviors, and even health trends within a specified population. Sutural morphology studies, for instance, underscore the extent to which developmental processes influence not only craniofacial stability but also resistance to stressors. By integrating knowledge from dental anthropology and craniofacial analysis, scientists can better trace the paths of human evolution and the implications for contemporary practices in human identification and forensic science (Figure 8.8).

8.3.1. Basic Structure of the Human Skull

The human skull is composed of two significant parts: the cranium and the facial skeleton, each serving a distinct purpose in sustaining life and enabling communication. The cranium, formed by eight bones, encloses and protects the brain and provides a firm framework for the sensory organs of vision, hearing, and equilibrium. On the contrary, the 14 bones that make up the facial skeleton supply the face with its structure, such as the nasal cavity, orbits, and maxillary regions. This two-part structure is crucial for numerous biological functions, such as respiration, phonation, and mastication. The overall morphology of the skull is shaped by complex interactions among genetic, environmental, and functional factors, underscoring the significance of studying craniofacial structures in dental anthropology and craniofacial analysis, as these features can provide insights into evolution and identity. Within the scope of craniofacial analysis, skull form and measurement are of primary importance, especially the understanding of variation among groups. Researchers have established numerous variables—such as the cephalic index, cranial breadth, and facial height—that provide insight into genetic diversity and adaptation tactics among different human populations. Variation in skull shape, for instance, is often associated with environmental pressures, indicating the influence of natural selection on craniofacial morphology. In accounting for these factors, studies use three-dimensional imaging equipment that enables accurate assessment of cranial and facial structures. Understandings of such morphological traits not only aid anthropological studies but also aid in uses such as forensic science, in which skull structure aids in identifying individuals or demographic information, demonstrating the far-reaching value of craniofacial examination across many different subjects. The relevance of the basic form of the human skull extends beyond mere anatomical classification; it becomes a critical component of forensic examination. Techniques such as craniofacial superimposition that are employed for human identification, where more traditional procedures, i.e., DNA testing, may be impossible, are illustrated to illustrate this utility. Research on both hand-calculated and computer-based methods for comparing skull images with identifiable photographs raises salient concerns for forensic anthropology, particularly regarding the validity of various imaging techniques (Lofthouse et al., 2025). With new methods, forensic experts are better equipped to overcome the challenges of human identification, continuing to bridge the gap between craniofacial analysis and dental anthropology. Finally, a full appreciation of the skull's anatomy further illuminates our understanding not only of human biology but also of identity issues in the forensic sphere, demonstrating the skull's significant contribution to many fields of study (Figure 8.9).

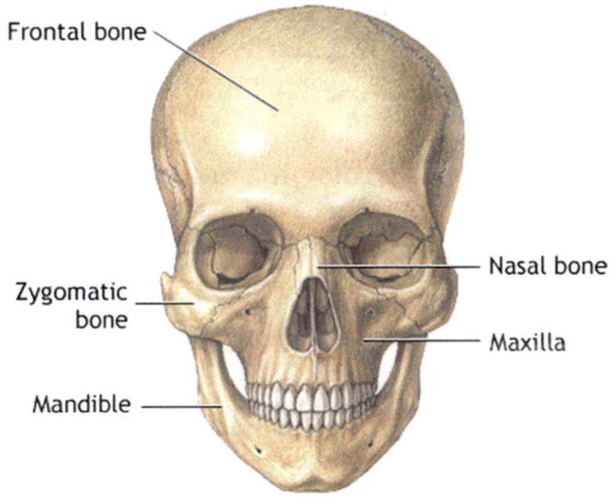

Figure 8.9. The human skull comprises two primary parts.

Source: https://medlineplus.gov/ency/images/ency/fullsize/8915.jpg.

8.3.2. Variations in Craniofacial Features

Intra- and interspecific differences in craniofacial characteristics are of key interest to dental anthropology, as they serve as markers of dietary adaptations and evolutionary history between species. Occlusal morphology of the dentition is characterized by great intra- and interspecific diversity, ultimately linked to the diet of organisms. A comparison of the occlusal surface profiles of hominins and non-hominins indicates this correlation and reveals that different dietary categories correlate with distinct dental variation patterns. To the researchers' surprise, the results showed that not all dietary adaptations correlated with the expected changes in tooth shape and size, particularly in Paranthropus robustus, which showed reduced variation despite its derived nature. This highlights the complexity of deconstructing craniofacial variation and further supports the need for more sensitive investigations that account for both dietary influences and phylogenetic affinities among species (O\\u27Neill et al., 2016). Aside from dietary considerations, craniofacial morphology is modulated by an intricate interplay of genetic and epigenetic events. Ongoing research has identified specific genes associated with craniofacial development, further informing our understanding of these variations. For instance, studies have focused on the FGFR1 gene and have identified its role in craniofacial skeletal formation. However, the relationship between FGFR1 variants and quantitative craniofacial characteristics remains unresolved, as shown by a large-scale study investigating 3D facial dimensions across a diverse sample. Crucially, no correlations were identified between specific FGFR1 single nucleotide polymorphisms (SNPs) and craniofacial dimensions. These findings highlight the complexity of interpreting the genetic basis of craniofacial features, underscoring the need for additional research to disentangle the multiple, overlapping forces that influence human face morphology (Kalra et al., 2015). The implications of craniofacial variation extend beyond mere anatomical measurement; they are windows into evolutionary forces and the adaptability of humankind. In particular, dental morphology and craniofacial research better inform us about ancient diets, environmental stress, and social life in early hominins. Craniofacial variation can also inform scientists about prehistoric nutrition and health. By comparing morphology and function, dental anthropologists can reconstruct past ways of life and ecological niches. As techniques and technology advance, including 3D imaging and DNA testing, so will our understanding of craniofacial differences, shining more light upon the interplay of environment and biology in human evolution assessment. The study of craniofacial traits is thus an essential coming together of anthropology, biology, and evolutionary theory.

8.3.3. Significance of Craniofacial Measurements

Craniofacial size is of particular significance when studying dental anthropology since they are important signifier of the function of both environmental and genetic factors in human growth. Craniofacial size provides significant information on the interrelationships among cranial components and other functional features, such as dexterity and intelligence. For instance, recent research has indicated that some aspects of craniofacial morphology are associated with skills such as hand preference and cognitive function, thus potentially being a link between skull shape and neurological development, especially under homeobox gene influence (Dayi et al., 2002). Understanding these associations not only broadens the scope of human evolution but also underlies clinical dentistry and orthodontic treatment, whose success depends on proper craniofacial analysis for diagnosis and treatment planning of malocclusion and other dental anomalies.

Craniofacial measurements are also at the heart of forensic anthropology and archaeology and are contributing critical information for identification purposes as well as for reconstruction of demographic profiles of ancient populations. By examining craniofacial morphology, anthropologists can infer ancestral origins, population movements, and environmental adaptations that have led to differences over time. Such an anthropological insight is complemented by the introduction of data collected using modern imaging modalities, which enable precise, non-invasive quantification of craniofacial measurements. These studies have established that facial width variation can reflect social and ecological circumstances that influenced ancestral human populations (Proença Heloísa Helena, 2016). These findings further elucidate craniofacial morphology's adaptation to specific the broader context of environmental pressures and cultural evolution. In addition, craniofacial measurements are not just clinically useful in anthropology alone but also have an integral role in contemporary medical practices, particularly orthodontics and maxillofacial surgery. Accurate craniofacial measurements are crucial for evaluating facial symmetry, identifying growth patterns, and planning surgical procedures. Clinicians use these measurements to diagnose malformations and predict developmental outcomes, thereby improving patient care management. The incorporation of craniofacial evaluation in custom treatment plans is increasingly emphasized. Accordingly, craniofacial dimensions offer not just historical and anthropological insight but also vital applications in present-day medicine, adding another level of importance to the topic within the overall context of dental anthropology and craniofacial assessment (Figure 8.10).

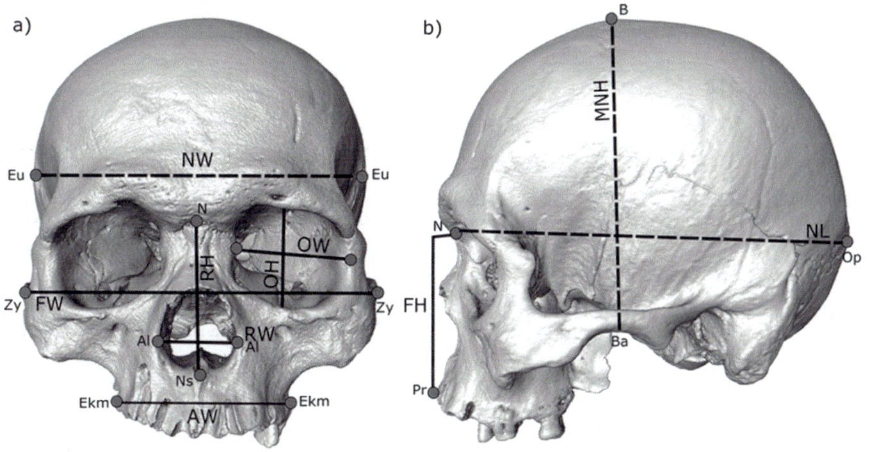

Figure 8.10. Craniofacial measurements hold significant importance in the field of dental anthropology.

Source: https://www.researchgate.net/publication/355609367/figure/fig3/AS:1083352979386368@1635302886681/Craniofacial-measurements-used-for-this-study-see-Table-3-in-frontal-a-and-lateral.ppm.

Test Your Knowledge

1. What are the main components of craniofacial anatomy in humans?
2. How does craniofacial anatomy help in understanding growth, development, and variation among populations?

8.4. Methodologies in Craniofacial Analysis

Learning Outcome

1. Traditional Measurement Techniques
2. Advanced Imaging Technologies
3. Statistical Analysis in Craniofacial Research

Methods of craniofacial analysis are central to the emerging sciences of forensic anthropology and forensic identification. Craniofacial superimposition is one of the most observable methods used in the discipline, allowing experts to superimpose facial features over skeletal remains to determine identity. Despite a history spanning more than a century, the technique remains contentious among scientists owing to inconsistencies arising from the lack of standardized protocols.

Recent studies highlight the need for systematic approaches yielding strong and reliable results, especially when ante-mortem and post-mortem data are presented in small quantities. Hence, the development of craniofacial analysis techniques is important not just for accuracy but also for enhancing confidence in forensic outcomes across the broader context of dental anthropology and craniofacial studies (Abramov et al., 2025). Identification through craniofacial superimposition has been subjected to extensive scrutiny regarding validity and usefulness. Variability in application, whereby practitioners use methodologies appropriate to their expertise and technological ability, challenges the value of the outcomes obtained. This range of approaches creates opposing material within the literature for craniofacial analysis, and it is numerous who call for empirical verification studies. Implementing rigorous protocols would not only standardize the methodology but also enhance overall confidence in forensic outcomes. Collaboration among experts to develop standardized protocols is intended to address such limitations. Through documenting best practices, avenues of error, and zones of uncertainty, practitioners are able to improve their method, ultimately enhancing the field's integrity of forensic identification (Abramov et al., 2025). Furthermore, the incorporation of emerging technologies into craniofacial analysis presents both opportunities and challenges. Advanced imaging techniques such as three-dimensional (3D) modeling and high-definition scanning offer unmatched precision in replicating craniofacial forms. However, such reliance on these technologies underscores the necessity of sound methodological approaches that seamlessly incorporate these advances into conventional practices. Cooperative endeavors, such as the recent undertaking towards a universal craniofacial superimposition standard, indicate shared efforts to overcome these technological hurdles with scientific precision. With the emergence of dental anthropology, the blending of evolving methodologies with traditional analytic protocols will not only enhance the validity of craniofacial analyses but also stimulate future investigations and simplify forensic methods in human remains identification (Abramov et al., 2025).

8.4.1. Traditional Measurement Techniques

Traditional measurement techniques have been at the heart of dental anthropology and craniofacial analysis, providing the foundation for many tests of craniofacial morphology. They primarily involve measurements recorded manually from skeletal samples, either *in situ* or from casts. They often use calipers or other measuring tools to systematically measure parameters such as skull size, dental arch form, and soft tissue thickness. This methodological construct allows for comparisons across populations, contributing to knowledge of biological variation and evolution. Despite advances in imaging technologies, the precision and reproducibility achievable with standard methods remain indispensable to anthropological research, providing reproducible datasets for follow-up studies and analyses, particularly in forensic anthropology. With technological advancements, earlier techniques have been combined with newer ones, making craniofacial analysis more accurate and practical. For example, lateral X-ray radiography has been used to measure facial soft-tissue thickness at various anatomical points and has achieved high inter- and intra-observer reproducibility. The use of Denta Pacs 8.1 software to compare these measurements is an excellent illustration of how outdated techniques are augmented by current technology to yield accurate data sets. Furthermore, outcomes from such procedures are reported to be particularly useful for craniofacial reconstruction and superimposition, indicating the ongoing relevance of outdated techniques in the constantly evolving field of dental anthropology. In a forensic context, the application of traditional measurement techniques is crucial, especially where modern identification methods are not possible or feasible. Skull-to-face comparison is predominantly used in human identification, as in mass disasters, where traditional identification processes are not functional. Research has highlighted a need for robust methods that combine manual and computerized craniofacial superimposition in such cases. Studies that , along with combined manual methods with computer-based approaches, stressed the importance of using multiple facial views for optimal identification success. The study reveals that while traditional methods remain effective, their integration with newer methods, such as frontal and profile facial images, is critical to accuracy and reliability in forensic use, a sign of the adaptive nature of classic methods to contemporary challenges (Lofthouse et al., 2025).

8.4.2. Advanced Imaging Technologies

While dental anthropology has evolved even further, advanced imaging technologies have played a key role in craniofacial analysis. Technologies such as three-dimensional (3D) imaging and computer-assisted morphometrics permit the registration of subtle details of craniofacial morphology with unprecedented precision. These technologies enable a more detailed understanding of human variation and developmental processes, enabling more refined craniofacial superimposition techniques. In instances such as disaster victim identification, where traditional methods fail, the utilization of these imaging technologies is crucial. Comparative studies indicate that profile and three-quarter views yield optimal reliability in craniofacial superimposition, highlighting the importance of diverse imaging approaches to enhance identification success rates beyond the limitations of frontal views, particularly in databases like the MPUB Interpol database, which typically rely on passport-like photos (Lofthouse et al., 2025). The application of 3D digital stereophotogrammetry to craniofacial anthropometry introduces a new dimension to the measurement and analysis of facial morphology. High-resolution imaging technologies enable investigators to produce robust 3D models with nuanced surface detail that may be overlooked by traditional methodologies. This holds deep significance for understanding genetic and environmental influences on craniofacial development. For instance, studies on the interaction between genetic markers, such as variants in FGFR1, and cranial and facial structure may have the potential to link genotype to phenotype. Although newer findings failed to replicate correlations between FGFR1 variants and some craniofacial measurements, judicious application of advanced imaging technology enables larger data sets and high-resolution analysis that can extend our knowledge of craniofacial traits molded by innumerable variables (Kalra et al., 2015). In addition to enhancing data capture, advanced imaging technology facilitates interdisciplinary collaboration across areas like genetics, archaeology, and forensic science. This intersection invites a whole-brain practice to craniofacial anthropology by bridging genetic data with cranial imaging to study the interplay between hereditary trends and environmental demands. As these technologies advance, the ability to conduct complex analyses of large sample sizes will become increasingly feasible, enabling revolutionary research in craniofacial morphology. The challenge is to make these technologies usable and relevant across various research environments, from academic research to forensic applications. Ultimately, the ongoing evolution of imaging sciences can transform dental anthropology and craniofacial analysis with significant advancements in theoretical frameworks and practical procedures needed for subsequent studies (Figure 8.11).

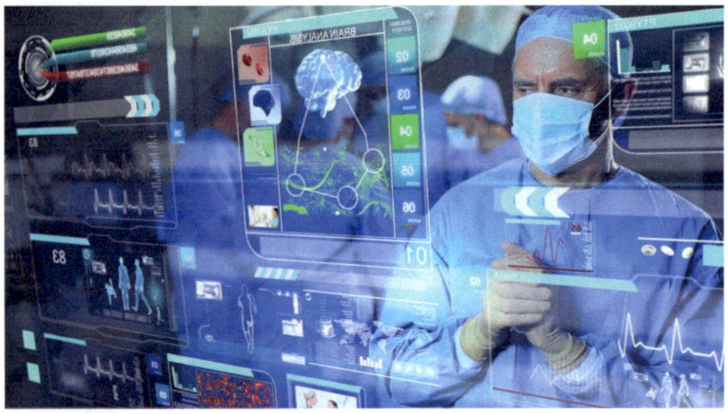

Figure 8.11. As dental anthropology continues to evolve, advanced imaging technologies.

Source: https://franchiseindia.s3.ap-south-1.amazonaws.com/uploads/content/wi/art/healthcare-automation-5094a4b2a4.jpg.

8.4.3. Statistical Analysis in Craniofacial Research

Statistical analysis employed in craniofacial studies provides a clear framework for understanding the complex interaction between dental morphology, dietary adaptation, and evolutionary processes. Quantitative methods enable scientists to investigate differences in dental structures in primate species and understand their environmental niches. For example, in occlusal surface characteristics, it is possible to determine clear patterns of differentiation between dietary life and evolutionary lineages. Using techniques such as Elliptical Fourier Functional Analysis and multivariate statistics, researchers have numerically compared occlusal surface shapes comprehensively across diverse taxa. Such comparisons allowed for a fine appreciation of dental variability associated with environmental stresses and dietary requirements, establishing a morphology-functionality correlation crucial in dental anthropology and craniofacial study (O\\\\u27Neill et al., 2016). Craniofacial science often uses advanced statistical analyses to clarify the genetic and epigenetic factors that govern morphological traits. Investigation of inbred genetic lines in model organisms, such as the mouse, provides a superior means to assess phenotypic variation in craniofacial structures induced by specific gene mutations. A detailed investigation of the Sprouty family of growth factor antagonists is an example of how gene interactions can profoundly affect craniofacial shape. By using multidimensional scaling and other quantitative measures, scientists can more effectively determine the interaction between genetic background and the severity of morphological variation. The findings substantiate the utility of statistical analysis for detecting the main genetic drivers of complex traits and highlight the interaction between genetics and craniofacial morphology (Hallgrímsson et al., 2017). Besides, integrating statistical analysis into craniofacial research enhances our understanding of the evolutionary significance of dental features across and within species. Consistency in methodology in this research opens the doors not just for comparisons across extant species but also for analyses of fossilized material in a paleoecological context. By analyzing contrasts and using robust statistical models, researchers can infer diet from dental form, connecting past and present species. This approach offers critical insights into the adaptation strategies of extinct hominins, as evidenced by studies examining occlusal surface variability. Moreover, the statistical examination of morphological traits reinforces the overarching narrative of human evolution in relation to environmental factors and dietary adaptations, underscoring the relevance of statistical methodologies in the broader domain of dental anthropology and craniofacial research (O\u27Neill et al., 2016).

Test Your Knowledge

1. What are the common methodologies used in craniofacial analysis in anthropology?
2. How do imaging and morphometric techniques contribute to the study of craniofacial variation and identification?

8.5. Applications of Dental Anthropology

Learning Outcome

1. Forensic Science and Identification
2. Archaeological Insights into Past Populations
3. Health and Disease Studies in Historical Contexts

The applications of dental anthropology are widespread across forensic science, archaeology, and medical studies, particularly because it can unlock human biological and cultural variation. By examining dental morphology, researchers can infer diets, health, and even the social structure of ancient populations, providing clues to their everyday lives. This analysis is vital in forensic cases where identification is based on dental records. Identification of characteristic features of dental structures would assist law enforcement units in solving crimes by enabling comparisons of skeletal remains with missing persons' dental records. Besides, dental anthropology provides illumination on the influence of environment and lifestyle on anthropometric traits, making our knowledge of human evolution and adaptation over time better. These vast applications only add value to the worth of dental anthropology as a crucial tool in both past and current understanding and resolution of human health issues. Dental anthropology plays a preeminent role in craniofacial analysis within craniofacial anomaly and variation study. Craniofacial shape and its study, particularly through in-depth analyses of dental shape and its integration with surrounding skeletal structures, provide an individual with an understanding of the genetic, environmental, and developmental controls on facial development. Research has established that inbred genetic backgrounds are significant in controlling craniofacial characteristics, and that several interactions between gene expression and external factors yield diverse phenotypes within populations (Hallgrímsson et al., 2017). The intricate interplay of genes controlling craniofacial morphology demonstrates not only dental anthropology's potential to study physical attributes but also its capacity to understand the principles governing craniofacial development. Such understanding thus enhances the application of dental anthropology in clinical contexts, including orthodontics and maxillofacial surgery, and even for genetic guidance. Secondly, with advancements in technology, dental anthropological analysis has become more efficient and more accurate, particularly in the measurement of craniofacial landmarks. New research has focused on developing low-cost, high-definition imaging systems for standardized facial photography to facilitate easy landmark detection for quantitative analysis (Payne et al., 2013). These methods contribute to the assurance of improved craniofacial measurement accuracy, illustrating landmark position reliability across imaging techniques. By determining which landmarks are more consistent, such developments not only optimize clinical utility but also improve research methods in anthropological research. The integration of state-of-the-art imaging technology into dental anthropology thus holds out the prospect of greater understanding of the complexity of craniofacial morphology—ultimately serving scientific understanding and practical applications in medicine.

8.5.1. Forensic Science and Identification

Forensic science plays a crucial role in identifying human remains, particularly when conventional methods such as DNA profiling are unavailable. Forensic anthropology is a subdiscipline that employs the skeleton's remains in a bid to deduce identity in case other techniques prove ineffective due to massive decomposition or severe destruction. The complexities of variation in the human skeleton require a thorough understanding of osteology and may involve techniques such as craniofacial superimposition, which require a unification of anthropological analysis and imaging technology. This combination enables the production of facial approximations, helping investigators establish identities when conventional identification methods fall short. By judiciously applying these techniques, forensic anthropologists can address gaps in identification procedures, ultimately resolving cases that would otherwise remain unsolved (Omari et al., 2019). Craniofacial analysis has been a valuable tool in forensic identification, employing advanced imaging technology in comparison between skulls and facial features. Experiments have shown that both computer-assisted and manual craniofacial superimposition techniques can be used successfully to identify remains with greater accuracy. Particularly during mass-casualty situations, such as natural disasters, where it is necessary to identify a large number of people with urgency, these techniques can prove invaluable. The literature comparing the effectiveness of photographic methods with 3D computerized methods indicates that, while both are beneficial, profile and three-quarter views most often yield consistent outcomes. This also suggests the importance of different image angles for the potential for positive identification in forensic use, especially with databases like the MPUB Interpol database (Lofthouse et al., 2025). In addition, the new dynamics of forensic science continue to include new approaches, with the consequence that identification of human remains is as impenetrable as possible. For example, three-dimensional (3D) imaging tools such as photogrammetry and laser scanning offer rapid, affordable means for reconstruction and comparison. These advancements not only reduce the need for invasive procedures but also provide digital records to be stored and accessed in the future. Forensic odontologists often collaborate with forensic anthropologists to ensure the highest possible identification accuracy, particularly when dental records are available. This fieldwork relationship is an example of cooperation between forensic specializations and how collaborative efforts can significantly enhance the identification process. As forensic science continues to develop, its fundamental aim is still precise: providing closure and justice through the verification of identification (Omari et al., 2019) (Figure 8.12).

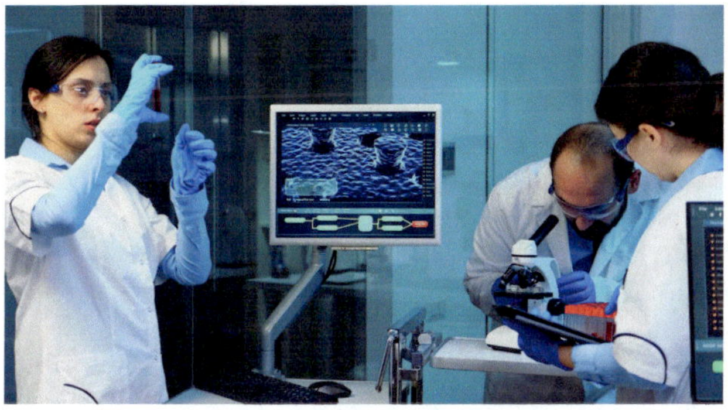

Figure 8.12. Forensic science plays a crucial role in the identification of human remains.

Source: https://external-content.duckduckgo.com/iu/?u=https%3A%2F%2Fwww.truthlabs.org%2Fwp-content%2Fuploads%2F2023%2F12%2Fsenior-chemist-analysing-blood-sample-while-coworkers-discussing-scaled-1.webp&f=1&nofb=1&ipt=f0adce7cab6604f915986bf032f2d8f0cbd51509be4d76ddc6e984dc392af812.

8.5.2. Archaeological Insights into Past Populations

Archaeological records of previous populations play an important role in offering historical backgrounds for the study of early human migration and human evolution. Archaeological records suggest that the early human migration into the Americas was likely more complex than previously thought. There is a new analysis refuting the Beringia model, which infers that all early migrations were conducted through the Bering Land Bridge. Instead, scientists propose that sea strategies enabled earlier populations to enter the Americas from Australasia via oceanic navigation. This argument, based on craniometric evidence, proposes that indigenous South American cultures were developed with contributions from Oceanic peoples, supporting a broader set of human migration and contact in the formation of the genetic and cultural existence of the Americas (Manley et al., 2018). This complexity of motion highlights the value of integrating evidence from all these disciplines, including archaeology, genetics, and dental anthropology, to determine the multifaceted histories of human populations. Other archaeological investigations have revealed specific cultural contexts that discuss the adaptation of ancient populations to differing environments. For example, analyses of paleoamerican cultures in Brazil during the early Holocene reveal unique subsistence patterns related to different ecological contexts. Tradição Nordeste and Tradição Itaparica illustrate how populations adapted to semi-desertic and high plain environments, respectively. Of interest is the excavation of the Capelinha sambaqui, which yielded well-preserved remains of a Paleoamerican individual named Luzio. In contrast to most marine-reliant coastal populations, the Luzios group had access to inland resources, as testified by stable isotopic analysis of their remains. This case not only detects dietary variation among ancient groups but also invites re-examination of their contact, producing a more nuanced image of their lifeways (Eggers et al., 2011). The application of archaeological data facilitates more expansive interpretation of craniofacial morphology and dentition among ancient groups. The dental anthropology framework can help identify the influence of environmental factors on physical characteristics and provide insight into diet and health conditions. For instance, differences in tooth wear between populations from coastal and interior regions help generate important information about food availability and dietary practices. Luxios outcomes provide an excellent opportunity to explore how various subsistence strategies may have led to distinct cranial and dental development and to shed light on the adaptive value of morphology in meeting environmental challenges. Last but not least, integrating archaeological information with dental and craniofacial studies enhances understanding of ancient human populations and their varied responses to environmental pressures, illuminating the dynamic relationship between culture, biology, and adaptation over time (Figure 8.13).

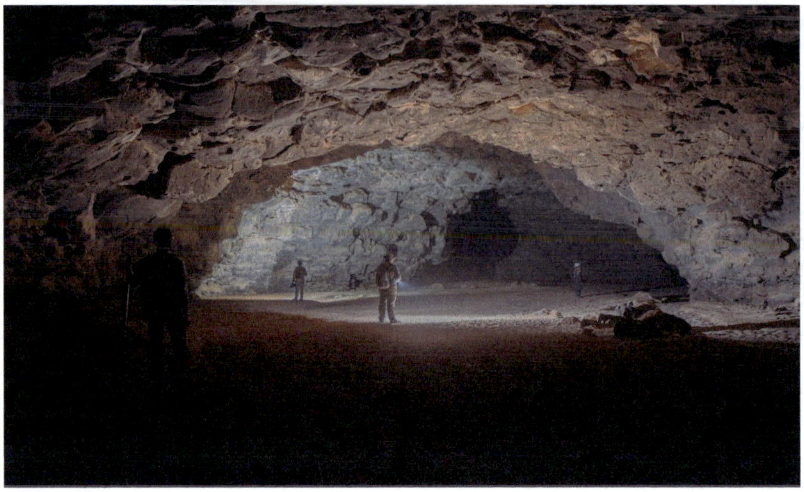

Figure 8.13. Archaeological insights into past populations.

Source: https://external-content.duckduckgo.com/i u/?u=https%3A%2F%2Fwww.gea.mpg.de%2F32986%2Foriginal -171576725 3.jpg%3Ft%3DeyJ3aWR0aCI6MTIwMCwiaGVpZ2h0IjpudWxsLC JmaXQiOm51bGwsIm9ial9p ZCI6MzI5ODZ9--8f33e09ced92a5836cdea7d043b3ad62992c1cf2&f=1&nofb=1&ipt=d6fc3811db0b32 255c93d749e69b946407387407b4001d2336417 04e64b4dd4a.

8.5.3. Health and Disease Studies in Historical Contexts

Health and disease, studied from the perspective of dental anthropology, reveal profound insights into the environments in which human populations lived in the past. By analyzing skeletal remains, such as dentition and craniofacial features, scholars can identify patterns in the health, diet, and social habits of past societies. For instance, at Tepe Hissar, bioarcheological analysis demonstrated impressive changes in oral health synchronous with economic and dietary changes throughout periods of history. The findings suggest not only that the occupants experienced altered subsistence strategies, but their overall well-being and health also reflected broader socio-cultural shifts over time, highlighting the value of considering dental health in its historical context (Afshar et al., 2014). Craniofacial examination also enhances the understanding of how social and environmental stressors affected the development and growth of individuals during ancient times. Research has confirmed that virtually any form of environmental stress can considerably hinder growth during development, and the effects may be observed within the cranial structure of such populations. A research analyzing Roman Catholic Girls' Orphanage crania demonstrated this by finding growth retardation in one sample that was a result of adverse living conditions in the late 19th century. By correlating craniofacial patterns with pathogenic characteristics, scientists can make informed associations between health outcomes and historical conditions within society, thereby adding valuable information to dental anthropology (Lombardi et al., 2017). Integrating information from both craniofacial growth and dental disease provides a comprehensive picture of how previous populations responded to their environmental and social challenges. The Tepe Hissar data on dental disease, for instance, revealed an abrupt decline in dental health in line with population change, whereas within the Maagdenhuis Orphanage, significant correlations between developmental pathologies and age provided clues into the social determinants sustaining these disease problems.

Together, these works show that the examination of health and disease in past environments through dental anthropology not only increases our understanding of human history but also places social organization and environmental parameters on an equal footing with other causes of health outcomes over time.

Test Your Knowledge

1. How is dental anthropology applied to study diet, health, and cultural practices in past populations?
2. In what ways does dental anthropology assist in forensic identification and age estimation?

8.6. Ethical Considerations in Dental Anthropology

Learning Outcome

1. Consent and Cultural Sensitivity
2. Implications of Research Findings
3. Responsible Use of Data

It is in dental anthropology that science and ethics collide, particularly when working in craniofacial analysis. As this discipline often involves the examination of human remains, ethical principles are particularly significant. Researchers must navigate complex issues of consent, respect for the dead, and the potential consequences of their findings. The application of very advanced technologies, such as active surface scanning, also complicates ethical issues because they provide unheard-of access to morphological data and historical information and raise concerns about privacy and the control of sensitive information. In their application of these methodologies, researchers must uphold ethical guidelines that place respect for the treatment of human remains at the forefront, to see their work contribute to the greater context of human history and health without compromising the dignity of those they are studying (Errickson et al., 2017). Relevance of the study to contemporary populations is a second grave ethical concern in dental anthropology. Research that entails the study of craniofacial morphology or dental conditions must account for potential socio-cultural sensitivities and misuse of data. Anthropometric data collected from certain demographic categories, such as the study on craniofacial dimensions in the Punjab province of Pakistan, may reinforce stereotypes or bias if not placed in context (Akhtar et al., 2023). Also, if results are applied in a legal or forensic environment, they must be carefully interpreted to avoid misrepresentation of groups or individuals. Hence, it is the responsibility of the researchers to present sophisticated interpretations attuned to the social context of their research, without losing sight of any practice that could amount to discrimination or misinterpretation. Finally, ethical dental anthropology practice also has its broader public health and educational aspects. As research uncovers significant findings on craniofacial variability and oral health, anthropologists must present their findings honestly and credibly. This means going out to local populations and stakeholders to provide information that helps shape public health policy and practice without stigmatizing particular groups. Moreover, integrating ethical teaching practices into anthropology programs has the potential to cultivate a new generation of scholars who are concerned with ethical considerations. By positioning ethical issues at the center of dental anthropology, scholars can initiate a process of field development that respects past context and current implications, thereby fostering a healthy and productive discussion of human diversity and health (Errickson et al., 2017).

8.6.1. Consent and Cultural Sensitivity

Consent and cultural sensitivity are more central in dental anthropology and craniofacial analysis, calling for a reflective approach to human remains. While researchers and practitioners work with historical and archaeological materials, they must address the intricacies of representing and analyzing these remains. Ethical considerations also arise, particularly when presenting post-mortem facial photographs, which could provoke intense emotions among descendant communities. As an example, misidentification of the deceased individuals, a familiar threat in forensic settings, highlights the importance of establishing precise protocols for obtaining informed consent from the family and communities dealing with the remains to be investigated (Achenbach et al., 2014).

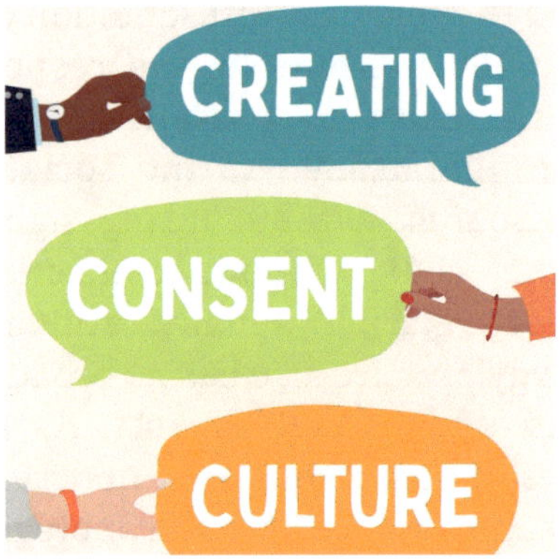

Figure 8.14. The principles of consent and cultural sensitivity.

Source: https://external-content.duckduckgo.com/iu/?u=https%3A%2F%2Fecdn.teacherspayteachers.com%2Fthumbuserbig%2FCreating-Consent-Culture-In-Your-Classroom%2F21478044.jpg&f=1&nofb=1&ipt=686cb2c504a5c5ca60cab6aae5299c8f3d7d718bbc1431283d95edaa45512b14.

This custom not only safeguards the deceased's dignity but also helps instill team spirit among researchers and relevant cultural communities. Respect for differing beliefs and customs about death and the management of human remains within societies extends beyond simply seeking permission; it signifies sensitivity towards culture. In dental anthropology, for example, the examination of craniofacial traits can yield information on ancestral relationships, cultural origins, and past health inequalities. Nevertheless, researchers need to be mindful that their interpretations have substantial implications for descendants who are still alive, especially when discussing features such as ethnicity and social class that may be based on craniofacial traits. The chapter employs inclusive approaches that incorporate indigenous voices and community knowledge to expand the applicability and acceptability of the findings. This is in accordance with contemporary ethical standards and encourages the incorporation of multiple voices into academic discourse, thereby enriching it through an enhanced sense of cultural context (Emerson et al., 2023). Lastly, advancements in digital reconstruction and modeling present both threats and opportunities regarding consent and cultural sensitivity. As evidenced in the application of digital hair construction to rebuild subjects such as George Dixon, the use of advanced methods in facial approximation raises ethical questions about the presentation and dissemination of these reconstructions. Digital reconstructions tend to perpetuate stereotypes or misrepresent individuals' identities merely based on superficial characteristics. Ethical guidelines must be followed to ensure that such reconstructions honor the cultural heritage of the respective communities and do justice to the historical context. Through its focus on consent and cultural sensitivity, dental anthropology and craniofacial analysis not only address historical gaps but also honor the complexity of identity in both previous and modern societies (Figure 8.14).

8.6.2. Implications of Research Findings

Dental anthropology and craniofacial analysis research findings carry meaningful implications, since they become more embedded in our knowledge of evolutionary biology and human development. For instance, studies on the cranial suture closure in animals such as the franciscana dolphin indicate that suture patterns may be indicative of adaptive requirements related to the evolutionary past. The lack of directional asymmetry in these sutures suggests a common evolutionary reaction across dolphin species and might inform us about functional demands and ecological adaptations appropriate to their habitats. These discoveries, in addition to advancing our understanding of mammalian craniofacial evolution, emphasize the importance of considering phylogenetic associations when comparing similar structures across taxa, helping fill some gaps in our understanding of craniofacial morphology in both non-human and human species (Cappozzo et al., 2015).

In addition, the study of craniofacial sex differences holds significant implications for medical and anthropological practices. Inferences deduced from analysis of craniofacial soft-tissue morphology confirm the existence of sexual dimorphism in early childhood and its continuous development with age. Such complexity demonstrates the necessity for measurements based on age in the case of investigation into craniofacial features. Understanding that certain features develop at rates different from others can be beneficial for clinical procedures such as reconstructive surgery or orthodontic treatment, thereby maximizing patient care outcomes by calibrating techniques to each patient's growth patterns (Cunningham et al., 2016).

These results provide a critical basis for the development of predictive models in facial reconstruction and forensic anthropology, indicating their practical applicability. Research syntheses in dental anthropology and craniofacial analysis have the potential to transform both academic research and practical applications. Since we appreciate the interconnectedness of craniofacial morphology and ecological adaptations, these findings could encourage further studies examining correlations among various human populations within geographic areas. Enhanced knowledge of the determinants of craniofacial morphology, both environmental and genetic, may lead to a substantial advancement in evolutionary anthropology, and inform discussion regarding human variation and health inequality. Lastly, these studies can better inform a synthesis of human diversity, informing anthropology of public health and creating cross-disciplinary collaborations highlighting the multidimensionality of craniofacial development across animals (Cappozzo et al., 2015; Cunningham et al., 2016).

8.6.3. Responsible Use of Data

Appropriate use of data in dental anthropology and craniofacial analysis is paramount to ethical practice and scientific integrity. Adopting rigorous data governance procedures ensures sensitive information about human subjects is handled with extreme care. Such measures include safeguarding informed consent, anonymizing data, and being mindful of data interpretation limits.

For instance, while facial presentations in forensic contexts can be useful for identification, caution is warranted against misidentification, especially when the physical condition of the remains may have been tampered with. This sensitivity is not only procedural but reflects a broader ethical duty to protect the dignity of individuals, even in death (Achenbach et al., 2014). By promoting a culture of responsibility in data handling and sharing, the field can more readily address the subtleties surrounding human remains and the implications of their analysis. Secondly, the incorporation of genetic data into craniofacial studies raises additional concerns about the proper use of this information. Research shows that there are correlations between genetic variants and craniofacial traits; therefore, caution should be used when using genetic information. For example, studies have identified various single-nucleotide polymorphisms (SNPs) responsible for normal-range facial structure, namely orofacial clefts (Claes et al., 2018). While such findings are a positive addition to the dental anthropology discipline, the scientists must balance the ethical considerations of genetic determinism without oversimplifying the relationship between genes and physical characteristics. Misinterpretation can further perpetuate stigmatization or even reinforce physical appearance-based social prejudices.

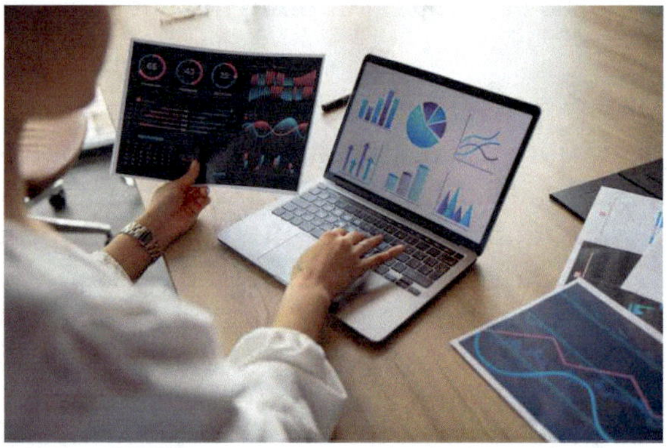

Figure 8.15. The responsible use of data in dental anthropology and craniofacial analysis.

Source: https://external-content.duckduckgo.com/iu/?u=https%3A%2F%2Fwww.bennett.edu.in%2Fwp-content%2Fuploads%2F2024%2F06%2FData-Ethics-The-Responsible-Use-of-Data.-An-Analysis.jpg&f=1&nofb=1&ipt=2890fe56cdd03d971c4c774951401c5540f27c715404c0f772b72f513dd16bc0.

Therefore, scholars must engage in open debate about the burdens of genetic information, so that knowledge can further develop responsibly without reinforcing harmful stereotypes. Lastly, interdisciplinary collaboration will provide room for an integrated perspective on responsible usage of data within dental anthropology and craniofacial analysis. Ethical considerations must be integrated into guidelines for research processes outside the scope of customary anthropology and genetics. Interdisciplinary collaborations with ethicists, legal experts, and community representatives can lay the foundations for well-integrated guidelines that safeguard the rights and welfare of living and deceased subjects. Moreover, such collaborations can enable a more responsive discussion of the role of data in representations of facial difference and its impact on identity. As the field evolves, a commitment to ethical data stewardship will not only increase scientific integrity but also ensure that the voices of those whose lives are affected by the research are heard and respected (Achenbach et al., 2014; Claes et al., 2018) (Figure 8.15).

Test Your Knowledge

1. Why is it important to follow ethical guidelines when studying human dental remains in anthropology?
2. What ethical issues must be considered in the collection, analysis, and display of dental specimens?

SUMMARY

It is worth noting the intricate relationship of dental morphology with the ecological and evolutionary past of both fossil and living species. Dental character studies, in particular the variability of the occlusal surface, yield valuable information regarding dietary adaptation and the behavior of various primate species. According to recent studies, this variation tends to reflect phylogenetic patterns rather than diet alone, contradicting earlier assumptions of direct dietary influence on dental form. The incorporation of analytical tools such as Elliptical Fourier Functional Analysis also provides more detailed insight into these patterns, enabling the interpretation of hominin and non-hominin dental morphology and its relationship to environmental factors (O\27Neill et al., 2016). Further, dental anthropological implications are not only anatomical but also serve as fundamental markers of population dynamics and migrations throughout history. As has been documented in recent research, the dental characteristics of populations can define important patterns of interaction and adaptation within various ecological contexts. This provides impetus for interdisciplinary approaches that utilize genetics, archaeology, and anthropology to construct a broader picture of human development. While previous paradigms of human migration, such as the Bering Land Bridge hypothesis, have been the prevailing explanation, recent evidence points to a more complex scenario of several rounds of migration and non-standard pathways, such as long-distance sea migration. This is conducive to an ongoing investigation that examines these multifaceted connections in correlation with craniometric data (Manley et al., 2018). In the end, the field of dental anthropology is a powerful means of reconstructing not only the biological history of our own kind but also the cultural and ecological histories that accompany it. By incorporating information from craniofacial analysis and fossil records alongside population science today, investigators can investigate questions of adaptation, diversity, and resilience in the human lineage. Future research must continue to use sophisticated analytical methods and undertake cross-disciplinary projects, thereby providing a more comprehensive picture of the dental features that characterize us. As our understanding grows, so does our respect for the intricacies that govern human evolution, laying the groundwork for further investigation in both anthropology and associated fields.

In analyzing craniofacial morphology in dental anthropology, it is important to highlight the role of genetic background in cranial development. Recent studies employing inbred mouse models illustrate how variation in genetic backgrounds can potentially affect the expression of craniofacial dysmorphologies. Notably, communication between an organism's genetic background and specific gene mutations, such as those in the Sprouty family of growth factor regulators, is responsible for significant craniofacial shape variation. These findings emphasize the nuances of epistatic interactions, with genetic resistance potentially varying wildly from one strain to another, as evidenced by the differential severity of craniofacial structures arising through genetic dysfunctions. These results have implications for informing the pathophysiology of human craniofacial malformations and highlighting the significance of extensive genetic testing in dental anthropological analysis (Hallgrímsson et al., 2017). A further key aspect of craniofacial assessment is the inquiry for sexual dimorphism during various developmental stages. Three-dimensional facial scanning studies revealed clear sex differences in craniofacial soft-tissue morphology that emerge early in childhood and persist into adulthood during puberty. The evidence revealed that specific distinctive characteristics begin to manifest even prior to three years of age, while others, particularly jaw and facial structure-related, manifest much later in life, following puberty. The quantitative interpretation of sexual dimorphisms captures the complex dance of interactions among biological and environmental determinants shaping craniofacial morphology. An awareness of the timing and nature of such changes is important for dental anthropologists, as it contributes to overall knowledge of growth patterns and the health conditions associated with craniofacial growth (Cunningham et al., 2016). Furthermore, integrating genetic and morphological data in craniofacial science enables a deeper understanding of the etiology of human variation. By studying the genetic underpinnings of craniofacial shape, as well as the phenomena observed, dental anthropologists can construct a unifying paradigm for explaining human variation. This integrated model not only aids in illuminating clinical examples of craniofacial abnormality but also influences best practice in reconstructive surgery and the conservation of orthodontics. Through ongoing innovation in research and the acceptance of new analytic methods, such as geometric morphometrics, empirical, rigorous methods further solidify their role in delivering insights into the interplay between genetic tendencies and phenotypic expression. In sum, the culmination of these significant findings exemplifies the intricate dimensions of craniofacial studies that are vital to the development of dental anthropology (Cunningham et al., 2016; Hallgrímsson et al., 2017).

KEY TERMS FROM THIS CHAPTER

- Caries
- Craniofacial Morphology
- Dental Anthropology
- Enamel Hypoplasia
- Facial Reconstruction
- Malocclusion
- Mandibular Torus
- Odontometrics
- Palatal Shape
- Periodontal Disease
- Tooth Morphology

CRITICAL THINKING QUESTIONS

1. **Dental anthropology primarily studies:**
   a. The development of dental tools
   b. The role of teeth in digestion
   c. Teeth as indicators of human variation, health, and evolution
   d. Genetic engineering of teeth
2. **Which of the following dental features is often used to assess ancestry in skeletal remains?**
   a. Dental caries
   b. Shovel-shaped incisors
   c. Root transparency
   d. Enamel hypoplasia
3. **Enamel hypoplasia is typically interpreted as a marker of:**
   a. Dental plaque buildup
   b. Excess calcium intake
   c. Physiological stress during development
   d. Postmortem damage
4. **Which part of the tooth is most durable and likely to survive in archaeological contexts?**
   a. Dentin
   b. Cementum
   c. Enamel
   d. Pulp
5. **In craniofacial analysis, the zygomatic bones are important for assessing:**
   a. Dental eruption
   b. Age
   c. Ancestry and facial projection
   d. Pathological lesions

Short Answer Questions

1. What is dental anthropology, and how is it used in the study of past populations?
2. Explain the significance of enamel hypoplasia as a marker of childhood health and stress.
3. What are shovel-shaped incisors, and how can they assist in ancestry estimation?
4. Describe two methods used to estimate age-at-death based on dental features.
5. Explain how cranial sutures are used to estimate age in adult skeletal remains.
6. Describe the role of the zygomatic bone in ancestry estimation.

Answers to Critical Thinking Questions

1. (c); 2. (b); 3. (c); 4. (c); 5. (c)

REFERENCES

1. Damas, S., Wilkinson, C., Kahana, T., Veselovskaya, E., Abramov, A., Jankauskas, R., Jayaprakash, P., Ruiz, E., Navarro, F., Huete, M., Cunha, E., Cavalli, F., Clement, J., Lestón, P., Molinero, F., Briers, T., Viegas, F., Imaizumi, K., Humpire, D., & Ibáñez, O. (2015). Study on the performance of different craniofacial superimposition approaches (II): Best practices proposal. *Forensic Science International*, *257*, 504–508. https://doi.org/10.1016/j.forsciint.2015.07.045Abramov, A., Campanones-Alvarez, C., Cavalli, F., Hardiman, M., et al. (2025). Study on the criteria for assessing skull-face correspondence in craniofacial superimposition. https://core.ac.uk/download/74237088.pdf (accessed on 21st July 2025).
2. Achenbach, R., Aitken, R., Algemeen, D., America's Most Wanted, Aries, P., Arnow, J., Barron, C., et al. (2014). A review of the changing culture and social context relating to forensic facial depiction of the dead. https://core.ac.uk/download/42477688.pdf (accessed on 21st July 2025).
3. Afshar, Z. (2014). Mobility and economic transition in the 5th to the 2nd millennium B.C. in the population of the Central Iranian Plateau, Tepe Hissar. https://core.ac.uk/download/30276436.pdf (accessed on 21st July 2025).
4. Akay, G., Bulut, Ö., Güngör, K., Kahraman, A., Gürcan, Y., et al. (2016). Repeatability of facial soft tissue thickness measurements for forensic facial reconstruction using X-ray images. https://core.ac.uk/download/228070379.pdf (accessed on 21st July 2025).
5. Akhtar, M. S., Khan, M. A., Nowak, O., Qureshi, A., et al. (2023). Anthropometric study of the human craniofacial morphology among different castes of Punjab Pakistan. https://core.ac.uk/download/578161554.pdf (accessed on 21st July 2025).
6. Bresin, A., Pepicelli, A., Rosas, A., Waltimo, A., Hannam, A. G., Ingervall, B., Ingervall, B., et al. (2018). Human mandibular shape is associated with masticatory muscle force. https://core.ac.uk/download/157728721.pdf (accessed on 21st July 2025).
7. Cappozzo, H. L., del Castillo, D. L., & Flores, D. A. (2015). Fusión de suturas craneales en el delfín franciscana, *Pontoporia blainvillei* (Gervais and D'Orbigny, 1844). https://core.ac.uk/download/159289136.pdf (accessed on 21st July 2025).
8. Claes, P., Feingold, E., Hens, G., Hoskens, M., et al. (2018). Six NSCL/P loci show associations with normal-range craniofacial variation. https://core.ac.uk/download/161527605.pdf (accessed on 21st July 2025).
9. Cucchi, T., Dobney, K., Evin, A., Larson, G., et al. (2015). Phenotype and animal domestication: A study of dental variation between domestic, wild, captive, hybrid and insular *Sus scrofa*. https://core.ac.uk/download/29151193.pdf (accessed on 21st July 2025).
10. Cunningham, M. L., Hecht, J. T., Heike, C. L., Kau, C. H., et al. (2016). Using the 3D Facial Norms Database to investigate craniofacial sexual dimorphism in healthy children, adolescents, and adults. https://core.ac.uk/download/43007792.pdf (accessed on 21st July 2025).
11. Curtis, N., Fagan, M. J., & Witzel, U. (2014). Development and three-dimensional morphology of the zygomaticotemporal suture in primate skulls. https://core.ac.uk/download/151157048.pdf (accessed on 21st July 2025).
12. Dayi, E., Okuyan, M., & Tan, U. (2002). Predictability of hand skill and cognitive abilities from craniofacial width in right- and left-handed men and women: Relation of skeletal structure to cerebral function. https://core.ac.uk/download/pdf/85076.pdf (accessed on 21st July 2025).

13. Duncan, W. N., Johnson, K., & Stojanowski, C. (2013). Geographic patterns of early Holocene New World dental morphological variation. https://core.ac.uk/download/519827302.pdf (accessed on 21st July 2025).

14. Eggers, S., Grupe, G., Parks, M., Reinhard, K., et al. (2011). Paleoamerican diet, migration and morphology in Brazil. https://core.ac.uk/download/12175538.pdf (accessed on 21st July 2025).

15. Emerson, R. (2023). Digital hair creation for archaeological facial approximation: George Dixon, the last captain of the *HL Hunley*. https://core.ac.uk/download/588290628.pdf (accessed on 21st July 2025).

16. Errickson, D., Gowland, R. L., Griffith, S. J., Grueso, I., et al. (2017). Towards a best practice for the use of active non-contact surface scanning to record human skeletal remains from archaeological contexts. https://core.ac.uk/download/322328997.pdf (accessed on 21st July 2025).

17. Fling, A. L., McAbee, K. R., Ravosa, M. J., Scott, J. E., et al. (2015). Chewed out: An experimental link between food material properties and repetitive loading of the masticatory apparatus in mammals. https://core.ac.uk/download/60580743.pdf (accessed on 21st July 2025).

18. Fornai, C. (2024). Por qué antropólogos y odontólogos deberían trabajar en coordinación para mejorar la salud bucodental (en América Latina). https://core.ac.uk/download/621964177.pdf (accessed on 21st July 2025).

19. Hallgrímsson, B., Klein, O., Marangoni, P., Percival, C. J., et al. (2017). The interaction of genetic background and mutational effects in regulation of mouse craniofacial shape. https://core.ac.uk/download/323072945.pdf (accessed on 21st July 2025).

20. Hubbe, M. (2024). Diversidad de la morfología craneofacial en América del Norte, Central y del Sur: Implicaciones para las discusiones sobre biología y salud oral. https://core.ac.uk/download/621964175.pdf (accessed on 21st July 2025).

21. Kalra, V., Karski, M. R., Leslie, E., Neiswanger, K., et al. (2015). The influence of FGFR1 variants on normal human craniofacial shape. https://core.ac.uk/download/33562722.pdf (accessed on 21st July 2025).

22. Lofthouse, A., & Wilkinson, C. (2025). The use of craniofacial superimposition for disaster victim identification. https://core.ac.uk/download/42477690.pdf (accessed on 21st July 2025).

23. Lombardi, K. M. (2017). Environmental stresses and its effect on craniofacial growth and development. https://open.bu.edu/bitstream/2144/23814/1/Lombardi_bu_0017N_12701.pdf (accessed on 21st July 2025).

24. Manley, D. E. (2018). Exploring an oceanic influence on the peopling of South America. https://core.ac.uk/download/159487642.pdf (accessed on 21st July 2025).

25. Nater, A., Wilting, A., Beynon, A. D., Russon, A. E., Russon, A. E., Zihlman, A. L., Badgley, C., et al. (2016). An enigmatic hypoplastic defect of the maxillary lateral incisor in recent and fossil orangutans from Sumatra (*Pongo abelii*) and Borneo (*Pongo pygmaeus*). https://core.ac.uk/download/46557792.pdf (accessed on 21st July 2025).

26. O'Neill, K. (2016). Dietary adaptations and intra- and interspecific variation in dental occlusal shape in hominin and non-hominin primates. https://core.ac.uk/download/79821503.pdf (accessed on 21st July 2025).

27. Omari, R. K. (2019). Virtual anthropology? Reliability of three-dimensional photogrammetry as a forensic anthropology measurement and documentation technique. https://core.ac.uk/download/286374092.pdf (accessed on 21st July 2025).

28. Payne, M. G. (2013). The reliability of facial soft tissue landmarks with photogrammetry. https://core.ac.uk/download/67758539.pdf (accessed on 21st July 2025).

9

METRIC AND NON-METRIC VARIATION

LEARNING OBJECTIVES

After studying this chapter, you will be able to:

1. Discuss the historical context
2. Understand applications of metric variation
3. Know applications of non-metric variation
4. Focus on advantages of metric variation
5. Learn about the advantages of non-metric variation
6. Know challenges of metric and non-metric variation

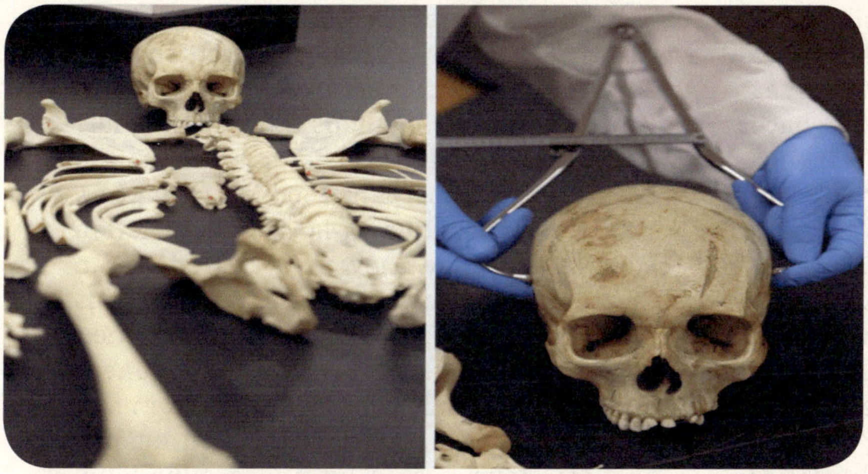

Introduction

In the exploration of patterns and contrast in data, the appreciation of both metric and non-metric variation becomes a critical framework. Metric variation accounts for changes that are measurable quantitatively via established measurement systems, hence providing a standardized means of comparing datasets. This type of variation is useful in domains such as statistics, where data measurements can influence conclusions drawn from research. In contrast, non-metric variation is associated with qualitative differences that may not be easily quantifiable, and at times may require a more advanced kind of analysis. This is an important distinction between the two types of variation, as it informs researchers about the kind of data involved and the methods to be employed in analyzing it. The relevance of metric and non-metric variation is extensive across a variety of disciplines, not merely impacting statistical techniques but also being common in fields like biology, sociology, and engineering. In biological research, for instance, metric variation would be observed in measurable features, and non-metric variation may be present in behavior patterns that cannot be numerically measured. An awareness of these differences enables more targeted data collection and interpretation, leading to more robust conclusions. The intersection between technological and methodological variation can often be complex, requiring more refined analytical procedures to deconstruct their effects. This complexity underscores the need to apply holistic analytical procedures, particularly as scholars seek precision in their results. To systematically examine these variations, sophisticated methods such as domain warping and Bayesian inference have become increasingly popular. Domain warping, for instance, enables researchers to represent horizontal and vertical variations in data more systematically. By using the Fisher-Rao metric to distinguish between these variations, researchers are able to discern underlying patterns that otherwise would go undetected. This is particularly crucial in functional data analysis, where distinctions among various forms of variation can significantly affect the analysis's outcome. Bayes inference, however, permits one to interpret how varying priors and data-generating distributions affect posterior findings, underscoring the need for appropriate model selection. Such advanced techniques lead to a deeper understanding of metric and non-metric variability, which is pivotal to accurate data interpretation across numerous applications (Lu et al., 2013; Owhadi et al., 2016).

Definition of Metric Variation

Metric variation theory is an essential framework in the differentiation of different types of data analysis methodologies in both metric and non-metric contexts. Essentially, metric variation is the measurable change in attribute values that can be detected along a predefined scale or metric space. This kind of variation is especially important, as it provides the mathematical underpinnings for comparing and contrasting data points, enabling researchers to identify patterns and trends necessary for decision-making based on data. The idea of metric variation is precisely captured by techniques such as domain warping methods, which partition horizontal and vertical variations in functional data with delicacy. By doing so, analysts can focus on the horizontal variation, which typically encapsulates latent patterns in their problem formulations, suggesting that a better understanding of complex data structures can be achieved by examining this metric variation (Lu et al., 2013). The methodology used to analyze metric variation tends to rely on advanced statistical methods that can untangle the intricacies of data sets. For example, the Principal Nested Spheres method, which appears to be a useful technique for horizontal variation decomposition, shows how metric variation can be successfully modeled and interpreted. This approach differs from conventional approaches, such as tangent plane principal component analysis, thereby underscoring the need for more accurate analytical frameworks when dealing with variations across advanced functional landscapes. These developments aid scientists in producing more interpretable results that will guide subsequent analyses and help drive the application of their outcomes across various research fields, for example, computational statistics and machine learning (Lu et al., 2013). Therefore, not only does the idea of metric variation describe variations in data, it also leads to methodological choices that enable good analysis. The relevance of metric variation extends even further in the broader context of understanding how variations impact larger systems, as in theoretical environments such as black hole physics. Black hole microstate analysis has brought new concepts into the statistical treatment of these astronomical phenomena. These studies demonstrate that, just like metric variations, understanding entropy and flux quantization between microstate geometries can provide enhanced insight into variability in very complex systems. In such a scenario, the intrinsic topological differences, just like data structure variations, illustrate how metric variation provides insightful parallels across an array of areas of study. Hence, an understanding of the definition of metric variation and its use is central not only to functional data analysis but also to the exploration of other scientific phenomena, thereby promoting the sharing of ideas between metrics and non-metrics in scholarly work (Figure 9.1).

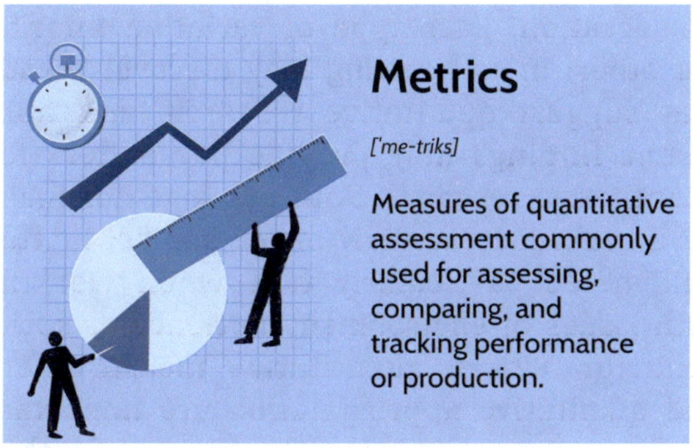

Figure 9.1. The concept of metric variation serves as a crucial framework.

Source: https://www.investopedia.com/thmb/3x0sL27fLZ1TrSyEjDdkDAkwL-I=/1500x0/filters:no_upscale():max_bytes(150000):strip_icc()/metrics.aspfinal-40312c5e32ab4aadbb522fa7566ebe40.jpg.

Definition of Non-Metric Variation

Among the pursuits of finding kinds of variation in a metric sense, non-metric variation is a significant concept that encompasses changes that cannot be measured in standard numerical value, such as organic form or unique aesthetic features. Non-metric variation is qualitative, not measured, compared to metric variation, which involves precise measures to indicate differences—e.g., lengths, sizes, or volumes. For example, it can be displayed as a series of unique morphological traits in biological specimens, and not necessarily in a linear sequence. These variations are essential to evolutionary biology, where they can signal adaptation, camouflage, or mating strategies between species. Non-metric variation thus requires an appreciation of the subjective qualities inherent in biological form, extending discussion beyond mere numbers to encompass the multidimensional meanings of diversity in natural selection. : The importance of non-metric variation extends across many scientific disciplines, especially anthropology and archaeology, where it helps explain cultural and temporal development. In these two fields, artifacts and human bones are typically assessed for non-metric attributes, which can give significant evolutionary or societal tendencies. For instance, cranial features can reveal variation associated with population movements or environmental adaptation, indicating lineage and migration lacking in broader quantitative evaluations. By employing techniques for analyzing non-metric variation, scientists can construct a more advanced picture of human history and behavior. This qualitative method is useful for addressing issues of identity, resilience, and cultural interaction that enrich the narrative of human evolution. Such integrative methods point towards the ever-increasing value of comprehensive study in the discipline, where metric data alone fall short of creating a complete description. The intersection of metric and non-metric variation calls for multidisciplinary dialogue and a richer methodology for balanced analysis. With various disciplines converging on the need for integrated methods, non-metric variation underscores the value of understanding qualitative distinctions alongside quantitative value. Recent advances in theoretical formalism, such as covariant phase-space formulations, reflect sound approaches to modeling these variations, underscoring their intricate interplay within dynamical systems. For instance, research on gravitational theories can determine non-metric variations that are essential for describing event horizons and conservation laws in black holes, as studied in recent work (Hertog, T., et al., 2006; Chandrasekaran et al., 2018).

These developments challenge the significance of combining both metric and non-metric techniques in refining theoretical understanding, ultimately leading to increasingly integrative models appealing to a range of scientific inquiry while further enhancing an appreciation for diversity of forms and meanings in nature (Figure 9.2).

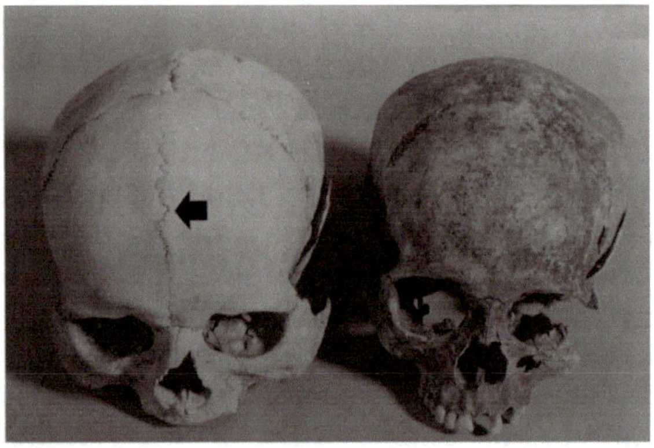

Figure 9.2. The exploration of variation types within the context of metrics.

Source: https://ebrary.net/htm/img/14/1312/90.png.

Importance of Understanding Both Types of Variation

It is crucial to understand both metric and non-metric variation in depth to advance research across various fields, particularly in disciplines such as mathematics, physics, and anthropology. Metric variation is measurable change that may be statistically quantified, typically employing numerical scales for expressing relationships and trends. With it, researchers can conduct rigorous tests, leading to valid outcomes grounded in empirical evidence. Conversely, non-metric variation addresses qualitative variation that may not be quantified so easily but is nonetheless essential to complete contextual understanding. Non-metric variation, for instance, can determine cultural forces that affect behavior or tendencies, whereas something numeric may not. Thus, a complete understanding of both types of variation not only aids our understanding of life's issues but also enhances our capacity to develop innovative problem-solving solutions in academic disciplines. Moreover, the interaction between metric and non-metric variation tends to expose the nuances of systems previously imagined to be homogeneous. For example, in population biology, capturing both variations enables scientists to observe patterns that differentiate between subspecies and assist conservation. Each type of variation informs the other; metric testing may discover trends that suggest qualitative research, and non-metric findings may provide parameters for quantitative research. Both put together make for a multi-faceted view of the subject matter. This holds particularly true when working with issues of environmental science or social behavior, where quantitative measurement and qualitative approximation are important to designing effective interventions. With a clear understanding of what both metrics and non-metrics mean, researchers can tighten their studies, leading to more stable, workable results. Finally, both metric and non-metric variation combined play a pivotal role in the construction of theoretical paradigms and applied methods. For instance, in theoretical physics, concepts formulated in expanded theories of gravity necessitate understanding both sides; understanding the dynamical equivalence between various gravity theories, as exemplified in scalar-tensor systems, is based on understanding gained from both metric and non-metric systems (Agnese et al., 2012). Similarly, while studying the gravitational field equations, one can observe that under either condition of non-zero torsion or zero nonmetricity, the outcomes differ greatly (Shahid-Saless et al., 1993). The situation demonstrates that both types of variation should be considered to yield revolutionary insights within theoretical structures. Lastly, the unification of metric and non-metric knowledge propels scholarly thinking forward, encouraging greater understanding of the complexity of variation within any system and enhanced interdisciplinary collaboration.

9.1. Historical Context

Learning Outcome

1. Development of metric systems
2. Evolution of non-metric systems
3. Impact of historical events on measurement systems

The background history behind metric and non-metric variation within measurement systems is crucial to understanding their applicability and evolution. Emerging from early cultures, early mathematical activity was geometric in nature, revolving around the need to survey land and construct architectural landmarks. The movement towards the use of algebraic techniques was a watershed, marking the shift in the mathematical paradigms that governed these variations. With the evolution of mathematical thinking, especially that of Persian and Arab philosophers, the forms proliferated, fostering a deeper appreciation of the complexities of measurement. This evolution of geometry, from the early rough measurement of space to a well-developed algebraic representation, essentially laid the foundations for both metric and non-metric systems, demonstrating their intricate interdependence as defined by Islami et al. (2017). Exploring the interaction between physics and mathematics further enriches the history of metric and non-metric variations. The philosophical implications of Einstein's Hole Argument explain the challenges in establishing the objectivity of measurement as they appear from the framework of general relativity. The argument taps into the idea of the physical individuality of points in space and time, thereby making it challenging to construct a metric system that can handle varied contexts uniformly. The solution to this issue from Leibniz's equivalence point of view means that it is not possible to derive a single geometric perception to account for the richness of physical existence, proving that the equivalence of measuring systems is dynamically fragile. Being aware of this philosophical debate, as discussed by Pauri et al. (2002), reinforces the historical richness and the evolution of thought that have shaped the development of both metric and non-metric forms. In the development of mathematical and physical theories throughout history, one discovers that the differences between metric systems stem from their respective cultural and context-dependent uses. Different societies have developed their own measurement systems tailored to their specific needs, values, and technological breakthroughs. Measurement is hence region-specific and turns into an integration of local and external factors. When scientific knowledge broadened, particularly through the syncretism of geometric and algebraic methods, the distinction between metric and non-metric means of measurement came to be not technical but epistemological. The discourse currently between various measurement systems reveals the evolution of common knowledge in the past and how society interacts with systems of mathematics, showing that these systems are far more than mere tools—they are a representation of the cultures that use them.

9.1.1. Development of Metric Systems

The metric system has transformed measurement and standardization in nearly all branches of science, engineering, commerce, and daily life. Created in France during the late 18th century, the metric system was a response to measurement systems that were highly variable by region and use during that time. Using a decimal system was revolutionary because it aimed to promote homogeneity and facilitate easier international cooperation. The system was founded on simplicity and uniformity so that conversion and utilization were easy across several fields. As nations began adopting the metric system, it gradually gained momentum, with a focus on the global shift towards a unified method of measurement to eliminate the ambiguity of its predecessors. As the metric system progressed, it sparked extreme political and cultural revolutions, particularly when it came to globalization. Use of metric units became the hallmark of modernity and scientific advancement, hand in hand with greater exchange of ideas and commodities between nations. Non-French nations were at first hesitant to embrace the metric system, for the most part clinging to traditional units of measurement rich in history and cultural significance. However, as empirical sciences advanced and global trade expanded, the benefit of standardization of measurement became more evident. This transformation allowed for better communication within industry and education, as well as provided the foundation for international standards bodies seeking to harmonize practices across borders and facilitate greater global cooperation. The resistance to metrication, particularly in countries with strong non-metric cultures, reflects broader trends in cultural inflexibility and the challenges posed by systematic reform. More significantly, the United States remains one of the only developed countries that have not adopted the metric system entirely because there is a large segment of the population who still apply customary units. The cultural preference highlights the tension between scientific progress and individual action, as the widespread adoption of non-metric systems can create disparities in education, engineering, and medicine. Thus, arguments regarding the metric system usually blur into debates over how best to educate, motivate, and transition societies to a universal metric system. As nations continue to grapple with these forces, the implementation of metric systems remains a pivotal point in discussions of measurement and standardization in our increasingly globalized world (Figure 9.3).

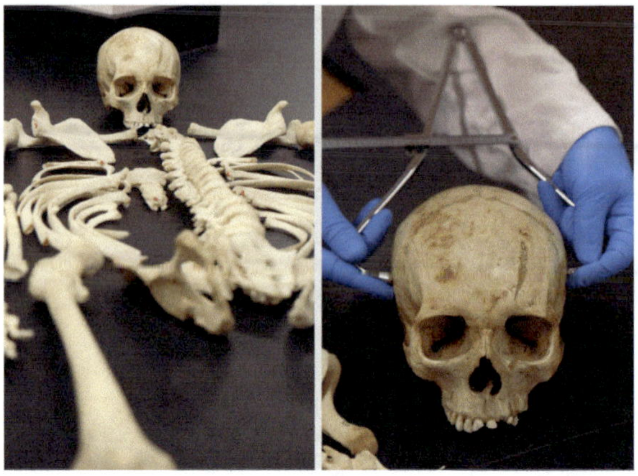

Figure 9.3. The development of metric systems.

Source: https://upload.wikimedia.org/wikipedia/commons/c/c1/FourMetricInstruments.JPG.

9.1.2. Evolution of Non-Metric Systems

The evolution of non-metric systems is a significant evolution in our understanding of gravitational theories and their application. Physics has always relied heavily on metric systems, primarily based on the theory of General Relativity. Non-metric systems evolved as alternatives that sought to explain gravitational phenomena without totally adhering to traditional metric conditions. These systems provide an alternative explanation of gravitational fields, particularly when conventional models are ineffective. One such system is the quasi-metric system, which provides a different way to explain the dynamics of systems such as planetary orbits and cosmological expansion, beyond the usual measures of time and space. This development shows evidence of an ongoing discussion among members of the scientific community regarding the essence of gravity and how various perceptions might have varying impacts on our understanding of the universe's structure and motion. Perhaps one of the most significant developments among non-metric systems is the quasi-metric system, which offers novel solutions to age-old gravitational puzzles. This model proposes that gravitational fields might operate independently of a fixed metric, thus accommodating the dynamic characteristics of cosmic objects. As argued in recent publications, the quasi-metric approach is intended to handle complex interactions between gravitational forces and cosmic expansion, providing a new degree of freedom in celestial mechanics. By developing equations describing the gravitational field outside and inside isolated bodies, scientists can predict inertial particle behavior under different gravitational conditions. These advancements reveal that non-metric systems hold potential for offering new insights into gravitational interactions that classical models might not otherwise capture, and providing a persuasive alternative to classical Newtonian dynamics. Although the quasi-metric structure has yet to be experimentally validated, it already offers significant potential for future research and development. More specifically, the ability to represent gravitational fields consistent with the expanding universe is significant for understanding galactic formations and structures. Experiments have begun to elucidate how non-metric theories can reconcile seemingly contradictory phenomena within classical frameworks, particularly regarding the interaction of motion and gravitational fields in a dynamical universe. For example, observations of planetary motions and their relation to cosmic expansion are self-evident within the quasi-metric framework, suggesting that the use of non-metric systems may be required for surmounting present pitfalls in gravitational physics. As scientists continue to probe these theories, their ability to reshape current paradigms is increasingly evident, foreshadowing a fundamental shift in our understanding of the cosmos.

9.1.3. Impact of Historical Events on Measurement Systems

History's evolution of measurement systems is a complex interplay of scientific innovation and socio-political circumstances. With the development of societies from feudal to more centralized governments, there arose an imperative requirement for standardized units of measurement. Standardization facilitated trade, economic progress, and the unification of scores from various cultures under one umbrella. History, such as the French Revolution, is a turning point in this process; the revolution had initiated not just the adoption of the metric system but also the Enlightenment's ideologies of reason and progress. The demand for reason led most nations to re-examine their measurement practices, creating standard and deployable measures across the board, an ongoing trend today as countries grapple with the duality of metric and non-metric approaches in globalized economies. Measurement systems in ancient times were typically local and based primarily on cultural idiosyncrasies and pragmatism. For example, ancient Egyptian cubits were defined by the physical dimensions of the Pharaoh, while Roman units borrowed from the human form, resulting in a variable system across regions and classes. This measurement variability made it difficult for societies to enable long-distance trade or cooperation. As events in history unfolded—wars, trade treaties, and the establishment of empires—the need for a consistent measurement system became more apparent. The 19th century witnessed universal acceptance of the metric system by other countries, spurred on by the acknowledgment that uniform methods of measurement could help spur economic growth and scientific research, creating the contemporary world in a manner that had previously been thought impossible. The measurement systems are often tested not only to demonstrate their mathematical precision but also to assess the social implications of their application. The invention of measurements in various domains has created immense advancement, but challenges in making these measurements practical. For example, in the context of social impact measurement, what organizations such as the Annie E. Casey Foundation achieve through their SI Program indicates the evolution and maturation of impact measurement. A critical review of the SI Programs practice supports the importance of rigorous methodologies and the social context in which they are being applied. The study aims to identify strengths and areas for improvement, with an emphasis on the observation that measurement not only records results but also influences strategic decisions, thereby shaping the future of impact investing and general societal well-being (N/A, 2016). The trajectory of the historical development of measurement systems thus reflects not only a quest for precision but also a continued interaction with the changing dynamic web of societal developments.

Test Your Knowledge

1. How did the study of metric and non-metric variation develop historically in anthropology?
2. Who were the key figures that contributed to the early research on metric and non-metric skeletal traits?

9.2. Applications of Metric Variation

Learning Outcome

1. Use in scientific research
2. Implementation in engineering and technology
3. Role in international trade and commerce

The applications of metric variation are inherently linked to the discipline of gravitational theories, wherein the understanding of spacetime's geometrical properties is imperative. Metric variation is a fundamental tool in obtaining field equations for gravitational actions, which helps physicists test gravity models. This process is particularly relevant in cases of disparate curvature tensors and their corresponding scalars, e.g., the Riemann or Ricci tensors. Varying the metric, it is possible to derive a master equation that encodes the relationships between the variational derivatives of generalized gravitational actions and those of their constituent curvature scalars. Such is an important technique that allows for investigations into advanced gravitational Lagrangian densities relevant to our ongoing research on gravitational phenomena in four-dimensional spacetime and, even further, as shown in recent research, this method can unify disparate gravitational theories (Abdelwahab et al., 2010). Furthermore, the amenability of metric variation allows for implementation across a variety of gravitational models with higher-order terms, such as the Gauss-Bonnet and Ricci-squared constructs. These terms, however, add additional complexity to the gravitational effect while providing better insight into the dynamics of spacetime. Through the use of the Lagrange multiplier method together with an orthonormal coframe, researchers are able to perform advanced variational processes that allow them to generalize Einstein's General Relativity. This unified account provides avenues for understanding a modified gravitational theory that could possibly describe phenomena such as cosmic acceleration or black hole thermodynamics. The use of algebraic generalizations, similar to those in generic f(R) theories, underscores the universality of metric variation methods in accommodating new theoretical ideas and enhancing gravitational theories (Abdelwahab et al., 2010). The applicability of metric variation extends beyond typical gravitational settings to theoretical problems in supergravity. By investigating asymptotic symmetry algebras, metric variations can explain boundary-condition implications in such advanced frameworks. For example, the study of boundary conditions in AdS_3 gravity can shed light on how they relate to supergravity theories, thereby facilitating a broader perspective on holographic principles in gravitational physics. The use of metric variation to test nonlinear extended superalgebras proves its ability to include elaborate theoretical architectures that arise in modern theoretical physics. This interdisciplinarity not only underpins the worth of metric variation but also renders it a crucial technique in the ongoing struggle to ascertain a unified explanation of gravity on varying scales and conditions within the universe (Figure 9.4).

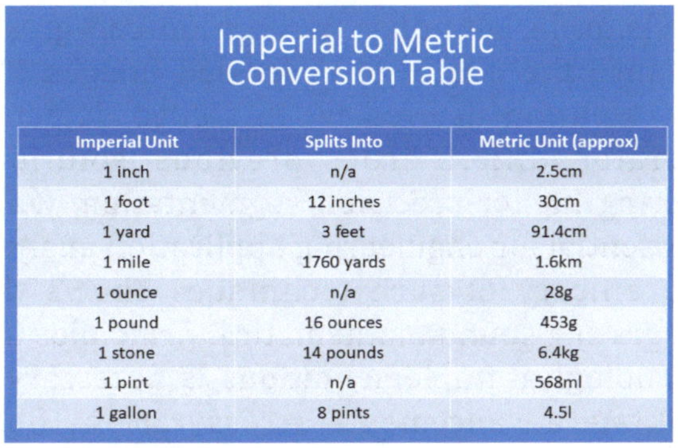

Imperial Unit	Splits Into	Metric Unit (approx)
1 inch	n/a	2.5cm
1 foot	12 inches	30cm
1 yard	3 feet	91.4cm
1 mile	1760 yards	1.6km
1 ounce	n/a	28g
1 pound	16 ounces	453g
1 stone	14 pounds	6.4kg
1 pint	n/a	568ml
1 gallon	8 pints	4.5l

Figure 9.4. The applications of metric variation.

Source: https://external-content.duckduckgo.com/iu/?u=https%3A%2F%2Fi0.wp.com%2Fvariationtheory.com%2Fwp-content%2Fuploads%2F2021%2F10%2FSlide2.png%3Ffit%3D960%252C720%26ssl%3D1&f=1&nofb=1&ipt=532918279d501098e9af81241a7085beaf7fcd2bc12d3f8084b80a09927bca8b.

9.2.1. Use in Scientific Research

In scientific studies, the application of both metric and non-metric methods is crucial for examining complex data and refining analytical techniques. Metric variation, typically quantified through statistical measurements, serves as the foundation for scientific analysis by allowing scholars to examine relationships and trends numerically. For instance, studies on implementing machine learning algorithms have demonstrated significant advancements in digital forensics, where the Random Forest technique enhances counterfeit NFT transaction detection by analyzing variables such as Detection Time and False Positive Rate. The integration of these measurements not only improves detection accuracy but also optimizes data use, thereby creating an increasingly secure digital transaction space, as demonstrated by Devaseelan et al. (2024). Non-metric variation has the same significance in scientific inquiry, particularly in disciplines such as archaeology and environmental science. The significance of qualitative measurements, such as the structural changes seen in corroded artifacts, highlights the need for intensive analysis to go beyond quantifiable information. Methods using neutron tomography and image registration, as demonstrated in recent studies, highlight the importance of non-metric fluctuations in depicting local changes in archaeological materials exposed to varying environmental conditions. By applying advanced imaging techniques and accurate registrations, scientists can delineate variations in moisture content and corrosive activity in samples, underscoring the complementary value of metric measurement and contextual analysis in advancing our understanding of material integrity and development, as shown in Shakoorioskooie et al. (2024). Moreover, the interfacing of metric and non-metric variation leads to a multidimensional methodology for scientific inquiry. By combining the two paradigms' capabilities, scientists can reach safer conclusions. The combination of broad-metric and qualitative observations allows for a richer understanding of phenomena, particularly in cross-disciplinary research. For instance, in fields where environmental factors affect material properties, quantitative and qualitative methods can be employed in combination to shed light that would be lost with the application of either method alone. As observed in studies that combine statistical techniques with experimental results, a complete analytical perspective emphasizes the growing tendency in scientific research to embrace complexity and diversity in interpreting data, thereby deriving more effective and meaningful results in today's dynamic research landscape (Figure 9.5).

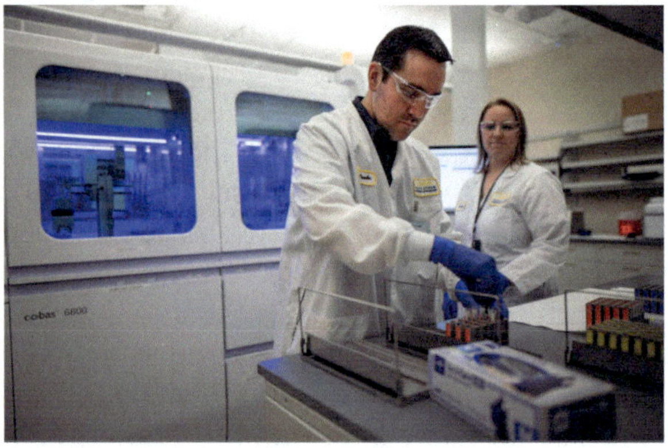

Figure 9.5. Use in scientific research.

Source: https://external-content.duckduckgo.com/iu/?u= https%3A%2F%2Fimg.particlenews.com% 2Fimg%2Fid%2F4T2EIY_11lkGf0000&f=1&nofb=1&ipt=f4ff0c38809b69ea5b5 8edecf8bdf8ef26d99beb7cf8fb3e5a27ac1d4ff370af.

9.2.2. Implementation in Engineering and Technology

Implementing engineering and technology solutions often involves overcoming metric and non-metric variance to optimize designs and processes. In mechanical engineering, for instance, employing vector-based algorithms can significantly enhance design accuracy. A good example is the use of multi-objective optimization methods, including the NSGA-II algorithm, enabling exploration across various parameters in nacelle design for aircraft. The approach employs computational fluid dynamics to model performance and optimize design under varying operating conditions, thereby highlighting the need for robust metric systems that can efficiently handle a variety of datasets. The results also demonstrate the potential impact of stringent selection of algorithm parameters, such as constraint handling and initial sample size, on optimization outcomes, highlighting the intricate relationship between metric precision and engineering effectiveness (Heidebrecht et al., 2017). In image processing, the use of edge detection techniques also illustrates the focal point of intersection between metric and non-metric variations. Technologies employed for segmenting vector-valued images always resort to applying nonlinear functionals to improve image quality. The edge-based technique presented employs geometrical features that are calculated from the image's metric tensor, yielding precise segmentation even under noisy environments. This method illustrates how mathematical precision in boundary description can greatly enhance the clarity of processed images. The new solution derived by this edge detection operator differs from previous solutions, offering higher-precision segmentation, which is essential for engineering application analysis. The efficacy of such techniques shows that integrating sound mathematical principles into technological implementations is necessary to facilitate advancements across various fields (Mahmoodi et al., 2007). The consequences of integrating metric and non-metric variations in technology and engineering are significant, affecting both function and effectiveness. With an increasing number of industries relying on superior algorithms and image processing techniques, the pursuit of the best solutions becomes the prime concern. The interaction among various methodologies, e.g., between genetic algorithms and functional optimization, indicates the varying environments where both metric and non-metric methods operate. As evident from nacelle design optimization and vector-valued image segmentation, technology professionals must accept such disparities to address the challenges posed by modern technology. The ability to switch between these paradigms provides high-level problem-solving techniques, positioning engineers to work with increasingly advanced design needs and optimize overall technical application performance (Figure 9.6).

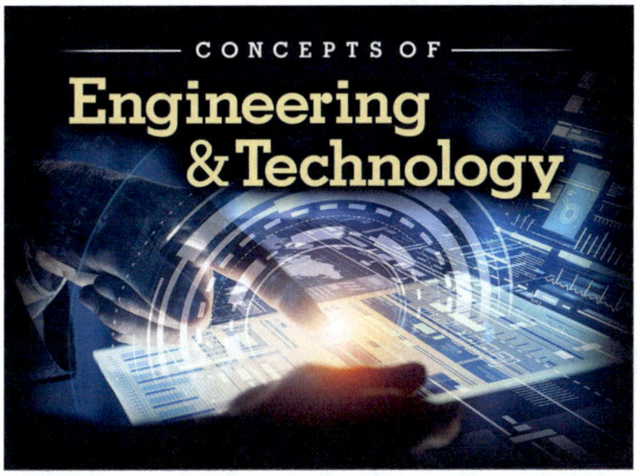

Figure 9.6. Implementation in engineering and technology.

Source: https://external-content.duckduckgo.com/iu/?u=https%3A%2F%2Fwww.edynamiclearning.com%2Fwp-content%2Fuploads%2F2019%2F04%2FEngineering-1024x768.jpg&f=1&nofb=1&ipt=d92981e31d30020e1e38fd8aa568b7dac244ce13cbfc99a2fafa7f09d777e886.

9.2.3. Role in International Trade and Commerce

International trade and commerce rely on the simultaneous use of metric and non-metric systems, particularly for countries navigating the complexities of cross-border regulation and standards. The worldwide use of the metric system promotes communication and transactions by reducing the potential for errors caused by the variability of conversions. For instance, for the dairy business, the U.S. experienced fluctuation in milk protein concentrate imports due to policies that encompass domestic pricing and international market dynamics. Such reliance points to the manner in which tariff frameworks and economic incentives, such as those under U.S. and EU dairy policies, significantly influence trade patterns, highlighting the need for uniformity across measurement systems to boost world trade (Babula et al.). Furthermore, the emergence of greenhouse tomato production is an example of how technological advancements in agriculture are interwoven with measurements in international commerce. As farmers in North America, particularly in Canada and the United States, shift to greenhouse cultivation, there is a measurable reorientation in market demand and product differentiation.

The change in market forces has introduced a new major player: greenhouse tomatoes capture 37% of all U.S. retail tomato sales, displacing the field tomato. The transformation is representative of cross-border trade relations and bears the traces of the need for standardized reporting and quality control measures, which are essential for maintaining competitive advantage in foreign markets (Calvin et al., 2025). Significantly, understanding of metric and non-metric changes goes beyond measurement at a quantitative level; it has implications for commercial planning and policy formulation. The dynamics of market dependencies, as illustrated in the case of the fresh tomato market, show that consumer preferences have instrumental effects on production and trading decision-making. As the mature green tomato market becomes more reliant on foodservice trends, growers are forced to adapt their operations to satisfy not only changing consumer requirements but also international practice and regulation. The widespread adoption of metrics—whether for quality, price, or quantity—across this sector serves as a key driver of enhanced market access and compliance in an ever-more globalized world, illustrating the strategic value of measurement systems in international business (Calvin et al., 2025) (Figure 9.7).

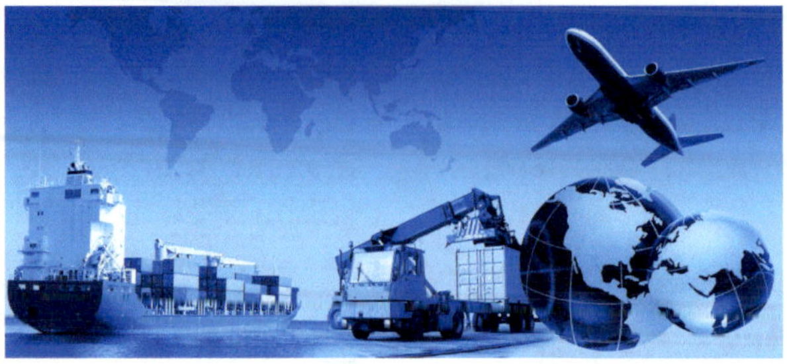

Figure 9.7. Role in international trade and commerce.

Source: https://external-content.duckduckgo.com/iu/?u=https%3A%2F%2Fwww.rakicc.com%2Fwp-content%2Fuploads%2F2019%2F09%2Ftrade-1030x470-1.jpeg&f=1&nofb=1&ipt=ab649c0e1ef2d371a1b27384a3647873bb586b68e4916a44745cd5881c26965a.

Test Your Knowledge

1. How is metric variation used to study population differences and biological diversity in anthropology?
2. What role does metric analysis play in forensic identification and ancestry estimation?

9.3. Applications of Non-Metric Variation

Learning Outcome

1. Cultural significance in various societies
2. Use in everyday life and local practices
3. Influence on art and design

Non-metric variation is at the core of the study of cosmology and gravity, particularly in the metric-affine theories. While the general metric structure assumes independence of the connection with respect to the metric, non-metric variations accommodate a richer understanding of gravitational forces. By treating the connection as a variable that can influence the dynamics of matter, scientists can investigate models that explain phenomena such as the growth of the universe. This has led to new possibilities in exploring generalized gravitational actions, with the highlight that non-metric formulations can provide analogous, if not better, information regarding the evolution of the cosmos than conventional methods. Scholars suggest a more specific research path for these non-metric theories, in the hope that they hold the solution to some of the issues still pending in gravitational physics, thereby broadening the horizon of gravity models beyond cosmological environments (Allemandi et al., 2006). Non-metric variations in field theories provide valuable information about the structure and pattern of energy-momentum tensors in a gravitational environment. The construction of a generic identity demonstrates the relationship between Lagrangian symmetry and the energy-momentum tensor to display how non-metric conditions can be employed to investigate symmetries in generally covariant classical Lagrangian theories. The context not only explains the various fields but also identifies limitations inherent in pursuing a gauge-invariant formulation of energy-momentum tensors for gravity. For instance, the linear gauge-invariant spin-2 field is a graphic illustration of how non-metric variance differs from the usual procedure, substantiating the claim that efforts to define gravitational energy density in terms of metric energy-momentum tensors are built upon flawed principles (Aragone et al., 2002). The consequences of non-metric variation extend far beyond theoretical study, having applications in many fields of physics, from cosmology to gravity. It is through non-metric methods that researchers can construct models that accommodate observational data for the cosmos's expansion without having recourse to the intricacies of curvature in spacetime. Further, it advances interdisciplinarity, closing theoretical physics loopholes with potential experimental tests in cosmology. As researchers continue to explore the implications of non-metric variation, it can become a vital tool in tackling some of physics'smost outstanding problems, such as dark energy and gravitational interactions on a cosmological scale. By fostering an integrated outlook that unites both metric and non-metric perceptions, the exploration of gravitational dynamics has the ability to shed light on the universe's most intimate secrets, demanding a paradigm shift in our knowledge of the texture of existence (Allemandi et al., 2006).

9.3.1. Cultural Significance in Various Societies

The cultural significance of various societies is closely tied to how populations express identity and heritage. The inquiry into cultural markers, such as tradition and language, reveals the distinctive characteristics that constitute each group's worldview. A good example is the Multigroup Ethnic Identity Measure (MEIM), which has been addressed in recent research, indicating the fluidity of ethnic identity formation in a multiculturally expanding society. This research emphasizes a three-factor framework of ethnic identity—encompassing Behavioral, Cognitive, and Affective domains—that encapsulates the multifaceted social dynamics and personal experiences of individuals across different cultural environments (Bunce et al., 2010). These conclusions emphasize that cultural meaning is not an invariant background but a fluid aspect of individuals' lives, shaping social interaction and collective memory. Understanding how cultural aspects manifest in different societies enables one to gain a greater appreciation of their respective identities and experiences. Language as a cultural signifier is more than communication; it is a tool through which society's values and norms are conveyed and transmitted. Language borrowing, the resultant standard product of social relationships and intercultural encounters, determines how societies transform and develop. New computational methods have demonstrated significant advances in identifying the likelihood that a word is borrowed in specific situations and in describing the porosity of language boundaries (Basu et al., 2017). The findings indicate that, in certain cases, annotators interpreted foreign words in mostly native contexts, reflecting a shift in how languages blend. This is a symptom of the cultural significance of language as an identity marker and a tool for cultural accommodation. These differences in language are the focus of further research into cultural accommodation and discourse negotiation among different social groups. Analysis of cultural meaning across societies also calls for a better understanding of how collective identity is constructed through shared history and experience. Every group has a narrative, fueled by divergent historical trajectories, that shapes its cultural expressions and intergroup relations. Given what can be witnessed in the UK's growing multiculturalism, it becomes imperative to distinguish among various ethnic identities to promote greater inclusivity and respect. Utilizing instruments such as the MEIM helps scholars disentangle these identities and the meaning that surrounds them in contemporary contexts (Bunce et al., 2010). Moreover, the tour can guide policymakers and educators in building environments that respect and celebrate diversity, thereby facilitating cohesion among mixed cultural groups. Thus, cultural significance in societies is not just a tool for analyzing human interactions but also a foundational element in building shared awareness and constructing identity (Figure 9.8).

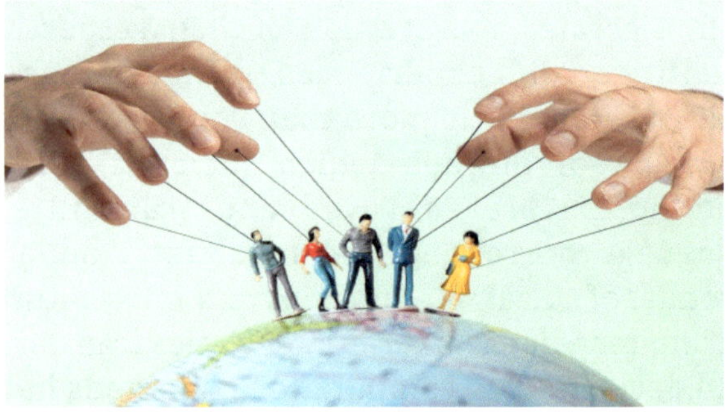

Figure 9.8. Cultural significance in various societies.

Source: https://www.pctiltd.com/web-assets/images/blogimage/202407121216310.jpg.

9.3.2. Use in Everyday Life and Local Practices

The integration of metric and non-metric systems in everyday life significantly influences local practices, particularly in activities such as cooking and agriculture. Recipes in households worldwide use non-metric units such as teaspoons and cups, which reflect culture, tradition, and preference. These standard units ensure an intuitive sense of quantity, facilitating the comfort of meals without compulsory education. By contrast, the metric system prevalent in scientific communities and gaining ground in schools promotes precision and standardized measurement. The coexistence of these systems within domestic routine thus indicates an even more substantial negotiation between convenience, convention, and technical accuracy, drawing on the tensions between customary practices and universal measures. Additionally, local conventions with regard to disposal of food wastes reflect the interest at stake in metric versus non-metric variation. While some regions emphasize the efficiency of the metric system, the majority still use non-metric household units when measuring portions and consumables. Such a concession can impact waste-reduction efforts in the community. Food waste diversion for meal preparation for food-insecure individuals, for instance, highlights the influence of indigenous measurement systems on community activities. In a pilot year for one convention food rescue program, avoiding over 24,000 kg of food translated into 45,383 meals provided, establishing the environmental and ethical benefits of local efforts (Coughenour et al., 2019). They can also be validated by the right metric that quantifies environmental impact, adding to the practical benefits inherent in an enlightened approach to food control. Additionally, raising awareness of energy efficiency in technology demonstrates that the metric system can trigger local practices across industries. Progress in software engineering has further reinforced the adoption of energy metrics to promote sustainability (Ardito et al., 2013). With energy efficiency encouraged as a core aspect of software quality models, developers can develop applications that are not only efficient but also consume minimal energy. This shift, with the application of metric principles, reflects a heightened ecological awareness in everyday activities. Numerous communities are increasing awareness of the impact of their technological choices, and the merging of local technological innovations with metric norms is an expedient way to propagate energy efficiency and conservation across the multifarious aspects of life.

9.3.3. Influence on Art and Design

The influence of technological innovation on design and art has been tremendous, particularly regarding metric and non-metric variation. As more artists and designers leverage new technologies, such as improved aircraft engines or advanced visual tracking devices, the processes of creativity change. For instance, iterative design choices in aircraft design maximize performance metrics such as specific fuel consumption (SFC) and facilitate visual changes that resonate with design (Grönstedt et al., 2020). The prospect of aligning utilitarian requirements with innovative art challenges traditional ideals of design, leaving artists to seek the possibilities offered by technological progress. Such interdependence endows creative products with a conversation between functionality and form, and provokes more integrated design thinking. Art and design are further assisted by approaches which overcome traditional perceptions of dimensionality. Methods such as online distance metric learning, for instance, reveal how artists can use computational operations to expand creativity. Through distance measures of knowing relationship between visual elements, designers can create responsive compositions that respond to alterations in context and viewer interaction (Dick et al., 2015). This can involve changing elements in response to audience interaction, leading to adaptive, time-based visual storytelling. Therefore, the designer's activity shifts from that of an individual author to that of an organizer of interactive events, constituting a dramatic shift in the art world transfigured by technological change. Furthermore, the exchange between metric and non-metric alters induces a new sensibility for aesthetic experience, such that the blending of the physical and the virtual becomes more relevant. Then the artists are free to use the measures derived from technology to inform their work, while also infusing it with more abstract themes that resonate at a cultural and emotional level. The variations allow space for narration that is rich in diversity, and they can accommodate both measurable gains and individual understandings of art. As seen in contemporary practices, the designer's interaction with technologies—not only in designing visually pleasing products but also in arranging utilitarian functions—illustrates a comprehensive appreciation of design that reunites functional needs with affective preferences (Grönstedt et al., 2020). In the end, this interaction expands the scope of art and design in contemporary society, revealing their fluid nature in measurement and artistic works (Figure 9.9).

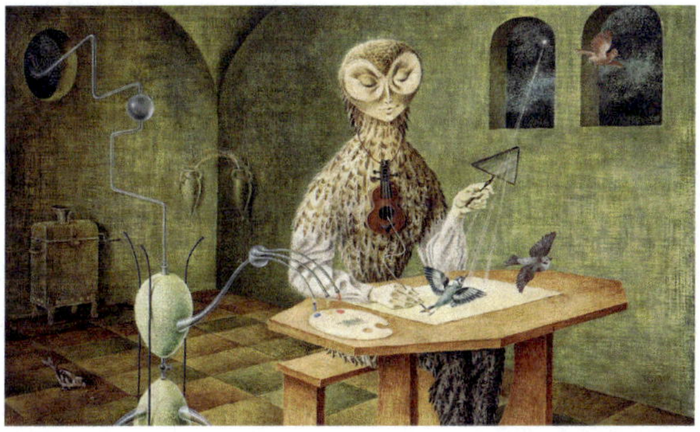

Figure 9.9. The influence of technological advancements on art and design.

Source: https://www.shutterstock.com/blog/wp-content/uploads/sites/5/2022/07/the_creation_of_birds_remedios_varo_editorial_5850819pp.jpg.

Test Your Knowledge

1. How is non-metric variation used to study population relationships and genetic affinities?
2. In what ways does non-metric variation assist in forensic identification and bioarchaeological research?

9.4. Advantages of Metric Variation

Learning Outcome

1. Standardization and consistency
2. Ease of conversion and calculation
3. Global acceptance and usage

The advantages of metric variation are evident in their ability to provide richer mathematical frameworks that justify elaborate physical theories. Using a method that involves the metric, physicists can capitalize on geometrical wisdom that is consistent with our elementary spacetime intuition. This opens the door to other higher-level theories, particularly gravitational physics. For instance, metric-Palatini compatibility allows for the possibility of studying higher-order curvature corrections, which is apparent in their uses for Einstein equations. The compatibility highlights the versatility of metrics, demonstrating that certain types of theories, such as those described by certain Lagrangians, yield viable solutions in this setup. Therefore, metric variation not only yields a richer theoretical framework but also enables sound studies of gravitational physics in high-dimensional settings, supporting traditional models in general relativity and cosmology to a considerable degree, thereby providing deep insights into gravity itself (Demir et al., 2008). Metric variation also plays the crucial role of enabling the unification of various physical fields with gravity. The study of gravitational theories, particularly those involving scalar or vector fields, is aided by metrics that briefly depict physical characteristics. For instance, introducing a dynamical vector field into gravitational theories allows for new conservation laws based on the separate symmetries of the involved fields. The covariant conservation of the energy-momentum tensor, as outlined in recent studies, reveals the intrinsic interrelations among different forms of energy-momentum within this formalism. The energy-momentum tensors, when expressed in terms of metrics, generate equations not only characterizing the gravitational interactions effectively but also fixing emergent properties and conservation laws for those interactions. Therefore, the positive connection between metric variation and other physical theories builds a cohesive image of the universe, leading to novel discoveries in cosmology and theoretical physics (Guendelman et al., 2009). Secondly, the advantages of metric variation include its introduction of degrees of freedom within gravitational theory, offering a more flexible system of describing the universe. How spacetime behaves under various conditions may provide crucial insights into the universe's underlying physical principles. By employing metric variation, scientists can fine-tune the framework to study varied situations, from cosmological models to particle trajectories. That kind of versatility is crucial when dealing with complex issues, such as the cosmological constant problem and other inconsistencies in general relativity. Moreover, the metric formalism leaves room for new models that can describe well such phenomena as string gas cosmology, which improve our understanding of the early universe without facing issues such as the horizon problem. Thus, through its own flexibility and generality, metric variation not only enhances theoretical models but also plays a significant role in the contemporary debate in modern physics, elevating our explanatory power over gravitational phenomena and the ground structure of space and time (Demir et al., 2008; Guendelman et al., 2009).

9.4.1. Standardization and Consistency

In the context of metric and non-metric variation, standardization and consistency are essential for ensuring comparability and accuracy across different measures. Standardization involves the creation of consistent criteria and procedures enabling comparable measurement and interpretation. Without such a framework, inconsistencies will emerge in the data, rendering analysis and the use of the results challenging. This is particularly true in medical imaging applications, where intensity differences between images can significantly affect interpretability and diagnostic performance. The inherent physiological intensity differences in MR images underscore the need for rigorous standardization protocols. As explained, acquisition-to-acquisition intensity differences may mask tissue characterizability, thereby inhibiting reproducible image analysis and segmentation (Bagci et al., 2010). Therefore, the use of a uniform intensity scale is required to ensure measurement consistency in clinical measurements and the derivation of valid conclusions. Secondly, the multidimensionality of measurement transcends mere data gathering; it entails the accurate design of measurement models linking observable symptoms to theoretical variables. Standardization here plays a critical role in ensuring that complexities involved in survey approaches and research designs are preserved. The process of construct definition and item generation must be approached with diligence to ensure that measurements are valid and reliable across heterogeneous populations. Cognitive resources and participant motivation can further influence variation in response behavior, complicating the results if not addressed systematically. Standardized procedures can address these issues by enhancing the comparability of measurements, enabling more robust interpretations of empirical results. As established by past studies, the quality of measurement across conditions not only affects findings but also enhances comprehension of theoretical constructs (Baumgartner et al., 2019). This dimension of standardization speaks to its applicability in guaranteeing consistency in qualitative and quantitative measures. In general, the pursuit of standardization and consistency creates a foundation for effective measures across disciplines, particularly where divergence may conceal necessary insights. The use of standardization techniques can make a significant contribution to measurement accuracy and reliability, ultimately driving empirical research and practical applications. In medical imaging, for instance, standardization operations designed to correct intensity inhomogeneities have been shown to improve registration accuracy, and the intricate relationship between intensity similarity and spatial consistency has been emphasized (Bagci et al., 2010). As the models of measurement continue to evolve and standardized procedures are embraced, the field will progress towards the development of more harmonized and comparable measures. Therefore, the value of standardization in addressing metric and non-metric variation cannot be overemphasized; it remains a focal point in developing sound, evidence-informed best practices that inform policy and decision-making across a range of fields (Figure 9.10).

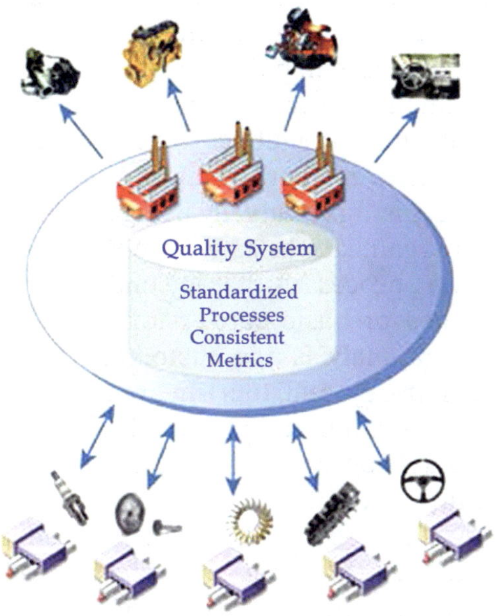

Figure 9.10. Standardization and consistency.

Source: https://www.qualitymag.com/ext/resources/QUAL/2004/02/Files/Images/100732.jpg.

9.4.2. Ease of Conversion and Calculation

Ease of calculation and conversion between metric and non-metric systems is a critical sector deserving significant focus, particularly as globalization continues to necessitate cross-system communication. The metric system, with its structured base-10 system, allows straightforward calculations and conversions. A unit conversion of millimeters to centimeters or vice versa is as simple as multiplying or dividing by ten. This rational model promotes effectiveness and accuracy, which are essential in fields ranging from science to engineering. The non-metric systems, such as the imperial system, however, are likely to be flawed by being reliant on arbitrary units, i.e., inches, feet, and yards, without a consistent base. This inefficiency can lead to larger calculation errors, particularly in the workplace where accuracy is paramount. Moreover, implications of ease of conversion extend beyond simple arithmetic calculations; they reach the very essence of businesses that rely on measurement for effectiveness. To use tourism as a case in point, conversion to metric measurement can lead to greater definiteness and efficiency of metrics that organizations apply to measure performance and outcomes. E-measurement is gradually being recognized by tourism organizations as vital to the evaluation of planning processes, thereby underscoring the importance of basic conversion practices for better data analysis and customer interaction. With a metric system, tourism organizations can standardize comparative statistics to be easily interpretable across a wide variety of markets, enabling more informed decision-making on strategy and growth. This not only enhances operational efficiency but also promotes regional integration within a global context, enabling nations to standardize measurement operations. Within school settings, the inherent qualities of metric systems improve learning and retention because students are able to comprehend underlying concepts of measurement and calculation better. Concepts such as area, volume, and weight become simpler to educate when taught with metric units based on multiplication and division for unit conversion. Moreover, this simplicity supports cross-disciplinary learning because students in fields such as mathematics and science can interact comfortably with measurement applications in the world. On the other hand, the complexities of non-metric systems make it difficult for students to learn from and apply formulas, and hinder their ability to interpret results across disciplines. As evidenced in various research products, both practical and theoretical roots, these education systems highlight the long-term benefits of adopting a metric approach throughout curricula globally, indicating an imperative need for reevaluation of the means of teaching measurement to address the needs of the times (Mazumdar et al., 2012; Ajzen et al., 2013).

9.4.3. Global Acceptance and Usage

Pressure towards global use of metric and non-metric systems of measurement is a two-way interaction between the standardization in today's world and cultural heritage. As global trade and globalization continue to rise, it has become increasingly evident that a common platform for measuring has become imperative. For instance, countries that adopt the metric system have easier scientific and technological communication, enabling collaboration and reducing errors. However, nations entrenched in non-metric cultures, such as the United States, are prevented from converting due to historical and cultural resistance. This situation reveals that acceptance is not merely a matter of preference but also closely connected to a country's identity and operating realities. The technological influence on the acceptance of measuring systems must also be taken into account. As digital tools and platforms become more ubiquitous, they facilitate a hybridization of measurement practices. An excellent illustration lies in Internet banking, as the Internet Banking Acceptance Model (IBAM) indicates that behavioral attitudes and intentions towards new technologies can differ substantially across cultures. These differences indicate that although technical standards are intended to promote homogeneity, application and acceptability may be tempered by local customs and traditions, further supporting the observation that international acceptance is not a one-way process but is often contested (Ajzen et al., 2010). This difference not only adds to the complexity of the standardization process but calls for tailor-made approaches that respect local usage and interpretation of measurement. In addition, the role of linguistic variation in global acceptance must be carefully scrutinized. Machine Translation (MT) systems, whose effectiveness depends on the accuracy of bilingual data, are a fine example. The nuances in translating measurement vocabulary across languages can lead to inconsistencies that further complicate the world to understand. Employing bi-sentence filtering techniques helps overcome such hindrances, enhancing translation quality while maintaining the subtleties of measurement language (Wołk et al., 2015). As these technologies continue to develop, their use will presumably become imperative for streamlining communication between non-metric and metric systems to ensure global communication and acceptance. This synergy of technology, culture, and language captures the fundamental aspects that define the new controversy over measurement systems in today's globalized world.

Test Your Knowledge

1. What are the main advantages of using metric variation in anthropological and forensic studies?
2. How does metric variation improve the accuracy of population and individual identification?

9.5. Advantages of Non-Metric Variation

Learning Outcome

1. Cultural relevance and identity
2. Flexibility in local contexts
3. Historical significance and storytelling

Research into non-metric variation offers several advantages that facilitate a more thoughtful understanding of biological systems. One of its greatest strengths is its ability to locate patterns of divergence that would be lost with metric measurement. Non-metric methods are simple to use in identifying exclusive evolutionary routes, and scientists can come to realize the complexity of speciation beyond such quantitative measures. For instance, these methods can illustrate the way environmental pressures determine species differentiation in incommensurable ways. With an emphasis on qualitative assessments, non-metric variation can reveal adaptive strategies and behavioral traits that define species' ecological niches. Ultimately, the flexibility of non-metric techniques provides avenues for interpretation better suited to the intricacies of evolutionary processes. Another advantage inherent in non-metric variation is the development of data analysis that is straightforward without compromising theoretical precision. Where a boundary is not clear-cut or where metric strategies are overly constraining and assign inaccurate labels, non-metric methodologies may offer a more adaptable context. These methods are more likely to eliminate the strict assumptions inherent in metric measurements, thereby allowing greater scope for data analysis. By employing methods that focus on patterns and relationships rather than exact metrics, researchers can engage with the data more actively. This flexibility delivers a richer assessment of complex interactions among species, generating an extensive picture of biodiversity and ecological interdependence that can be best achieved through metrics. In addition, the utilization of non-metric variation adds strength to speciation rate estimates, particularly with its emphasis on biological meaning rather than numerical simplicity. Studies have shown that model-free non-metric approaches yield more accurate estimates of speciation than rates of net diversification, thereby confirming their practical utility for evolutionary biology. For example, studies have shown that non-metric measures can effectively account for environmental variables and ecological controls influencing adaptations in species (Rabosky et al., 2019).

These approaches can detect patterns that reflect fundamental evolutionary dynamics rather than mathematical artifacts. With the utilization of these non-metric variations, scientists can make biologically meaningful interpretations and hypotheses about the relationship between a species and its environment and thus reach enhanced and applicable scientific conclusions (Figure 9.11).

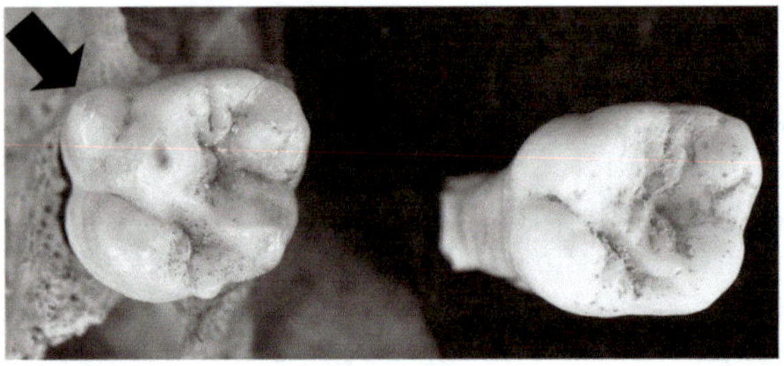

Figure 9.11. The exploration of non-metric variation.

Source: https://ebrary.net/htm/img/14/1312/98.png.

9.5.1. Cultural Relevance and Identity

Cultural identity and relevance are crucial for understanding how people perceive themselves and their environment, especially in settings of metric and non-metric variation. For the sake of establishing an important identity, individuals would tend to adopt cultural symbols and practices that represent their values and origins. This is particularly noticeable when facial structures and expressions are taken into account, as they convey special cultural messages. Computational models of the face suggest direction towards which these attributes become markers of identity that continue to evolve and thus influence perceptions of age and kinship. By modeling these factors, researchers can better appreciate the complexity of cultural identity in relation to physical characteristics. Such an appreciation is important for developing consistent identity validation systems that are sensitive to human variation and cultural differences, hence making these technologies more applicable in multicultural communities (Georgopoulos et al., 2018). Also, cultural identity is influenced by personal and social variables that shape responses to both foreign and domestic brands. The intersection of identity and consumer behavior highlights the concept of favoritism, which can mirror cultural attachments and societal values at the macro level. By drawing on social identity theory and categorization theories, researchers can illuminate the processes underlying brand preference and loyalty across different populations. For instance, attitudes toward foreign versus domestic products are likely to reveal underlying identity processes that affirm cultural salience. This illustrates how cultural contexts impact not only individual choice but also how groups create identities around specific brands, leading to a richer understanding of the measures embedded in consumer preferences (Stathopoulou et al., 2019). Lastly, cultural significance and identity go beyond beauty concerns, with significant effects on broader social exchange and collective self-conceptions. In the context of metric and non-metric differences, awareness of this dynamic is significant for understanding how various cultural narratives converge and mesh across varied forms of expression. By uniting data visualization with the nuance of cultural context, scholars are increasingly able to address issues of identity authentication and representation. The conclusions of this study have broad implications beyond the academic world, suggesting applications in applied contexts such as marketing, design, and social science, thereby validating the call for further research into technological paradigms of cultural identity. In conclusion, there is an urgent need to maintain an integrated perspective that recognizes the multidimensional nature of identity, thereby respecting and accepting cultural diversity across various societal constructs (Georgopoulos et al., 2018) (Figure 9.12).

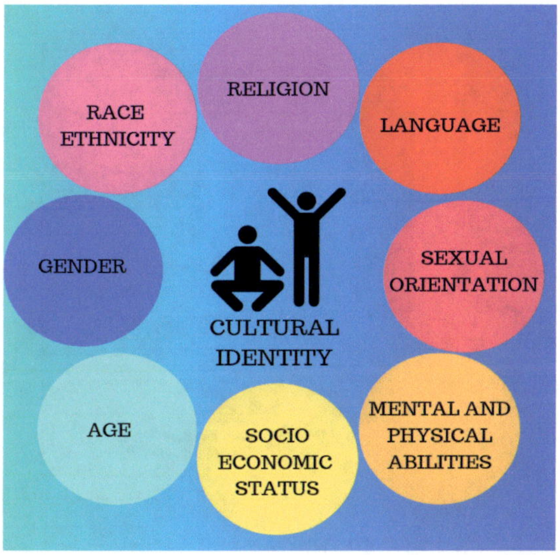

Figure 9.12. Cultural relevance and identity.

Source: https://media.licdn.com/dms/image/v2/C4D12AQHuZv8UeQGI6w/article-inline_image-shrink_1000_1488/article-inline_image-shrink_1000_1488/0/1559884222951?e=1755734400&v=beta&t=t3dH5h3a1mv9xeH3YAcspaFonuGkXkQvtIbpUR46Tzs.

9.5.2. Flexibility in Local Contexts

The concept of flexibility in local contexts is key when defining metric and non-metric variation. Understanding how local environments and cultural traditions influence the application of metrics can inform broader discourses of adaptability across disciplines. Learning spaces, for instance, generally require tailored practices attuned to specific values and cultures of learning in communities. This flexibility allows institutions to integrate local knowledge so that not only are measures of success inclusive, but they are also meaningful and available to students of diverse backgrounds. This flexibility within the education system is a fine example of how it is possible to respect local contexts and create standards that would otherwise appear stiff or over-prescriptive. In addition, local environments also provide a setting in which metric and non-metric differences may be measured to suit a community's needs. A notable challenge is the appropriate granularity of measures, as reflected in the variation of word senses expounded in contemporary linguistic studies. Notably, Amplayo et al. (2018) emphasize that sense granularity variability is crucial to identify the complex meaning words may convey in contexts suitably. Such specificity is particularly crucial when working with technical terms that may vary based on application by location or context. The ability to adapt measurement to local language and cultural orientation thus not only enhances comprehension but also fosters inclusivity in communication. Apart from linguistic adaptation, the body of scientific theory itself demonstrates flexibility across local contexts, as seen in advancements in gravitational theory. The research documented in Gruzinov et al. (2011) shows that the wide-ranging uses of theoretical models are bound to yield varying interpretations depending on local environmental factors. Research on gravitational potentials and their local modifications in condition is proof of the urgency of contextual flexibility. Such flexibility is evident in the ability to develop a range of theories that meet specific astrophysical or cosmological needs, thereby forming an interconnected network of theoretical frameworks and empirical applications. Such an endeavor to search for an understanding of metric and non-metric variation through flexible spectacles leaves a broad scope of inquiry in its implications across the spectrum.

9.5.3. Historical Significance and Storytelling

The intersection of historical importance and narrative is found across most cultures, demonstrating how stories inform our understanding of history. Storytelling as a means of passing on values, belief systems, and lessons accumulated over time is found in societies. The craft of narrative is as ancient as society itself, evolving through forms and technologies. As stated, "Interaction Design, which is essentially story-making and storytelling, is at once both an ancient art and a new technology" (Harvey et al., 2007). This dichotomy reflects the importance of narrative in informing both historical time and technological development. Through compelling narratives, communities are able to remember significant events in a manner that keeps their communal memory alive.

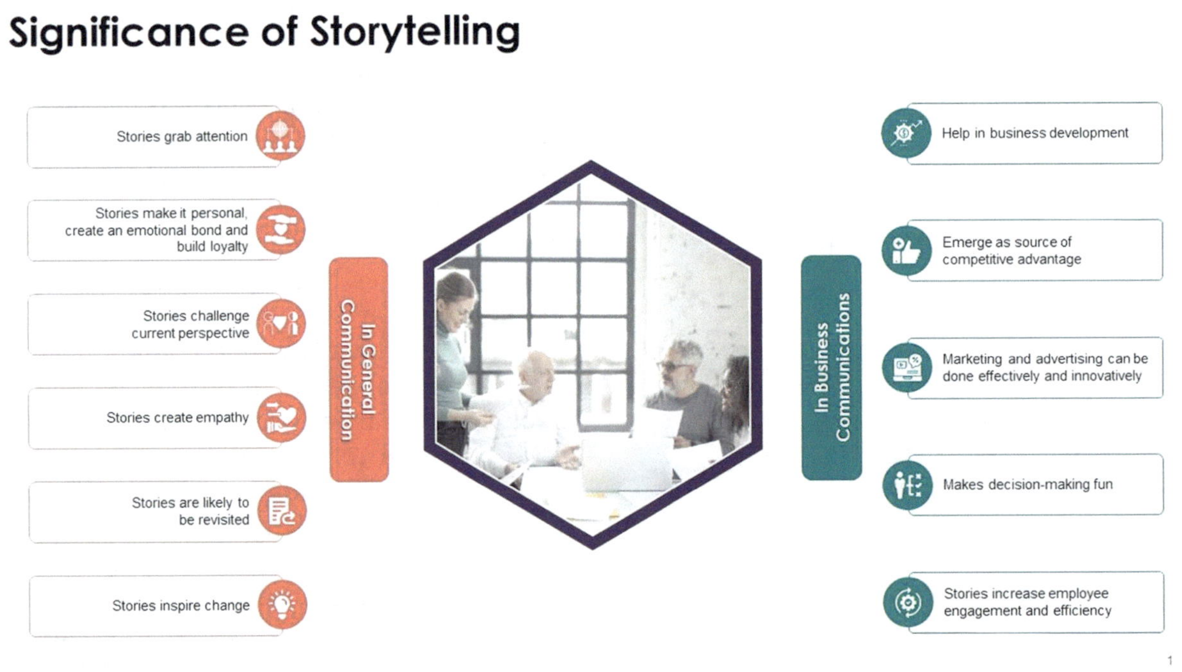

Figure 9.13. The interplay between historical significance and storytelling.

Source: https://www.slideteam.net/media/catalog/product/cache/1280x720/s/i/significance_of_storytelling_in_general_and_business_communication_training_ppt_slide01.jpg.

As narrative evolves, it remains central to conveying the intricacies of human experience, enabling a richer understanding of both history and its impact on contemporary society. Different forms of telling, ranging from oral societies to modern-day digital media, shape how people understand and interpret history. This variation in medium and form may impact the framing of historical narratives, building collective memory and identity. The way an event is told, either visually or in text, can highlight some points over others. For instance, advances in visual narration through broadcast design have allowed for improving the storytelling in re-enactments of historical events, and as such, the events become more accessible and engaging to the audience (Harvey et al., 2007). By integrating several sources of information into storytelling forms, the narrator can establish connections between what has happened and what is current, furthering an understanding of history's relevance. To these ends, the evolution of storytelling techniques informs not only the aesthetic value of history but also its comprehension and memorization of essential realities. Further, an examination of differences in language across stories emphasizes the realities of conveying historical significance. For instance, research on rhythm measures between different dialects, such as Australian English and Barunga Kriol, shares understandings of how language informs stories and influences comprehension. The rhythm and pattern of storytelling can enhance the intelligibility and emotional resonance of historical narratives. These differences, in contributing to the overall cultural narrative fabric, also address the multilingualism that provides societies with diverse forms of expression. The exploration of rhythm and vowel reduction demonstrates storytelling's ability to serve as a vehicle for both the significance of history and the presentation of cultural identity. By examining these aspects of language, we can appreciate how storytelling is an active practice of preserving and interpreting history that enriches our social story space (Figure 9.13).

Test Your Knowledge

1. What are the main advantages of using non-metric variation in anthropological and forensic studies?
2. How does non-metric variation complement metric analysis in understanding population and individual differences?

9.6. Challenges of Metric and Non-Metric Variation

Learning Outcome

1. Resistance to change in non-metric systems
2. Confusion in international communication
3. Balancing tradition with modernization

Issues inherent to metric and non-metric variation are key to understanding how these forms of variation influence research outcomes in the sciences, particularly in biology and anthropology. Metric variation, or measurable differences, is likely to yield straightforward statistical analysis. However, scientists face the challenge of selecting appropriate scales and measurement methods. The degree of precision required in these measurements can be sophisticated, demanding advances in equipment and technology. Alternatively, non-metric variation entails qualitative variation that resists numerical expression. This is a major analytical problem because the lack of quantifiable information could mask valid data on kinship or phenotypic features. Hence, both forms of variation need to be unified while making exhaustive inferences from high-dimensional data that reflect the complexities of the real world. New advances in computational models present promising solutions to these challenges. Computational facial model building and its refinement, for instance, offer effective approaches for recording age progression and verifying kinship based on facial features. As suggested, researchers can use geometric, hand-crafted, and learned facial representations to examine these features (Georgopoulos et al., 2018). The use of these models, however, requires knowledge of metric and non-metric variation, as the researchers must critically examine the datasets used to train them. Furthermore, the test protocols and procedures used to assess the efficacy of these models are equally flawed, calling for robust frameworks that can accommodate variability in the accuracy of representation. Thus, the relationship between technological innovation and theoretical variation remains a subject for exploration. Further, the role of technologies such as Generative Adversarial Networks (GANs) illustrates the evolution in metric and non-metric variation issues. These deep generative models capture high-level data distributions but are afflicted by serious issues such as mode collapse and training instability (Cao et al., 2020). The feasibility of these issues is directly related to modeling variation, both non-metric and metric, because the underlying algorithms require precise optimization to generate reliable outputs. Thus, solving these problems not only fuels GANs but also strengthens methodologies for learning variation across all lines of inquiry. By integrating theoretical principles and cutting-edge technology, researchers can gain a better understanding of variation, creating opportunities for novel solutions to address sophisticated problems (Figure 9.14).

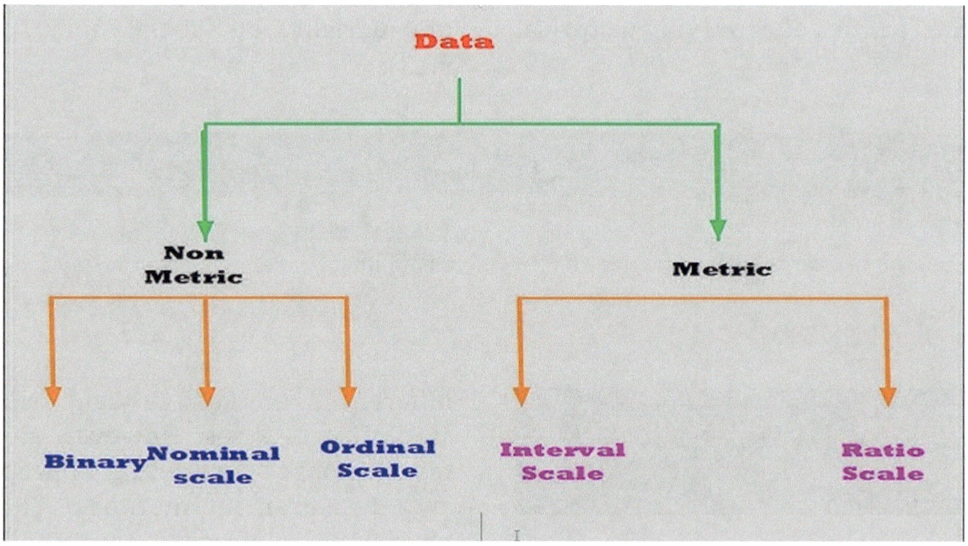

Figure 9.14. The challenges inherent in metric and non-metric variation.

Source: https://i.ytimg.com/vi/MK_P6mnurX8/hq720.jpg?sqp=-oaymwEhCK4FEIIDSFryq4qpAxMIARUAAAAAGAElAADIQj0AgKJD&rs=AOn4CLBUqga_e1AFeBUxrlC8GbBRND1bwQ.

9.6.1. Resistance to Change in Non-Metric Systems

Resistance to change in non-metric systems derives from various social, cultural, and practical factors. Individuals and societies prefer to be comfortable with their heritage systems that have existed for centuries. This is the case with measurement systems, where familiarity brings about a sense of reliability and effectiveness. Non-metric systems, such as the imperial units of everyday experience and usage, are embedded in culture and in everyday use. Converting from miles to kilometers, or from ounces to grams, for example, might not be a purely numerical challenge but a psychological one, since it involves a significant shift in thinking and behavior. The ingrained nature of such units leads to a general reluctance to adopt metric systems when the benefits are obvious, thereby creating a pattern of inertia in measurement practice. Another significant factor for resistance to change is the implications for industries and commerce based on non-metric systems. Businesses, particularly those in manufacturing and commerce, will appreciate efficiency and standardization in operation. Conversion to a metric system could entail enormous retraining, reassessment of production functions, and even potential interference with the supply chain. According to different research, stakeholders could be skeptical about change due to fear of additional costs and inefficiencies in operations. This could be substantiated by a perceived sense of non-urgency for such a transformation, resulting in a culture where things remain as before due to an overall sentiment of risk aversion. Therefore, resistance to abandoning non-metric systems not only suppresses innovation but also hinders broader economic cooperation with metric-using nations. Furthermore, the process of resisting change in non-metric systems crosses over with school structures and government policy programs. Schooling systems tend to favor traditional approaches to instruction using non-metric units, further entrenching students within the system. As students learn about imperial measures, they may become less flexible to a metric system, ensuring the continued use of measurement preferences from generation to generation. Public policy also plays an important role; without legislative support for promoting metric systems, attempts to drive change can be thwarted. Implementing metric units in the public sectors—education, transport, and health—requires effective communication to overcome existing biases and gain acceptance. Overall, resistance is reduced by a strategy that addresses the cultural, economic, and educational bases for non-metric systems.

9.6.2. Confusion in International Communication

With an increasingly interconnected world, international communication complexities often create immense confusion. This uncertainty is most evident when one considers the inconsistency between metric and non-metric systems. Different measurement systems may cause misinterpretations that compromise communication. For example, an international project may fail if members work with different units, e.g., meters or feet. In the absence of a common foundation for understanding variations, there is a higher likelihood of miscommunication, which can lead to decision-making and project management issues. Not only does the miscommunication of measurements present functional issues, but it also emphasizes the existence of a profound difference in culture regarding information handling and transmitting. Understanding metric and non-metric systems is thus imperative in the facilitation of , more transparent communication across borders. Moreover, technological advancement in communication has not necessarily exempted all these challenges. As automated platforms and programs enhance real-time interactions among global participants, measurement differences in interpretation still persist. For example, automated speech recognition research has shown that linguistic context and language play significant roles in shaping error rates in recognition systems. As observed in existing research, traditional metrics for evaluating ASR performance overlook issues inherent to varying linguistic backgrounds, leading to increased miscommunication in findings. This incompatibility is symptomatic of a broader picture in which variations between measurement systems can impede technology's ability to bridge cultural differences. By not making sufficient effort to address these issues, technology development risks perpetuating rather than reducing the obstacles to international communication. Finally, of utmost importance in overcoming confusion in global communication is developing metrics that appeal universally across cultures. Because metric and non-metric differences pose difficulties, researchers are currently advocating other assessment frameworks that better reflect usability and comprehension across varied users. For instance, a new metric specifically for captioning that prioritizes the user experience for Deaf and Hard of Hearing users has been proposed, which demonstrated substantial usability improvement compared to conventional metrics—the shift in focus in metric mirrors the significance of looking towards user-centered approaches when assessing communication effectiveness. By prioritizing measures that capture cultural and contextual variation, stakeholders can increase involvement in worldwide settings and, ultimately, enhance understanding and collaboration beyond differences in measurement. Thus, measurement differences become a prime area of inquiry in the creation of a more universal global narrative (Figure 9.15).

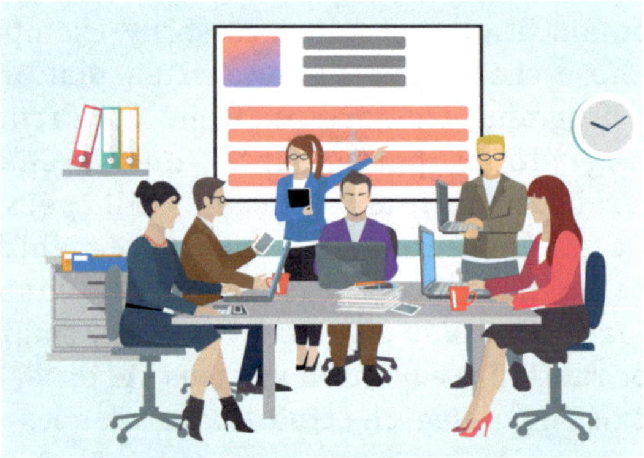

Figure 9.15. Confusion in international communication.

Source: https://www.cdi-usa.biz/wp-content/uploads/2021/12/Workplace-Communication.png.

9.6.3. Balancing Tradition with Modernization

Synchronizing tradition with modernization typically occurs across a broad spectrum of domains, particularly in the development of measurement systems—both non-metric and metric. Pre-modern measurement systems rooted heavily in cultural heritage are not only functional tools but also symbols of identity. However, as globalization accelerates, standardized measurement systems such as the metric system become more unnecessary. The metric system promotes efficiency, facilitates international trade, and enhances scientific communication. Societies are therefore forced to balance the precision and universality of the metric system with the cultural symbolism introduced by conventional units simultaneously. It involves educational efforts and policy changes that raise awareness of the advantages of modernization without erasing the historical context that underpins local identity. Public administration regimes research exhibits the same dilemma of balancing tradition and modern forms of governance. Countries vary in their adherence to traditional administrative designs and to modern market-economy principles. For instance, Anglo-American, French/German, and Scandinavian regimes exhibit distinctive characteristics that describe how tradition shapes governmental processes. The application of market-based instruments in public administration is a step toward modernization, but must be managed with care to avoid the demolition of the institutional harmony that underpins public confidence. It is the general need to balance existing public administration practices with the needs of the contemporary era, as reforms along traditional paradigms can create windows for preserving democratic principles even in the face of pressures from modernization (Gottschall et al., 2010). Lastly, tradition and modernization are polarizing themes that reflect significant societal changes, also evident in discourses on food production capacity. Food security is not just interpreted through the technological but rather the socio-cultural dimensions that govern patterns of consumption and production. Environmental and economic stress, combined with the need to support a growing population, necessitates that the solution be sensitive to traditional agriculture while seeking more advanced solutions. Technologies with potential to increase food production must be developed through an environmentally and socially responsible approach, ensuring sustainability without undermining local lifestyles and knowledge systems. The evolving nature of human interaction with food demonstrates the capability for harmony in the coexistence of traditional ways and modernity, ensuring a sustainable future (Heilig et al., 1993).

Test Your Knowledge

1. What are the main challenges in analyzing metric and non-metric variation in skeletal studies?
2. How can observer bias and population diversity affect the interpretation of metric and non-metric traits?

SUMMARY

The research on metric and non-metric variation has revealed deep insights into underlying structures and relationships in data. It should be emphasized that both types of variation serve distinct functions in analysis: metrics provide quantitative information enabling explicit comparisons, while non-metric methods offer qualitative insights that can capture the finer shades often missed by strict numerical analysis. By identifying such distinctions, researchers can make more significant interpretations and ultimately enhance their decision-making process across various areas. Such a two-sided perspective not only enhances our insight into intricate datasets but also yields innovative approaches that leverage the strengths of both methods. The implications of the findings, in practice, in terms of metric and non-metric variation extend beyond theories, impacting applications across areas such as statistics, data science, and machine learning. One example is the understanding gained from research on the gravitational field of black holes, as illustrated by Giulini et al. (2007), to show how metric variation can be used to explain astrophysical observations. Similarly, advances in domain warping methods, as discussed in Lu et al. (2013), underscore the importance of exposing differences in functional data. The ability to represent horizontal as well as vertical differences allows researchers to approach intricate datasets with a higher level of sophistication, such that analyses can be both encompassing and explanatory. Overall, the convergence of metric and non-metric differences can influence upcoming studies and more analytical models. By integrating these approaches, researchers can construct robust methodologies that not only help address the specific complexities of data variation but also advance the broader debate on data analysis. This organized approach calls forth interdisciplinarity, through which greater understanding and innovative problem-solving tools are shared across the social sciences and the natural sciences. As we progress toward an ever-more data-driven world, it will be essential that we embrace both metric and non-metric variations to broaden our knowledge and develop effective problem-solving strategies.

Summary of Key Points

In exploring the definition of metric and non-metric variation, a critical step is to present key points that articulate the distinction between the two frameworks. Metric variation, based on quantitative data, provides an accurate measurement of variance for a given dataset or phenomenon. The mathematical foundation provides firm comparisons and analyses with significant insights into the underlying patterns and trends. Non-metric variation incorporates qualitative aspects such as terms and categories that prioritize context over numeric data. This approach tends to draw attention to subjective experience and cultural nuance, which could be overlooked by measures, thereby complicating the argument. This dichotomy between the two approaches underscores the importance of a balanced trend in research activity among scholars, where metric and non-metric perspectives can coexist to provide greater insight into the topic at hand. The other key area to discuss is the real-world applications of both the metric and non-metric approaches in the natural and social sciences. For instance, in automatic speech recognition systems, the use of metric measures provides a standardization that enhances performance evaluations across diverse algorithms. The audio adversarial examples recognition work, pointing to the need to develop more sensitive and comprehensive methods, is an excellent demonstration of how metric diversity can drive technological advancement (Ding et al., 2020). Conversely, non-metric methods can assist us in understanding users' experience and how they are perceived, perhaps not fully achieved with metrics alone. This dual use shows how conflicting methodologies can coexist and support one another, ultimately yielding a more enriching synthesis of data and interpretation that can better inform practice and policy. Furthermore, the interdisciplinary status of metric and non-metric variation underscores its importance across theoretical frameworks and applications. As revealed by the examination of variational principles in metric general relativity, the marriage of mathematical form and intuitive understanding is of profound importance to theoretical physics (Brown et al., 2002). By exploring variational principles in spacetime and gravitation, scientists can reveal new ways to understand complex interactions in the universe. This complementarity between the two strategies in stimulating innovation and fostering inquiry in scientific disciplines demonstrates synergy. Consequently, the following detailed summary of these key points not only synthesizes our understanding of metric and non-metric variation but also encourages their existence together and, therefore, advances scholarly debate and practical outcomes in diverse ways.

KEY TERMS FROM THIS CHAPTER

Metric Traits
Principal Component Analysis (PCA)
Metric variation theory
Non-metric knowledge
Phase-space formulations
Principal Component Analysis (PCA)
Non-Metric Traits
Morphological traits
Morphological traits
Non-metrics
Planetary motions

CRITICAL THINKING QUESTIONS

1. **Metric traits are defined as:**
   a. Discrete traits scored as present or absent
   b. Genetic mutations found in soft tissue
   c. Continuous measurements of skeletal features
   d. Traits observable only in children
2. **Non-metric traits are often used to assess:**
   a. Height
   b. Ancestry and population affinity
   c. Age-at-death
   d. Stature estimation
3. **An example of a non-metric trait in the cranium is:**
   a. Maximum cranial length
   b. Bizygomatic breadth
   c. Supraorbital torus presence
   d. Femoral head diameter
4. **Which of the following is a metric trait used in forensic anthropology?**
   a. Carabelli's cusp
   b. Mastoid process length
   c. Metopic suture presence
   d. Third molar agenesis
5. **What is a key limitation of non-metric traits?**
   a. They cannot be observed in adults
   b. They are always symmetrical
   c. Their expression can be subjective and vary among observers
   d. They require expensive equipment

Short Answer Questions

1. Define metric and non-metric traits in skeletal analysis.
2. What are the advantages and limitations of using metric traits in population studies?
3. How can craniometric data be used in forensic identification?
4. Explain the importance of standardization when collecting metric data from skeletal remains.
5. What is the role of non-metric dental traits in understanding population relationships?
6. Describe a scenario where non-metric traits may be more useful than metric traits in skeletal analysis.

Answers to Critical Thinking Questions

1. (c); 2. (b); 3. (c); 4. (b); 5. (c)

REFERENCES

1. Menden, M. P., Wang, D., Mason, M. J., Szalai, B., Bulusu, K. C., Guan, Y., Yu, T., Kang, J., Jeon, M., Wolfinger, R., Nguyen, T., Zaslavskiy, M., Abante, J., Abecassis, B. S., Aben, N., Aghamirzaie, D., Aittokallio, T., Akhtari, F. S., Al-Lazikani, B., . . . Fourches, D. (2019). Community assessment to advance computational prediction of cancer drug combinations in a pharmacogenomic screen. *Nature Communications, 10*(1), 2674. https://doi.org/10.1038/s41467-019-09799-2Abdelwahab, M., Ahmedov, H., Aliev, A. N., Ahmedov, H., Aliev, A. N., Baykal, A., Ayón-Beato, E., Barrow, J. D., Benn, I. M., et al. (2010). A unified approach to variational derivatives of modified gravitational actions. http://arxiv.org/abs/1012.4246 (accessed on 21st July 2025).
2. Agnese, A. G., Boehmer, C. G., Coule, D. H., Page, D. N., Darabi, F., Accetta, F. S., Lobo, F. S. N., et al. (2012). Classical Euclidean wormhole solutions in Palatini $f(\dot{R})$ cosmology. http://arxiv.org/abs/1110.5485 (accessed on 21st July 2025).
3. Ajzen, I., Ajzen, I., Ajzen, I., Bagozzi, R. P., Bagozzi, R. P., Bajaj, A., Alsajjan, B., et al. (2010). Internet banking acceptance model: Cross-market examination. https://core.ac.uk/download/336208.pdf (accessed on 21st July 2025).
4. Ajzen, I., Albrecht, K., Attaran, M., Barua, A., Bogner, A., Boyatzis, R. E., Bremser, W. G., et al. (2013). Performance measures of net-enabled hypercompetitive industries: The case of tourism. https://core.ac.uk/download/76188.pdf (accessed on 21st July 2025).
5. Allemandi, G., Allemandi, G., Barrow, J. D., Barrow, J. D., Benn, I. M., Birrell, N. D., Buchbinder, E. I., et al. (2006). Metric-affine $f(R)$ theories of gravity. http://arxiv.org/abs/gr-qc/0604006 (accessed on 21st July 2025).
6. Amplayo, R. K., Hwang, S., & Song, M. (2018). AutoSense model for word sense induction. http://arxiv.org/abs/1811.09242 (accessed on 21st July 2025).
7. Amsel, A., Hertog, T., Hollands, S., Marolf, D., Ashtekar, A., Bombelli, L., Reula, O., Berkooz, M., Chrusciel, P. T., Marolf, D., Fefferman, C., Graham, C. R., Hertog, T., et al. (2006). Asymptotic generators of fermionic charges and boundary conditions preserving supersymmetry. https://core.ac.uk/download/44150583.pdf (accessed on 21st July 2025).
8. Aragone, C., Aragone, C., Baryshev, Y., Bel, L., Boulware, D., Brown, J. D., Deser, S., et al. (2002). Symmetry properties of the metric energy-momentum tensor in classical field theories and gravity. http://arxiv.org/abs/gr-qc/0103072 (accessed on 21st July 2025).
9. Ardito, L., Morisio, M., Procaccianti, G., Vetrò, A., et al. (2013). Introducing energy efficiency into SQALE. https://core.ac.uk/download/pdf/11432455.pdf (accessed on 21st July 2025).
10. Asadifard, M., Bradski, G., Reimer, B., Gaur, R. P., Lee, J., King, D. E., Klauer, S. G., et al. (2016). Owl and Lizard: Patterns of head pose and eye pose in driver gaze classification. http://arxiv.org/abs/1508.04028 (accessed on 21st July 2025).
11. Babula, R. A., Coleman, J. R., & Gehrke, B. C. (2025). An analysis of the impact of European Union and United States dairy policies on EU-U.S. trade in milk protein concentrate. https://core.ac.uk/download/pdf/7055674.pdf (accessed on 21st July 2025).
12. Bagci, U., Bai, L., & Udupa, J. K. (2010). The influence of intensity standardization on medical image registration. http://arxiv.org/abs/1002.1285 (accessed on 21st July 2025).
13. Basu, A., Choudhury, M., Mukherjee, A., Mukherjee, A., et al. (2017). All that is English may be Hindi: Enhancing language identification through automatic ranking of likeliness of word

borrowing in social media. http://arxiv.org/abs/1707.08446 (accessed on 21st July 2025).

14. Bauer, F., Demir, D. A., Janssen, B., Borunda, M., Calcagni, G., Exirifard, Q., Sheikh-Jabbari, M. M., Iihoshi, M., Ketov, S. V., et al. (2008). Palatini versus metric formulation in higher curvature gravity. http://arxiv.org/abs/0804.4440 (accessed on 21st July 2025).
15. Baumgartner, H., & Weijters, B. (2019). Measurement in marketing. https://core.ac.uk/download/287939809.pdf (accessed on 21st July 2025).
16. Brants, T., Favre, B., Garofolo, J. S., Gaur, Y., Gray, S. S., Lei, X., Mishra, T., et al. (2017). Evaluating the usability of automatically generated captions for people who are deaf or hard of hearing. http://arxiv.org/abs/1712.02033 (accessed on 21st July 2025).
17. Brown, J. D., Lau, S. R., & York, J. W. (2002). Action and energy of the gravitational field. https://core.ac.uk/download/475610234.pdf (accessed on 21st July 2025).
18. Buchel, D., Berenstein, G., Milanesi, H., Lin, H., Bena, I. R., Klebanov, M. M., Caldarelli, M., et al. (2005). Black hole statistics from holography. http://arxiv.org/abs/hep-th/0507260 (accessed on 21st July 2025).
19. Bunce, D., Gaines, S. O., Robertson, T., Wright, T., et al. (2010). Evaluating the psychometric properties of the Multigroup Ethnic Identity Measure (MEIM) within the United Kingdom. https://core.ac.uk/download/336721.pdf (accessed on 21st July 2025).
20. Busse, J. E., Gwiazda, P., & Marciniak-Czochra, A. (2016). Mass concentration in a nonlocal model of clonal selection. http://arxiv.org/abs/1401.6043 (accessed on 21st July 2025).
21. Calvin, L., & Cook, R. L. (2025). Greenhouse tomatoes change the dynamics of the North American fresh tomato industry. https://core.ac.uk/download/pdf/6418211.pdf (accessed on 21st July 2025).
22. Cao, J., & Saxena, D. (2020). Generative adversarial networks (GANs): Challenges, solutions, and future directions. http://arxiv.org/abs/2005.00065 (accessed on 21st July 2025).
23. Chaisson, E. J. (2015). Energy flows in low-entropy complex systems. http://arxiv.org/abs/1512.04981 (accessed on 21st July 2025).
24. Chandrasekaran, V., Flanagan, E. E., & Prabhu, K. (2018). Symmetries and charges of general relativity at null boundaries. http://arxiv.org/abs/1807.11499 (accessed on 21st July 2025).
25. Chapelle, O., Lefortier, D., & Vasile, F. (2017). Cost-sensitive learning for utility optimization in online advertising auctions. http://arxiv.org/abs/1603.03713 (accessed on 21st July 2025).
26. Coughenour, C., Pharr, J., & To, S. (2019). The environmental impact and formation of meals from the pilot year of a Las Vegas Convention food rescue program. https://core.ac.uk/download/223094777.pdf (accessed on 21st July 2025).
27. Devaseelan, S., & Praveen, B. M. (2024). Random forest-based forensic investigation of non-fungible tokens: For enhanced detection and anomaly identification. *International Journal of Scientific Research in Science and Technology*. https://www.semanticscholar.org/paper/7872641da8216ea1336c7dad8b758ed9dca71370 (accessed on 21st July 2025).
28. Dick, A., Li, X., Shen, C., Zhang, X., et al. (2015). Online metric-weighted linear representations for robust visual tracking. http://arxiv.org/abs/1507.05737 (accessed on 21st July 2025).
29. Ding, Y., Liu, X., Wan, K., Zhang, H., et al. (2020). Weighted-sampling audio adversarial example attack. http://arxiv.org/abs/1901.10300 (accessed on 21st July 2025).

30. Druet, A., Elhadad, N., Li, K., Shea, S., et al. (2020). Characterizing physiological and symptomatic variation in menstrual cycles using self-tracked mobile health data. http://arxiv.org/abs/1909.11211 (accessed on 21st July 2025).
31. Georgopoulos, M., Panagakis, Y., & Pantic, M. (2018). Modeling of facial aging and kinship: A survey. http://arxiv.org/abs/1802.04636 (accessed on 21st July 2025).
32. German, A. (2018). A description of the rhythm of Barunga Kriol using rhythm metrics and an analysis of vowel reduction. https://core.ac.uk/download/351828798.pdf (accessed on 21st July 2025).
33. Giulini, D., Huisken, G., Bray, H. L., Jezierski, J., Kijowski, J., Kijowski, J., Jezierski, J., et al. (2007). Energy-minimizing two black holes initial data. http://arxiv.org/abs/0706.0129 (accessed on 21st July 2025).
34. Gottschall, K., Kittel, B., & Tepe, M. (2010). A structural fit between states and markets? Public administration regulation and market economy models in the OECD. https://core.ac.uk/download/71738879.pdf (accessed on 21st July 2025).
35. Grönstedt, T., Thoma, E. M., & Zhao, X. (2020). Quantifying the environmental design trades for a state-of-the-art turbofan engine. https://core.ac.uk/download/389670587.pdf (accessed on 21st July 2025).
36. Gruzinov, A., Vainshtein, A., Vainshtein, A. I., Petrov, A. N., Marzban, C., de Rham, C., Boulware, D. G., et al. (2011). Universally coupled massive gravity, II: Densitized tetrad and cotetrad theories. http://arxiv.org/abs/1110.2077 (accessed on 21st July 2025).
37. Guendelman, E. I., Einstein, A., Ng, Y. J., Ng, Y. J., Page, D. N., & Wilczek, F. (2009). Gravitational theory with a dynamical time. http://arxiv.org/abs/0911.0178 (accessed on 21st July 2025).
38. Harvey, J. A. (2007). Telling the market story through organic information interaction design and broadcast media: Submitted to the College of Creative Arts as requirement for the degree of Master of Design, Massey University, Wellington, New Zealand, 2007. https://core.ac.uk/download/162617417.pdf (accessed on 21st July 2025).
39. Heidebrecht, A., MacManus, D. G., & Robinson, M. (2017). An optimization method for nacelle design. https://core.ac.uk/download/74410891.pdf (accessed on 21st July 2025).
40. Heilig, G. K. (1993). *How Many People Can Be Fed on Earth?* https://core.ac.uk/download/33895244.pdf (accessed on 21st July 2025).
41. Islami, A., & Longo, G. (2017). Marriages of mathematics and physics: A challenge for biology. https://core.ac.uk/download/186330579.pdf (accessed on 21st July 2025).
42. Lu, X., & Marron, J. S. (2013). Principal nested spheres for time warped functional data analysis. http://arxiv.org/abs/1304.6789 (accessed on 21st July 2025).
43. Mahmoodi, S., & Sharif, B. (2007). Geometrical-based algorithm for variational segmentation and smoothing of vector-valued images.
44. Mazumdar, A., Starobinsky, A. A., Starobinsky, A. A., Cheung, C., Herzog, C. P., Byrnes, C. T., Byrnes, C. T., et al. (2012). Local non-Gaussianity from rapidly varying sound speeds. https://core.ac.uk/download/29586351.pdf (accessed on 21st July 2025).
45. N/A. (2016). *Aligning Capital with Mission: Lessons from the Annie E. Casey Foundation's Social Investment Program.* https://core.ac.uk/download/80511019.pdf (accessed on 21st July 2025).

46. Østvang, D. (2020). Quasi-metric relativity. http://arxiv.org/abs/gr-qc/0112025 (accessed on 21st July 2025).

47. Østvang, D. (2020). Spherically symmetric, metrically static, isolated systems in quasi-metric gravity. http://arxiv.org/abs/gr-qc/0201097 (accessed on 21st July 2025).

48. Owhadi, H., & Scovel, C. (2016). Qualitative robustness in Bayesian inference. https://core.ac.uk/download/33126595.pdf (accessed on 21st July 2025).

49. Pauri, M., & Vallisneri, M. (2002). Ephemeral point-events: Is there a last remnant of physical objectivity? https://core.ac.uk/download/11920273.pdf (accessed on 21st July 2025).

50. Poojary, R. R., & Suryanarayana, N. V. (2018). On asymptotic symmetries of 3D extended supergravities. http://arxiv.org/abs/1712.09221 (accessed on 21st July 2025).

51. Rabosky, D. L., & Title, P. O. (2019). Tip rates, phylogenies and diversification: What are we estimating, and how good are the estimates? http://deepblue.lib.umich.edu/bitstream/2027.42/149536/1/mee313153-sup-0001-FigS1-S10.pdf (accessed on 21st July 2025).

52. Shahid-Saless, B., Dirac, P. A. M., Einstein, A., German, G., Green, M. B., & Berthias, J. P. (1993). Torsion and nonmetricity in scalar-tensor theories of gravity. https://core.ac.uk/download/25334085.pdf (accessed on 21st July 2025).

53. Shakoorioskooie, M., Granget, E., Cocen, O., Hovind, J., Mannes, D., Kaestner, A., & Brambilla, L. (2024). Neutron tomography and image registration methods to study local physical deformations and attenuation variations in treated archaeological iron nail samples. *Applied Physics A: Materials Science & Processing, 130*. https://www.semanticscholar.org/paper/e6b5a47b69802db36b8624b537b7e16cc5789aaf (accessed on 21st July 2025).

54. Stathopoulou, A., Balabanis, G., Qiao, J., Uzma, K., Magnusson, P., Micevski, M., Muthén, L. K., et al. (2019). Favoritism toward foreign and domestic brands: A comparison of different theoretical explanations. https://core.ac.uk/download/286356795.pdf (accessed on 21st July 2025).

55. Wołk, K. (2015). Noisy-parallel and comparable corpora filtering methodology for the extraction of bi-lingual equivalent data at sentence level. https://core.ac.uk/download/229289332.pdf (accessed on 21st July 2025).

IMAGING AND DIGITAL TECHNOLOGY IN OSTEOLOGY

10

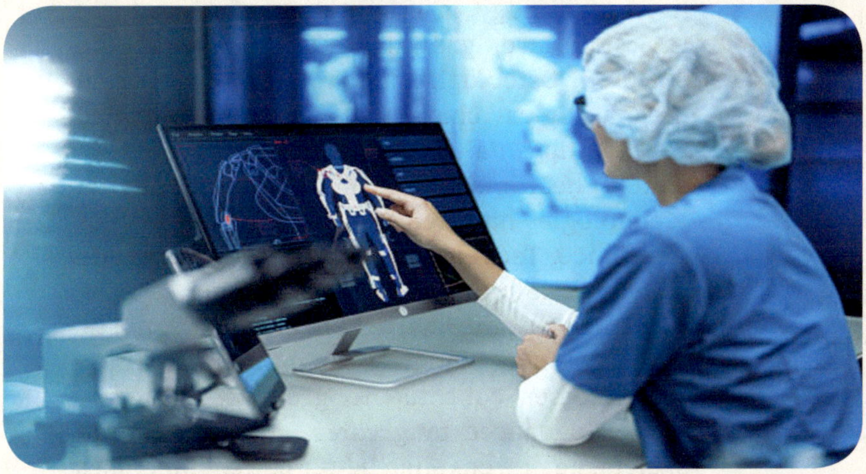

LEARNING OBJECTIVES

After studying this chapter, you will be able to:

1. Describe the historical development of imaging techniques
2. Define the X-ray imaging in osteology
3. Explain the computed tomography (CT)
4. Understand magnetic resonance imaging (MRI)
5. Know digital imaging techniques
6. Learn about future trends in osteological imaging

Introduction

Improvements in imaging technology and digital technology have greatly impacted osteology, enabling scientists and practitioners to study bone architecture and intricate pathologies with high precision. The synergy of techniques such as computed tomography (CT), magnetic resonance imaging (MRI), and digital radiography has further enhanced visualization of skeletal systems in three dimensions. These technologies not only allow for the recognition of fractures and disease but also the detailed analysis of fossilized remains, as it is critical to anthropological research and medical applications. The innovation of these techniques marks a dramatic shift from traditional to advanced digital imaging, transforming the way osteologists conduct investigations and analyze findings in their respective areas. Besides this, the inclusion of multi-modal imaging technologies has opened new avenues for inter-disciplinary research among scientists in paleoanthropology and forensic anthropology. As clearly highlighted in recent literature, computed tomography has provided unprecedented information for the conservation and analysis of ancient human remains, establishing its place as more than a simple diagnostic instrument. Virtual osteological analysis is one such example of the trend towards non-invasive techniques that maintain the integrity of biological material while providing the necessary forensic data. This indicates the necessity of standard methodology in procedures that rely on the reliability and accuracy of imaging technologies, particularly in legal and ethical considerations of human remains analysis (Uldin et al., 2017). Furthermore, the future of osteology is poised to benefit from further advances in imaging and digital technology, with potential for both educational and practical applications. With private groups and institutions increasingly investing in high-resolution imaging facilities, the need for innovative research and accurate educational outreach programs expands exponentially. Projects like ToScA North America are focusing on key scientific areas, such as multimodal imaging and educational outreach, to foster collaboration between academia and industry (Ahmed et al., 2017).

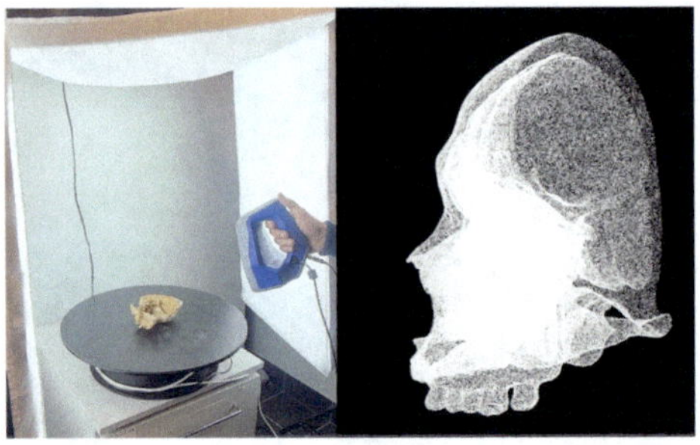

Figure 10.1. Imaging and digital technology in osteology.

Source: https://media.springernature.com/lw1200/springer-static/image/art%3A10.1186%2Fs12909-022-03408-5/MediaObjects/12909_2022_3408_Fig1_HTML.png.

These developments bear testament to ongoing efforts to embrace emerging technologies in osteology, and doors are now open to further insight into bone biology and to safeguarding its heritage. The importance of such advances is vast, influencing both current forensic science practice and the preservation of our archaeological record (Figure 10.1).

Definition of Osteology

Osteology, the scientific study of bone, spans a wide interdisciplinary spectrum encompassing anatomy, pathology, and anthropology. This field of biology is essential to the study of the structure, growth, and disease of the skeleton. Osteologists do not only investigate morphological characters of bones but also their functional implications and roles in general health issues. New imaging and digital technologies have led to tremendous advances in science. Techniques such as X-ray, MRI, and CT scan allow non-destructive examination of bone health and, hence, enhanced diagnostic and treatment planning capabilities. As these technologies continue to grow, osteology is further advanced by greater understanding of skeletal health, enabling better patient outcomes through prompt intervention and detection. The integration of these new methodologies in osteological practice illuminates the interconnected nature of bone health and total health. Osteology is also described as the pathology of bone, such as osteoporosis, a disease characterized by reduced bone density and increased fracture risk. Osteoporosis has been recognized to be a multifactorial and heterogeneous disease encompassing a rapidly growing number of, particularly, post-menopausal women and older adults. Although the foundations of osteology were laid more than 250 years ago, the establishment of comprehensive clinical and epidemiological knowledge has only occurred in the past seven decades. Studies of ancient populations with osteoporosis provide a diachronic perspective, offering pertinent historical insights into age-related, lifestyle-, and sociocultural-related alterations in the skeleton. Since osteology informs paleopathology, it provides rich insights into past bone diseases. This cross-fertilization of fields strengthens modern osteology, enabling practitioners to apply insights from the past to today's healthcare challenges related to skeletal well-being, as highlighted in studies examining the biographical paradigm of bone illness (Curate et al., 2014). In the modern era, the field of osteology is increasingly shaped by the influence of imaging technologies and digital media. These innovations allow for visualization of bone structures previously impossible, enabling accurate analysis of bone morphology, integrity, and disease. Digital platforms have also transformed how osteologists collect and analyze data, enabling more accurate diagnoses and treatments. The educational role of osteology has also been enhanced by digital technologies, with learning tools such as virtual reality simulation and 3D modeling aiding training and comprehension of skeletal anatomy. The integration of imaging technology has further enhanced research capabilities, enabling more thorough studies of various bone diseases, such as osteoporosis, that require comprehensive evaluation for effective management (Bashutski et al., 2015). With the evolution of osteology, the integration of digital innovations and traditional approaches is set to enhance the field's contributions to healthcare, as diagnostic accuracy and patient care planning improve.

Importance of Imaging in Osteological Studies

Advances in imaging have dramatically transformed the science of osteological studies, enabling scientists to analyze the skeleton with unparalleled precision. CT and other digital imaging methods have enabled the non-destructive analysis of living and fossilized remains, thereby providing greater insight into morphological innovations throughout evolutionary history. Scientists can see detailed internal structures in specimens without destructive procedures by applying CT imaging. This capacity is particularly valuable in studying unusual or rare fossils, where preservation is crucial. The three-dimensional reconstructions obtained from CT scans display a range of skeletal morphology features, including bone density and structural integrity, required to understand an organism's biological and ecological roles. Imaging technology is thus at the heart of ongoing attempts to unravel the complexity of bone morphology and its evolutionary significance. Imaging techniques in osteological studies illuminate not only structural data but also facilitate the analysis of functional morphology. Analysis of muscle attachment sites, joint configurations, and the interconnectedness of skeletal elements through imaging allows scientists to infer the locomotion, diet, and ecological interactions of long-extinct animals. The history of jaw evolution in mammals, for instance, has been an area of active inquiry, and CT imaging has provided precious insights into the jaw adductor musculature, which are significant for understanding the evolution of diet and behavior over time. New evidence derived from recent studies suggests that jaw musculature changes played a pivotal role in mammalian jaw biomechanics and stability, a significant part of its evolution (Abdala et al., 2016). Imaging technologies thus play the leading role in the emergent understanding of evolutionary pressures that constructed skeletal adaptations and survival modes in various taxa. Moreover, imaging technology in osteological analysis extends its applications to forensic anthropology and paleoanthropology, where accuracy and preservation are equally essential. The process of "virtual anthropology" illustrates how imaging has been the central driving force, enabling the study of human remains without damage (Uldin et al., 2017). As virtual osteological analysis becomes an increasingly common practice among forensic anthropologists, the standardization of imaging parameters ensures that results are reproducible and can prove helpful in court cases. Moreover, these methods promote collaborative studies across disciplines to advance shared knowledge of human evolution and bone biology. Thus, the value of imaging in osteology extends beyond theoretical application, and these technologies become necessary tools that fill the chasm between ancient and modern biological sciences (Figure 10.2).

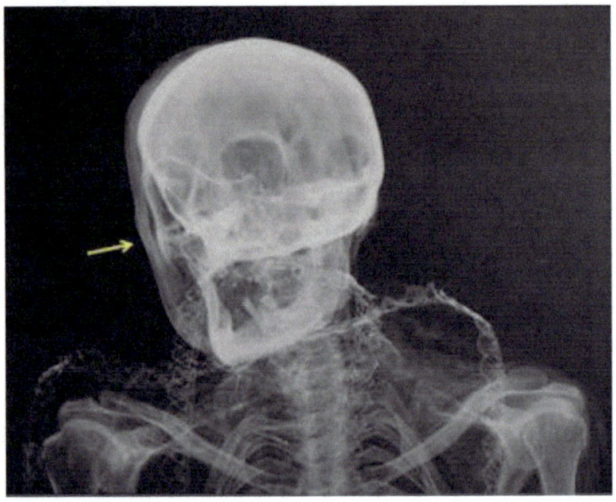

Figure 10.2. Advancements in imaging technology have fundamentally transformed the landscape of osteological studies.

Source: https://media.springernature.com/lw685/springer-static/image/chp%3A10.1007%2F978-3-319-51726-1_157-2/MediaObjects/184254_0_En_157-2_Fig23_HTML.jpg.

Overview of Digital Technology's Role in Osteology

The use of digital technology in osteology has revolutionized the methods used in the analysis of bone and skeletal remains. Resolution-based imaging techniques, such as CT and MRI, have been employed to depict internal anatomy without the need for invasive intervention. Such imaging modalities enable high-quality 3D reconstructions of skeletal components, which can enhance understanding of anatomical variation and pathology. These developments are significant not only for forensic analysis but also for archaeology, be preserved where they can be. The process of examining bones on digital platforms is free from the danger of contaminating fragile remains, thus protecting the integrity of archaeological findings and facilitating valuable information is maintained to be used by future researchers. In addition to complementing imaging resources, digital technology enhances interdisciplinary communication in osteology. The development of specialized software to analyze skeletal data promotes interdisciplinarity among disciplines such as anthropology, archaeology, and forensic science. For instance, the use of digital modeling in facial approximation techniques is employed alongside archaeological evidence in the reconstruction of historical person features, as illustrated in facial approximation studies of individuals such as George Dixon (Emerson et al., 2023). This interdisciplinarity triggers sharp controversies among specialists, effectively bridging knowledge gaps and methodological gaps in osteology. Moreover, digital media enable data storage and transmission, which are essential for multi-author collaboration and education, thereby democratizing access to osteological resources. Furthermore, the ethical considerations of applying digital technologies in osteology cannot be downplayed. While new revelations can prove an asset, issues regarding the exploitation of human remains for technology are worth debating seriously. Digital technology, by expanding research capacity, raises ethical questions about the representation of the dead, particularly in archaeological contexts. Critics argue that the use of evolving computing tools could lead to insensitivities toward cultural heritage and ancestral remains (Valentine et al., 2017). As such, navigate these complexities judiciously, making sure that technological applications are performed in deference to the people whose remains are being examined. In the end, the further evolution of digital technology in osteology can only be promising, provided it is balanced with a strong ethical framework that safeguards the cultural significance of skeletal remains (Figure 10.3).

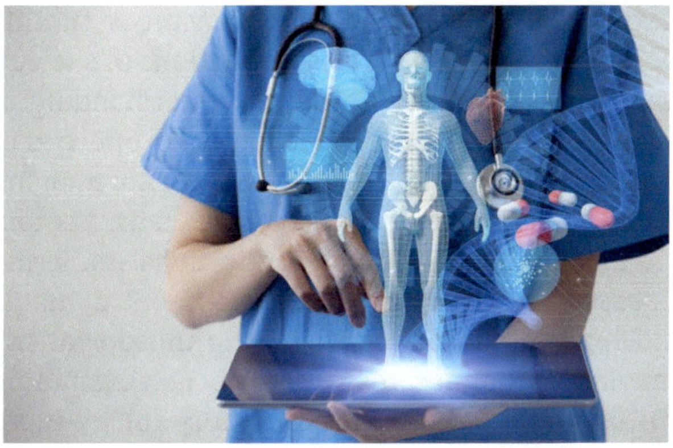

Figure 10.3. The integration of digital technology in osteology.

Source: https://media.springernature.com/lw725/springer-cms/rest/v1/content/18831618/data/v2.

10.1. Historical Development of Imaging Techniques

Learning Outcome

1. Early methods of bone imaging
2. Evolution of X-ray technology
3. Introduction of advanced imaging modalities

The history of imaging modalities has significantly transformed the field of osteology, enabling better understanding of bone structure and developmental history. Early methods, such as radiography, enabled two-dimensional imaging of bone structures but were limited by superimposition and decreased detail. The arrival of computed tomography (CT) marked the peak of imaging technology, enabling three-dimensional reconstructions that exposed more than ever before the morphology of skeletal remains. The technology not only helped analyze specimens that are available but also assisted in reconstructing the anatomical features of extinct groups. Specifically, CT scans of the jaw adductor muscles in fossil cynodonts have elucidated evolutionary patterns towards the modern mammals with an emphasis on how CT scanning is able to contribute to filling gaps in osteological transition (Abdala et al., 2016). Beyond CT, three-dimensional scanning technology has also enhanced the documentation and reconstruction of fossil bones.

This technique is instrumental in the cultural heritage field because it allows for the meticulous conservation of fossils and artifacts while allowing digital analysis to take place without the actual physical contact. For instance, 3D scanning of Roman sculptures has provided scientists with quantifiable data on facial structures, enabling them to connect individual portraits based on style and formal qualities. This interdisciplinary approach entwines classic archaeology, forensic anthropology, and computer science to illustrate the adaptability of 3D imaging in human osteological analysis. The potential to create accurate, detailed digital models of skeletal morphology enables comparative examination and aids preservation of cultural heritage (Anderson et al., 2012).

Osteological imaging techniques follow a historical path towards greater precision and interdisciplinarity. While initial imaging technologies offered limited solutions, the transition to advanced technologies such as CT and 3D scanning has fueled innovations that enhance our understanding of skeletal anatomy while aiding the fields of archaeology and forensic science. As imaging procedures continue to evolve, so too will our knowledge of bone morphology, evolutionary relationships, and functional implications of skeletal anatomy. This broad vista of imaging in osteology highlights the need for continued research and innovation in science, demonstrating how technological advances can significantly alter our perception of the past and guide future research into skeletal biology (Figure 10.4).

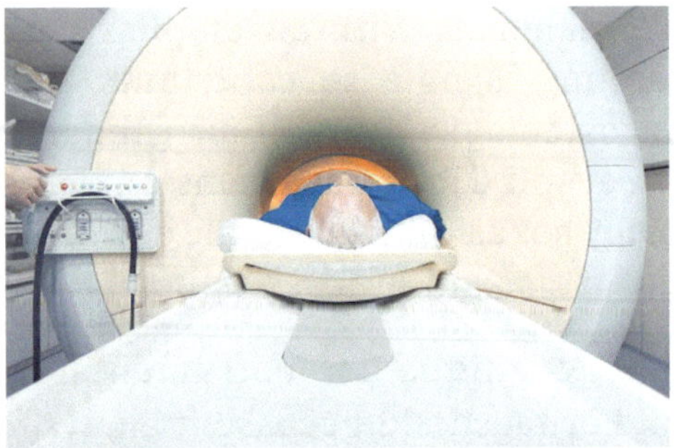

Figure 10.4. The evolution of imaging techniques.

Source: https://www.theglobeandmail.com/resizer/v2/YNNSCKFOFNBC3N7Q6WJ3BOGDDU.jpg?auth=544933328e3fab85c43037c63fa4b2895496931e9a7c7f2cbc8b037b36ab8c21&width=600&height=400&quality=80&smart=true.

10.1.1. Early Methods of Bone Imaging

The early methods of bone imaging were the foundation of modern osteology and the examination of skeletal anatomy. These methods initially relied on basic methods such as visual inspection and palpation by experienced individuals. Bone courses could be qualified assessed by external examination, but it was not extensive, especially concerning the internal anatomy. With the advent of radiography in the early 20th century, osteologists gained access to a very useful tool for visualizing the interior of bones. The use of X-rays enabled them to diagnose fractures, pathologies, and developmental abnormalities. This was a breakthrough, providing scope for non-invasive diagnosis and playing a massive role in the discipline of osteological research. Computed tomography (CT), introduced in the second half of the 20th century, transformed bone imaging. CT scans provided detailed cross-sectional images that enhanced the representation of intricate bone anatomy over what was possible with plain X-rays. The technique allowed the evaluation of subtle bone lesions and fine morphological features, thereby optimizing diagnostic accuracy. Further advances in this technology enabled 3D reconstructions of skeletal structures, enhancing in-depth understanding of the spatial patterns and mechanical properties of bones. Technologies derived from digital imaging addressed several of the earlier constraints and laid the foundation for new applications, rendering research into osteological development dynamic and multidisciplinary. Integrating these evolving imaging techniques, researchers began examining evolutionary changes in bone morphology more precisely. For instance, the application of digital imaging tools like CT and 3D modeling has made it possible to conduct in-depth analysis of osteological traits during critical stages of evolution, as in the case of the evolution from non-mammalian synapsids to mammals. The tools have provided insight into the organization and modification of the jaw joint, enhancing our understanding of functional morphology in extinct taxa. Furthermore, interdisciplinary partnerships, such as the University of Texas High-Resolution X-ray CT Facility and other establishments, have enabled the study of vertebrate and invertebrate fossils, thereby demonstrating how early bone imaging methods have evolved into highly sophisticated equipment that powers existing osteological studies (Abdala et al., 2016; Ahmed et al., 2017) (Figure 10.5).

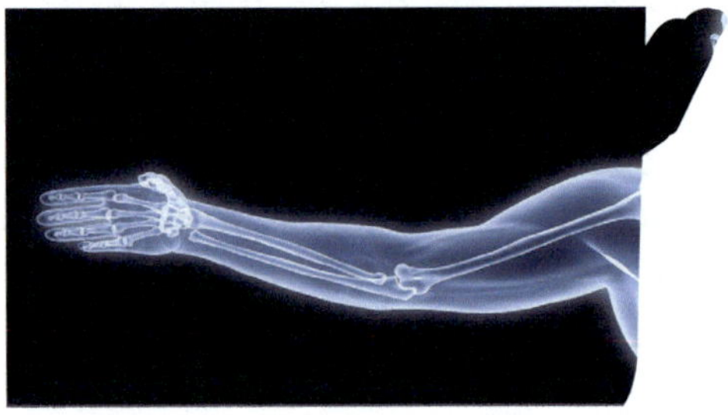

Figure 10.5. The early methods of bone imaging.

Source: https://external-content.duckduckgo.com/iu/?u=https%3A%2F%2Fpmrxcontent.com%2Fwp-content%2Fuploads%2FWhat-Is-A-Bone-Scan.jpg&f=1&nofb=1&ipt=4162a23eb05118a604557cae044ceb2b09443e6c0e8645920c7a22638c3b8ae8.

10.1.2. Evolution of X-ray Technology

The evolution of X-ray technology has significantly transformed the field of osteology, providing invaluable insights into bone disease and structure. X-rays were first discovered by Wilhelm Conrad Röntgen in 1895 and represented a groundbreaking innovation that enabled the visualization of internal structures without invasive procedures. Initial applications were rudimentary, primarily used for foreign body detection within the body or for fracture diagnosis. Over time, technology grew better, with developments in film and image processing further enhancing the resolution and sharpness of X-ray images. Not only did this improve diagnostic processes, but it also led to an entire line of research exploring the uses of X-ray imaging for identifying various osteological conditions. Furthermore, integrating digital and traditional X-ray technologies has enhanced image capture, enabling accurate interpretation of complex skeletal structures (Kivell et al., 2016). With advanced digital imaging technology in development, it has filled the gaps in traditional X-ray technology, hence strengthening the diagnostic capabilities in osteology. The transition from digital to analog X-rays made the retrieval and manipulation of assessment images possible at the same time, thereby improving the reliability of bone assessment. There are many advantages of digital X-rays, such as reduced radiation dosimetry and the ability to enhance images for precise assessment of fractures or abnormalities. Furthermore, modern imaging systems increasingly rely on computer-aided diagnosis, enabling algorithms and artificial intelligence to assist osteologists in interpreting complex cases. This technological advancement not only streamlines the workflow in clinical settings but also provides direction for new areas of study, including the possibility of advancing knowledge of bone disease and disorders (Valentine et al., 2017). Advances in high-technology imaging modalities, including computed tomography (CT) and magnetic resonance imaging (MRI), have progressively advanced the practice of osteology beyond the conventional X-ray technology. These modalities provide three-dimensional imaging of bone morphology with greater detail than standard X-rays. For the osteologist, this means an enhanced capacity to examine the subtler features of bone morphology and disease, particularly relevant in surgical planning and the management of complex cases. The integration of these technologies with standard X-ray imaging provides an interdisciplinary diagnostic armoury that underpins improved clinical outcomes. Additionally, continual improvements in imaging technology imply that future technologies may introduce even more advanced techniques, which would further develop the discipline of osteology and have profound implications for patient treatment and care planning (Kivell et al., 2016) (Figure 10.6).

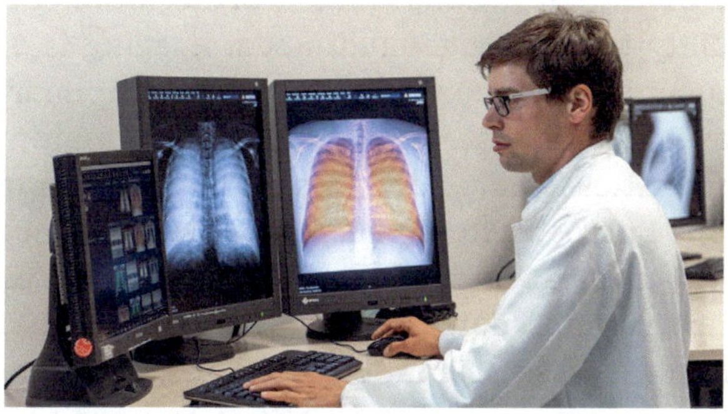

Figure 10.6. The evolution of X-ray technology.

Source: https://external-content.duckduckgo.com/iu/?u=https%3A%2F%2Fwww.healthcareradius.in%2Fpublic%2Fimages%2F2021%2F10%2F27%2FMunich-3.jpg&f=1&nofb=1&ipt=ae8e5604ef2bc1e6823feb76d714006d3a437037ea089ec76877cd488da7119b.

10.1.3. Introduction of Advanced Imaging Modalities

The development of advanced imaging modalities has significantly advanced the discipline of osteology, accelerating the pace of research and application in clinics and academe. Advanced technology, such as high-resolution X-ray computed tomography (HRCT) and magnetic resonance imaging (MRI), permits non-invasive, detailed visualization of osseous structures, which is necessary in the diagnosis of disorders, surgical intervention planning, and study of bone biology.

Facilities like the University of Texas High-Resolution X-ray CT Facility are among the leaders in applying such cutting-edge imaging techniques, producing data that educate scientists on skeletal anatomy and disease, and vice versa. By incorporating such cutting-edge modalities into routine practice, researchers and clinicians can enhance the accuracy of their analyses and interventions, thereby ultimately leading to better patient outcomes and contributing to a better understanding of osteological conditions. Furthermore, the ability to undertake multimodal imaging is an unparalleled opportunity for cross-disciplinary research in osteology. Emerging imaging modalities enlarge the capability to monitor bone microstructure, mechanical performance, and interfaces with neighboring tissues. Such copious data becomes invaluable when shared across scientific disciplines, including geosciences and material science, signaling the possibility of making revolutionary discoveries in osteological research. For instance, the intersection of specialties can be used to deepen understanding of bone development and bone remodeling processes, which are crucial to the progress of treating osteoporosis and other skeletal diseases. The Natural History Museum and the Royal Microscopical Society are among the institutions pushing the boundary on these interdisciplinary efforts and advancing the interface between advanced imaging techniques and their variety of applications in osteology and other fields. The consequences of newer imaging modalities even extend to educational outreach, enhancing the impact of osteological work on the next generation of scientists and the public at large. Educational efforts that highlight the power of imaging technologies, such as virtual dissections and 3D reconstructions, can facilitate a better understanding of bone structure and pathology. These educational programs, made possible through advances in imaging technology, are vital to demystifying the complexities of osteology for the public. By engaging students and the public with simple-to-understand visualizations and interactive presentations, the programs build a heightened appreciation of skeletal disease and health. As advanced imaging evolves, its application in educational settings will be critical for inspiring the next generation to innovate in the field, ensuring that advances in osteological imaging are successfully transferred to both research and public education (Figure 10.7).

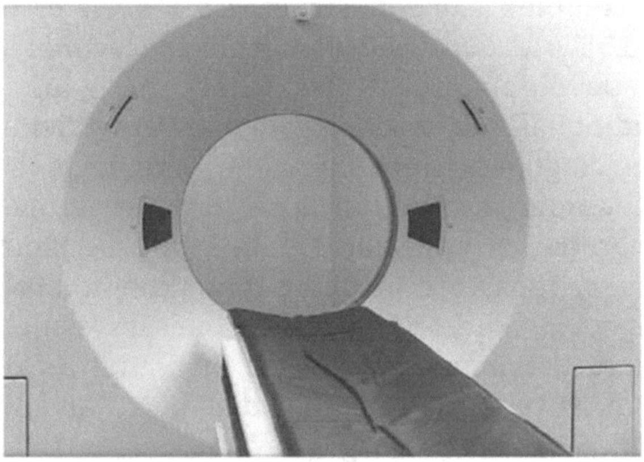

Figure 10.7. The introduction of advanced imaging modalities.

Source: https://external-content.duckduckgo.com/iu/?u=http%3A%2F%2Fradiologykey.com%2Fwp-content%2Fuploads%2F2019%2F05%2FC18-FF4.gif&f=1&nofb=1&ipt=fa7124a3e59a42c67eb0de4b8dee53083440f44ba2200cba3e2be994e558c141.

Test Your Knowledge

1. How have imaging techniques historically developed in medicine and anthropology?
2. Who were the key contributors to the advancement of imaging technologies, and what were their contributions?

10.2. X-ray Imaging in Osteology

Learning Outcome

1. Principles of X-ray technology
2. Applications in diagnosing bone diseases
3. Limitations and challenges of X-ray imaging

The application of X-ray imaging in osteology has significant advantages in terms of diagnosis as well as forensic applications. The technique is the cornerstone of bone structure assessment, offering accurate visualization of hard tissues without any invasion. X-rays enable the interpretation of bone integrity and fractures, and the detection of pathological conditions such as osteomyelitis or tumors. Besides, high-contrast imaging facilitates osteologists in the interpretation of skeletal morphology and anthropometric characteristics of past populations. The integration of various imaging techniques, for instance, CT and digital radiography, enhances the quality of X-ray analysis and expands opportunities for study and use in osteology. In forensic science, X-ray imaging plays a role in identifying unknown individuals through skeletal remains analysis. A method of significance is the comparison of antemortem and postmortem X-ray; however, there are constraints since few antemortem records are accessible. This paucity of information can be addressed by panoramic dental radiographs, which provide unobscured imaging of the maxillary sinus region, a feature also present in antemortem records. Through visual observation and geometric morphometric analysis of the maxillary sinus outline, researchers have shown that these anatomical features can be used to establish identification of missing persons in forensic contexts.

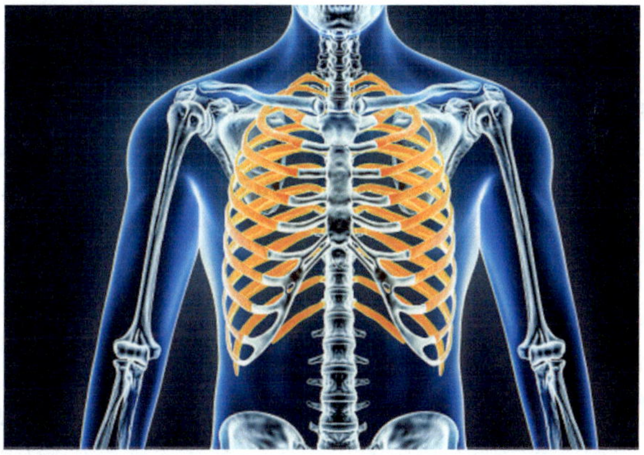

Figure 10.8. The application of X-ray imaging in osteology.

Source: https://external-content.duckduckgo.com/iu/?u=https%3A%2F%2Fmedia.istockphoto.com%2Fid%2F1437537934%2Fphoto%2Fribs-x-ray-osteology-of-the-human-skeleton-thorax-bones-and-rib-or-thoracic-cage-3d-rendering.jpg%3Fs%3D170667a%26w%3D0%26k%3D20%26c%3D-2LaX4ayF5MNxJrDRpe3V7zZfOwxacG8N2ctJkeZCjM%3D&f=1&nofb=1&ipt=06106177646d36993ea6564d6a6770691107dd2f8ac2a406c1d8ce099c766094.

These advances point to the suitability of using X-ray technology in medicolegal practice to enhance the effectiveness of forensic anthropologists and other professionals in identification (Collins et al., 2014). Further, the intersection of X-ray imaging with advanced digital technologies is revolutionizing osteology, particularly skeletal reconstruction from sample remains. Traditional methods for restoring original morphology after physicochemical or biomolecular testing are likely to yield inaccurate results. However, employing computed microtomography (microCT) alongside reverse engineering and computer-aided design techniques allows for the creation of accurate digital models. This is not only beneficial in reconstructing missing portions of bones or teeth, but also in ensuring that the resultant models exhibit a high degree of resemblance to the original shape. The technology is critical in archaeological contexts, in which the integrity of fossil human bones must be preserved throughout scientific analysis, thus optimizing the potential utility of X-ray imaging and digital technology in osteological research (Benazzi et al., 2022) (Figure 10.8).

10.2.1. Principles of X-ray Technology

The X-ray technology is based on the intersection of physics and medicine on ionizing radiation to render invisible structures inside the human body visible. The technology's foundation is the production of X-rays by colliding high-energy electrons with a target material, such as tungsten. The collision generates X-rays that are directed toward the body, passing through various tissues to varying degrees depending on their density. For instance, denser bones absorb more X-rays and appear radiopaque in the final image, while softer tissues allow greater passage of X-rays and less contrast.

This straightforward principle of differential absorption has its most tremendous significance in osteology, permitting detailed imaging of the skeleton, which is the bedrock of clinical diagnosis and research. The development of imaging technologies has significantly enhanced the capabilities of traditional X-ray systems. Digital radiography, a key technological advancement in the field, employs digital sensors to capture and transmit images more effectively than traditional film-based systems. This shift not only raises image quality but also reduces radiation exposure, an important consideration in the medical field. In addition, the images are manipulated for better visualization and diagnostic use, such as adjusting brightness and contrast to reveal minute skeletal details. Inclusion of computerized imaging modalities, such as CT, further enhances diagnostic ability by providing cross-sectional images that offer better insight into complex skeletal disease. As highlighted by recent studies, the application of these technologies has enhanced knowledge of osteological analysis, leading to more efficient methods for the conservation and reconstruction of modern and fossilized remains (Uldin et al., 2017).

In forensic anthropology, the application of X-ray technology has been greatly advantageous for the identification of unknown individuals. Standard protocols, such as matching antemortem and postmortem radiographs, primarily suffer from the absence of complete antemortem records. Advances in imaging technology have introduced more accessible methods of identification, such as the utilization of panoramic dental radiographs. Dental autopsy examines these radiographs to reveal structures such as the maxillary sinus in unobstructed detail, enabling close visual and geometric inspection for identification. A study of such approaches employed survey-based methods and statistical analysis to assess the effectiveness of identifying individuals through variation in the shape of the maxillary sinus, highlighting the importance of X-ray technology in forensic analysis (Collins et al., 2014). This fusion of X-ray basics with advanced imaging protocols not only enhances osteological research but also reinforces forensic techniques for identifying remains effectively (Figure 10.9).

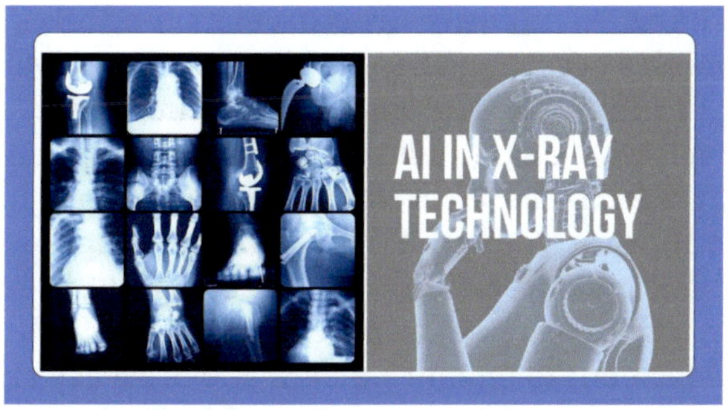

Figure 10.9. The principles of X-ray technology.

Source: https://external-content.duckduckgo.com/iu/?u=https%3A%2F%2Ftheradiologictechnologist.com%2Fwp-content%2Fuploads%2F2023%2F06%2FBlue-White-Practical-Uses-of-AI-in-EFL-Presentation-1024x576.png&f=1&nofb=1&ipt=a5aaadec6f4bf237aa6d47260c6f2bad91b042a4479b450c152b23660fa8a6ce.

10.2.2. Applications in Diagnosing Bone Diseases

In osteology, the diagnosis of bone diseases has been transformed by the application of new imaging and digital technology. The most notable among the three-dimensional (3D) imaging technologies are photogrammetry and laser scanning, which are used extensively to create precise models of skeletal material. These methods are instrumental in forensic anthropology, where biological profiles derived from 3D images must be as precise as is humanly possible. Research indicates that although 3D imaging has the potential to supplement traditional methods, interobserver variation and the need for standardized protocols remain hurdles to widespread adoption. Therefore, despite its promise, the efficacy of 3D imaging in the diagnosis of bone diseases needs further research to maximize these approaches (Valenzuela et al., 2016). Furthermore, micro-computed tomography (μCT) has also proven to be a valuable instrument for examining skeletal health in archaeology and currently. μCT enables researchers to quantitatively determine bone density and morphology, providing evidence for diseases such as osteoporosis. For instance, studies using μCT scans of the first metatarsal (MT1) have shown substantial variation in osteovolumetric density across various demographic groups, thereby improving our understanding of skeletal health in the past. The presence of sexual dimorphism and age-related changes in bone anatomy can be used to validate the need for bone disease and condition diagnoses via advanced imaging in a non-invasive manner. As demonstrated by the MT1 data, μCT effectively reveals the minute details required to generate individualized health profiles (Teeter et al., 2017).

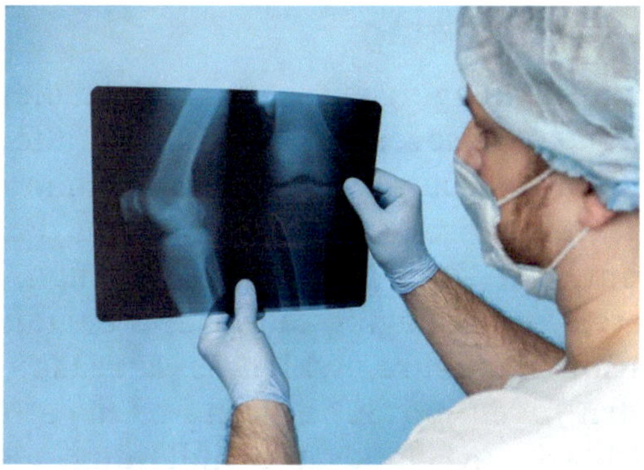

Figure 10.10. Applications in diagnosing bone diseases.

Source: https://external-content.duckduckgo.com/iu/?u=https%3A%2F%2Fst5.depositphotos.com%2F6537122%2F64872%2Fi%2F450%2Fdepositphotos_648724850-stock-photo-diagnosis-bone-disease-doctor-traumatologist.jpg&f=1&nofb=1&ipt=fb10295d8c1d733a7361d6a57da6f35d106bf0b15b322b9dceb8d2500f605408.

Lastly, digital imaging technologies not only facilitate proper diagnostics but also enable the creation of inclusive databases that could further clarify research on bone disease. In digitizing skeletal collections, researchers can now broaden their application to historical and current populations, as well as to current clinical cases. This enhanced resource can be used to help create population-specific standards needed to clarify variability in bone health across populations. As greater data are produced, the integration of imaging sciences with bioarcheological research will facilitate more effective diagnostic approaches in diagnosing bone diseases, eventually leading to better management and treatment options in clinical practices. The future of osteological research, therefore, relies on the ongoing development and growth of such digital applications (Valenzuela et al., 2016) (Figure 10.11).

10.2.3. Limitations and Challenges of X-ray Imaging

While X-ray imaging is essential in osteological research, it has several drawbacks that affect its efficacy and accuracy. The primary limitation lies in the inherent ionizing radiation dose of conventional X-ray technology. Though tiny, repeated X-ray imaging can lead to cumulative radiation exposure, which is a reason for concern over potential long-term effects, particularly in vulnerable individuals, such as children. In addition, X-ray images do not provide much information about surrounding soft tissues, which can overshadow diagnoses of conditions involving both hard and soft tissues. This can impair detailed analyses necessary for the development of effective treatment plans, thus necessitating the application of complementary imaging methods offering more extensive visualization of soft tissues in addition to X-ray results. In addition, the reader may face difficulty interpreting the X-ray images due to numerous potential complicating factors, such as operator inexperience and patient positioning during the procedure. Inconsistency in image quality stems from technical issues, such as inappropriate X-ray machine settings, resulting in inadequate detail in the final images. Additionally, overlapping anatomy can make it challenging to discern pathologies, making it hard to identify fractures or underlying illnesses accurately. This is particularly relevant in multifurcate regions such as the pelvis or spine, where multiple structures converge on a single area. Therefore, reliance on X-ray imaging alone can predispose to missed diagnoses or misinterpretation, underscoring the need for an expansive approach to osteological assessment to enhance diagnostic accuracy and patient care. The limitations of X-ray imaging are also its applicability in specialized areas, such as forensic anthropology, where precision is paramount. While methods such as multi-detector CT have transformed imaging in this field, the transition from traditional X-rays to sophisticated imaging systems presents both opportunities and dilemmas.

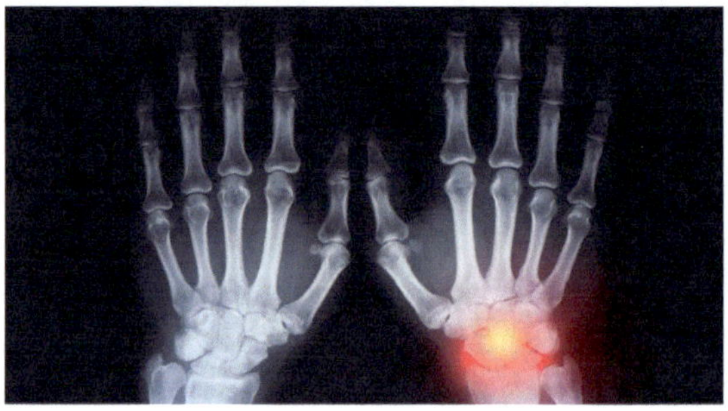

Figure 10.11. X-ray imaging, while pivotal in the study of osteology.

Source: https://external-content.duckduckgo.com/iu/?u=https%3A%2F%2Fcentersurgentcare.net%2Fwp-content%2Fuploads%2F2025%2F03%2FWhat-Can-X-Rays-Detect-6-2.jpg&f=1&nofb=1&ipt=7b8659e8042362235433f2208fdd3b0ae9064d7b6d6ddeb9c51e2873c5347f1a.

For instance, fragmented bone remains may escape characterization by traditional X-ray imaging methods, leading to identification difficulties. Forensic science is increasingly applying high-end imaging techniques, such as micro-CT, to facilitate exact comparisons, for example, between species based on microstructural data. Through new applications of imaging technologies, researchers aim to overcome limitations of standard X-ray imaging, enabling more accurate osteological examinations and expanding the field's capacity for informative analysis and reconstruction (Uldin et al., 2017; Stephen et al., 2018) (Figure 10.11).

Test Your Knowledge

1. How is X-ray imaging used to study bone structure and pathology in osteology?
2. What are the advantages and limitations of X-ray techniques in osteological analysis?

10.3. Computed Tomography (CT)

Learning Outcome

1. Mechanism of CT imaging
2. Advantages of CT in osteological research
3. Case studies showcasing CT applications

CT has revolutionized the field of osteology by providing unrivalled access to the internal bone structure without the need for invasive surgery. This technology applies X-ray measurements to produce high-resolution cross-sectional images of the skeletal system, allowing researchers and practitioners to see anatomical complexities that were not visible before. The non-destructive nature of CT imaging is beneficial in osteology, as it preserves the integrity of valuable specimens while providing high-resolution data for research and clinical purposes.

Notably, CT enables the detection of subtle pathologies and facilitates assessment of bone density, which is critical for diagnosing osteoporosis and metabolic bone diseases. Additionally, the versatility of CT technology has made it a valuable tool in forensic anthropology and palaeoanthropology, where it is used to analyse and interpret human remains. As stipulated in current studies, computer-aided osteological analysis has become more prevalent, boosting the ability to perform non-invasive analysis of skeletal and fossilized remains. With its capacity to produce detailed three-dimensional models, CT allows forensic specialists to produce information on the demographic features of deceased individuals, including age and sex estimation and trauma analysis. This new approach not only aids the investigatory process but also addresses ethical issues in the processing of human remains in forensic and archaeological contexts (Uldin et al., 2017).

Furthermore, CT imaging continues the growing emphasis on multimodal imaging methods and the integration of various technologies to provide comprehensive analyses. Cooperative applications, such as centers like the University of Texas High-Resolution X-ray CT Facility, emphasize the critical convergence of imaging technology and scientific inquiry in osteology (Ahmed et al., 2017). As technology improves through enhanced computational power and algorithmic design, CT is at the forefront of expanding our understanding of the skeleton. The combination of machine learning and artificial intelligence with CT imaging protocols will further hone diagnostic capability and enable more sophisticated analysis of complex bone structures, solidifying its role in accelerating education and research in osteology (Figure 10.12).

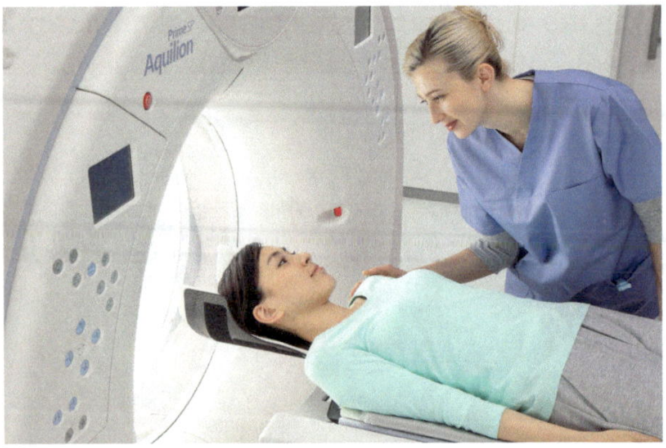

Figure 10.12. The advent of computed tomography (CT).

Source: https://external-content.duckduckgo.com/iu/?u=https%3A%2F%2Fwww.hudson-imaging.com%2Fwp-content%2Fuploads%2F2022%2F11%2FHudson_imaging_CT_SCAN_3.jpg&f=1&nofb=1&ipt=809fd1e02c5aa347f8916b428d00b5be28ec5368d41f4a2dbbad632b5f0fed23.

10.3.1. Mechanism of Computed Tomography (CT) Imaging

The CT imaging process is a significant advance in osteology, particularly in the enhanced visualization of bone anatomy and pathology. CT employs a series of X-ray measurements from a group of various angles around a single axis of rotation, which the computer coordinates to create cross-sectional images of the body. The capability to generate detailed three-dimensional reconstructions permits the observation of complex anatomical relationships. The ability to capture both hard and soft tissues with accuracy provides an advantage of CT over traditional radiographic imaging, especially in evaluating osseous structures. Furthermore, high-resolution micro-computed tomography has revolutionized research in osteology by providing extreme detail at the microanatomical level, thereby allowing for better appreciation of skeletal morphology and development. The precision and versatility of CT imaging have made it an important tool for clinical and research applications in bone research. The inclusion of digital technology in CT imaging has significantly expanded the range of functions in osteological research. Advances in image reconstruction algorithms and image processing have enhanced the resolution and precision of CT images, enabling researchers to detect subtle details previously unseen. Further, the application of multimodal imaging techniques, such as combining data from different modalities, enables deeper investigation of bone structure and function.

For instance, multi-body dynamics analysis (MDA) can accurately explain the complex interactions between muscle attachments and movement within skeletal systems (Curtis et al., 2009). The sophisticated technique, when applied to CT datasets, enables scientists to construct three-dimensional anatomically correct models. These 3D models further elucidate the deeper biomechanics of skeletons and interactions within the osteological framework, thereby propagating the field significantly. In addition, the educational value of CT imaging in osteology cannot be overemphasized. The high-resolution visualizations generated by CT not only augment diagnostic capabilities but also serve as pivotal instructional tools in educational environments. Centers such as the University of Texas High-Resolution X-ray CT Facility are vital for sharing access to advanced imaging technology for research and education (Ahmed et al., 2017). Access to high-resolution imaging for students and researchers enhances their understanding of bone anatomy and pathology, thereby promoting experiential learning. As technology advances, the addition of CT imaging to osteology is a classic demonstration of the digital era's ability to enhance methods in research and teaching alike, ultimately leading to smarter clinical interventions and improved understanding of skeletal science (Figure 10.13).

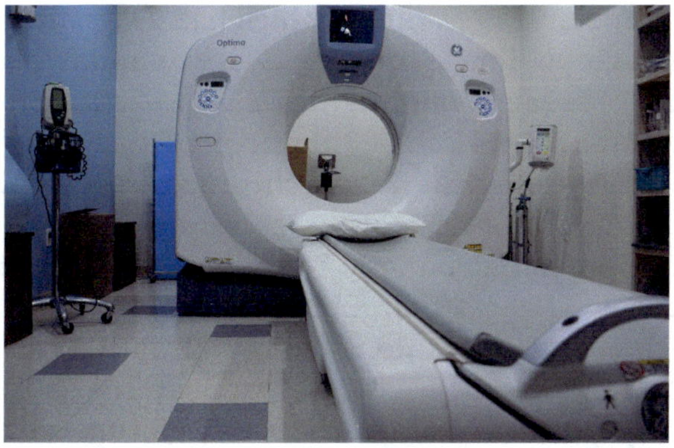

Figure 10.13. The mechanism of computed tomography (CT).

Source: https://external-content.duckduckgo.com/iu/?u=https%3A%2F%2Foptimumimaging.com%2Fwp-content%2Fuploads%2F2019%2F09%2FOptimum-520-CT-Scanner-OIC-Mission.jpg&f=1&nofb=1&ipt=799f77ed28f8e21e8d620e3150907940680b47bd84787ca349fb3dd49b2f16ef.

10.3.2. Advantages of Computed Tomography (CT) in Osteological Research

Application of CT in osteological science presents many groundbreaking advancements in the examination of skeletal remains. In contrast to traditional radiographic techniques, CT provides high-resolution three-dimensional reconstructions that enable unprecedented detail of bone structure. This capability not only enhances the interpretation of anatomical features but also facilitates the precise reconstruction of skeletal morphology. This level of specificity can be particularly valuable in forensic anthropology, where the creation of a biological profile for an unidentified individual is at a premium. Research indicates great potential for 3D imaging in making valid assessments, though research as it stands displays the need for more training in using anthropological methods to interpret such images, as referenced in the work by Valenzuela et al. (2016). Moreover, CT technology enables improved visualization of internal anatomy without damaging specimens that are typically irreplaceable and one-of-a-kind. Since CT scans are non-destructive, scientists can analyze fragile or rare bones without risking damage to these artifacts, preserving them for further research. Furthermore, CT scans can be stored in digital format, which significantly improves accessibility and collaboration among scientists. This digitization opens opportunities for longitudinal studies and comparative analysis that were previously challenging due to the logistics of handling physical specimens. Further, the use of high-tech CT centers, as noted by Ahmed et al. (2017), is expanding the reach of osteological work by enabling institutions to share their resources and methodologies that can deliver joint standards in the field. The application of CT to osteological work also holds out the prospect of population-specific standards required for contemporary anthropology. The ability to generate and examine large datasets through CT imaging bridges gaps in skeletal data finding applications in demographic studies and evolutionary biology. As more research is applied to optimizing scan protocols, as emphasized by Valenzuela et al. (2016), CT's capacity to derive biological profiles accurately will expand. Such advancement is not just applicable to research being carried out within the academic environment, but also to enhance educational outreach where interactive digital models can be employed as an educational tool. Lastly, through the adoption of CT technology, osteological research places itself at the forefront of scientific inquiry as well as applied use, infusing human history and biological diversity with powerful insights.

10.3.3. Case Studies Showcasing Computed Tomography (CT) Applications

CT applications in osteology have opened new frontiers in the investigation of skeletal form, most significantly through meticulous case studies. One such instance is the investigation into fossilized ancient remains, in which CT scans provided unprecedented insight into the morphology of extinct species. Scientists were able to non-invasively examine the internal structure of bones using high-resolution CT, enabling a full appreciation of evolutionary features and phylogenetic relationships. Such case studies not only deepen our understanding of extinct creatures but also legitimize CT as a key tool in paleontology. It uncovers aspects not visible to more traditional methods (Ahmed et al., 2017). Moreover, such non-invasive methods reduce the risk of damaging precious samples, highlighting the ethical considerations in current osteological research. The utility of CT extends beyond paleontological studies to modern herpetological research, providing a new methodology for examining developmental stages in amphibians. A compelling case study examined the vertebrae of tadpoles using microcomputed tomography (micro-CT), juxtaposing traditional bone-cartilage double-staining techniques with CT imaging. Results showed that micro-CT was a precise, efficient, and non-surgical method for finding and enumerating vertebrae, with no outliers in the results compared to traditional procedures. Notably, in the case study, the vital scanning parameters, e.g., voltage, which had a significant impact on image quality, were emphasized. This research highlights the potential for additional applications of micro-CT technology in herpetological research, encouraging its use in vertebrate morphological diversity and developmental biology research across other species (Jiang et al., 2018). Furthermore, CT technology applications are significantly crucial in forensic anthropology, particularly in the analysis of skeletal human remains from crime scenes. A notable case study demonstrated how CT scans unraveled intricate patterns of trauma in bones, providing essential information for legal analysis. Forensic anthropologists employed CT imaging to produce 3D replicas of skeletal evidence, enabling close visual inspection and proof of injury mechanisms. Not only did this enhance analytical potential, but it also increased the lucidity of forensic evidence during court proceedings. As can be seen from these case studies, not only is CT technology employed as a research instrument, but it also powerfully promotes interdisciplinary collaboration among biology, medicine, and legal studies. The interdisciplinary incorporation of CT into forensic analysis reflects its revolutionary potential, providing a higher level of accuracy and ethical research design in anthropology (Ahmed et al., 2017).

Test Your Knowledge

1. How is computed tomography (CT) used in osteological and forensic investigations?
2. What are the advantages of CT scans over traditional X-rays in analyzing skeletal structures?

10.4. Magnetic Resonance Imaging (MRI)

Learning Outcome

1. How MRI works in imaging bones
2. Benefits of MRI over traditional imaging methods
3. Specific osteological conditions diagnosed with MRI

MRI revolutionized the field of osteology by enabling precise images of bone and soft tissue without using ionizing radiation. This non-invasive imaging technique is particularly beneficial for imaging delicate anatomical structures and pathological conditions related to the skeletal system. Its pronounced increase in soft-tissue contrast is one of the most important advantages of MRI, allowing very detailed assessment of bone marrow lesions, cartilage injuries, and tumors. MRI allows improved characterization of soft tissue compared to traditional imaging techniques such as X-ray or CT scan, beneficial for diseases like osteomyelitis or inflammatory arthritis. With advancing technology, MRI has become a useful tool for research and clinical applications, capable of probing bone structure and function with greater precision and depth. Of particular interest is the application of gadolinium-based contrast agents (GBCAs) in MRI, as they markedly enhance the detectability of certain pathological processes within bone. GBCAs, which contain gadolinium in the chelated form, increase MRI contrast by altering adjacent water molecules' magnetic properties. While the blood elimination half-life of these drugs is about 90 minutes, recent studies demonstrate that gadolinium may accumulate in bone tissue, with implications for long-term health consequences. Cutting-edge synchrotron radiation-induced micro- and submicro-X-ray fluorescence spectroscopy (SR-XRF) experiments have been used to image gadolinium distribution in bone, as in patients with idiopathic osteoporosis. Results like these underscore the importance of gadolinium pharmacokinetics, as they can affect the safety and efficacy of MRI during osteological studies (Burghammer et al., 2020). Moreover, MRI's capacity to create detailed three-dimensional (3D) models of skeletal structures has taken osteological research to new heights. By integrating MRI data with advanced imaging techniques, researchers can generate interactive 3D representations that facilitate a deeper exploration of anatomical systems. For instance, 3D modeling enables visualization of complex morphological features that are often obscured in traditional imaging methods. This technique not only documents anatomical variations but also enables the sharing of results between clinicians and researchers. The ability to manipulate these models offers significant advantages in both education and the clinical environment, as clinicians can visualize and discuss intricate anatomical relationships in real time. By bridging the imaging-digital technology interface, MRI has established its vital place in further understanding bone pathology and biology (McHenry et al., 2014) (Figure 10.14).

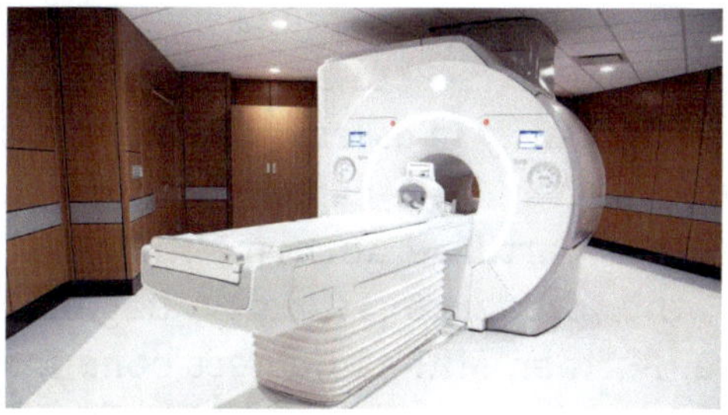

Figure 10.14. Magnetic resonance imaging (MRI).

Source: https://external-content.duckduckgo.com/iu/?u=https%3A%2F%2Fwww.columbiaradiology.org%2Fsites%2Fdefault%2Ffiles%2Fstyles%2Fcola_media_800_16_9%2Fpublic%2Fmedia%2Fimages%2F2020-02%2F211a7317-edit.jpg%3Fitok%3DrnA-mUVB&f=1&nofb=1&ipt=a0f636cea2aa644c8dcbfba737b2327c9c688d4fb93cc1b0dfc21c7aadf99b3f.

10.4.1. How Magnetic Resonance Imaging (MRI) Works in Imaging Bones

MRI has emerged as a significant weapon in bone imaging due to its non-invasive nature and ability to create high-quality images. In contrast to conventional X-rays, which primarily depict bone density and structure, MRI uses strong magnetic fields and radio waves to generate high-resolution images of bone and adjacent tissues. The method takes advantage of the natural magnetic properties of hydrogen atoms, which are primarily contained in water and fat, thereby enabling MRI to image based on differences in the magnetic resonance signals produced by these atoms. The generated pictures provide detailed information not only about the bones' morphology but also about adjacent soft tissues, which is particularly helpful in diagnosing diseases such as tumors, fractures, or infections that cannot be seen with other imaging methods.

One of the impressive advantages of MRI in osteology is that it has improved contrast resolution, which provides better vision of soft tissues such as cartilage, ligaments, and muscles around the bones. This proves to be of immense utility in assessing joint-associated pathology, with MRI capable of diagnosing even minor cartilage abnormalities that may signal the presence of early degenerative disease. Further, MRI can detect bone marrow edema, providing invaluable information about underlying pathologies such as osteomyelitis or stress fractures that may be missed with routine X-ray imaging. The use of more sophisticated MRI technology, including diffusion-weighted imaging and three-dimensional reconstructions, has also enhanced diagnostic sensitivity, allowing clinicians to direct treatment more rationally based on accurate anatomical data. Progress in MRI technology over the past decade has also introduced functional imaging modalities that measure bone metabolism and perfusion. These methods, when combined with traditional imaging sequences, enhance the overall understanding of bone health and disease progression. For instance, MRI's role in assessing bone response to therapies in conditions like osteoporosis is increasingly recognized, as it can monitor changes in bone density and structure over time. The integration of these new imaging modalities into clinical practice not only ensures accurate diagnosis and treatment of skeletal disorders but also improves the overall quality of osteological care. With improvements in imaging and digital technology, MRI plays an important role in maximizing patient outcomes in osteological assessment, underscoring its indispensable role in modern medicine (Jayapala et al., 2024; Gulhan et al., 2017) (Figure 10.15).

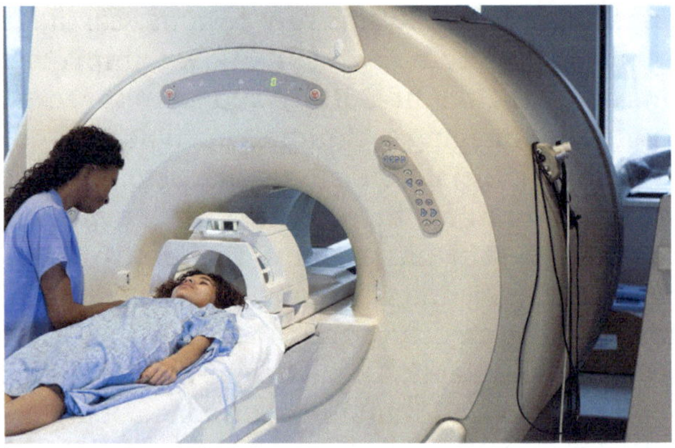

Figure 10.15. How magnetic resonance imaging (MRI) works in imaging bones.

Source: https://external-content.duckduckgo.com/iu/?u=https%3A%2F%2Fwww.verywellhealth.com%2Fthmb%2Fc9Uu7YK--wzxNW2ssfyvlrD5V5U%3D%2F1500x0%2Ffilters%3Ano_upscale()%3Amax_bytes(150000)%3Astrip_icc()%2FGettyImages-103919304-44ca865113b449fcb59574cd99fcf9a4.jpg&f=1&nofb=1&ipt=d58028d26034a937efba70d8c94404ff41f4fb976c9a3ddaa250136496255656.

10.4.2. Benefits of Magnetic Resonance Imaging (MRI) Over Traditional Imaging Methods

Technological progress in imaging has revolutionized osteological practice, particularly by the use of MRI. Compared to traditional imaging modalities such as X-ray or CT, MRI offers superior soft-tissue contrast and visualization of complex structures, with no ionizing radiation. The non-invasive nature of MRI is particularly valuable for analyzing intricate bone-soft tissue relationships, which are important for a complete understanding of skeletal anatomy and disease. Tissue differentiation ability contributes to the diagnostic power of investigators and clinicians by enabling them to make more accurate assessments of conditions such as arthritis or tumors, which involve both bone and soft tissues. Thus, MRI use can significantly improve the effectiveness and precision of osteological studies and care of patients. Moreover, the multi-planar imaging capability of MRIs allows for visualization in a variety of planes, which is not feasible with standard imaging techniques. This versatility is significant when studying anatomical variation or diagnosing in complex cases. Three-dimensional reconstruction of MRI data enables more detailed analysis of skeletal morphology and yields insights that could be overlooked with traditional techniques. Because MRI provides images with acceptable spatial resolution, it enables researchers to investigate small changes in morphology over time, which is essential for following diseases, assessing treatment response, and conducting longitudinal studies in osteology. Such overdetail is intended to enhance the reliability of information and ultimately help in knowledge creation in the discipline. While MRI offers many advantages, it should be recognized that traditional imaging methods remain significant in some cases. While MRI has excellent ability in imaging soft tissues, methods like X-rays offer fast, low-cost solutions for initial assessments or when MRI is not possible. In addition, specific research highlights the benefits of combining modalities in imaging, underscoring the synergistic advantages of alternative techniques for comprehensive morphological comparison. A synergy between MRI and conventional imaging can result in a holistic appreciation of osteological samples at the expense of budgetary and temporal constraints typical to researchers. By recognizing such dynamics, it is clear that MRI is a useful technology. However, its optimal use resides in an environment that harmoniously weaves together novel and traditional imaging modalities, thereby leading to depth as well as breadth in osteological pursuit (Ahmed et al., 2017; Albert et al., 2023).

10.4.3. Specific Osteological Conditions Diagnosed with Magnetic Resonance Imaging (MRI)

MRI has revolutionized the diagnosis of most osteological conditions, providing hitherto unattainable detail in the demonstration of osseous and soft-tissue anatomy. MRI can detect early changes in osteoarthritis, such as cartilage loss and subchondral bone changes, that are not visible on plain X-rays. An MRI can capture the subtle details of the morphology of joints, depicting morphologies such as Schmorl's nodes, a pathological morphology with intervertebral disc compromise, in which nucleus pulposus herniates into adjacent vertebral bodies. Additionally, because MRI is non-invasive, clinicians can assess pathological conditions without exposing patients to ionizing radiation, thus it is a diagnostic modality of choice in clinics and research work. MRI's capability of producing high-resolution images raises the accuracy of disease formation determination, enabling early intervention that improves patient outcomes. Moreover, MRI's role extends beyond imaging, venturing into quantitative measurement and morphometric analysis. In osteoarthritis research, MRI plays a crucial role in measuring cartilage thickness and detecting bone marrow edema, generating valuable data on disease symptoms. Single osteological abnormalities, such as osteomyelitis and stress fractures, can also be accurately diagnosed on MRI because it can differentiate more effectively among various tissue types. This ability is necessary for planning treatment and evaluating the disease's course. The integration of MRI results with high-technology imaging, like three-dimensional reconstruction, enables orthopedists and radiologists to work with complex cases effectively. Multidimensional approaches of this type are paving the way for precision medicine, with treatments designed according to each patient's unique profile. Furthermore, digital technology is increasingly penetrating osteology, opening up a broader scope for research and clinical application. The use of geometric morphometrics offers a deep way of understanding the correlation between skeletal structure and various pathological conditions. For instance, bone shape change measurement, as in conditions like osteoporosis and leprosy, illustrates the potential of new imaging technologies to illuminate the disease process. This integration of MRI technology with morphometric analysis has a high likelihood of enhancing diagnostic potential and enabling preventive interventions in osteological health. As research continues, the integration of such technology could enable universal protocols for constructing biological profiles, thereby improving diagnostic accuracy across different osteological conditions, as highlighted by recent studies (Plomp et al., 2013; Valenzuela et al., 2016).

Test Your Knowledge

1. How is magnetic resonance imaging (MRI) used to study bones and soft tissues in osteology?
2. What are the advantages of MRI compared to other imaging techniques in skeletal analysis?

10.5. Digital Imaging Techniques

Learning Outcome

1. Introduction to digital radiography
2. Role of 3D imaging in osteology
3. Impact of digital technology on data analysis

Computer imaging techniques have transformed the field of osteology, providing us with a superior means of visualizing and comprehending skeletal remains than previously possible. Among these techniques, computed tomography (CT) has proven particularly useful for investigating bone structures non-invasively. By producing cross-sectional images, CT not only helps identify and document osteological attributes but also reconstruct three-dimensional anatomical features. The ability to visualize within without physically dissecting significantly benefits forensic anthropology and palaeoanthropology, as researchers can thoroughly analyze specimens without causing them any damage. Additionally, advances in multi-detector CT have improved image resolution, providing greater insight into the detailed skeletal morphology necessary for age, sex, and ancestry estimations in osteological analysis (Uldin et al., 2017). Apart from CT, other imaging modalities have become essential tools in osteology. Digital radiography and MRI are two methods that provide complementary information and enable multidimensional analysis of the skeleton. MRI, for example, is highly effective in assessing soft tissue and can provide valuable information about the status of adjacent structures, which is often lost when using only traditional imaging methods. Digital radiography has also improved imaging processes by using digital sensors, which not only enhance image quality but also reduce radiation exposure. With the growing demand for accuracy in skeletal analysis, integrating these heterogeneous imaging modalities offers a comprehensive framework for understanding the complexity of human remains (Uldin et al., 2017). Digital imaging techniques are not only gaining prominence in research and forensic applications but also in educational research and public engagement. With further development of multimodal imaging technologies, institutions can create accurate, interactive models that support richer learning experiences for students and society at large.

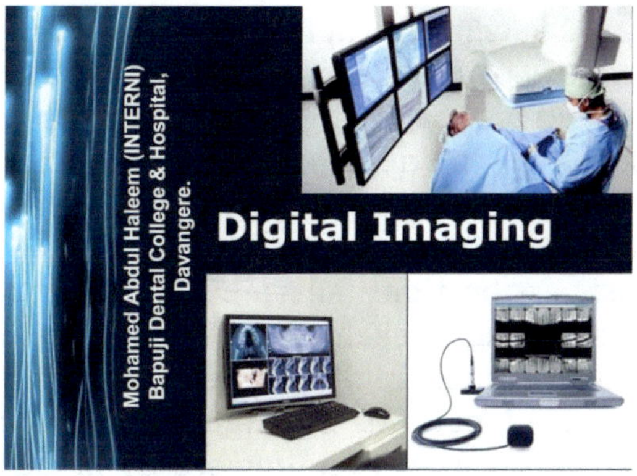

Figure 10.16. Digital imaging techniques.

Source: https://cdn.slidesharecdn.com/ss_thumbnails/digitalimaging-161130050256-thumbnail.jpg?width=640&height=640&fit=bounds.

The access to high-quality digital models encourages greater understanding of osteological principles and the significance of human remains as a historical and cultural phenomenon. In addition, institutions such as those operated by the University of Texas High-Resolution X-ray CT Facility are showcasing how digital imaging is being utilized to bridge the gap between academic research and educational outreach, thereby promoting broader knowledge of osteological study and its importance to our understanding of human history (Ahmed et al., 2017) (Figure 10.16).

10.5.1. Introduction to Digital Radiography

The introduction of digital radiography has changed the practice of osteology significantly and given scientists and practitioners better imaging capabilities than those available with conventional radiographic methods. Digital radiography uses sophisticated electronic sensors to capture images, enabling instant access to high-resolution visual information. This speed enables instantaneous diagnostics, an important aspect in both clinical and forensic applications. Such manipulation and analysis of images, easily, in the digital format, further augment their application in osteological assessment. For instance, researchers would use computer software to evaluate and measure skeletal morphology more accurately, thereby enabling a more reliable assessment of sex and stature from digitized skeletal material. This has profound applications in forensic anthropology and human variation, particularly in victim identification in mass fatality contexts, where accurate skeletal analysis is of paramount importance (Gulhan et al., 2017). Compatibility with three-dimensional imaging technologies such as computed tomography (CT) is one of the principal attributes of digital radiography. Whereas digital radiography provides excellent 2D images, CT imaging allows accurate 3D reconstructions that reveal finer details of skeletal morphology. It has been demonstrated that the accuracy of osteometric data extracted from digital images is as good as, if not better than, that achieved through traditional direct measurement, thereby also vindicating its application in clinical and forensic situations alike (Beckett et al., 2019). The ability to create digital models from CT scans also increases the precision of anatomical measurements, thereby enhancing the validity of osteological interpretations. Moreover, such a relationship between digital radiography and CT indicates the interdependence of current imaging modalities, that is, their synergistic potential to enhance the science of osteology. Despite the various advantages of digital radiography, there are limitations that the practitioners will have to consider. Most importantly, magnification errors can compromise measurement precision and lead to misinterpretation if left uncorrected. Research has demonstrated that while digital radiography is less expensive and more convenient than PMCT, the inherent magnification must be strictly calibrated to ensure measurements are valid (Beckett et al., 2019). The use of correction factors for magnification will enhance the validity of information gathered through digital radiography, thus a promising component in osteometric studies. As technology evolves, more empirical studies are needed to finalize standardized procedures for corrections, thus paving the way for digital radiography to be a component of forensic anthropology and general osteology.

10.5.2. Role of 3D Imaging in Osteology

The evolution of 3D imaging has completely transformed osteology, thereby improving the precision and timeliness of skeletal analysis. Technology allows precise visualization of the bone's structure without invasive procedures, hence the integrity of specimens is preserved. Among the greatest uses of X-ray microcomputed tomography (micro-CT) is that it generates high-resolution images that reveal fine details of osseous and cartilaginous tissues. Scientists can visualize complex anatomical configurations and assess variations in bone pathology, morphology, and density with great accuracy. So, not only does 3D imaging enhance our understanding of typical osteological characteristics but also enable the diagnosis and treatment planning of certain skeletal disorders. The introduction of 3D imaging in osteology is a fine example of how digital technologies can effectively close the gap between conventional methods and changing scientific demands. Beyond its analytical role, 3D imaging significantly improves the learning environment of osteology. By offering interactive models that can be virtually manipulated, instructors have access to unparalleled teaching tools to instruct students on bone anatomy and function. This visual approach benefits diverse learning styles and makes complex structures more accessible and comprehensible. Also, 3D imaging can enable virtual dissections and simulations, providing experiences that may not be attainable with real specimens. Such types of improvements to learning methods can enhance student motivation and retention. As mentioned, schools are tapping into equipment such as the University of Texas High-Resolution X-ray CT Facility to explore the latest imaging technology. This trend is a move toward a more active, technology-centered approach to osteology instruction. Third, 3D imaging does not stop at teaching and research; it is important in applied osteology in clinical and forensic applications. Micro-CT, for instance, is used to examine skeletal remains in forensic investigations, enabling non-destructive testing of the evidence. As highlighted in ongoing research, the utilization of micro-CT in tadpole and adult samples demonstrates its relevance in different osteological subdisciplines. In the clinical environment, this imaging modality aids surgical planning and the evaluation of bone-healing processes, significantly improving patient treatment. As the evidence continues to mount for the utility of such digital technologies, it is crucial that the science of osteology continues to evolve, embracing 3D imaging technologies as shared probes for research and application to maintain further advances in the understanding of skeletal biology.

10.5.3. Impact of Digital Technology on Data Analysis

The transformational impact of digital technology on data analysis in osteology cannot be overstated. The introduction of advanced imaging techniques, such as X-ray microcomputed tomography (micro-CT), has dramatically altered the process of obtaining and analyzing skeletal data. This technology enables non-invasive observation of complex internal anatomy, thereby enabling a better understanding of osseous anatomy. The invention of high-resolution imaging has played a crucial role in acquiring enormous volumes of data, enabling analyses previously unimaginable. With facilities like the University of Texas High-Resolution X-ray CT Facility implementing measures to enhance imaging capabilities, researchers can delve deeper into complex osteological matters, leading to significant advances in paleontology and comparative anatomy (Ahmed et al., 2017). Moreover, computerization of data analysis enables one to conduct comparative studies across taxa. For instance, the application of micro-CT in the analysis of adult amphibians and larval stages allows scientists to investigate vertebral structures effectively. Evidence suggests that this imaging technology can efficiently quantify the number of tadpole vertebrae, filling an essential knowledge gap on amphibian development (Jiang et al., 2018). Digital technology also enhances data handling, where scientists can better store, share, and process large amounts of data. This feature ensures coordination among scientists and further enhances the multidisciplinary aspect of osteological studies, where findings are applicable in other disciplines such as herpetology and evolutionary biology. Furthermore, digital technology enables the development of analytical tools for data, offering deeper insights into morphological variations that occur over time in the skeletal system. Researchers can employ sophisticated software to run statistical analyses on data gathered from imaging studies, thereby uncovering patterns and trends previously concealed. Precision and accuracy of digital data analysis allow for more refined information on how the development of bones is influenced by evolutionary forces. Thus, as technology continues to advance, digital tools are certain to have an even stronger impact on osteological work, enabling researchers to uncover subtle details of skeletal anatomy and providing insight into the evolutionary history of vertebrates (Ahmed et al., 2017) (Figure 10.17).

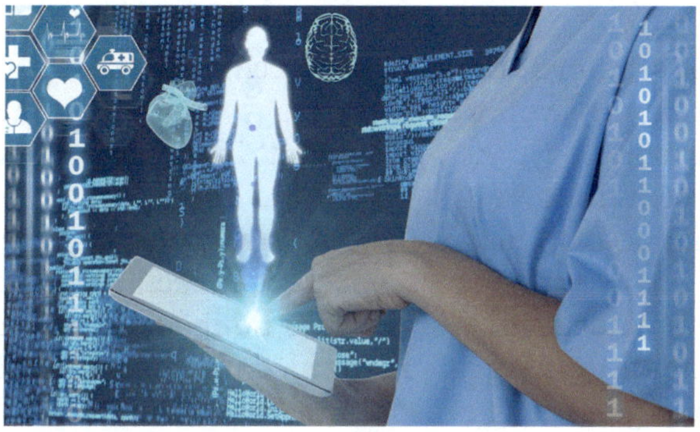

Figure 10.17. The transformative effects of digital technology on data analysis in the field of osteology cannot be overs.

Source: https://i0.wp.com/sidgs.com/wp-content/uploads/2023/02/The-Role-of-Data-and-Analytics-in-Digital-Transformation-in-Health-Care-1500-x-914.png?fit=1500%2C914&ssl=1.

Test Your Knowledge

1. How are digital imaging techniques applied in the study and documentation of skeletal remains?
2. What advantages do digital imaging methods offer over traditional imaging in osteology and forensic analysis?

10.6. Future Trends in Osteological Imaging

Learning Outcome

1. Emerging technologies in imaging
2. Integration of artificial intelligence in imaging
3. Potential for personalized medicine in osteology

The discipline of osteological imaging is evolving rapidly, particularly with the use of advanced digital technologies that enable more precise, less intrusive examination of skeletal fossils. Among the trends to watch is the increasing application of high-resolution computed tomography (CT) and three-dimensional reconstruction techniques. Such techniques enable researchers to view complex osteological structures in greater detail than ever before, thereby enhancing discovery in areas of evolutionary biology and functional morphology. As illustrated in more recent research, for example, on the evolution of the mammalian jaw, CT and digital modeling offer a robust way to reconstruct musculoskeletal characteristics, pushing the boundaries of our understanding of anatomical transformation over geological timescales (Abdala et al., 2016). Having the ability to image fossils without the hazards of traditional techniques can greatly assist preservation, and such present imaging methods are priceless for both scholarly investigation and heritage conservation. With advances in imaging technology, the potential for interdisciplinary collaboration in osteology is increasingly evident. The integration of disciplines such as palaeoanthropology, forensic anthropology, and bioarcheology is no longer rare, especially with each of these fields employing the same imaging modality in research. In forensic anthropology, for instance, the use of multi-detector CT has introduced an open door to a standardized process of virtual osteological analysis that assures similarities of parameters across studies (Uldin et al., 2017). This convergence of methodologies not only enhances the validity of research findings but also fuels a dynamic debate among scientists from diverse backgrounds. Consequently, with this convergence of specialties, the range of osteological imaging is widened, and more information on modern and ancient human and animal populations is obtained. Future directions in osteological imaging will likely focus on integrating artificial intelligence (AI) and machine learning to enable more sophisticated analysis of existing imaging technologies. Both technologies can automate the identification of skeletal system anatomical landmarks and pathological conditions, accelerating data interpretation and analysis. With increasing digitalization of osteology, machine learning software can be employed to find patterns and anomalies that the human researcher may not perceive. Such research, driven by data, could lead to ground-breaking findings in the evolution of disease, biomechanics, and adaptation as a response to the stress of the environment. The implementation of these innovative instruments will push the limits of osteological research, permitting a more refined understanding of the evolutionary past and how it echoes through contemporary sciences.

10.6.1. Emerging Technologies in Imaging

The emergence of new imaging technologies has transformed the field of osteology, offering researchers and practitioners unprecedented tools for analyzing and interpreting skeletal remains. Among these innovations, 3D imaging is one very significant development. Trends in thought within the osteological profession today promote the integration of 3D imaging with traditional practices to enhance educational outcomes. Evidence supports that the use of collaborative online resources alongside conventional cadaveric resources efficiently boosts students' performance in anatomy courses, as evidenced by a 6% rise in laboratory grades following the implementation of digital libraries and quizzes in learning environments (Massa et al., 2016). This demonstrates not only the enhanced learning capabilities enabled by 3D imaging technology but also how it can create a more engaging and interactive learning space. It has been used in forensic anthropology to reconstruct biological profiles from human remains. It is one such recent study utilizing 3D images derived from Computed Tomography (CT) scans that found it possible to make reliable estimates of age and sex from skeletal morphology (Valenzuela et al., 2016). The study also highlighted issues with interobserver error magnitudes when applying traditional testing protocols to 3D models. The challenge lies in the need to use standardized procedures and to provide further training in 3D visualization skills among practitioners. By resolving these concerns, the field of forensic science can enhance the accuracy of biological profile creation through 3D imaging and thereby increase the scope and effectiveness of osteological analysis in scholarly and professional realms. With the constant development of new technologies, the integration of innovative imaging technologies into osteology is expected to further elucidate skeletal biology and its applications in both medical and archaeological fields. The potential to digitize skeletal collections enhances access to these valuable resources, facilitating collaborative research and extrapolating osteological information to living populations (Valenzuela et al., 2016). Population-specific guidelines derived from 3D analysis and imaging might be valuable in a clinical context. These advances create an engaging new frontier in osteology, whereby technology and innovation join to enable the continued pursuit of knowledge in human anatomy and its concomitant impacts on health and heritage. The possible applications of these technologies to teaching within academia, as well as practical uses, solidify the transformative role of new imaging technologies in osteology (Figure 10.18).

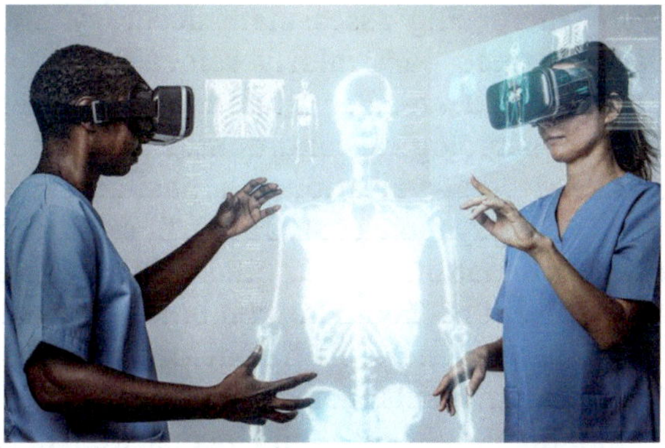

Figure 10.18. The advent of emerging technologies in imaging.

Source: https://www.softcath.com/wp-content/uploads/2021/06/doctors-wearing-vr-simulation-with-hologram-medical-technology_53876-98566.jpg.

10.6.2. Integration of Artificial Intelligence (AI) in Imaging

The incorporation of AI into imaging has transformed the practice of osteology by enhancing the accuracy and speed of skeletal examination. AI techniques such as machine learning enable high-speed processing of large volumes of imaging data, enabling the identification of subtle pathological conditions that may escape the human eye. In the area of osteology, where precise imaging plays a crucial role in disorders like fractures, tumors, or degenerative diseases, machine learning techniques can be employed to make the detection process automated, thus providing clinicians with important insights that lead to timely interventions. With advancements in these AI technologies, their ability to learn from enormous amounts of data enables them to adapt to new challenges in skeletal imaging, optimizing diagnostic outcomes and shaping future approaches in this specialized field. Moreover, AIs' role in imaging extends beyond detection to classification and prognosis. Advanced algorithms can classify various bone conditions based on their radiological features, thereby increasing assessment accuracy. Such usage becomes particularly relevant in light of the intricate vascular anatomical variations that affect osteological conditions, such as those associated with variations in basilar artery termination (Jayapala et al., 2024). Classification process automation that has otherwise remained subjective opens doors to combined research and clinical practices. AI has helped scientists optimize their results using emerging scientific data and taxonomy, resolving inconsistencies in classification that define current osteological research (Nunes et al., 2020). Such AI approach enables enhanced understanding of bone pathologies to enhance evidence-based practice in patients. The application of AI in osteological imaging has broad implications for clinical diagnosis, as well as for training and education. With future healthcare professionals working with increasingly sophisticated imaging technologies, exposure to AI-generated results is unavoidable. Education programs must adapt to include AI literacy, teaching students to read classifications generated by machines and to leverage these technologies to deliver enhanced patient outcomes. Also, the moral implications of AI's role in medical imaging cannot be overlooked; ensuring the integrity of AI algorithms and protecting the data of patients are of utmost importance in placing trust in these technologies. Therefore, as AI becomes increasingly entrenched within the matrix of imaging, it not only promises to augment clinical practice but also recasts the educative model for osteology and beyond.

10.6.3. Potential for Personalized Medicine in Osteology

The advent of digital technology and imaging has opened the door to significant technological advances in personalized medicine, including osteology. Personalized medicine is centered on tailoring treatment approaches based on individual anatomical, biological, and health variations. In osteology, this is particularly critical where bone density, geometry, and biomechanics can significantly determine the success of treatment for conditions such as osteoporosis or fractures. Modern imaging methods, such as high-resolution CT and MRI, allow more precise assessment of bone health and morphology, facilitating the creation of highly customized treatment plans. The convergence of these technologies can maximize the precision of diagnosing bone disease and tracking the course of interventions over time, making it an invaluable component of personalized care in osteology. In addition, the application of three-dimensional (3D) printing technology has proven to be one of the most promising technologies in personalized osteological treatment. As explained, three-dimensional printing is remarkable in that it enables the production of complex geometries and high-precision models, which is crucial for creating personalized prosthetics and bone grafts suitable for the specific anatomical structure of every patient. This capability also significantly facilitates pre-surgical planning, enabling physicians to develop patient-specific bone structure models for simulation and improved surgery. Also, 3D printing enables the development of biocompatible implants that enhance bone tissue integration, ultimately resulting in shorter recovery periods and reduced complications. In this context, 3D printing is among the most significant resources in advancing individualized solutions that can transform osteological patient treatment (Benchabane et al., 2023). Finally, the scope of personalized medicine extends beyond treatment methods and influences prevention methods for osteoarthritis. By applying innovative imaging technologies, medical professionals are better positioned to assess risk factors for bone density loss and fractures much earlier. For example, by combining genetic and imaging test results, it is possible to obtain a comprehensive picture of one's vulnerability to osteoporosis. Subsequently, evidence-based treatment plans are developed, including tailored dietary counseling and targeted exercise regimens for bone strengthening. Consequently, the strategy becomes shifted from reactive treatment to proactive prevention, thereby reducing the incidence of skeletal complications. This paradigm shift towards individualized methods emphasizes the revolutionary potential of integrating imaging and digital technologies into osteological condition prevention and treatment, foretelling a forward-looking direction for research and clinical response (Ahn et al., 2019).

Test Your Knowledge

1. What emerging technologies are shaping the future of osteological imaging?
2. How might advancements in imaging improve the accuracy and efficiency of skeletal analysis?

SUMMARY

In short, the integration of imaging and digital technology into osteology has revolutionized the field, providing unprecedented insights into ancient and contemporary skeletal remains. As demonstrated by numerous applications, these technologies enable scholars to document anatomical features and reconstruct biological histories meticulously. A good example is three-dimensional scanning, which has been applied to the minute examination of objects such as artifacts and bones, thereby allowing closer scrutiny of human osteological variation and evolution over time. Technology enables not only enhanced scholarly research but also applications in real life in forensic inquiry and conservation of cultural heritage. Through the application of these new imaging technologies, osteologists are able to tell more detailed stories about the lives and societies of populations in the past, creating a richer picture of human history. Additionally, the interdisciplinary context of this technological advancement indicates its importance beyond documentation. As shown in projects that use three-dimensional scans of Roman works of art, digital imaging naturally combines disciplines such as archaeology, anthropology, and computer science, enabling multifaceted examinations. Through the integration of methods from these multidisciplinary areas, scholars are not only able to analyze formal and stylistic aspects of ancient depictions but also derive biometric measurements that broaden our understanding of individual identities through time. The interplay among disciplines highlights the cooperative potential of these breakthroughs and, with it, efforts to provide more comprehensive overall views of the collected information. This incorporation of data ultimately serves the science of osteology, paving the way for new research and interdisciplinary efforts. In general, the evolution of imaging and computer technology presents an exceptional opportunity for ongoing expansion in osteology and related sciences. With continued refining of techniques, the potential for expanded analysis capacity and access to information will continue to increase. Emphasizing the need to keep investing in such technology will be key to advancing basic research and informing today's applied practice in the forensic sciences and the cultural heritage world. By embracing technologies that capture multidimensional data, like those revealed by the study of Roman portrait statues, osteology will be able to progress considerably in both the understanding of human anatomy and the interpretation of the tale that skeletons provide. It is thus imperative that those interested in scholarship, technology, and the conservation of culture unite to determine the true potential of these digital technologies, so that the richness and depth of our shared human heritage are not only documented but also celebrated.

Integration of imaging and digital technologies in osteology offers revolutionary possibilities for research and clinical practice. The most significant of these developments is the application of 3D CT imaging, which allows for high-resolution skeletal morphology images. The technology has been valuable in forensic applications, especially in sex determination, by providing critical measurements from femur bones. It has been discovered that the use of 3D reconstructions can yield reproducible data, which helps derive discriminant function equations for populations. The reproducibility and reliability of such methods were accentuated by a study underscoring the accuracy of measurements obtained from volume-rendering models compared to traditional dry bone assessment, paving the way for better forensic endeavors in establishing biological identity in criminal cases, particularly in jurisdictions with limited access to documented skeletal histories like Turkey (Gulhan et al., 2017). Reproducibility of imaging methods is necessary for accurate sex estimation, as highlighted by recent femoral measurements derived from CT analyses. A preliminary reliability study conducted prior to the primary data collection revealed no significant differences across repeated measurements of the same variables. Evidence supports 3D volume rendering techniques utilized via special software to ensure high intra-observer reliability, a parameter that attests to their application in forensic practice. These image technology improvements not only enhance the skeletal analysis procedure but also contribute to the field of forensic anthropology, which enhances methodologies for victim identification in mass fatality events. The validity of different rendering methods provides evidence for the need for continuous evolution of standardized protocols that yield similar and accurate results across different populations, a requirement for forensic use (Gulhan et al., 2017). In addition to their benefits in forensic use, imaging technologies also extend to understanding bone-muscle interactions, and this is proof of the multidisciplinary nature of modern osteology. Research suggests that osteocyte-secreted factors greatly influence muscle function and myogenesis. For instance, WNT3a secreted by osteocytes is a potent enhancer of muscle contractile strength, with effects even observed at low doses. This correlation demonstrates that image improvements not only enhance skeletal assessment but also expand our understanding of the biological interactions between bone tissue and muscle. These findings highlight the potential of osteocyte signaling in myogenesis and musculoskeletal health, showing that technological developments in imaging techniques can stimulate cross-disciplinary scholarship and application to osteological and physiological understanding of musculoskeletal health.

KEY TERMS FROM THIS CHAPTER

- 3D Reconstruction
- Computed Tomography (CT)
- Digital Modeling
- Laser Scanning
- Micro-CT
- Photogrammetry
- Virtual Anthropology
- 3D Scanning
- CT Imaging (Computed Tomography)
- Geometric Morphometrics
- Magnetic Resonance Imaging (MRI)
- Osteology
- Radiography

CRITICAL THINKING QUESTIONS

1. **What is the primary purpose of digital imaging in osteology?**
   a. To extract DNA from bones
   b. To enhance visualization and analysis of skeletal structures
   c. To preserve soft tissues
   d. To identify muscle attachments
2. **Which imaging technique provides detailed 3D visualizations of internal bone structures?**
   a. X-ray
   b. MRI
   c. CT scan (Computed Tomography)
   d. Ultrasound
3. **In forensic and bioarcheological contexts, 3D scanning is most commonly used for:**
   a. Recording and replicating skeletal features
   b. Determining bone density
   c. Measuring blood flow
   d. Enhancing DNA extraction
4. **Which of the following technologies is most suitable for non-invasive analysis of ancient remains?**
   a. Histological sampling
   b. CT imaging
   c. Bone biopsy
   d. Chemical staining
5. **Photogrammetry in osteology involves:**
   a. Laser scanning of bone cross-sections
   b. Capturing DNA from photos
   c. Using photographs to create 3D digital models
   d. Measuring bone weight

Short Answer Questions

1. What is the role of CT (Computed Tomography) scanning in osteological analysis?
2. How does 3D scanning benefit the documentation and preservation of skeletal remains?
3. What are the advantages of using non-invasive imaging techniques in the study of ancient human remains?
4. Explain how digital technologies enhance the accuracy and reproducibility of osteological measurements.
5. Describe one way that imaging technology can help differentiate between antemortem and postmortem trauma.

Answers to Critical Thinking Questions

1. (b); 2. (c); 3. (a); 4. (b); 5. (c)

REFERENCES

1. Lautenschlager, S., Gill, P., Luo, Z., Fagan, M. J., & Rayfield, E. J. (2016). Morphological evolution of the mammalian jaw adductor complex. *Biological Reviews/Biological Reviews of the Cambridge Philosophical Society*, *92*(4), 1910–1940. https://doi.org/10.1111/brv.12314Ahn, H. S., Al-Ardah, A., Bottino, M. C., Chia, H. N., Draenert, F. G., Dyke, T. E., Edwards, S. P., et al. (2019). Personalized scaffolding technologies for alveolar bone regenerative medicine. http://deepblue.lib.umich.edu/bitstream/2027.42/149271/1/ocr12275.pdf (accessed on 21st July 2025).
2. Albert, J. S., Chakrabarty, P., Evans, K., Ford, D., et al. (2023). A new era of morphological investigations: Reviewing methods for comparative anatomical studies. https://core.ac.uk/download/565799822.pdf (accessed on 21st July 2025).
3. Anderson, M., Davy-Jow, S., Lorenz, K., Schofield, C., et al. (2012). Roman portraiture and biometric identification. https://core.ac.uk/download/42505482.pdf (accessed on 21st July 2025).
4. Bashutski, J. D., Cobb, C. M., Cochran, D. L., Lin, Z., et al. (2015). Emerging regenerative approaches for periodontal reconstruction: Practical applications from the AAP regeneration workshop. http://deepblue.lib.umich.edu/bitstream/2027.42/141131/1/cap0040.pdf (accessed on 21st July 2025).
5. Beckett, S., Carew, R. M., Conlogue, G. J., Márquez-Grant, N., et al. (2019). Accuracy of computed radiography in osteometry: A comparison of digital imaging techniques and the effect of magnification. https://core.ac.uk/download/286350604.pdf (accessed on 21st July 2025).
6. Benazzi, S., Bernardini, F., Bettuzzi, M., Bondioli, L., Bortolini, E., Collina, C., Di Domenico, G., et al. (2022). High-accuracy methodology for the integrative restoration of archaeological teeth by using reverse engineering techniques and rapid prototyping. https://core.ac.uk/download/577166287.pdf (accessed on 21st July 2025).
7. Benchabane, A., Kaidi, R., Khelef, D., Marouf, A., et al. (2023). Primjena 3D pisača u veterinarstvu–pregledni članak. https://core.ac.uk/download/541412117.pdf (accessed on 21st July 2025).
8. Bonewald, L. F., Brotto, L., Brotto, M., Dallas, S., et al. (2017). Crosstalk between MLO-Y4 osteocytes and C2C12 muscle cells is mediated by the Wnt/β-catenin pathway. https://core.ac.uk/download/129148778.pdf (accessed on 21st July 2025).
9. Burghammer, M., Fox, O. J. L., Hofstaetter, J. G., Pichler, M., et al. (2020). Detection and imaging of gadolinium accumulation in human bone tissue by micro- and submicro-XRF. https://core.ac.uk/download/347160714.pdf (accessed on 21st July 2025).
10. Collins, K. M. (2014). Visual and geometric analysis of maxillary sinus region variability for identification of unknown decedents. https://core.ac.uk/download/267571339.pdf (accessed on 21st July 2025).
11. Curate, F. (2014). Osteoporosis and paleopathology: A review. https://core.ac.uk/download/pdf/151538188.pdf (accessed on 21st July 2025).
12. Curtis, N., Evans, S. E., Fagan, M. J., Jones, M. E., et al. (2009). Visualizing muscle anatomy using three-dimensional computer models–An example using the head and neck muscles of *Sphenodon*. https://core.ac.uk/download/1876869.pdf (accessed on 21st July 2025).

13. Emerson, R. (2023). Digital hair creation for archaeological facial approximation: George Dixon, the last captain of the *HL Hunley*. https://core.ac.uk/download/588290628.pdf (accessed on 21st July 2025).

14. Garcia de Leon Valenzuela, M. J. (2016). Three-dimensional image technology in forensic anthropology: Assessing the validity of biological profiles derived from CT-3D images of the skeleton. https://open.bu.edu/bitstream/2144/15358/1/GarciadeLeonValenzuela_bu_0017N_10802.pdf (accessed on 21st July 2025).

15. Gulhan, O. (2017). Skeletal sexing standards of human remains in Turkey. https://core.ac.uk/download/84591371.pdf (accessed on 21st July 2025).

16. Jayapala, D., & Mathangasinghe, Y. (2024). The prevalence of termination variations of the basilar artery: A systematic review and meta-analysis. https://core.ac.uk/download/642711585.pdf (accessed on 21st July 2025).

17. Jiang, J., Li, C., Shu, G., Xie, Y., et al. (2018). A rapid, non-invasive method for anatomical observations of tadpole vertebrae *in vivo*. https://core.ac.uk/download/199410535.pdf (accessed on 21st July 2025).

18. Kivell, T. L., Lemelin, P., Richmond, B. G., Schmitt, D., et al. (2016). The primate wrist. https://core.ac.uk/download/46164637.pdf (accessed on 21st July 2025).

19. Massa, H. M., Bakr, M. M., & Massey, W. L. (2016). Digital cadavers: Online 2D learning resources enhance student learning in practical head and neck anatomy within dental programs. https://core.ac.uk/download/208034039.pdf (accessed on 21st July 2025).

20. McHenry, C. R., Barnes, D. G., Quayle, M. R., & Kaluza, O. L. (2014). An interactive three-dimensional approach to anatomical description—The jaw musculature of the Australian laughing kookaburra (*Dacelo novaeguineae*). https://core.ac.uk/download/pdf/26815232.pdf (accessed on 21st July 2025).

21. Nunes, C. V. da S. (2020). A machine learning taxonomic classifier for science publications. https://core.ac.uk/download/395835684.pdf (accessed on 21st July 2025).

22. Plomp, K. A. (2013). Quantifying palaeopathology using geometric morphometrics. https://core.ac.uk/download/16280720.pdf (accessed on 21st July 2025).

23. Stephen, H. (2018). Inferring species origin through virtual histology: A comparison of third metapodials from *Homo sapiens* and *Ursus americanus* using micro-computed tomography. https://core.ac.uk/download/232684509.pdf (accessed on 21st July 2025).

24. Teeter, M. A. (2017). The human first metatarsal in bioarcheological research: New insights into human variation and bone health research from Kellis 2, Dakhleh Oasis, Egypt (50–450 CE). https://core.ac.uk/download/215380959.pdf (accessed on 21st July 2025).

25. Uldin, T. (2017). Virtual anthropology–A brief review of the literature and history of computed tomography. https://core.ac.uk/download/149207482.pdf (accessed on 21st July 2025).

26. Valentine, A., & Valentine, A., Jr. (2017). Archaeology and the computing age. https://core.ac.uk/download/143838323.pdf (accessed on 21st July 2025).

27. Ahmed, F., & Maisano, J. (2017). *ToScA North America (6–8 June 2017, The University of Texas, Austin, TX) Program*. https://core.ac.uk/download/211334283.pdf (accessed on 21st July 2025).

ETHICS AND REPATRIATION IN OSTEOLOGICAL RESEARCH

11

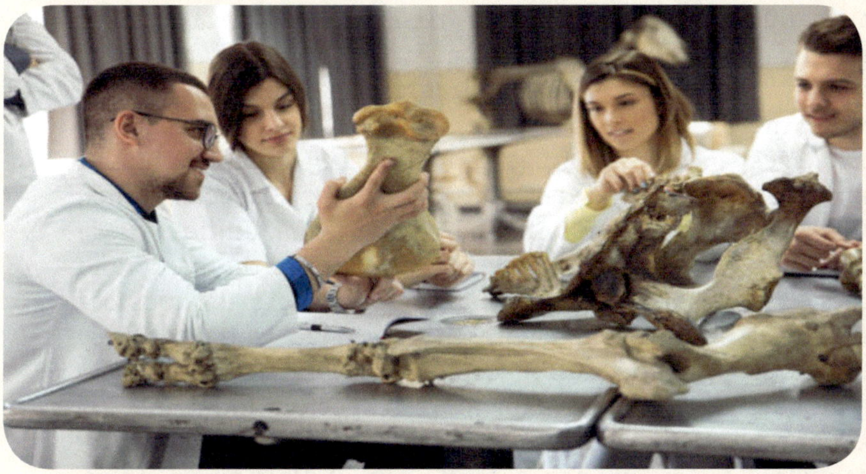

LEARNING OBJECTIVES

After studying this chapter, you will be able to:

1. Discuss the historical context of osteological research
2. Understand ethical considerations in osteological research
3. Explain the legal framework surrounding repatriation
4. Evaluate perspectives of indigenous communities
5. Differentiate scientific value vs. Ethical responsibility
6. Know current trends in repatriation practices

Introduction

Increased sophistication in osteological research has heightened the demand for basic ethical concerns, given their relevance to repatriation. For decades, the study and examination of skeletons have been involved in controversial practices that constitute broader society debates on race, heritage, and identity. Previously, indigenous exhumations and desecration of remains symbolized a racially symbolic theme that defined academic discourse, most notably anthropology and archaeology. As such practices have increasingly fallen under the radar, legal frameworks like the Native American Graves Protection and Repatriation Act (NAGPRA) have given indigenous people power to reassert their cultural selves. This has transformed the context for archaeological study, providing indigenous voices with a voice to challenge historical wrongdoing and redefine stories around their ancestral remains (Bourgault et al., 2011). Contemporary controversies in osteological research are polarized, with the tensions lying beneath between indigenous rights and scientific endeavor. While proponents of repatriation argue that it encourages ethical scholarship and respects cultural sovereignty, they argue that scientific access to human remains is essential for knowledge building. This epistemological divide reflects divergent philosophies about the value of human remains, as Western scientific paradigms typically oppose indigenous notions in which ancestral spiritual and historical connections are of most significant importance. The complexities are compounded by the fact that, despite two decades of legal repatriation efforts, thousands of indigenous peoples continue to exist in the face of institutional denial by government and academic institutions, thereby complicating the discourse on rights and ethical responsibilities in research processes (Kakaliouras et al., 2012). Navigating these complex ethical issues, it is imperative to establish a framework that balances recognition of indigenous peoples' rights with a recognition of the benefits of osteological work. The search for knowledge must never constitute the predominant aspect over respect for cultural values and historical preservation; instead, it should instill cooperative frameworks that entwine indigenous worldviews into the research process. As such discussions are undertaken, researchers and anthropologists are in immediate need of engaging in serious consultation and dialogue with indigenous peoples, so that ethical issues would become the focal aspect of their work. Ultimately, success in repatriation within osteological research may lie in bridging cultural gaps and in creating cooperative partnerships that value both scientific inquiry and indigenous sovereignty.

Definition of Osteological Research

Osteological study is the scientific analysis of bones and skeletons in order to learn about human past behavior, health, and cultural practices. It is an interdisciplinary subject that derives from anthropology, archaeology, and medicine by applying methodologies such as bioarcheology and forensic examination in order to make inferences about the lives of individuals and populations. As scientists excavate bones, they try to reconstruct population and social structures, health status, and even potential causes of death in ancient societies. The significance of osteological research lies not only in what it can inform us about the human past, but also in its ethical considerations, particularly regarding the treatment and handling of human remains and the responsibilities researchers have to descendants and Indigenous communities whose ancestors' remains may be at risk for research and display. Despite the intellectual merit of osteological research, delicate handling is required when negotiating the ethical concerns of excavating and analyzing human remains. Cultural sensitivity is necessary, especially when working with Indigenous communities whose cultural beliefs may be against the study and display of their ancestors. These tensions are concerned with the so-called colonial legacy embedded in osteological practice, which has raised calls for more respectful and respectful involvement that is respectful of traditional knowledge systems and Indigenous peoples' rights to their ancestors' remains. Ethical frameworks are essential to the study of osteology, both to right the historical wrongs and to ensure that the knowledge gained through such research does not supersede the ethical obligation of researchers to the communities upon which they work. In addition, the convergence of osteological research with international legal instruments makes the controversies over repatriation and Indigenous peoples' rights a matter of contention. With legal instruments evolving to recognize the unique status of Indigenous peoples and ethnic minorities, such as the Māori in Aotearoa and the Aboriginal people of Canada, increasing pressure is on academic institutions and museums to reconsider their collections of human remains and associated items. This adjustment emphasizes the value of dialogue among researchers and Indigenous people, as it encourages the discussion of ethical practices that prioritize repatriation and the return of ancestral remains. As there is a growing established law protecting traditional knowledge and cultural heritage, the merit of ethical concerns continues to escalate in the world of osteological studies, compelling researchers to examine their practices and the impact their research will have on ancestral genealogies and community identities (Morse et al., 2011; Bourdieu et al., 2014) (Figure 11.1).

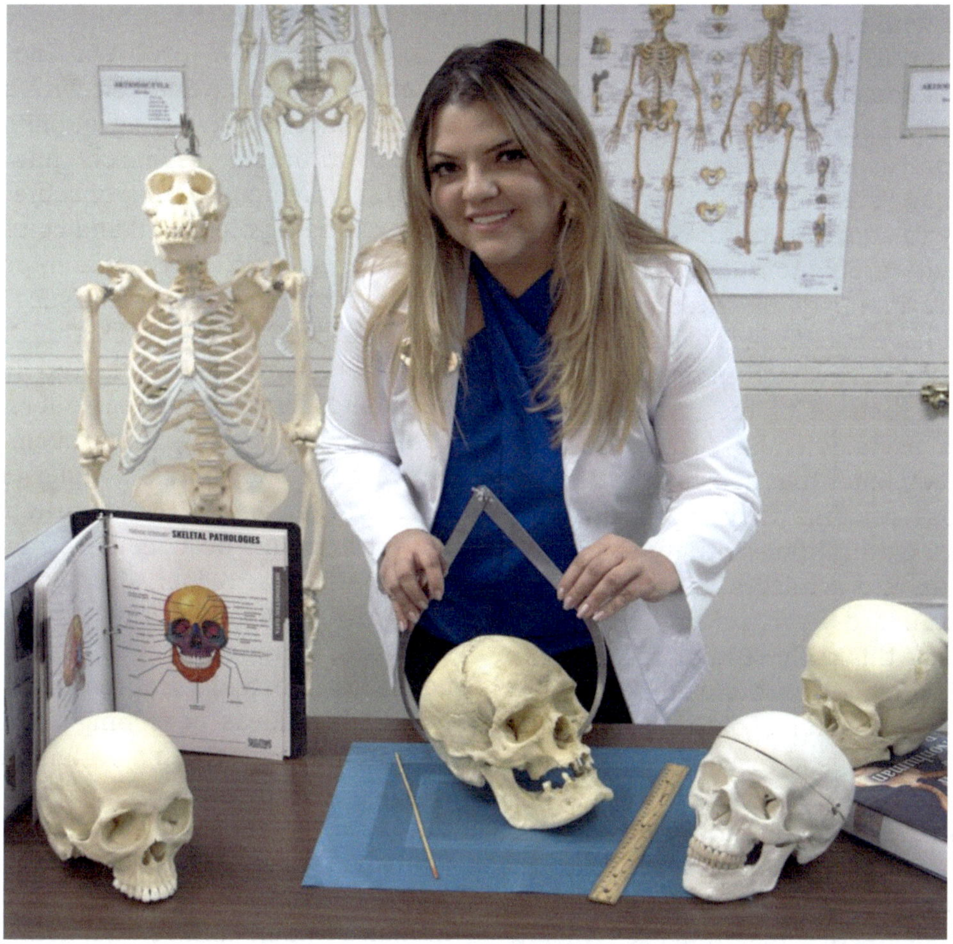

Figure 11.1. Osteological research refers to the scientific study.

Source: https://external-content.duckduckgo.com/iu/?u=https%3A%2F%2Fwww.marylandnature.org%2Fwp-content%2Fuploads%2F2023%2F08%2FAshley-Forensic-Osteology-975x975.jpeg&f=1&nofb=1&ipt=8b8ea3e5c114598eb85a46198d4fef36b7abdc15f2e60fe19e42a3d06d98117c.

Importance of Ethics in Scientific Research

The importance of ethics in scientific research cannot be overstated, particularly in osteological research. Ethics are the foundation of scholarly integrity, and they guide researchers toward knowledge while carefully honoring the individuals and populations from which the biological specimens are drawn. With osteologists utilizing documented human osteological collections (DHOCs), the ethical challenges of collecting, managing, and researching human remains become more complex. This has prompted anthropologists to review their roles in using these collections, particularly regarding their scientific value and the history of the involved remains (Belcastro et al., 2022). Prioritizing ethical concerns not only enables researchers to establish trust and collaborations with descendant groups, but also to a more culturally responsive and respectful science. Ethical considerations must also move beyond the compliance model of legal regimes to capture the moral aspects of research practice. In cremated human remains studies, for instance, it is necessary to address ethical concerns that are traditionally rarely mentioned in scholarly literature. The majority of osteologists and archaeologists have noted a lack of standardized ethical processes, particularly in the excavation, analysis, and exhibition of the remains (N/A, 2025). These exclusions have the effect of precipitating outcomes that demean the dignity of those whose remains they represent, and may constitute cultural insensitivity to groups associated with the artefacts. Emphasized as ethical best standards, particularly in training and consultancy, this truly readies researchers to operate through these demanding arenas, advocating for the position of ongoing education in the field of osteological research. Finally, the implications of ethical research encompass the emerging controversy surrounding repatriation. Repatriation of human remains and artifacts to their original communities is an essential, ethically driven practice that reflects growing sensitivity to the rights of local and indigenous peoples. The ethical imperative for repatriation remains a testament to the responsibilities of researchers to acknowledge historical injustices perpetrated through scientific practices under colonial legacies. In these conditions, reconciling scientific investigation with the preservation of cultural heritage requires sensitivity. Through adherence to ethical practice, researchers can advocate for measures that accommodate both the scientific community's need for information and individuals' entitlement to reclaim their shared heritage. This dual allegiance underscores the foundational role of ethics in shaping a responsible and just future for osteological science.

Overview of Repatriation Issues in Osteological Studies

The repatriation problem in osteological research is also interlinked with ethical issues that impact the handling of human remains. Anthropological research has long used DHOC, which are indispensable sources for understanding biological and cultural diversity. However, such reliance raises important ethical issues, more particularly on issues of ownership and treatment of these remains. The scientific value of research on osteological materials must be balanced with ethical considerations in their collection, especially when such remains can be traced to indigenous peoples. Scholars who have worked on DHOC have noted that such matters should be considered ethical issues, highlighting the responsibility that researchers have both in conducting the research and disseminating the findings. With ongoing advances in osteological research, the need for ethical standards governing the treatment of human remains remains paramount (Belcastro et al., 2022). Additionally, repatriation of ancestral remains has been a focal point in the controversy between indigenous peoples and scientific communities. Attempts to repatriate human remains and related artifacts to Native Americans and other indigenous peoples usually encounter a system that is multilayered and multifaceted in its complexity of cultural heritage concerns. Despite legal structures for repatriation being in place for more than two decades, ongoing tensions persist between anthropologists and repatriation advocates. The epistemological divide between Western scientific and indigenous traditions makes it difficult to negotiate mutually beneficial agreements that account for the handling of human remains. Anthropologists are thus obliged to reconcile discrepant worldviews, with a dialectic that gives dignity to indigenous people's values while enhancing scientific inquiry. This silent interplay is critical in forging a more moral alignment between the scientific community and indigenous peoples, as the value of respecting the remains of ancestors becomes increasingly recognized (Kakaliouras et al., 2012). In considering repatriation issues in osteological research, technological innovation also plays a critical role. New imaging techniques and non-destructive technologies have revolutionized how scientists can analyze human skeletons without physically interfering. This technological innovation enables more respect for ethical concerns such that bone materials can be scrutinized with less destruction of cultural heritage. With these new techniques, scientists can achieve their scientific objectives while resolving the ethical problems associated with traditional osteological research. The use of new technologies not only enhances our understanding of biological profiles but also aligns scientific practice more closely with ethical requirements, ultimately resulting in a more respectful and fair debate around repatriation and the treatment of human remains (Belcastro et al., 2022) (Figure 11.2).

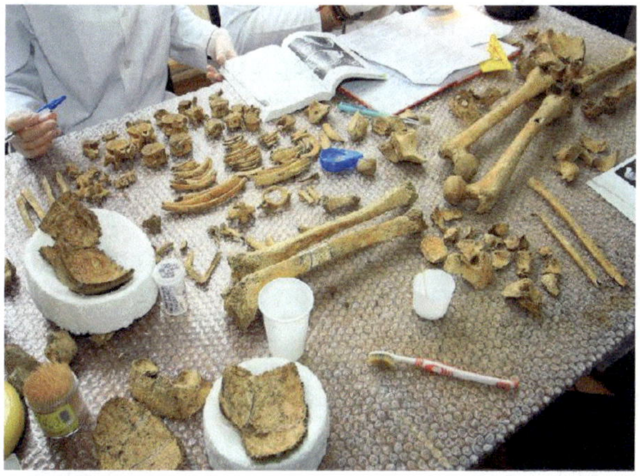

Figure 11.2. The issue of repatriation in osteological studies.

Source: https://www.archaeological.org/wp-content/uploads/2019/03/lab1_0.jpg.

11.1. Historical Context of Osteological Research

Learning Outcome

1. Development of osteological research practices
2. Historical treatment of human remains
3. Case studies of repatriation in different cultures

A history of osteological research is characterized by a complex equilibrium between scientific research and ethical practice, in particular, how people are treated. The discipline started at a period when colonialism was dominant, and so were overarching hypotheses regarding races, which simplified the natives by dehumanizing them. Early archaeologists and anthropologists would dig up and excavate human skeletons without the consent of the descendants, seeing only such relics as items of interest and not respecting their cultural and spiritual significance. Such a lack of care was the foundation for present ethical controversies regarding human remains repatriation, calling for the recognition of past injustices and cultural sensitivities. As researchers study the history of osteological studies, the need for an equitable approach comes with a priority of referring to native peoples in determining the fate of their ancient remains. The signing into law of the Native American Graves Protection and Repatriation Act (NAGPRA) of 1990 was a significant milestone toward solving the ethical shortcomings of osteological studies and the treatment of human remains. NAGPRA not only gave a legal framework to the repatriation of ancestral human remains to Native American communities but also raised the indigenous voice to participate in discourses about their cultural heritage. This legislative attempt was an effort to end the historical injustices resulting from anthropological procedures that tended to overlook indigenous rights and perspectives.

Additionally, NAGPRA led the researchers to rethink how they engage with communities from which remains are being extracted, fostering a more respectful and collaborative relationship. Although the legislation is favorable, continued discussions reveal that the legacy of institutional racism and pillaging continues to jeopardize the anthropology field (Bourgault et al., 2011), and more information about ethics in osteological research must be known despite the advances that have come with NAGPRA, the relationship between indigenous people and anthropologists is characterized by conflict and misunderstanding to this day. Problems typically arise from divergent perceptions of cultural heritage, where Western scientific practice is at odds with indigenous expectations of the sacredness of human remains. Scholars must navigate the epistemological divide because the repatriation process and the construction of cultural heritage remain sources of controversy (Kakaliouras et al., 2012). The issue is not merely repatriating remains but providing a space in which indigenous narratives are valued and incorporated into research methodology. In order to introduce transformative change to the discipline of anthropology, researchers must take the initiative to be involved with indigenous stakeholders, assuming moral ethics that advocate for respect, cooperation, and mutual understanding. Finding equilibrium between scientific interest and cultural sensitivity is important in reconstructing osteological research in a post-colonial world.

11.1.1. Development of Osteological Research Practices

The practice of osteological research has changed significantly in response to ethical concerns and increasing repatriation demands. Conventional osteology, as an anthropological field of study, used to work with human remains with a utilitarian orientation, giving little consideration to the remains' accompanying cultural background. But growing awareness of past injustices experienced by indigenous people was prompting academics to re-evaluate their methods and the implications of their work. Lawful contexts, such as the Native American Graves Protection and Repatriation Act (NAGPRA), have also encouraged the shift, prompting researchers to forge collaborations with indigenous peoples. Through recognition of profound cultural and religious connections that connect living descendants and ancestors, osteological practice began integrating ethical concerns into its paradigms of research, opening the way for a more socially responsible and respectful methodology for researching human remains (Bourgault et al., 2011). Informed by changing values in society, osteological research has begun to embrace a more holistic valuation of cultural heritage, leading to innovative practices that blend scientific investigation and ethical stewardship. Encounters with indigenous knowledge systems have raised issues around ownership and interpretation of the skeleton and related artifacts. For instance, acknowledgment of different worldviews has brought insight to the complexities in repatriation, with many indigenous groups asserting control over ancient remains. Debate among anthropologists and indigenous representatives challenges hegemonic academic norms, compelling scholars to close the epistemological gaps that tend to hinder reciprocal understanding. The ongoing debates regarding repatriation rights highlight the importance of osteologists critically assessing their roles as custodians of cultural heritage while engaging in an enriching, multidisciplinary discussion that respects diverse perspectives (Kakaliouras et al., 2012). Second, the development of osteological practices is marked by a dynamic legal and ethical climate that encourages proper treatment of human remains. Repatriation campaigns not only put indigenous rights and needs into the limelight but also compel researchers to adopt practices of responsibility and transparency. Ethical research requires osteologists to adopt collaborative approaches, often involving consultation with affected communities. Such a paradigm shift is evidence of recognition that scientific knowledge production occurs within social contexts, with cultural values given priority. As the field works to continue addressing its past legacies, the integration of ethical values into osteological practice must remain a priority for a fairer future—where indigenous peoples are heard and valued as part of the broader cultural heritage (Bourgault et al., 2011) (Figure 11.3).

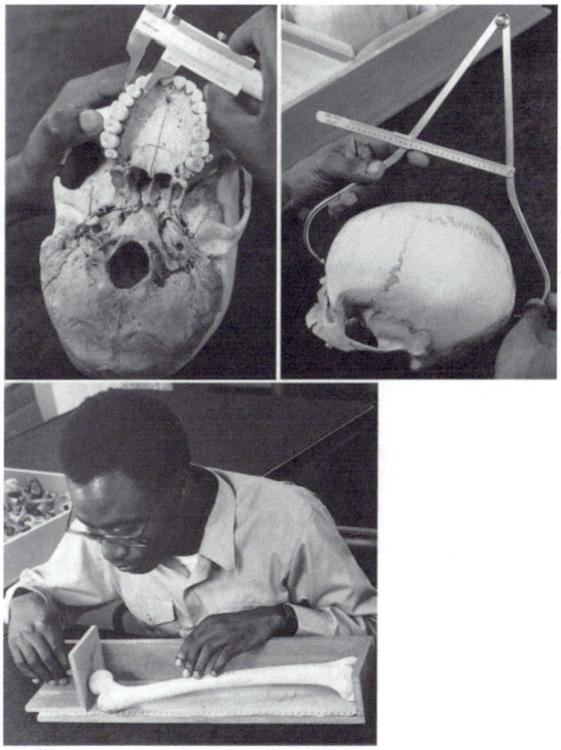

Figure 11.3. The evolution of osteological research practices.

Source: https://ars.els-cdn.com/content/image/3-s2.0-B9780120884674500211-f18-05-9780120884674.jpg.

11.1.2. Historical Treatment of Human Remains

Historically, the treatment of human remains is rich with cultural contradictions and ethical challenges, particularly in osteological investigation. For centuries, osteology has been under the grip of Western scientific epistemologies that tend to treat skeletal materials solely as objects of research. It tends to disregard the religious and cultural significance that these remains have in common with the indigenous people and thus leads to worldwide practices of non-consensual disinterment and study. The heritage of colonialism in anthropological practice has fashioned a complex dynamic between scientists and the peoples whose human remains are being removed. It has generated deeply ingrained insecurities that emphasize the need for ethical strategies in osteological research, because any technique that does not consider the cultural contexts of such remains will be obligated to imitate historical oppressions and disenfranchise descendant groups (Kakaliouras et al., 2012). With legislation such as the Native American Graves Protection and Repatriation Act (NAGPRA) on the horizon, the debate regarding the repatriation of human remains has shifted toward an ever-more inclusive paradigm recognizing the rights of indigenous peoples. NAGPRA has resulted in the repatriation of ancestral remains to Native American tribes so that indigenous peoples can reclaim their heritage and take control of the treatment and display of their ancestors. This legal system has not only reformed archaeological practice but also prompted researchers to rethink their methodologies and approach in dealing with human remains. Anthropologists' collaboration with indigenous peoples sheds light on a paradigm shift towards the treatment of human remains, with more focus on honoring cultural identity and historical narrative within scholarly discourse (Bourgault et al., 2011). Despite advancements towards equitable treatment of human remains, there remain significant problems in overcoming the conflicting perceptions of Western science and indigenous societies. There remains an epistemological divide between these practices that creates barriers to comprehension of one another and respect for each other's perspectives, particularly in repatriation of remains discussions. The legacy of racism and mistreatment within archaeology has created continuing suspicions from indigenous individuals regarding the intentions of anthropological inquiry. While repatriation is a critical tool for redressing past wrongs, at times it does not significantly shift the dynamics of researcher-indigenous people relationships. Integrating these worldviews is essential to developing an ethical path for osteological research, enabling a dialogue that honors the richness of cultural heritage while facilitating scholarly advancement (Kakaliouras et al., 2012).

11.1.3. Case Studies of Repatriation in Different Cultures

Repatriation case studies across cultures illuminate the ethical challenges and moral complexities of osteological research. The repatriation of Native American skeletons in the United States via the Native American Graves Protection and Repatriation Act (NAGPRA) is a quintessential example of the problematic relationship between indigenous groups and anthropological institutions.

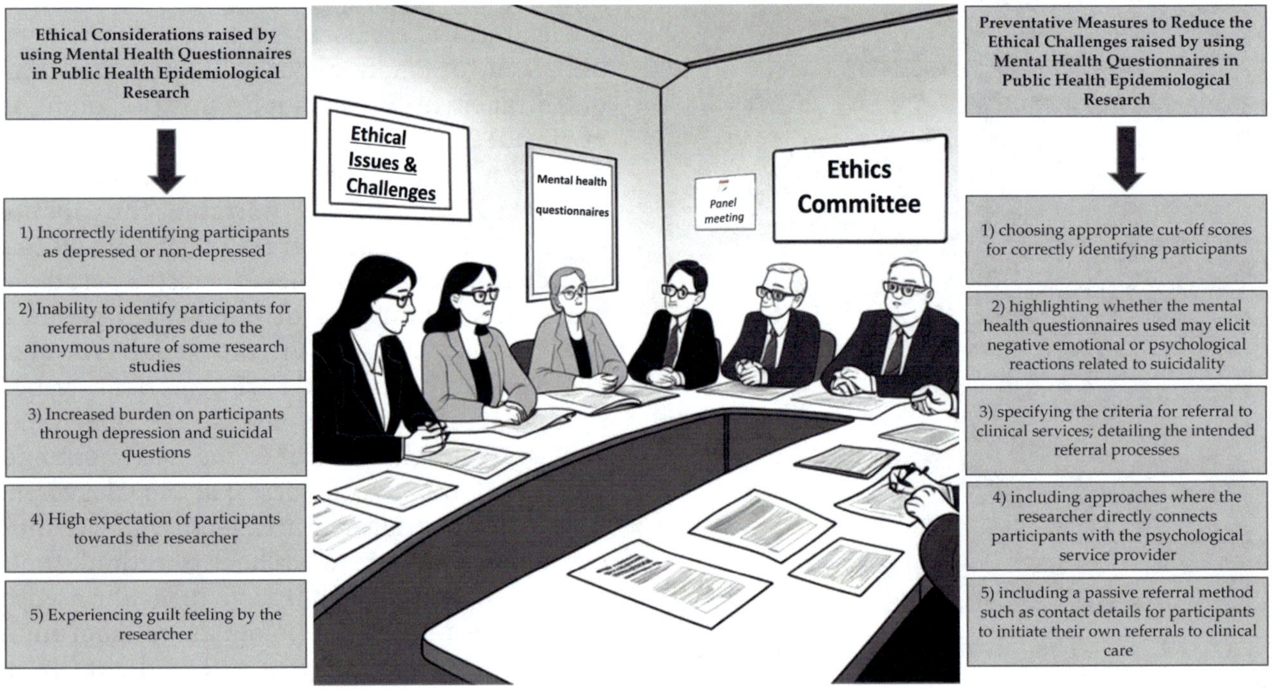

Figure 11.4. The moral complexities and challenges inherent in osteological research.

Source: https://pub.mdpi-res.com/nutrients/nutrients-17-00715/article_deploy/html/images/nutrients-17-00715-ag.png?1739860166.

The act is a testament to the enduring legacy of colonialism's impact on indigenous cultures and identities. While NAGPRA has been around for over two decades, there are still many conflicts, in part due to the various world vision's regarding ancestral remains between Western anthropologists and Native Americans. Such persistent conflict points to the necessity of cooperation and communication as well as recognition of indigenous peoples' rights to their heritage. As noted in the relevant literature, bridging this epistemological gap is important for fostering mutual understanding and respect in repatriation processes (Kakaliouras et al., 2012). International repatriation processes also introduce dynamic legal frameworks that acknowledge indigenous rights worldwide. In countries like Aotearoa New Zealand and Canada, the juridical status of Māori and Aboriginal people has dramatically shifted, impacting how institutions operate through the intricacies of cultural heritage and osteological investigation. The systems have ensured an environment in which indigenous people have been able to exercise their right to repatriate biological and cultural material. For example, in Aotearoa, the repatriation of Māori remains has involved not only legal procedures but also cultural reconciliation between institutions and communities. The legal recognition of self-determination by indigenous peoples has driven museums, libraries, and archives to redefine their operations, thereby becoming more sensitive and respectful towards repatriation (Morse et al., 2011). This shift reflects growing awareness of the importance of indigenous perspectives in anthropology. In addition, the repatriation practices case studies reflect broader ethical considerations for osteological research in a multicultural society. Consideration of these cases shows that effective repatriation requires advanced sensitivity to the cultural values of human remains in various societies. Although scientific analysis of osteological material is informative regarding the human past, the determination of such remains as lived performances of ancestral identities necessitates a shift in the ethical framework governing research practice. Scientists must grapple with the responsibility of honoring the wishes of descendant groups and the repercussions of laying bare their personal histories in their work. Being involved in collaborative research that is respectful of the cultural dimensions of repatriation can significantly enhance the ethical framework of osteological research as well as promote a more comprehensive model for studying human history and identity (Kakaliouras et al., 2012) (Figure 11.4).

Test Your Knowledge

1. How has osteological research developed historically from early studies to modern practices?
2. Who were the key figures in the historical development of osteology, and what were their contributions?

11.2. Ethical Considerations in Osteological Research

Learning Outcome

1. Respect for cultural heritage
2. Informed consent and community involvement
3. The role of ethical guidelines and institutional review boards

The ethical issues in osteological research are paramount, particularly regarding the repatriation of human remains. Researchers must navigate a complex matrix of historical injustices and cultural sensitivity when handling skeletal collections, particularly documented human osteological collections (DHOC). These data aggregates are critical for understanding human cultural and biological diversity, yet their ethical application must be weighed extremely carefully. The University of Bologna's DHOC case study emphasizes the need for anthropologists to factor not only scientific value but also ethical considerations into their research methodology. The need for a balance between advancing the horizons of knowledge and respect for cultural heritage is of utmost importance because individuals only trust the research community if they can be assured that human dignity is not offended at any point during the research (Belcastro et al., 2022). The renewed interest in the study of archaeological cremated human remains introduces one more ethical aspect. While such labor puts another layer of knowledge about the communities of earlier times, it also raises questions about the excavation, examination, and preservation of these remains. Ethical concerns also result from the manner in which cremated remains are handled, but by virtue of the type of damage that misrepresentation or incompetence can do to descendant communities.

As seen in today's literature, a lack of open debate on the ethical treatment of cremated remains further clouds these matters (N/A, 2025). Practitioners of archaeology and osteology, thus, must incorporate ethics training into their professional development to develop a culture of respect and accountability when dealing with human remains of cultural importance. Finally, establishing uniform ethical standards for osteological research is essential in upholding sound care for human remains. Professional organizations should set the pace in developing particular guidelines that demystify the intricacies surrounding the excavation, storage, and display of cremated and non-cremated human remains.

These guidelines should incorporate intensive ethics training for researchers and practitioners alike, prioritizing cultural sensitivity and cooperative engagement with communities connected to the remains. Emphasis on ethical practice in osteological research can engender trust and facilitate more equitable conversation between scientists and cultural stakeholders. This approach, in addition to enhancing the integrity of research, also contributes to the broader agenda of reconciliation and respect for human dignity in scientific practice (N/A, 2025).

11.2.1. Respect for Cultural Heritage

Respect for cultural heritage is at the forefront of the debate regarding ethical issues in osteological study, as regards repatriation. The prehistory of archaeology and anthropology is marked by a cycle of looting and cultural insensitivity that has all too often disregarded the wishes and sentiments of indigenous peoples. The passage of the Native American Graves Protection and Repatriation Act (NAGPRA) is a turning point, which allows indigenous peoples to reclaim their cultural artifacts and ancestors' remains. This legislation not only provides a place to heal through culture but also emphasizes the value of cooperation among archaeologists, anthropologists, and Native American people, thereby making archaeology an ethical and respectful practice that honors cultural heritage (Bourgault et al., 2011). Furthermore, the ongoing complexities of repatriation highlight the necessity of balancing alternative worldviews regarding cultural heritage. The conflict between anthropological research goals and indigenous people's rights highlights an inherent ethical conundrum of osteological research. Since repatriation movements have been legally warranted for more than two decades, controversies remain regarding the consequences of such activities for scientific research and cultural conservation. The closure of the epistemological divide between Western scientific methods and indigenous wisdom requires a radical shift in how anthropologists frame their endeavors. About the significance of ancestral remains and artifacts as symbols of social power and identity, it is vital to guarantee a more inclusive culture of cultural heritage in research settings (Kakaliouras et al., 2012). Ultimately, the discussion of respect for cultural heritage in osteological research must transcend legal concepts and encourage genuine collaboration between researchers and indigenous peoples. This would mean not just meeting the near-term needs of repatriation but also opening space for listening to indigenous voices within the research process itself. By actively promoting Native Americans' involvement in determining their cultural heritage, the discipline of anthropology can transform itself into a more responsible, informed, and responsive science. By doing so, the discipline can engage in a mutually respectful conversation, appreciative of the cultural heritage, to ensure that the heritage of the past does not dominate the rights and beliefs of the current indigenous people (Bourgault et al., 2011; Kakaliouras et al., 2012) (Figure 11.5).

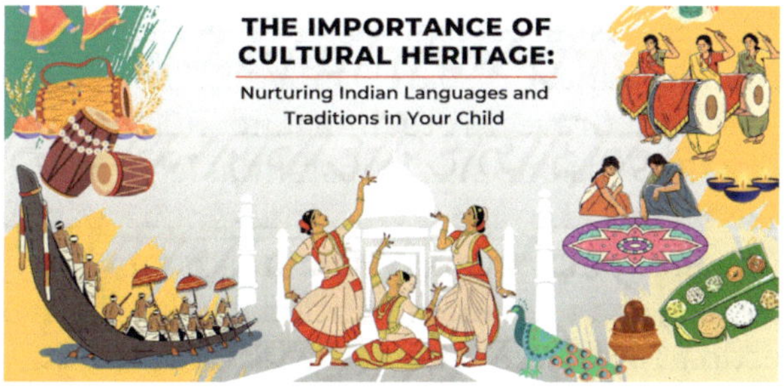

Figure 11.5. Respect for cultural heritage.

Source: https://k-12experts.com/wp-content/uploads/2024/07/The-Importance-of-Cultural-Heritage-Nurturing-Indian-Languages-and-Traditions-in-Your-Child.png.

11.2.2. Informed Consent and Community Involvement

In osteological research, informed consent is a core component that prioritizes ethical practice, particularly the return of human remains. Obtaining informed consent is not merely a legal procedure; it requires active engagement and communication with affected populations. These populations are likely to have strong cultural affinities with the remains, and it is important that they be consulted to ensure that decisions based on their values and customs are followed. Since the law continues to evolve, particularly regarding Indigenous peoples' rights, researchers must keep pace with this by recognizing the unique legal position of Indigenous peoples, such as the Māori in Aotearoa and Aboriginal peoples in Canada. By assigning high value to informed consent, researchers not only adhere to ethical standards but also have a working style rooted in mutual respect and understanding (Morse et al., 2011). Community involvement broadens the concept of informed consent into a general context of participation and collaboration. Active participation of local communities in decision-making allows researchers to establish more meaningful and respectful partnerships. The different aspects of research, such as study design, data interpretation, and the final treatment of remains, should be integrated. The interdisciplinarity approach to working with human remains by contemporary researchers allows for a plurality of perspectives, incorporating the expertise of archaeologists, anthropologists, conservators, and the indigenous people themselves. In addition to refining the research, this cooperation facilitates a full appreciation of cultural sensitivities and moral issues, ensuring that the treatment and exhibition of remains align with the wishes of local stakeholders (Clark et al., 2010). Lastly, the integration of informed consent and community involvement has the potential to reshape the landscape of osteological scholarship by creating ethics attentive to the complexity of cultural heritage. As institutions wrestle with historical grievances surrounding the taking of human remains, such concepts formalize a shift toward restorative practice. By enforcing a robust framework of consent and community engagement, researchers can help promote healing processes among traumatized communities and provide a platform for recognizing and respecting cultural histories. This paradigm shift affects not only the repatriation of remains but also sets the tone for ethical research practices across every field, as it establishes the paramount need for collective action to reverse historical injustices in osteological research (Clark et al., 2010; Morse et al., 2011).

11.2.3. The Role of Ethical Guidelines and Institutional Review Boards (IRBs)

The complexity of osteological research necessitates a well-defined framework of ethical guidelines and IRBs to ensure responsible practice in the collection and handling of human remains. This framework is a safeguard not only for the dead's dignity but also for living populations associated with the remains. Since educational institutions are struggling to comprehend the ramifications of their possessions, ethical governance is vital for formulating effective strategies that remain sensitive to cultural interests. IRB decisions are predominantly influenced by changing moral norms, and their work is to examine proposals for research in accordance with ethical principles. With heightened sensitivity to the handling of human remains, IRBs are obligated to scrutinize the procurement methods and purposes of such material, thereby maintaining respect, accountability, and integrity in research. Furthermore, the incorporation of ethical standards has emerged as a top priority in defining the dynamics of interaction between researchers and Indigenous groups, especially about repatriation attempts. Historical practices have excluded mainly the voice and rights of such groups, including widespread ethical abuses in the treatment of their ancestors' remains. There is growing pressure on institutions to incorporate Indigenous stakeholders' voices into decision-making regarding osteological collections. The standards written by the American Association for Anatomy within its Legacy Anatomical Collections Task Force are evidence of this shift in focus through the institution of ethical guidelines that set forth the importance of provenance research and community engagement in the management of legacy collections (Champney et al., 2024). By such measures, ethical standards provide a framework for researchers to tread sensitive terrain in osteological analysis, promoting respect and cooperation with individuals whose remains are directly affected. For North American bioarcheology, legal frameworks and cultural resource legislation have begun to redefine ethical research practice. The Native American Grave Protection and Repatriation Act of 1990 is one such substantial legal change that values the agency of Indigenous people over ancestral remains (Hamilton et al., 2004). This act, and the more intentional application of Section 106 of the National Historic Preservation Act, illustrate how altered regulation can impose controls necessary to scientific practice, challenging scientists to reconsider their ends and means. The dialogue between Indigenous peoples and bioarcheologists is key to resolving historical injustices and reconfiguring the terms of the cultural heritage-science relationship. Compliance with these shifting ethical norms requires researchers to create collaborative strategies that prioritize the voices and wills of living Indigenous people and the dead individuals they hold in respect from an ethical standpoint.

Test Your Knowledge

1. Why is it important to follow ethical guidelines when conducting osteological research on human remains?
2. What ethical issues must be considered in the collection, analysis, and display of skeletal specimens?

11.3. Legal Framework Surrounding Repatriation

Learning Outcome

1. National laws regarding the treatment of human remains
2. International treaties and agreements
3. Case law examples influencing repatriation efforts

In the contemporary discourse on the repatriation of osteological remains, a robust legal framework has emerged that addresses the complex interplay among indigenous rights, cultural heritage, and ethical considerations. At its foundation are international agreements such as the United Nations Declaration on the Rights of Indigenous Peoples, which articulates the rights of indigenous peoples to their cultural heritage and self-determination. This legislative trend reflects a growing acknowledgment of the particular legal status of indigenous peoples, including the Māori in Aotearoa and Aboriginal peoples in Canada, as evidenced by recent research on their rights in their respective nations. This recognition portends not only legal rights but also a shift in the moral landscape, compelling institutions like museums and archives to contend with the implications of their collections and policies for the remains of indigenous forebears (Morse et al., 2011).

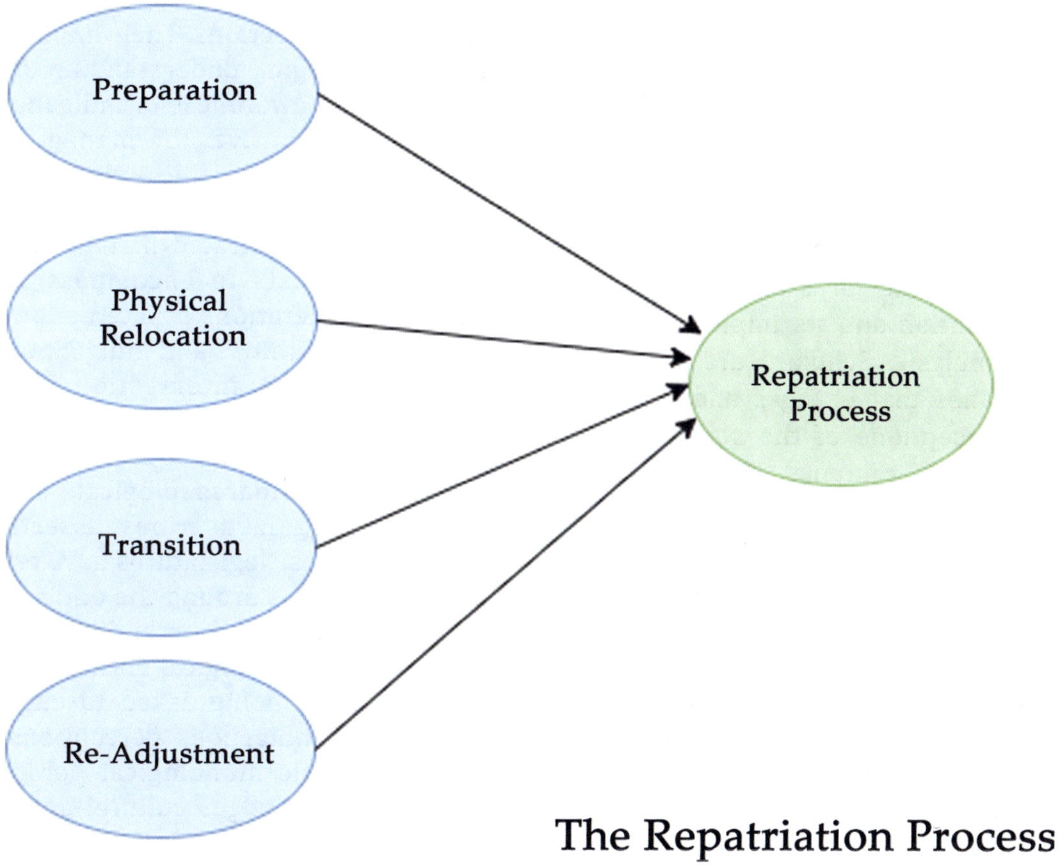

Figure 11.6. The contemporary discourse surrounding the repatriation of osteological remains.

Source: https://i0.wp.com/theintactone.com/wp-content/uploads/2019/02/11.2-r-1.png?resize=414%2C341&ssl=1.

The laws of repatriation are further complicated by divergent worldviews among indigenous peoples and anthropological professionals. While the majority of legal frameworks encourage repatriation as a means to rectify historical injustices, there is also a tension between the scientific world's motives and the spiritual and cultural requirements identified by the indigenous peoples. For instance, the United States' repatriation laws have continually attempted to bridge the gap of epistemology between Western scientific practice and the indigenous worldview. Proponents of repatriation argue that the repatriation of remains to their populations honors both the dead and living generations, thereby promoting reconciliation and healing. However, altering anthropology's long tradition of work with indigenous peoples is difficult, as its relationship with them is typically extractive rather than collaborative (Kakaliouras et al., 2012).

Moreover, with the law constantly changing, new theoretical frameworks are emerging to redefine repatriation and its implications for osteological analysis. Scholars are urging a dynamic response that engages and respects indigenous conceptions of the social power and subjectivity of remains. This emergent discourse seeks to address the imbalance between academic fascination with osteological research and the cultural significance of remains within indigenous societies. Through the negotiation of these alternative frames, scholars and indigenous representatives can partner to develop an inclusive and ethically sound repatriation process. The issue is one of balancing legal principles with cultural values so that repatriation meets legal standards but also addresses the ethical needs of indigenous knowledge systems (Kakaliouras et al., 2012) (Figure 11.6).

11.3.1. National Laws Regarding the Treatment of Human Remains

The treatment of human remains is greatly influenced by national law, which reflects society's values regarding cultural heritage and ethics. In America, the Native American Grave Protection and Repatriation Act (NAGPRA) of 1990 is a landmark law that informs the repatriation of ancestral remains of Native Americans and their associated cultural objects. This legislation helped federally recognized tribes regain human remains and objects currently held by museums and educational institutions. NAGPRA not only addresses the physical return of remains but also opens up a broader ethical discussion that involves respect for indigenous cultural histories and perspectives, and the honoring of ancestral connections. Their implementation shows an emerging understanding of heritage and increasing awareness of indigenous rights in national narratives of managing human remains, aligning scientific activity with ethical responsibility. National treatment of human remains is a complicated matter that extends beyond legal texts to encompass the socio-political considerations of interaction between scientific communities and indigenous peoples. For instance, the intersection of NAGPRA and Section 106 of the National Historic Preservation Act has put more stringent regulations on bioarcheological study. With federally recognized tribes asserting their sovereignty, these legislatures have established new controversies around the ethical effects of human remains collection and research within the discipline of biological anthropology. Thus, researchers are being asked to engage more actively with indigenous perceptions, moving from a scientific monological perspective to one that acknowledges cultural and historical context. These tensions between obtaining knowledge and honoring cultural heritage are considered in current debates over ownership, identity, and moral responsibilities that researchers owe the indigenous peoples when researching osteological studies (Hamilton et al., 2004). Additionally, the application of domestic legislation creates a complicated landscape that shapes the practices of human remains. Scholars assert that, despite achieving significant legal milestones through repatriation initiatives, these initiatives fail to remold the core relations between indigenous peoples and anthropological sciences. The intransigent epistemological contrasts between the Western scientific tradition and indigenous cognition undermine the implementation of repatriation programs. Furthermore, the problem persists that, even where legal frameworks are favorable to cooperation, far too many indigenous cultures remain excluded from participation in issues about their ancestral remains. Closing this gap requires compliance not only with existing law but also an intention to respect and include indigenous epistemological models within osteology. This collaboration can help to build a more equitable relationship that honors the social power and cultural significance of human remains (Kakaliouras et al., 2012).

11.3.2. International Treaties and Agreements

International agreements and treaties are significant components of the ethical framework for osteological research, particularly regarding the repatriation of human remains and cultural items. These legal regimes are likely to reflect overall societal norms regarding respect for Indigenous rights and cultural heritage. Multilateral treaties, for instance, the United Nations Declaration on the Rights of Indigenous Peoples (UNDRIP), emphasize the need to consult Indigenous peoples when dealing with their heritage and cultural artifacts. These agreements facilitate interactive debates between researchers and those populations whose ancestors are represented in osteological assemblages, such that an environment is created where ethical issues are afforded greater significance than apathetic scientific inquiry. In these respects, adherence to international covenants is not merely a legally binding obligation but also an ethical imperative that requires institutions to revisit their obligation to Indigenous peoples.

The evolution of international law concerning Indigenous rights has continued to emphasize the demand for self-determination and cultural sovereignty. Morse et al. (2011) note that Indigenous peoples are increasingly recognized as having a particular legal status that confers greater autonomy in deciding how their cultural knowledge and remains are handled. This shift has important implications for museums and research institutions, which must navigate the respective legal intricacies of repatriating remains and artifacts in ways that respect the desires and customs of the communities. Its incorporation into osteological research practice demands ongoing dialogue between stakeholders, including policymakers, Indigenous leaders, and researchers.

By adhering to international standards, institutions can enhance their ethical obligation and participate effectively in the repatriation process, thus acknowledging the historical injustices committed against Indigenous peoples. Furthermore, repatriation generally occurs through formal treaties and voluntary agreements that attempt to facilitate the return of cultural property to First Nations. As outlined in N/A (2010), these are not just guidelines for negotiation but a commitment to reasserting cultural self-determination and facilitating reconciliation. However, such a process is a complex one and can be subject to various challenges, including clashing legal interpretations and trust problems within the communities. Repatriation of osteological collections is therefore an exercise that must be guided by a nuanced examination of the ethical considerations as well as the legal imperatives involved. Besides this, to ensure repatriated items can be integrated into cultural practice without restriction, institutions must be ready to place the practices and interests of Indigenous people first in their work. By doing this, they can contribute to healing and justice and make the repatriation process supportive of broader cultural revitalization efforts (Figure 11.7).

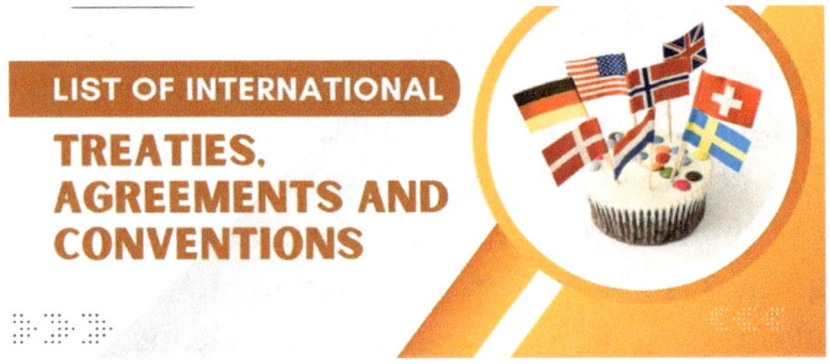

Figure 11.7. International treaties and agreements.

Source: https://pwonlyias.com/wp-content/uploads/2024/11/list-of-international-treaties-agreements-and-conventions-67349fba0573e-1568x882.webp.

11.3.3. Case Law Examples Influencing Repatriation Efforts

The evolving case law landscape reveals the complex dynamics between repatriation activities and the law governing osteological remains. The precedent-setting cases have exposed the ethical dilemmas institutions face in their handling of human remains. Significantly, the Native American Graves Protection and Repatriation Act (NAGPRA) has set out the legal foundation for the repatriation of Native American ancestral remains and cultural items. Through a series of legal proceedings, this legislation has identified the requirement to reconcile scientific interest with Indigenous people's rights to recover their heritage. Legal rulings have been inclined to uphold the requirement for consultation with Indigenous peoples, illuminating persistent conflicts within the field of anthropology, since the necessity for ethical stewardship comes into conflict with scientific interests in investigation and conservation (Kakaliouras et al., 2012). Case law similarly reflects the broader ramifications of Indigenous rights across cultural heritage and traditional knowledge. The application of contemporary judicial precedent has acknowledged that Indigenous peoples possess unique rights that must be respected in national systems. Such cases, invoking the self-determination of Indigenous peoples, have begun to transform the working practices of research institutions and museums. For instance, setting out the legal position of Māori in New Zealand and of Aboriginal peoples in Canada prompted museums to reassess their collections and their ethical responsibilities in the context of repatriation claims. The complexity of these legal narratives reveals the need for museums and anthropologists to engage with repatriation with caution and Indigenous group cooperation, mediating between oppositional epistemologies (Morse et al., 2011). Thus, the role of case law in establishing repatriation efforts is both key and multifaceted, constituting a significant milestone toward the recognition of Indigenous rights in osteological research. Law precedents not only shape the process of repatriation but also compel institutions to adopt an ethical mindset that emphasizes Indigenous perspectives and norms. This evolving legal context complicates the traditionally embedded scientific discourses prioritizing scholarly investigation over Indigenous rights, encouraging more equitable engagement between parties. In addition, ongoing evolution in legal interpretations of repatriation underscores the need for flexibility and responsiveness in research methods. Emerging case law is thus both a force for change and a necessary beacon for addressing ethical concerns in repatriating human remains for osteological research (Kakaliouras et al., 2012; Morse et al., 2011).

Test Your Knowledge

1. What legal frameworks govern the repatriation of human remains and cultural artifacts?
2. How do national and international laws influence the process of returning skeletal remains to descendant communities?

11.4. Perspectives of Indigenous Communities

Learning Outcome

1. Cultural significance of ancestral remains
2. Impact of osteological research on Indigenous identities
3. Voices and advocacy from Indigenous groups

Indigenous communities have been grappling with the repatriation of ancestors and cultural items for centuries. The historical evidence about looting and institutionalized silencing of Indigenous voices in archaeological literature indicates the necessity to undo these injustices. The National Museum of the American Indian Act and the Native American Graves Protection and Repatriation Act (NAGPRA) provide a framework for correcting these wrongs, enabling Indigenous peoples to restore their patrimony. By promoting dialogue and cooperation, these legislative measures not only account for past mistakes but also enable Indigenous perspectives to reshape the discourse surrounding archaeological research. As anthropologists increasingly recognize the significance of these perceptions, ethical scholarship opportunities arise, and a culture emerges in which Indigenous nations are involved in determining the future of their cultural heritage, thereby reorienting fields that have long worked against their rights and assumptions (Bourgault et al., 2011). The need to overcome the epistemological gap between Indigenous worldviews and Western scientific approaches stands as central in repatriation. While NAGPRA has served as a legal response to justice, the social and cultural significance of repatriation extends far beyond legal considerations. Native people possess unique worldviews that shape their definition of cultural heritage, which diverges appreciably from Western paradigms. This raises problematic issues of ownership and stewardship of remains and artifacts. Thus, Indigenous activists and anthropological experts must collaborate so that better appreciation of Indigenous knowledge systems can be developed. This can potentially yield new theoretical instruments that cross conventional anthropological work, ultimately enabling a more equitable repatriation debate that honors Indigenous beliefs and practices (Kakaliouras et al., 2012). As Indigenous voices increasingly dominate conversations about cultural heritage, the potential for reconfiguring anthropological methods and orientations is within reach. Recognition of the active social agency of cultural remains necessitates reconsidering research design and ethical regulation in osteological research. By putting Indigenous voices at the forefront of research design, researchers can develop additional understanding of how cultural heritage shapes identity, history, and kinship. This approach also speaks to contemporary calls for ethical guidelines that prioritize consent, respect, and cooperation. Ultimately, positioning the repatriation process from an Indigenous perspective not only honors the past but also creates opportunities for future generations to reconnect with their heritage on worthwhile terms. These shifts in perspective are crucial in trust and reparative relationship building between the Indigenous communities and the broader academic and scientific communities (Bourgault et al., 2011) (Figure 11.8).

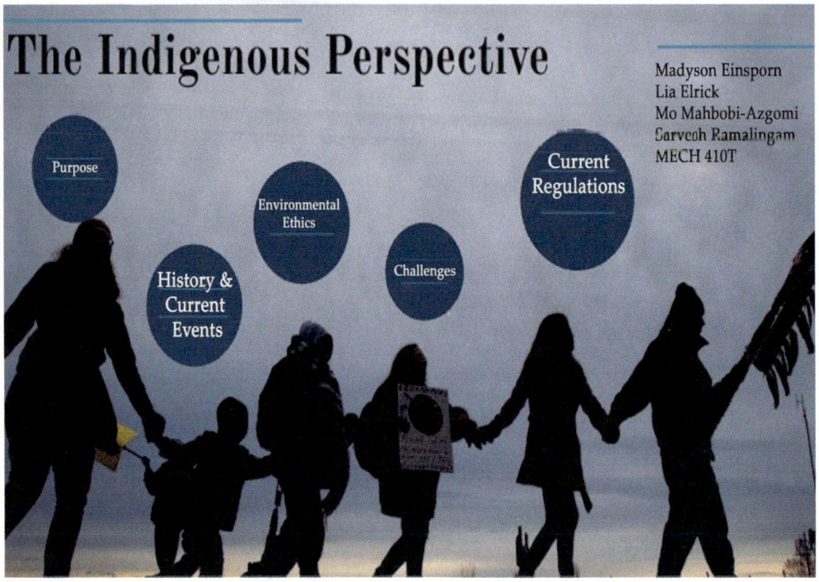

Figure 11.8. Perspectives of indigenous communities.

Source: https://external-content.duckduckgo.com/iu/?u=https%3A%2F%2F0901.static.prezi.com%2Fpreview%2Fv2%2F63txg6alvoihxadtcbvfmfyaql6jc3sachvcdoaizecfr3dnitcq_3_0.png&f=1&nofb=1&ipt=302655628a9642d116f18329bd0d5f06add4946b9c5e3b16899219ea0ed5ed01.

11.4.1. Cultural Significance of Ancestral Remains

The cultural significance of ancestral remains is deeply embedded in the heritage and identity of Indigenous communities. Ancestral human remains are more than skeletal remains; they encompass the legacies, traditions, and cosmologies of the ancestors. For many Indigenous peoples, the remains are a tangible connection to the ancestors, serving as containers of cultural memory that frame their contemporary identities. The ethical issues at play in the repatriation of these remains are increasingly compounded when considering the potential emotional and spiritual impacts for communities that do not view these people as a part of history but rather as family with whom they have a shared history. This perception is one of calling scientific practice into question in the context of osteological research, demanding a dialogue on respect, collaboration, and the recognition of the intrinsic value that ancestral remains hold for Indigenous peoples. The passing of bills, such as the Native American Grave Protection and Repatriation Act (NAGPRA) of 1990, has had a significant influence on the situation of osteological research and bioarchaeology in North America. This legislation was a turning point in the bioarcheologists ' engagement with Indigenous peoples, requiring ethical practice and respect. As painted in the current scholarship, this new dynamic demands scientists alter their practices to honor the cultural integrity of the ancestor remains, most commonly by practicing within collaborative contexts among tribal groups. The increased legal restrictions on the scientific gathering and exploration of these remains reinforce a broader scholarly recognition of Indigenous rights and perspectives. These practice developments highlight the importance of cultural awareness in research, in which the need to probe the past must be balanced with respect for the traditions and beliefs of modern-day communities, as exemplified by the case of the Eastern Band of Cherokee Indians (Hamilton et al., 2004). Also, the encroachment of international law into Indigenous affairs significantly enters into the repatriation processes of ancestral remains and cultural artifacts. Legal frameworks increasingly see the special status of Indigenous peoples, supporting their rights of self-determination and the protection of their traditional knowledge and culture. In Aotearoa and Canada, this has shifted the working protocols of museums, archives, and research institutions, compelling them to respond to Indigenous voices as they manage ancestral remains. Thus, the ethical considerations of osteological research exceed academic interest; they demand recognition of historical injustice and a commitment to make amends through the repatriation of remains. This new context emphasizes the ethical responsibility of scholars and institutions to respect the cultural significance of such remains, vindicating the histories and identities they support in the contemporary world (Morse et al., 2011) (Figure 11.9).

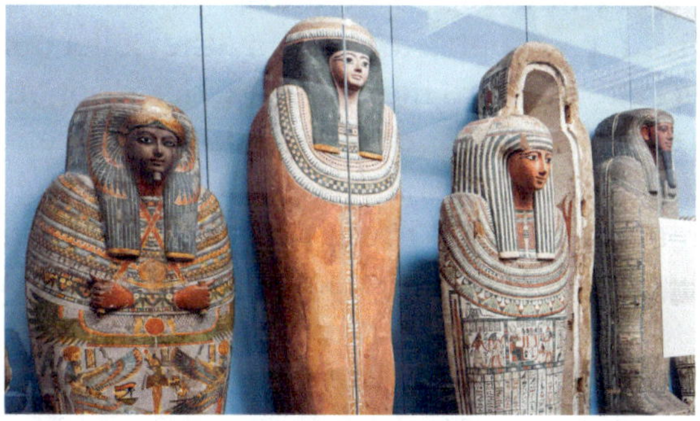

Figure 11.9. Cultural significance of ancestral remains.

Source: https://i.guim.co.uk/img/media/605df9dc3205c5eff80898c28e08b549f1bf46b2/0_0_4031_2419/master/4031.jpg?width=1200&quality=85&auto=format&fit=max&s=36469a1746e83ee9dc86d324d12a3648.

11.4.2. Impact of Osteological Research on Indigenous Identities

The intersection of Indigenous identities and osteological research is a complex and contentious area, most notably within the scope of repatriation. The repatriation of ancestral remains and objects to Indigenous peoples over the past two decades has revealed multiple perspectives regarding cultural heritage. These repatriation endeavors have the propensity to unsettle prevailing Western scientific paradigms, revealing a disconnect between Indigenous epistemology and anthropological knowledge bases. It remains a relevant challenge that while various stakeholders have been in conversation, anthropology's transformative relationship with Indigenous peoples remains yet to be fully actualized. This disparity highlights the imperative of ongoing advocacy and cooperation, representing a turning point in the recognition of Indigenous identities, in that the process of repatriation not only restores remains but also energizes cultural accounts that have been historically silenced (Kakaliouras et al., 2012). In addition, osteological inquiry offers an important framework for considering Indigenous identities in complex ways beyond representation. For instance, studies of skeletal remains can yield dietary evidence, health and demographic trends in Indigenous communities. Scientific examination of this sort can yield a deeper insight into the pre-colonial way of life and the socio-cultural transformation that occurred over time. In some cases, as in ongoing research on African American burial grounds such as the Avondale Burial Place, osteological findings can link living descendants of communities to their ancestors, thereby complementing genealogical data and reinforcing collective identity (Vanderpool et al., 2011). That said, the knowledge obtained through this kind of study must be received with a keen eye towards ethical issues related to information ownership and sensitivity towards Indigenous individuals. Within the general discussion of repatriation, osteological work is a double agent in that it is both a source of information and a point of issue in the debate around ethics. Indigenous people are often in positions where they must reclaim not only their physical remains but also the histories and scientific narratives that accompany them. This reclamation is necessary for the creation of Indigenous identities, which are significantly entangled with ancestral histories and relationships. As guidelines for working together between scientists and Indigenous people become more established, there is growing potential for a more effective exchange of knowledge. This publication is a significant contribution to the recognition of the social power of skeletal remains and material culture, and to the need for respectful cooperation commensurate with Indigenous concepts of heritage and identity (Kakaliouras et al., 2012).

11.4.3. Voices and Advocacy from Indigenous Groups

The voice and advocacy of Indigenous groups are central to the current debate surrounding osteological research and the ethics of repatriation. Historically, the removal of Indigenous ancestral remains has been a manifestation of colonial endeavors, whereby scientists have pursued research at the cost of the cultural significance that such remains hold for Indigenous communities. Presently, the demand from Indigenous people is to recognize their rights to ownership and guardianship of their ancestral remains. Such demands call for ethical principles that challenge traditional scholarly literature and are in favor of reciprocity, respect, and collaboration. By moving forward with their views, Indigenous groups not only reassert agency in the discourse of their heritage but also bring the ethical obligation of researchers and institutions into play to responsibly and reflectively engage with the histories that these remains embody, as can be seen in many scholarly arguments over multidisciplinary practice in the management of human remains (Clark et al., 2010). Moreover, integrating Indigenous perspectives into osteological research enriches the research approach by not only enhancing understanding of human remains but also making it more ethical. It is only through an integrated approach that a more ethical system is achieved about both scientific inquiry and Indigenous heritage. For instance, initiatives like the African Collections Futures project demonstrate how collaborative efforts can illuminate the histories and narratives surrounding collected objects, yielding valuable insights into their origins and cultural significance. By incorporating Indigenous peoples into the decision-making processes for these materials, institutions can create channels for respectful engagement guided by the needs and desires of the peoples, ultimately fostering a more just and equitable research culture (N/A, 2024).

These approaches can establish a model for osteological research, confirming the position of Indigenous advocacy to direct ethical practice. The evolving nature of museum collections and scholarly research underscores the importance of ongoing dialogue between researchers and Indigenous peoples. The interdisciplinary nature of osteological research requires ethical reflection that integrates the perspectives of all stakeholders, particularly minority and Indigenous peoples affected by the collections. This action toward inclusive practice recognizes the significance of combining both science and culture in the examination and reporting of human remains. Through consultation with Indigenous peoples, researchers can ensure that these communities' cultural context and history are permitted to shape the proper management of their ancestors. This is significant, as not only does it enable the process of repatriation but also works to disempower the colonial legacies that have long dominated the discipline of osteology, representing a significant stride toward redemptive justice in terms of heritage management (Clark et al., 2010) (Figure 11.10).

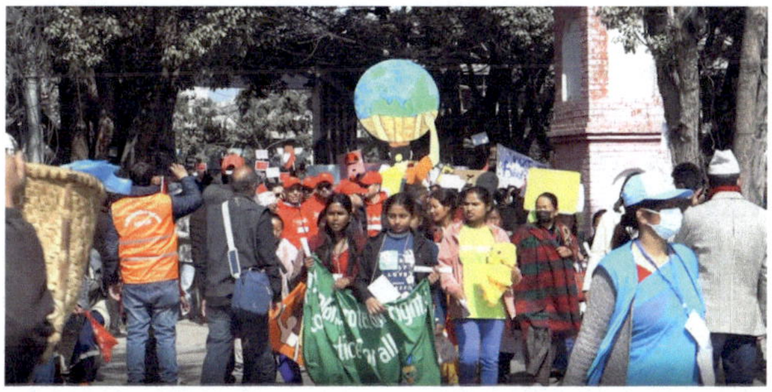

Figure 11.10. The voices of Indigenous groups are pivotal in the ongoing discourse.

Source: https://www.culturalsurvival.org/sites/default/files/inline-images/426720651_264723316661272_565345822577138649_n.jpg.

Test Your Knowledge

1. How do Indigenous communities view the study and handling of ancestral human remains?
2. Why is it important to consider the perspectives of Indigenous communities in repatriation and osteological research?

11.5. Scientific Value vs. Ethical Responsibility

Learning Outcome

1. Balancing research benefits with ethical obligations
2. The role of scientific inquiry in understanding human history
3. Consequences of disregarding ethical standards

In osteological research, the tension between scientific excellence and ethical duty is increasingly pressing. On the positive side, bioarcheological research provides valuable data on the history of human beings, population patterns, and health conditions. The ability to access the analysis of human bones can inform us regarding ancient civilization and inform current medical practices. However, as explained in conversation on the Native American Grave Protection and Repatriation Act, the scientific enterprise generally conflicts with the ethical imperative to respect the dignity and cultural wealth of these remains. It has transformed the character of scientists doing fieldwork from a distance into involvement with Native American tribes to integrate cultural understanding into the science narrative (Hamilton et al., 2004). Thus, ethical considerations have become absolutely paramount to ensuring that research does not exploit past injustices but rather honors the communities from which these remains derive. A further complication in the conflict between scientific worth and ethical obligation arises from the historical process by which human remains have been assembled and deposited. Numerous collections were amassed over time in the absence of the people or their descendant communities, hence raising ethical issues concerning ownership, identity, and respect (Champney et al., 2024). With growing awareness among individuals of the consequences of these collections, researchers are now under greater ethical scrutiny and are therefore considering proper stewardship of legacy anatomical collections. The development of guidelines, such as the Recommendations for the Management of Legacy Anatomical Collections, reflects a general recognition of the ethical obligations researchers have toward affected communities. They prioritize accountability, inquiry into provenance, and working with communities, and, as a result, seek a balanced approach sensitive to ethical issues while also aiming to retain scientific integrity. To balance scientific inquiry with ethical considerations, it is crucial that osteological scientists interact directly with descendant populations at every stage of research, from initial study conception to the ultimate repatriation of the remains. This involvement not only helps to render investigations more culturally appropriate but also permits the incorporation of traditional knowledge that can enhance and complement scientific knowledge. Moreover, an investment in these relations can actually restore trust, which has long been ruined through exploitation in the discipline. Emphasizing openness and dialogue between indigenous groups and researchers can eventually lead to greater morally accountable practice that simultaneously upholds the scientific value of osteological study and the paramount importance of ethical responsibility (Champney et al., 2024; Hamilton et al., 2004). By foregrounding these interactions, the field can become one that honors the richness of human remains and their cultural significance and pursues genuine scientific advancement.

11.5.1. Balancing Research Benefits with Ethical Obligations

The interaction between research gains and ethical obligations in osteological research is necessary, particularly as technology continues to advance and further our methods. The entrance of 3D printing into the field is a good example of this precarious balance. While up to 3D-printed replicas of skeletons have been highly promising for complementing education and forensic work, including within the UK criminal justice system, there are as yet no acceptable solutions to the ethical questions surrounding their use. Without empirical testing of the replicas, outcomes can be misleading of human remains in pivotal legal cases. Consequently, researchers must find structures that give utmost priority to the dignity and respect of the deceased while ensuring that these advancements in technology yield tangible results in other fields, such that they advance a more ethically grounded stance of osteological research (Carew et al., 2021). As the subject of ethical obligations remains a heated topic, it is critical to examine how research practices can have unforeseen impacts on the conservation of skeletal remains. A detailed analysis of the conservation of stored skeletal remains in English museums discovers that access for study can cause deterioration but often less than environmental factors or inadequate storage. This underlines the gravity of the necessity of osteological research with two priorities: obtaining knowledge and maintaining the integrity of the collections. In fulfilling this dual function, researchers not only contribute to the academic community but also strive to advance preservation techniques and secure robust funding to ensure skeletal remains are preserved for possible future use. This equilibrium approach can help reduce ethical dilemmas arising from the meeting of preservation and research (Hughes et al., 2022). As they navigate the complex world of osteological research, researchers are constantly reminded in their attempts to balance the search for knowledge with ethical considerations. This responsibility to ethics extends beyond mere passive adherence to ethical guidelines to active involvement with descendant communities and interested individuals who may hold deep cultural and affective attachments to the remains in question. With cooperation and dialogue, researchers can work towards consent-based research that upholds the wishes of such communities while not forsaking scientific pursuit. All osteological research should ultimately be driven by an ethic of responsibility to ensure that the acquired knowledge does not occur at the expense of dignity or cultural integrity. This ongoing dialogue is at the core of reshaping how osteological research is conducted in response to ethical demands to provide a more equitable and empathetic learning environment.

11.5.2. The Role of Scientific Inquiry in Understanding Human History

Scientific investigation plays a key role in dismantling the complexities of human history, if anything, through the lens of osteological research. By analyzing skeletal remains, scientists can determine vital information about ancient populations, including their health, diet, and social structure. An inquiry of this nature not only illuminates the biological history of humankind but also enlightens us regarding the cultural values and belief systems of ancient societies. However, the ethical issues of this kind of research particularly arise in repatriation contexts, where indigenous peoples often grapple with the scientific construct that has for centuries dominated their histories. The challenge is balancing the scientific value of osteological data with the cultural and religious significance placed on ancestral remains by contemporary indigenous peoples, thereby reasserting the need for an ethical framework when conducting research that respects both scientific inquiry and indigenous ontologies. The passing of such legislations as the Native American Grave Protection and Repatriation Act (NAGPRA) has revolutionized the scope of bioarcheological studies in the United States. According to the act, ancestral remains, along with any related artifacts, must be repatriated to Native American tribes, which provided a significant boost to the ethical aspects of osteological studies. As noted in the shifting dynamics between tribal communities and bioarcheologists , collaboration is increasingly a requirement of ethical research that honors both scientific practice and native knowledge. Researchers are increasingly being asked to generate new scientific paradigms, as in encounters with tribes such as the Eastern Band of Cherokee Indians. Integration of local perspectives into scientific thought not only helps bridge epistemological distances but also recasts the debate on the human past to include neglected voices that would otherwise have been excluded from discourse (Hamilton et al., 2004; Kakaliouras et al., 2012).

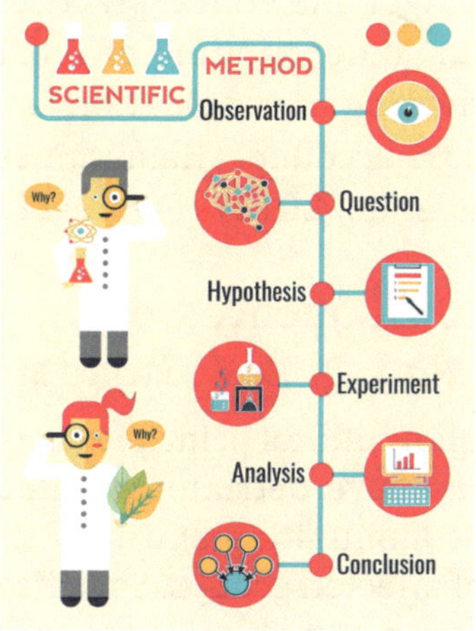

Figure 11.11. The role of scientific inquiry in understanding human history.

Source: https://blogger.googleuse rcontent. com/ img/b/R29vZ2xl/AVvXs EhqHd 2psUTAVqytbN HWPtDf1yfH-G4XzsguUTEQejSKe7x3 RayK5gzoQY6Jlhh6je7zJ5MRGG807kBbT MFo_rFwEHolhMnP6J uyJNvvuRtJcHz9 FbLMeVpvcS2k2F /s2000/scientific- method. webp.

Besides this, the consequences of such ethical factors extend beyond mere compliance with legal frameworks; they confront the very methodologies of anthropology as a discipline. In light of past conflicts between scientific investigation and the human rights of indigenous peoples, a paradigm shift is required to establish genuine partnerships. Scientific practices in the classical sense, long perceived as exploitative, must change to include community consent and cultural sensitivity. By enabling collaborative research practices, bioarcheologists have access to a wider understanding of the circumstances that lie with the skeletal remains and offer a more complete reading of human history. This approach not only benefits the scientific community but also provides richer, more detailed data and helps address long-standing indigenous grievances regarding their cultural heritage and the legacies of their ancestors. Creating dialogues that meet both the demands of scientific rigor and ethical practice ultimately enriches our understanding of human history while cultivating reconciliation and respect across diverse accounts (Hamilton et al., 2004; Kakaliouras et al., 2012) (Figure 11.11).

11.5.3. Consequences of Disregarding Ethical Standards

Failing to follow ethical principles in osteological analysis may have detrimental effects beyond scholastic communities and into the cultural existence of affected groups. Specifically, ethical misconduct can compromise the trust between Indigenous groups and bioarcheologists that is most crucial when they collaborate. The Native American Grave Protection and Repatriation Act of 1990 was a turning point in this relationship that put legal guidelines under which the bioarcheologists work. These guidelines not only restrict the scientific collection of skeletal material from American Indian locations but also highlight the need to respect cultural heritage. Bypassing such ethical guidelines could trigger a backlash from Indigenous populations, leading to the suspension of research opportunities and loss of reputational integrity within the academic community, thereby endangering the future of North American osteological studies (Hamilton et al., 2004). In addition, the balance between ethical requirements and scientific advancements is essential because the progress of fields such as paleopathology relies on a foundation established through mutual respect and understanding. Ignoring ethical standards can negatively impact research results, highlighting the importance for bioarcheologists to accept and address these problems ahead of time. By adopting an ethical standard that foretells cooperative interaction with tribal communities, researchers can formulate a more equitable platform for knowledge sharing. This cooperative framework not only enhances the credibility of research but also honors the cultural standing of the remains studied. Consequently, avoiding ethical practice can yield shallow results, even misrepresenting history and perpetuating scholarly disengagement with groups with ancestral ties to the remains in question (Grauer et al., 2022). In the end, the effects of ignoring ethical practices in osteological research reaffirm the extensive repercussions for academic integrity and social accountability. Dealing with Indigenous populations and adhering to ethical guidelines is not only an educational obligation; it is an ethical requirement that invites reconciliation and acknowledgment. Bioarcheology is at a crossroads where researchers must critically evaluate their practices and effect of their work. By ethical adherence and sensitive collaboration alonecan the field , the field can make a positive contribution to the history books and cultural heritage of Indigenous populations. Therefore, disrespect for ethical values not only impedes scientific advancement but also undermines the profession's credibility, triggering an irrevocable fissure in the faith that is a prerequisite for multilateral endeavors (Hamilton et al., 2004).

Test Your Knowledge

1. How do researchers balance the scientific value of studying human remains with ethical responsibilities?
2. What ethical dilemmas arise when scientific research conflicts with cultural or community values?

11.6. Current Trends in Repatriation Practices

Learning Outcome

1. Successful repatriation cases and their implications
2. Evolving policies in academic institutions
3. The influence of public opinion on repatriation efforts

The evolving climate of repatriation policy is prompted by growing recognition of the ethical issues involved in the handling of human remains in osteological science. Current developments run counter to the exclusive accrual of anthropological data and instead move toward greater sensitivity that honors the wishes and cultural requirements of descendant peoples. This shift indicates broader acknowledgment of historic injustices done to many Indigenous and marginalized groups, particularly with respect to their forebears' remains. As illustrated by such human osteological collections (DHOC) at the University of Bologna, researchers now face the dual challenge of upholding scientific research while respecting the rights and faith of the communities whose remains are being researched. These balancing acts underscore the necessity of open, inclusive communication between researchers and descendant groups to provide mutual understanding and trust in repatriation (Belcastro et al., 2022). Moreover, contemporary repatriation processes have been shaped by legal practices and ethical principles that inform osteological research. Policy implementation involving consultation with Indigenous peoples prior to excavation of remains shows a prominent acknowledgement of rights to claim ownership of the story of their forebears. Over recent years, bioarcheological studies have sought more and more to integrate multi-disciplinary approaches with regard to the cultural significance of remains, as with the multi-isotopic bioarcheological investigation of the Avondale Burial Place. Such research not only restores the past lifestyles but also engages descendant populations to provide them with valuable information regarding their heritage. This shift mirrors the fact that repatriation is no longer a personal decision; instead, it emerges from thoughtful collaboration and a shared purpose among researchers, institutions, and community stakeholders (Vanderpool et al., 2011). The increasing trend towards repatriation is also facilitated by technology's impact on osteological research, which enhances the ability to investigate human remains without physically bringing them into the lab. Advances in imaging techniques, for example, make detailed analysis possible that can act as an alternative to physical desecration of graves. This adaptive research approach aligns with ethical best practice, encouraging minimal damage to ancestral remains during inquiry. In addition, it opens up avenues for training programs that instruct the scholarly community and public on the significance of preserving cultural heritage. As institutions adopt these progressive approaches, the limits of repatriation extend past straightforward return of remains; they encompass a greater commitment to rectifying past wrongs and constructing a more inclusive history of human beings (Belcastro et al., 2022) (Figure 11.12).

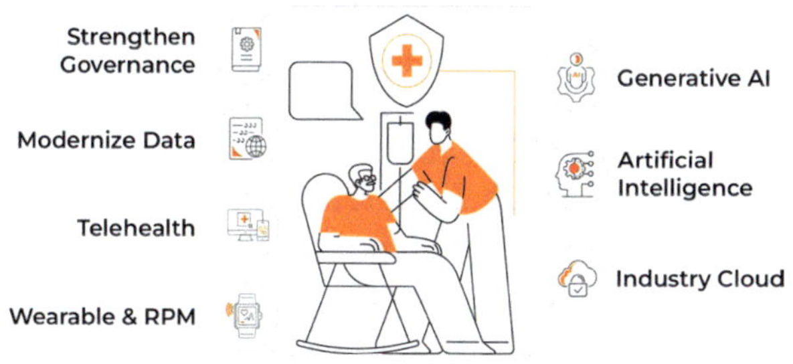

Figure 11.12. The evolving landscape of repatriation practices.

Source: https://automationedge.com/home-health-care-automation/wp-content/uploads/2025/01/Top-7-Healthcare-Trends-to-Watch-for-in-2025_info.webp.

11.6.1. Successful Repatriation Cases and Their Implications

Discourse concerning successful repatriation cases reveals a pivotal confluence of ethics and cultural heritage, particularly in osteological studies. First among these cases is the repatriation of ancestral remains previously held by academic centers or museums. The Native American Graves Protection and Repatriation Act of 1990 was a sea change, forcing the repatriation of such remains to their people. Repatriations that succeed not only redress historical injustices but also serve as potent symbols of indigenous peoples' agency, allowing them to reestablish control over their cultural narratives and spiritual practices. The intricate negotiations of repatriation represent an ethical responsibility to acknowledgment of historical injustice, as well as to the creation of relationships based on mutual respect and understanding. As such, these cases are paradigmatic of repatriation's power to transcend epistemological faultlines and foster social justice in osteological inquiry. In addition, the results of such successful repatriation cases reach beyond local levels to shape national and international policy in bioarcheology and anthropology. The changing legal landscape—demonstrated by the actions of federally recognized tribes under Section 106 of the National Historic Preservation Act—has fundamentally changed the practice of archaeology. As suggested by Hamilton et al. (2004), the development poses risks and opportunities for bioarcheologists to adapt to new legal restrictions and ethical considerations. Cooperation with tribal societies not only enhances the scientific understanding of indigenous societies but also promotes the development of culturally sensitive research protocols. Thereafter, instances of successful repatriation appeal for reconsidering institutional bioarcheological approaches, prompting scholars to engage indigenous voices with active social agency and subjectivity of ancestral remains. In addition, instances of successful repatriation represent a critical shift toward reconceptualizing academia-indigenous peoples' relations. While challenges inherent in bridging the epistemological gap between Western scientific models and indigenous worldviews persist, these positive examples demonstrate the importance of meaningful dialogue and collaboration. Kakaliouras et al. (2012) emphasize the necessity to create theoretical foundations for repatriation that respect the autonomy and heritage of indigenous peoples. Continuing this discussion provokes the reconceptualization of osteological material not only as scientific specimens but also as a vital link to community heritage and identity. Lastly, the process of responding to the consequences of winning repatriation cases creates a critical conversation that can revolutionize both the practice of anthropology and the cultural contexts that it seeks to comprehend.

11.6.2. Evolving Policies in Academic Institutions

Policy reform within academic institutions has been strongly spurred by the growing awareness of moral considerations surrounding the repatriation of osteological material. The reform can generally be attributed to changing sociopolitical forces, in which Indigenous individuals are increasingly demanding the repatriation of ancestral remains and cultural items. As universities face such demands for repatriation, the controversies highlight the imperative of aligning Western scientific practice with Indigenous concepts of cultural heritage. The controversies also reflect a more profound appreciation that science is not immune to cultural bias, and the policies guiding osteological research must change to accommodate such complex worldviews. As such, academic institutions are challenged to restructure their research paradigms to facilitate ethical engagement with Indigenous peoples and uphold their rights to their culture, thereby promoting greater collaborative involvement in osteological research. In an attempt to address emerging global standards and Indigenous activism, academic institutions are adopting significant changes to their osteological research policies. The Native American Grave Protection and Repatriation Act was codified in 1990, marking a turning point with a legal mandate to repatriate human remains to Native American tribes. This legislative shift is a significant turning point in the anthropology-Indigenous people dynamic because it began pressuring schools to question their practices of collecting and the ethics of their own research. As outlined in recent studies, the enactment of new cultural resource legislation reflects mounting calls for higher education institutions to adopt more ethical and respectful research methods with Indigenous peoples.

By upholding these legal guidelines, institutions are not only safeguarding Indigenous rights but also closing the intellectual gap between researchers and tribal peoples, thereby enriching both fields. Moreover, the form of the encounter between Indigenous peoples and bioarcheologists is evolving due to the nature of scholarly policies that prove a collaborative model in osteological analysis is necessary. The use of Section 106 of the National Historic Preservation Act demonstrates that federally recognized tribes are taking greater control over archaeological data and remains, challenging traditional scientific practice. Consequently, bioarcheologists are urged to rethink their research strategies and work with cooperative structures that respect tribal sovereignty and cultural values. The paradigmatic shift mandates adopting new scientific paradigms that respect Indigenous knowledge and public engagement in research activities. By becoming more inclusive, educational institutions are not only conforming to evolving policies but also enhancing the overall quality of research and showing respect for the cultural value of osteological materials (Hamilton et al., 2004; Kakaliouras et al., 2012) (Figure 11.13).

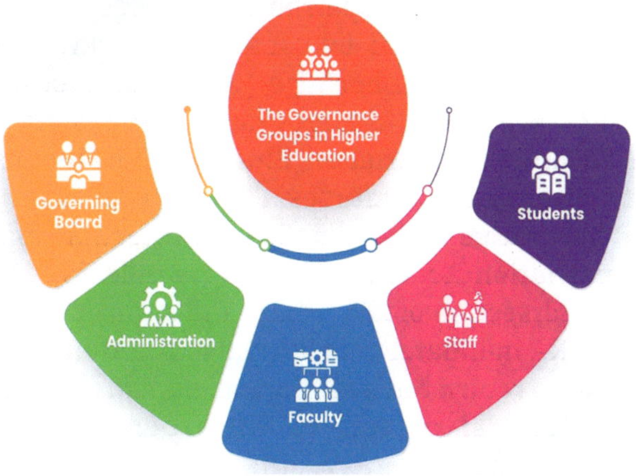

Figure 11.13. The evolution of policies within academic institutions.

Source: https://external-content.duckduckgo.com/iu/?u=https%3A%2F%2Fcdn.azeusconvene.com%2Fwp-content%2Fuploads%2Fimage-4_What-is-Shared-Governance-in-Higher-Education.jpg&f=1&nofb=1&ipt=2ee950f1fa2b7750706fe56b818dc09588259ec735e64241ba0c4ce39686343a.

11.6.3. The Influence of Public Opinion on Repatriation Efforts

Public opinion and repatriation are interdependent, influenced by cultural history, historical conditions, and evolving legal landscapes. As society continues to focus on the recognition of indigenous peoples' cultural heritage and rights, public opinion has become a significant force propelling the movement supporting the repatriation of ancestral human remains and cultural artifacts. Protests by indigenous communities and their allies have drawn much publicity, most often gaining the support of the general public, which contradicts the dominant narratives advanced by scientific and academic institutions. This shift in public attitude not only reshapes discourse on osteological research but also forces institutions to reconsider their ethical obligations to indigenous peoples. Such forces underscore the importance of engaging indigenous voices in the ongoing debate on repatriation, as evidenced by the problems posed by competing worldviews regarding cultural heritage (Kakaliouras et al., 2012). Legislative changes have been essential to advancing repatriation, illustrating the impact of shifting public attitudes. The 1990 enactment of the Native American Grave Protection and Repatriation Act (NAGPRA) was a milestone in the intersection of law, ethics, and anthropology. NAGPRA mandates that federal institutions and agencies return Native American human remains and cultural objects to their descendants, typically due to increasing public pressure. Additionally, the successful use of Section 106 of the National Historic Preservation Act by recognized tribes has produced limitations on the scientific recovery of bioarchaeological data, an evolution consistent with a broader societal trend toward respecting the desires and rights of native peoples. These legal frameworks demonstrate that public opinion has not merely led to legal reform but also to a rethinking of conventional academic protocols and moral priorities across the discipline (Hamilton et al., 2004). Moreover, the role of public opinion within repatriation efforts demonstrates a growing recognition of the necessity for collaborative relationships between indigenous peoples and bioarcheologists . Increasingly, public debate is encouraging a shift away from a single scientific explanation toward a broader discourse that acknowledges indigenous people's agency and cultural significance. By advocating to advance focus on partnerships and participatory processes, repatriation groups urge bioarcheologists to change their practices and theoretical frameworks to reflect more closely indigenous voices. Such collaborative ventures can help facilitate mutual understanding, build trust, and bridge the epistemological distances that have long characterized the partnership between anthropology and indigenous communities. The transformation elicited by public opinion helps to cement the moral imperative of repatriation, encouraging continued debate that is sensitive to the social power embodied in skeletal and cultural remains (Kakaliouras et al., 2012).

Test Your Knowledge

1. What are the current trends in repatriation practices for human remains and cultural artifacts?
2. How are modern policies and collaborations shaping ethical and legal approaches to repatriation?

SUMMARY

The intersection of repatriation and ethics in osteological research emphasizes a significant transformation in how societies treat and perceive human remains. Cultural sensitivity only partly establishes the necessity of ethical responses; it is also underscored by histories that shape present discourses. Scholars must walk a delicate line between historical injustices and silenced narratives to ensure their work facilitates a more inclusive narrative. As demonstrated in case studies like this analysis of the Avondale Burial Place, questioning the history of a community established during emancipation, an ethical framework sharpens our understanding of ancestral traditions. Such questions facilitate respectful and educational repatriation, enabling descendants to reclaim their heritage without challenging prevailing paradigms sustained in osteological research (Vanderpool et al., 2011). In addition, interdisciplinary osteology is vital to resolving ethical issues arising from repatriation. By integrating knowledge from anthropology, archaeology, and paleopathology, researchers can adopt a multidimensional approach that focuses on source community views. This engagement, aside from contributing to the development of scientific discourse, breaks the prevailing narratives that seek to remove the ethical dimensions of human remains investigation. With the expansion of the discipline, there is a need to address and acknowledge the ethical issues arising, particularly on the representation and agency of the deceased and their lineage. The expansion in methods and techniques of paleopathology highlights a holistic approach in enhancing ethical clarity alongside scientific pursuit (Grauer et al., 2022). Lastly, the role of osteological researchers is not only research itself; it is also the advocacy of the rights and representations of historically suppressed groups. As the ethical debate and repatriation struggle progress, scholars must continue to be mindful of the needs of the communities affected through their endeavor. By establishing an atmosphere of transparency, accountability, and discussion, researchers can establish trust and cooperation with descendant populations and ensure that repatriation initiatives heal, not exacerbate, historical wounds. The moral framework behind osteological research must seek not just to comprehend the past but also to seek to remedy its injustices, representing a commitment to honor the dignity of the deceased as well as their living descendants.

The repatriation and ethics debates in bioarcheological scholarship point towards significant shifts in interactions between indigenous communities and bioarcheologists . Central to the debate is the passage of legislation such as the Native American Graves Protection and Repatriation Act (NAGPRA) in 1990, which was a milestone for biological anthropology. It not only established a basis for the repatriation of ancestral remains to federally recognized tribes but also created new ethical responsibilities for researchers regarding the treatment of human remains. These modifications serve to illustrate the necessity for bioarcheologists to revisit their ways and ensure that they meaningfully involve indigenous individuals. By integrating the perspectives of such groups, researchers are then in a better position to comprehend cultural heritage within an ethical framework that respects ancestors' remains and the beliefs of their descendants, a shift that reflects broader changes within the field towards inclusiveness and responsibility (Hamilton et al., 2004). Furthermore, the impact of altering cultural resource legislation extends far beyond legal spheres; it raises questions about the scientific trajectory of osteological research. Section 106 of the National Historic Preservation Act is a case in point regarding how tribes are increasingly exercising sovereignty over archaeological resources, complicating traditional research patterns. As bioarcheologists navigate these legal landscapes, they encounter unforeseen constraints necessitating a reformulation of data gathering and research objectives. This legal context has witnessed bioarcheologists engaging more with the living descendants of their populations of study, forming collaborations that are sensitive to indigenous systems of knowledge. Such collaborations have the potential to inform innovative methodologies better suited to capture more integrative perceptions of ancestral occupation and burial contexts, thereby bridging gaps between scientific research and cultural conservation (Hamilton et al., 2004). The dialogue traverses public mortuary archaeology to highlight the broader implications of death and burial culture being examined in society today. As in dialogue regarding public mortuary archaeology, there is a strong correlation between the treatment accorded skeletal remains and community sentiments regarding death and remembrance. Looking at the implications of ancient and modern DNA research only makes this debate more complicated, placing osteological work in the context of public engagement and ethical duty. Researchers must consider the voices of affected communities, especially when repatriation of remains raises ethical concerns about consent and representation. Such an open-minded strategy is not only necessary for constructing better relationships with descendant communities but also necessary for constructing a fuller understanding of the overlap between archaeology, ethics, and public opinion regarding death, burial, and commemoration.

KEY TERMS FROM THIS CHAPTER

- Accountability
- Consultation
- Cultural Sensitivity
- Descendant Communities
- Human Remains
- Informed Consent
- Provenience
- Research Permissions
- Stakeholder Engagement
- Bioethics
- Cultural Heritage
- Curation Ethics
- Ethical Stewardship
- Indigenous Rights
- Institutional Review Board (IRB)
- Repatriation
- Respectful Treatment

CRITICAL THINKING QUESTIONS

1. **What does the term "repatriation" refer to in osteological research?**
   a. Shipping human remains to museums
   b. Returning human remains to descendant communities or countries of origin
   c. Storing human remains in laboratory freezers
   d. Disposing of unidentifiable skeletal remains
2. **The Native American Graves Protection and Repatriation Act (NAGPRA) is a law in the United States that:**
   a. Allows unrestricted study of indigenous remains
   b. Prohibits the excavation of all burial sites
   c. Facilitates the return of cultural items and human remains to Native American groups
   d. Requires DNA testing on all skeletal remains
3. **Which of the following is a key ethical principle in osteological research?**
   a. Maximizing data at all costs
   b. Anonymity of skeletal remains
   c. Respect for human dignity and cultural beliefs
   d. Avoiding contact with local communities
4. **Which action would most likely be considered unethical in osteological research?**
   a. Gaining informed consent for study
   b. Sharing data with affiliated indigenous communities
   c. Publishing photos of human remains without permission
   d. Collaborating with descendant groups on excavation
5. **Which of the following is a goal of ethical repatriation policies?**
   a. Retaining all skeletal collections for future science
   b. Promoting cultural healing and justice
   c. Avoiding bureaucratic procedures
   d. Ignoring religious perspectives

Short Answer Questions

1. What are the primary ethical concerns in conducting osteological research on human remains?
2. Define repatriation in the context of osteological and archaeological research.
3. Why is informed consent important in the study of recently deceased individuals or descendant communities?
4. What role do indigenous communities play in decisions about the study and display of ancestral remains?
5. Explain the difference between legal ownership and ethical stewardship of human remains.

Answers to Critical Thinking Questions

1. (b); 2. (c); 3. (c); 4. (c); 5. (b)

REFERENCES

1. Belcastro, M. G., Pietrobelli, A., Nicolosi, T., Milella, M., & Mariotti, V. (2022). Scientific and ethical aspects of identified skeletal series: the case of the documented human osteological collections of the University of Bologna (Northern Italy). *Forensic Sciences*, *2*(2), 349–361. https://doi.org/10.3390/forensicsci2020025Bourdieu, P., Carey, N., Caruth, C., Cohen, A., Interpol, Lessig, R., Marshall, R. D., et al. (2014). Who knows who we are? Questioning DNA analysis in disaster victim identification. https://core.ac.uk/download/30704511.pdf (accessed on 21st July 2025).
2. Bourgault, A. (2011). The changing understanding of North American archaeology and Native American heritage. https://core.ac.uk/download/215536375.pdf (accessed on 21st July 2025).
3. Carew, R. M. (2021). An investigation into 3D printing of osteological remains: The metrology and ethics of virtual anthropology. https://core.ac.uk/download/480393497.pdf (accessed on 21st July 2025).
4. Champney, T. H., Cornwall, J., de la Cova, C., DeLeon, V. B., et al. (2024). American Association for Anatomy recommendations for the management of legacy anatomical collections. https://core.ac.uk/download/640944293.pdf (accessed on 21st July 2025).
5. Clark, J. (2010). Towards a multidisciplinary practice for human remains: The conservation, collection, and display of human remains and objects made from them. https://core.ac.uk/download/2778549.pdf (accessed on 21st July 2025).
6. Grauer, A. (2022). Introduction. https://core.ac.uk/download/614446076.pdf (accessed on 21st July 2025).
7. Hamilton, M. D. (2004). Seeking after empire: Bioarcheologists and American Indians in the new millennium. https://core.ac.uk/download/268795320.pdf (accessed on 21st July 2025).
8. Kakaliouras, A. M. (2012). An anthropology of repatriation: Contemporary physical anthropological and Native American ontologies of practice. https://core.ac.uk/download/337304555.pdf (accessed on 21st July 2025).
9. Morse, B. W. (2011). Indigenous human rights and knowledge in archives, museums, and libraries: Some international perspectives with specific reference to New Zealand and Canada. https://core.ac.uk/download/29200136.pdf (accessed on 21st July 2025).
10. N/A. (2010). Breaking copper: Legislating the repatriation of First Nations cultural property to restore self-determination and promote reconciliation. https://core.ac.uk/download/84871854.pdf (accessed on 21st July 2025).
11. N/A. (2024). *African Collections Futures*. https://core.ac.uk/download/630300673.pdf (accessed on 21st July 2025).
12. N/A. (2025). *Cremated Bone in Archaeology: Ethical Considerations in The Excavation, Analysis, Storage, And Display of Cremated Bone in the United Kingdom*. https://core.ac.uk/download/635797915.pdf (accessed on 21st July 2025).
13. Vanderpool, E. (2011). Bioarcheological investigations of community and identity at the Avondale Burial Place (McArthur Cemetery), Bibb County, Georgia. https://core.ac.uk/download/71421738.pdf (accessed on 21st July 2025).
14. Williams, H. (2018). Introduction: Public archaeologies of death and memory. https://core.ac.uk/download/233924689.pdf (accessed on 21st July 2025).

CURRENT CHALLENGES AND FUTURE DIRECTIONS IN OSTEOLOGY

12

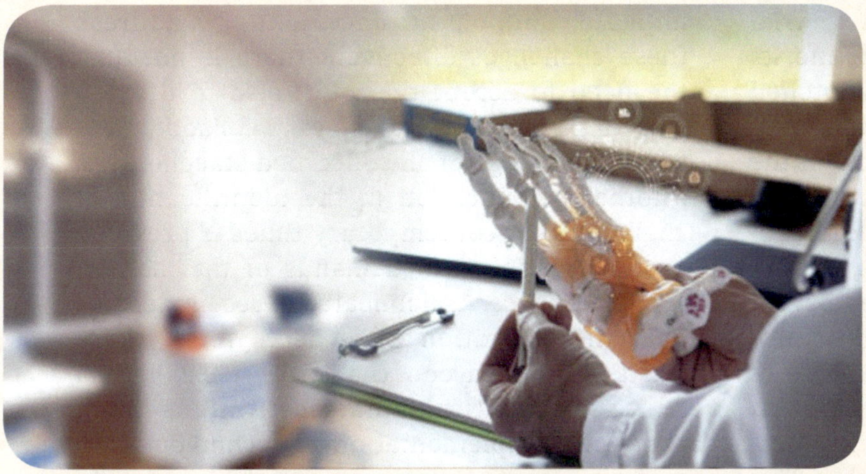

LEARNING OBJECTIVES

After studying this chapter, you will be able to:

1. Discuss the economic challenges
2. Focus on environmental issues
3. Explain the technological advancements
4. Understand social and cultural challenges
5. Evaluate political landscape
6. Focus on the education system

Introduction

In exploring the dense themes of today's challenges and future visions across many fields, it is necessary to establish a fundamental understanding of the issues at hand. The complexities regarding convergence among computational systems and social sciences emphasize the necessity of sound methodologies that are able to advise research findings effectively. Most relevant here is the new application of social norms to multi-agent systems, mirroring human social life. As the nature of these systems evolves, so too must the advice from researchers, necessitating an evaluation of the latest literature. This process of iteration is not only responsible for the advancement of knowledge but also paves the way towards solving the issues of social control inherent in dynamic multi-agent systems, which will be delineated in detail within this essay (Wu et al.). Similarly, in the field of healthcare, in the context of non-pharmacological interventions (NPTs) for the elderly afflicted with dementia, the requirement of stringency in methodology becomes increasingly apparent. Although the potential of NPTs to enhance the quality of life of vulnerable populations is significant, research is frequently hampered by inconclusive findings, making actionable evidence rare. The meeting of experts to delineate treatment targets, objectives, and ingredients through an umbrella system such as the Rehabilitation Treatment Specification System is an innovative step that attempts to unify research efforts. This synthesis not only identifies the current knowledge gaps but also highlights the importance of prespecified protocols in trial execution. In consideration of both the merits and the deficits in this regard, an enlightened understanding of NPTs will be achieved, paving the way for more effective interventions in the future (Bahar-Fuchs et al., 2020). To integrate these findings, one must adopt a forward-looking perspective that acknowledges both successes and ongoing challenges in the relevant areas. Conforming to social standards in multi-agent systems includes an understanding of the model of interaction complexity as well as an appreciation of the centrality of empirical evidence in informing healthcare practices. This essay attempts to demystify the tension between theory and practice, demonstrating that by drawing on both schools of opinion, researchers can more effectively negotiate the complexities of their fields. Through a critical examination of current issues and the identification of potential future studies, this investigation will contribute importantly to the conversation on emerging methodologies, reasserting the role of interdisciplinarity in solving current problems. Ultimately, the goal is to foster an environment for increasingly innovative research to better society.

Definition of Current Challenges

Definition of current challenges of the current academia is, on the whole, multifaceted, as per the paradigm shift of education and research. One of the challenges is the need for international cooperation for Scholarship of Teaching and Learning (SOTL). As institutions strive to enhance the delivery and effectiveness of education, collaborative action across different geographical points is of utmost significance. Importantly, as Mackenzie et al. (2012) define, more scholarly activities are increasingly requiring transnational collaboration that crosses geographical boundaries. However, collaborations most often confront issues such as disparities in educational quality, cultural differences, and institutional policies that might impede common advancement. To address these challenges effectively, there is not only the need to accept them but also to develop structures that facilitate effective collaborations to the advantage of all concerned stakeholders. Another complication in the identification of challenges for contemporary times is provided by the technological demands of the modern academic space. As delineated in recent debates over the federation Edge deployment, there exists a twofold layer of challenge—technological and socio-political—that institutions must overcome. Implementation of technology into pedagogical models is essential in order to facilitate new learning paradigms and research operations. However, as testified by Baktir et al. (2018), networking facilities and resource management issues usually complicate such intentions. Furthermore, legal and geopolitical factors hinder the smooth implementation of advanced technologies, hindering successful communication and cooperation. While institutions are working to create a global network of educational resources, overcoming these technical and structural limitations is at the core of realizing the potential benefits of integrating technology in higher education. Lastly, scarce funding and limited support for collaborative efforts further complicate the identification of today's challenges in higher education. Financial constraints often limit the ability of institutions to invest in necessary resources, including technology, training, and human resources, that facilitate effective collaboration. In addition, changing funding priorities can lead to an uneven distribution of resources, unequally affecting smaller or less well-known institutions. The results of Mackenzie et al. (2012) indicate that, in the absence of strategic investment in collaboration-based programs, the potential for innovation in teaching practice remains largely untapped. Hence, overcoming these financial issues is crucial to enabling effective collaboration and innovation in academe, underscoring the need for collective efforts to create an environment where problems can be turned into opportunities for growth (Figure 12.1).

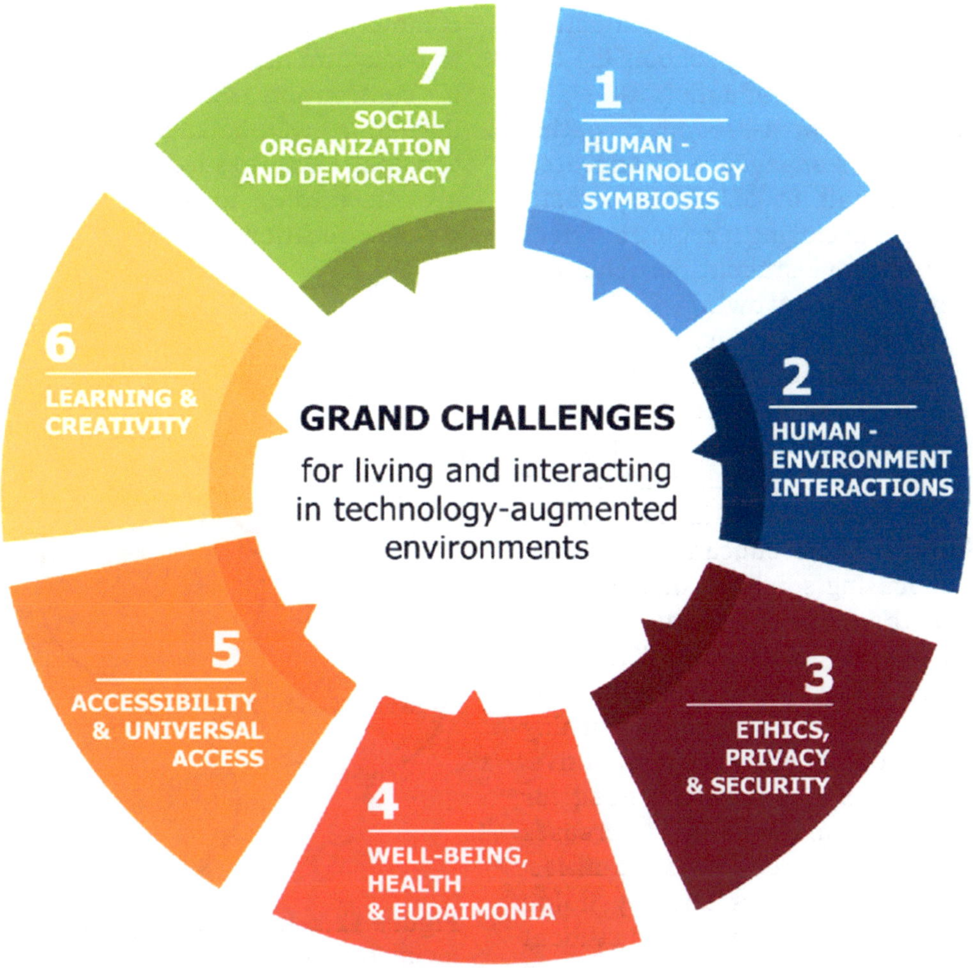

Figure 12.1. The definition of current challenges.

Source: https://external-content.duckduckgo.com/iu/?u=https%3A%2F%2Fwww.researchgate.net%2Fprofile%2FConstantine-Stephanidis%2Fpublication%2F334164083%2Ffigure%2Ffig1%2FAS%3A775928540041217%401562007188119%2FThe-Seven-Grand-Challenges.png&f=1&nofb=1&ipt=c4d7ea27b6b339e43896142ee0a4f7bca2c3d67d1ed6a776af786e0a67877111.

Importance of Addressing These Challenges

In addressing the myriad problems faced by public schools, it is crucial to identify the inherent link between these problems and the goal of providing equal opportunity for quality education to all students. The very issues of narrowing the achievement gap and improving student motivation underscore the absolute necessity of systemic reform. Procrastination in solving these problems has the effect of perpetuating disadvantage cycles, blocking the potential of underprivileged groups, and limiting socioeconomic mobility. By taking bold action to provide equal opportunities, schools lay the foundation for improved graduation rates and smooth transitions to post-secondary paths, thereby educating an engaged and educated citizenry. As Adelman et al. (2018) posit, significant progress in closing learning barriers is imperative to effective student participation and retention, finally growing individual students and society as a whole. Additionally, limits on traditional school reform approaches depict the necessity for innovative solutions beyond pedagogical advantage. Recognizing that effective teaching cannot bypass the multifaceted barriers learners face is essential to building inclusive solutions. Some educational leaders have said that focusing solely on instructional quality, rather than on environmental and emotional factors, is insufficient. Thus, the value of this challenge extends to support structures that facilitate individualized learning opportunities. Keeping that in perspective, Adelman et al. (2018) mention the need for an interconnected framework that increases the co-engagement of educators, families, and community stakeholders and, by doing so, produces a supportive context for student learning. Reconciling these interdependent issues provides the foundation for deep reform and school sustainability, enabling them to address their diverse constituencies more effectively. Finally, addressing the issues that overwhelm the current education landscape ensures reforms not only work but also persist in the long run. To achieve long-term impact, schools must adopt an integrated approach that strategically reallocates resources and implements innovative learning pedagogies. For example, enhancing school climate and strengthening family engagement are fundamental in developing robust support systems for all students, particularly those in marginalized communities. Furthermore, proactive crisis management at the educational level can effectively reduce learning interruptions. In accordance with Adelman et al. (2018), a collaborative effort among educators, community leaders, and policymakers is required to ensure an inclusive education system. Lastly, by confronting these challenges head-on and developing well-balanced strategies, instructors can open doors to success wider than individual growth, leading to a revolutionary impact on public education in the future (Figure 12.2).

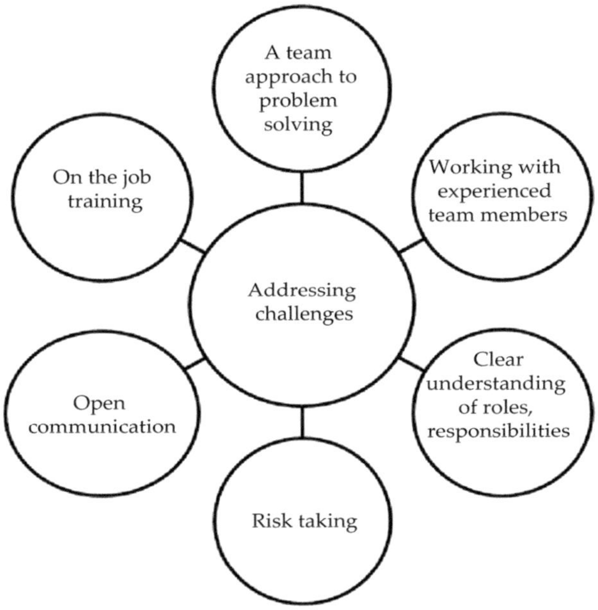

Figure 12.2. In addressing the myriad challenges facing public education.

Source: https://external-content.duckduckgo.com/iu/?u=https%3A%2F%2Fwww.researchgate.net%2Fprofile%2FDonna-Mcghie-Richmond%2Fpublication%2F284273838%2Ffigure%2Ffig4%2FAS%3A391482176491524%401470348032208%2FAddressing-the-challenges.png&f=1&nofb=1&ipt=a55492ed2e89316b8f4141c265c204ff3e932d41f4bb9e9b70b9965535cc896a.

Overview of Future Directions

Gazing into the future of technology, particularly in the field of brain-computer interfaces (BCIs), record the decisive directions these technologies can take. The direction from the laboratory to practical applications of BCIs is a pivotal turn, signaling a forthcoming revolution in the way humans, especially people with disabilities, engage with technology.

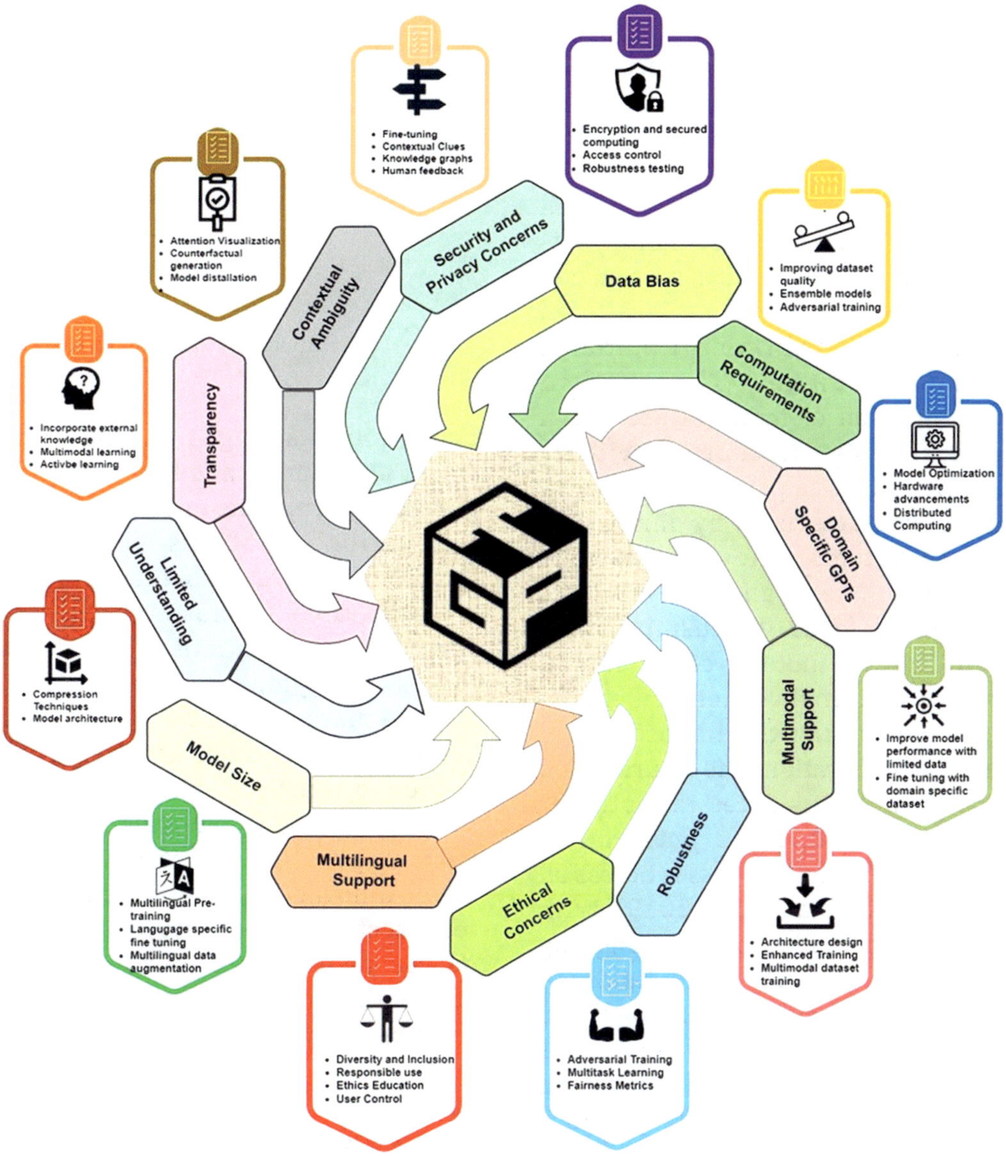

Figure 12.3. As we look towards the future of technology.

Source: https://external-content.duckduckgo.com/iu/?u=https%3A%2F%2Fwww.researchgate.net%2Fpublication%2F370869544%2Ffigure%2Ffig3%2FAS%3A11431281159745677%401684465614579%2FChallenges-and-Future-Directions.jpg&f=1&nofb=1&ipt=b3ddf399fc41ce59db313ca36923ea7d1fee831ac29ae17ffa7637aaf6789a25.

Central issues in practical field detection and analysis of brain activity must be addressed, driving innovation in device usability and functionality. As BCIs integrate into diverse user experiences, their naturalness and sensitivity are expected to increase, enabling more intuitive interaction. Lastly, the future of BCIs is characterized by stark dynamics and unremitting growth, presenting challenges and opportunities for the construction of future interactions with interfaces (Allison et al., 2012). Similarly, the future of additive manufacturing (AM) holds abundant exciting possibilities that will reshape industries. 3D printing technology has ushered in an era in which complex, customized designs are produced with unparalleled efficiency, radically transforming traditional manufacturing paradigms. The method allows for optimization of material use and a certain degree of design freedom previously unimaginable. With AM as a part of the Industry 4.0 framework, characterized by innovative manufacturing systems, the implications for product development and delivery are enormous. With its focus on sustainability, innovations in AM technology could extend economic, social, and environmental benefits even further, underscoring the importance of interdisciplinary collaboration. The future of AM is highly dependent on advances in materials and applications that have the potential to revolutionize manufacturing processes across all sectors (Dehghanghadikolaei et al., 2019). With this rapidly evolving landscape, the ongoing convergence of BCIs and AM could hold key insights into the trajectory of technology. The coupling of newer manufacturing techniques can potentially accompany the advances in BCI technology, making it easier to produce more advanced and customized applications. As both disciplines continue to develop, they will inevitably converge, creating greater user experiences that emphasize accessibility and eco-friendliness. Through ongoing investigation and empirical quantification, exploring synergies among these technologies could yield new solutions to many of the most significant challenges being encountered today. Overall, the future promise of BCIs and AM represents a tableau awaiting exploration upon which technological innovation could redefine human interaction and production processes to make them more efficient and inclusive in diverse settings (Figure 12.3).

12.1. Economic Challenges

Learning Outcome

1. Global recession impacts
2. Income inequality and its effects
3. Unemployment trends and solutions

Economic challenges in the contemporary world are compounded by the acceleration of globalization and the intricacies of technological innovation. Nations are increasingly interconnected, and therefore their economies are vulnerable, as shocks in one nation tend to spread to other nations. This interdependence forces policymakers to adapt quickly to shifting market conditions, often prompted by external factors such as foreign trade policy, economic sanctions, and emerging industries. In biotechnology, countries such as China are reshaping their roles, not only as manufacturers but as innovators pushing frontiers in the high-tech sector. These developments mirror the degree to which nations' ability to weather economic challenges is interconnected with their capacity to harness economic innovation sustainably, a correlation highlighted in the examination of the biotech innovation system and its social sustainability (Chen et al., 2011). The labor market, a key indicator of economic prosperity, is under intense pressure amid chronic macroeconomic uncertainty. Employment trends are increasingly subject to rapid fluctuations, reflecting broader global economic changes. As economies grapple with challenges stemming from technological disruption and market shifts, the focus on labor market adaptability becomes paramount. Understanding how to forecast and analyze labor market states helps formulate effective state policies to mitigate economic risks. In such cases, issues such as rising unemployment and skill mismatches require collaborative action by governments, schools, and industries to prepare the workforce to meet future demands. For example, a pressing need is the projection of the technology and skills that will be required, which can transform job patterns significantly (Maryna, 2019).

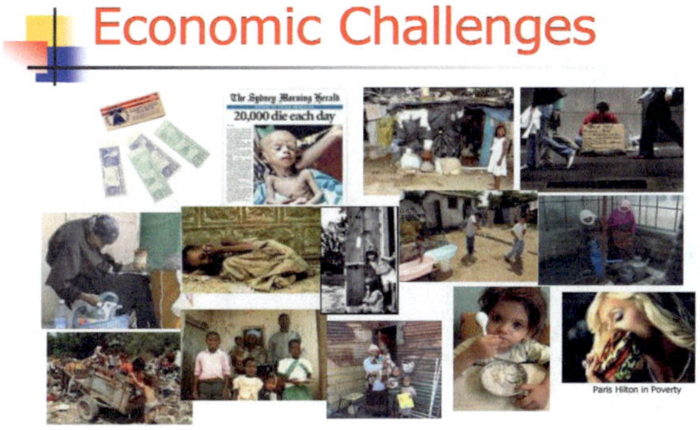

Figure 12.4. Economic challenges in the contemporary world.

Source: https://external-content.duckduckgo.com/iu/?u=https%3A%2F%2Fimage.slideserve.com%2F16413%2Feconomic-challenges5-l.jpg&f=1&nofb=1&ipt=1e2dbe03c2f023df0208934f929d165c6673759bba8ac90591dcedbac9e7386b.

These financial challenges also emphasize the importance of sustainable growth to ensure that development mechanisms are inclusive and consider social factors. As economies strive to recover and restructure, the distribution of economic gains and risks must be addressed openly. Policymakers must walk the tightrope between increasing innovation and safeguarding public interest to avoid creating widening disparities. The distribution of opportunities, technology, and resources must be managed with a dedication to equity and social sustainability to avoid reinforcing current inequalities. Understanding the future directions through harmonizing lessons learned from current economic challenges can lead to comprehensive frameworks that not only pursue economic development but also pursue the betterment of society as a whole, enriching the connection between innovation, risk management, and social responsibility (Chen et al., 2011; Maryna, 2019) (Figure 12.4).

12.1.1. Global Recession Impacts

The global recession has far-reaching effects that extend beyond immediate economic instability and into other realms of society and international relations. Because monetary crises tend to begin in economically developed nations, their effects filter into developing countries, heightening vulnerability among such populations. One of the major problems is that reduced demand and smaller export prices significantly erode the ability of such nations to stabilize their economies. Furthermore, diminished private financial flows and a remittance withdrawal increase inherent imbalances, which compound the risk that prevents countries already struggling to escape poverty from reaching their growth potential. This fact ultimately underscores the interdependence of the world economy and the need for collective international action to build resilience in vulnerable markets (Addison et al., 2025). Overall, the agricultural sector is highly susceptible to the effects of a global recession. Market variations can result in sudden drops in agricultural supply and demand, and therefore food insecurity, especially in rural societies. Relying on past experience from crises, as highlighted in a recent assessment of the impact of the COVID-19 pandemic on rural economies, it is evident that consumer behavior changes significantly during economic recessions. Out-of-home consumption-based firms suffer from severe setbacks, while consumption-based firms that lie in the home can possess fresh routes for growth and development. Gendered considerations also play a significant role in understanding how families deal with financial constraints, as women generally put in additional effort to provide household income. The complexity implies that any measures taken should address both economic and social considerations (Aitken-McDermott et al., 2020). Against the backdrop of such challenges, the need for creative policies to mitigate the impact of a global economic downturn becomes obvious. Climate change, food security, and social welfare are the only issues an all-embracing economic strategy has to address. The overlapping of these crises gives rise to a multi dimensional problem, which will demand policy intervention with a synergic impact. Efforts towards economic recovery should include sustainable approaches that not only restore financial stability but also build environmental and social resilience. Using the available vulnerabilities in various societies, especially in the global South, inclusive and sustainable economic systems will play a significant role in forging a more resilient world. Thus, cooperation among governments, civil society, and international institutions is necessary to address these intersecting problems successfully and achieve a sustainable path forward (Addison et al., 2025) (Figure 12.5).

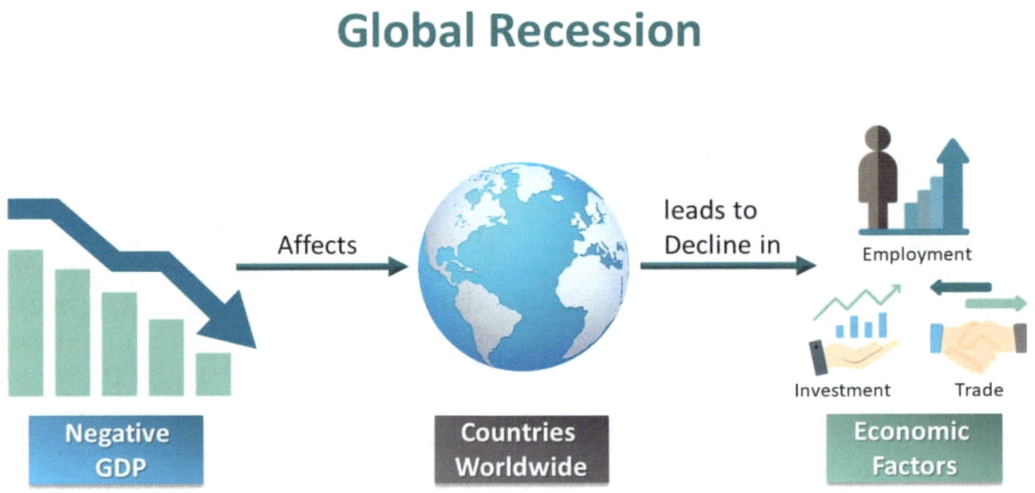

Figure 12.5. The global recession has far-reaching impacts.

Source: https://external-content.duckduckgo.com/iu/?u=https%3A%2F%2Fcdn.educba.com%2Facademy%2Fwp-content%2Fuploads%2F2023%2F02%2FGlobal-Recession-1.jpg&f=1&nofb=1&ipt=4db3b5d1ea2c8957e332479c1813bcf1e6a130f6e2a8729db192eca89aa2c294.

12.1.2. Income Inequality and Its Effects

Income inequality remains a significant issue in contemporary society, posing critical challenges for policymakers and social scientists alike. The growing disparity between the rich and the economically disenfranchised not only undermines social stability but also stains the pillars of democratic rule. With wealth concentrated in a narrow segment of the population, disenfranchisement by ever-larger segments of the poorer classes leads to mounting disillusionment and resentment. Those tensions can fuel social discord and exacerbate disparities across demographic groups; therefore, it becomes important to develop a more nuanced investigation of economic disparities. Rather than focusing solely on poverty alleviation, research suggests that social policy must broaden its scope to adequately address income inequality and consider the role of wealthier residents in the broader economic context (Orton et al., 2006). Moreover, with nations experiencing globalization and technological pressures, the implications of income inequality are more acute. Economic policies that lack solutions to this menace threaten the cycle of vulnerability entrenchment for marginalized communities, thereby stifling aggregate economic growth and innovation. For instance, in Germany, policymakers face the challenging task of designing an economic environment conducive to inclusive growth amid ongoing demographic transformation and pressure from digitalization (Barišić et al., 2017).

The urgency of an inclusive growth agenda is to highlight that economic growth should translate into higher opportunities for all sections in society, and not only the benefit of the elite. A lack of tangible plans to curb income inequality can put at risk not just social disintegration but also the country's capacity to withstand future economic stresses. To achieve sustainable development in addressing income disparity, policy frameworks must be reassessed. Policies should target increased access to quality education, progressive wage policies, and social protection schemes that ensure equal distribution of resources. Policymakers must prioritize implementing comprehensive social policies to bridge gaps across economic strata, making upward mobility and improved living standards for marginalized communities a reality. These programs can reduce economic disparities but also increase social confidence and community strength, key components of a thriving society. Though the debate about income inequality continues, subsequent research and policy initiatives must explore new solutions and innovative approaches that solve these systemic issues in a comprehensive fashion. By doing so, societies can create the best platform to have a more just and equitable future for all.

12.1.3. Unemployment Trends and Solutions

Unless all the diverse causes of unemployment are considered in their full impact, trends in unemployment cannot be comprehended. Over time, unemployment levels across the world have experienced tremendous fluctuations, largely dependent upon the growth of economies, changes in population, and technological innovation. For example, in 2004, world unemployment fell by a narrow margin, from 185.2 million to 184.7 million. This slight improvement is credited to strong economic growth at a growth rate of 5%, which highlights the nexus between economic strength and the performance of the labor market. However, though a decline in unemployment is to be hailed, it must be done with caution, as fundamental issues such as employment quality and underemployment still loom over the labor market. The interfacing of such variables necessitates ongoing research and policy development that prioritize not only employment growth but also working conditions, as evidenced by issues across various labor markets in recent studies (International Labour Office, 2005). In addressing unemployment, it is imperative to identify solutions that effectively address existing issues. Policymakers and stakeholders must join forces to address the structural and systemic barriers that are slowing job creation. This may include investments in education and labor development programs for equipping individuals with the skills required for rapidly evolving job markets. Furthermore, measures that improve the job matching between employers and job seekers can help reduce unemployment rates. Furthermore, the importance of not forgetting to consider labor market participation dynamics, particularly among vulnerable groups such as youth and the poor, should not be overlooked. As the study highlights, a comprehensive, unified approach to addressing workforce issues is most likely to lead to successful policy implementation and foster a conducive environment for meaningful employment prospects (Horn et al., 2011). Finally, the future of unemployment solutions should be founded on an emergent framework capable of responding to evolving trends in the labor market. To this end, it is important to enhance coordination among national, state, and local agencies to develop plans that reflect the unique needs of different areas. According to extended workforce research, drawing on concepts from a broad range of stakeholders, including community organizations and philanthropic foundations, can help highlight gaps in current employment and training programs. Further, the ability to predict the impacts of potential future job-market disruptions, such as automation and outsourcing, plays a critical role in opening the door for the workforce of the future. Policymakers, in the future, will have to put priority on sustainable approaches that not only meet short-term job requirements but also consider long-term worker resilience (Horn et al., 2011) (Figure 12.6).

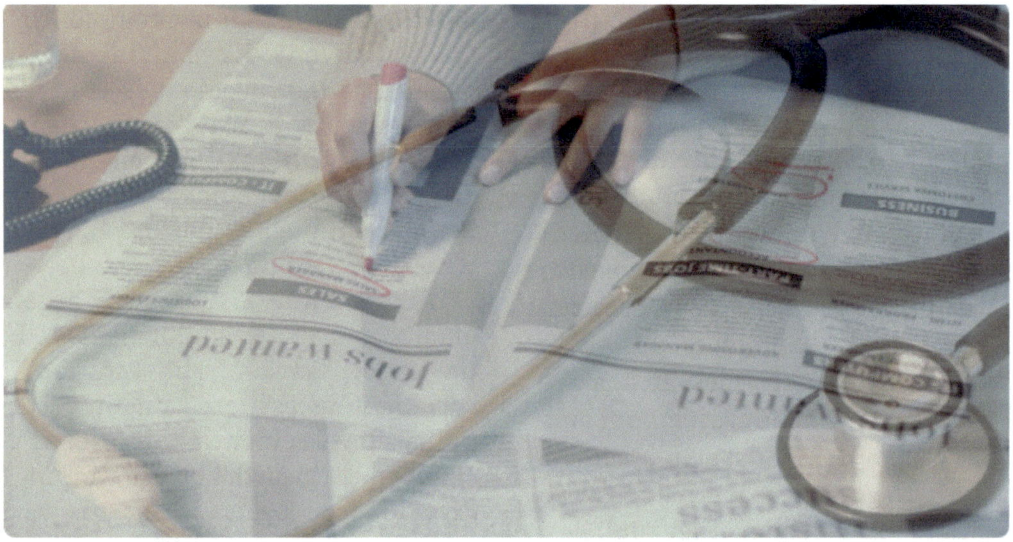

Figure 12.6. Unemployment trends and solutions in health.

Source: https://media.licdn.com/dms/image/v2/D5612AQGHIM73-DLe1A/article-cover_image-shrink_720_1280/article-cover_image-shrink_720_1280/0/1692971865466?e=2147483647&v=beta&t=5sX2P_0uQBZzryGxaJBAYWX7XbMoT0f2y8WUmgp2cj8.

Test Your Knowledge

1. What are the common economic challenges faced in conducting research or implementing projects in osteology and bioarchaeology?
2. How can limited funding impact the scope, quality, and ethical considerations of scientific studies?

12.2. Environmental Issues

Learning Outcome

1. Climate change and its consequences
2. Pollution and public health
3. Sustainable practices and innovations

The convergence of technology and environmental management grows ever more essential as global challenges reach their peak. AI has been a revolutionary force in environmental engineering, delivering groundbreaking solutions to complex challenges, particularly in air and water quality monitoring, waste management, and biodiversity conservation. The use of machine learning and neural networks enhances environmental modeling and forecasting, thereby facilitating more efficient management of resources. The research states that these technologies can facilitate improved conservation outcomes as well as valuable insights on climate change mitigation efforts. With this, AI enables an active approach to environmental issues, allowing stakeholders to implement strategies that are not only effective but also sustainable. However, ethical concerns and energy consumption associated with the deployment of AI systems must be addressed critically within any comprehensive strategy that suggests general application (Kamyab et al., 2024). Although technological progress provides ample opportunities, it leads to some issues at present, focusing on environmental degradation. Traditional methods of pest control, particularly against vector species such as ticks, have become ineffective due to growing resistance and adverse environmental effects. The application of chemical substitutes, including pyrethroids and organophosphates, raises strong issues of sustainability and environmental integrity. The need for alternative approaches has sparked renewed interest in plant-derived acaricides, which offer effective, environmentally friendly solutions. The integration of nanotechnology with these plant materials enhances their efficacy, overcoming stability and bioavailability issues. The intersection of plant science and nanotechnology offers a promising approach to pest control and demands the development of sustainable approaches that can continuously adapt to the shifting dynamics of environmental complexity (Bechara et al., 2025). To properly manage the intricate web of environmental complexities, a multidisciplinary approach is needed. Coordination among sectors, including academia, industry, and government ministries, can lead to cutting-edge research and development of technologies for environmentally friendly applications.

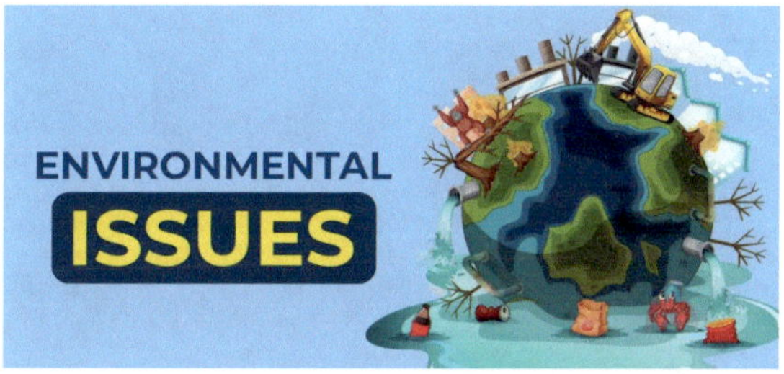

Figure 12.7. The intersection of technology and environmental management.

Source: https://external-content.duckduckgo.com/iu/?u=https%3A%2F%2Fmedia.geeksforgeeks.org%2Fwp-content%2Fuploads%2F20230620175013%2FEnvironmental-Issues-.webp&f=1&nofb=1&ipt=bd37b6851a3f9c8e13cf34dea01b5de43c9baa9de13afcb602cc8145d5b7f732.

The intersection of biotechnology, nanotechnology, and artificial intelligence holds prospects for breakthroughs in the future to address key environmental challenges. These interdisciplinary methods not only create an appreciation for the intricacy present in ecological systems, but they also promote the development of strong policies that balance ecological integrity with human needs. As world awareness shifts towards sustainability, sustained investment in research and integration of new-age technologies will go a long way towards shaping the ecologically resilient future, such that future generations inherit a healthy world capable of supporting a range of life forms (Kamyab et al., 2024; Bechara et al., 2025) (Figure 12.7).

12.2.1. Climate Change and Its Consequences

As global warming intensifies, the effects of climate change are becoming increasingly evident across ecosystems and human populations. Extreme weather events such as hurricanes, droughts, and floods are becoming more frequent, causing widespread devastation.

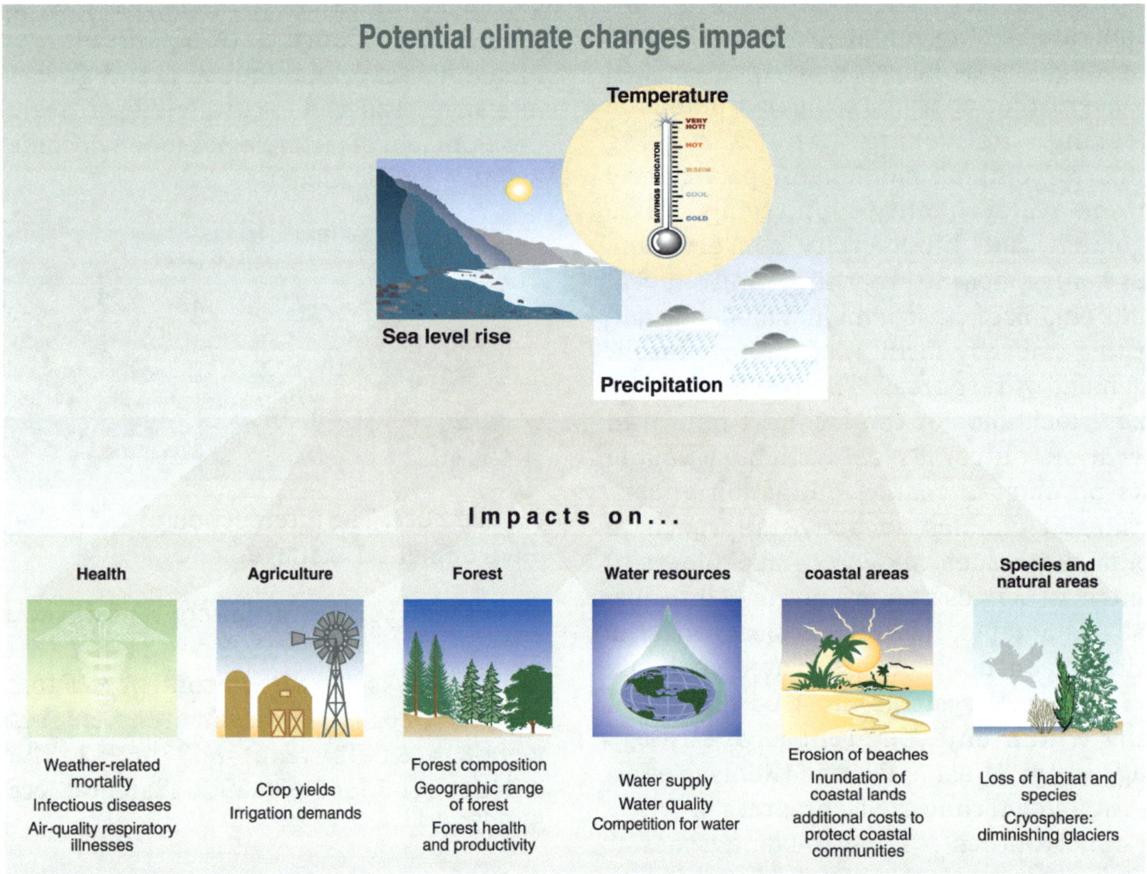

Figure 12.8. Climate change and its consequences.

Source: https://external-content.duckduckgo.com/iu/?u=http%3A%2F%2Fsites.ehe.osu.edu%2Fbeyondweather%2Ffiles%2F2011%2F12%2Fpotential_climate_change_impacts.png&f=1&nofb=1&ipt=9b9e0a7be6e1b755f13e4f0bd90a2939b08a719c1cb3f33dc1207b98cc7a9809.

The economic cost of such natural disasters is overwhelming, as they destroy infrastructure, displace people, and destabilize local economies. Further, the decimation of natural habitats threatens biodiversity and leads to the extinction of numerous species. Destruction magnifies past inequalities in society, as poor and marginalized groups possess the least capacity to adapt to the changes that are being imposed upon them. An aggregate global response is necessary because not reducing these effects will not just halt current development plans but also render future generations' ability to thrive in a safe environment futile. Climate change also poses serious hazards to human health, apart from its impact on nature. Rising temperatures bring with them numerous health issues, including heat illnesses, respiratory ailments brought on by poor air quality, and the spread of infectious diseases. The elderly and those with pre-existing medical conditions are the most susceptible. Food security is also threatened by agricultural production becoming less reliable due to shifting weather patterns and an increasing number of pests. The intersection of climate change and health underscores the imperative of an integrated, comprehensive approach to addressing these risks. As the public health systems are not able to handle these rising threats, we must invest in preventive interventions and resilient health infrastructures so that all populations have access to the care that they need during these changes. Addressing the multifaceted issues of climate change demands innovative solutions that infuse equity and cooperation. As envisioned in recent reports, emerging new technology assessment models that factor in people's participation and technical expertise can best inform policy and strategy development in this area. The "new models" suggest a transnational solution, recognizing that climate change is a global issue that transcends frontiers and requires cooperative action. Additionally, investments in training and capacity-building in the affected countries will further enhance local governance and empower communities to address their respective challenges. An understanding of the interconnectedness of social, environmental, and technological systems is essential in creating sustainable solutions. Stakeholders must foster open dialogue that explores diverse perspectives and collaboratively determine the most significant ways to address the omnipresent consequences of climate change, opening the door to a more resilient future (Adelman et al., 2018; Ely et al., 2011) (Figure 12.8).

12.2.2. Pollution and Public Health

The intricate dynamics between public health and pollution pose daunting challenges that must be addressed with utmost urgency in contemporary society. With growing urbanization, the waste disposal problems created increased environmental pollution, with serious health consequences for the population. In developing nations, open dumping and incineration are widely used as the primary waste treatment options, leading to air and land pollution. Inadequate waste management practices not only lead to environmental degradation but also pose hazardous situations for vulnerable populations, especially waste pickers, who are directly exposed to hazardous materials. This creates a vicious cycle under which contamination enhances health issues, making it imperative the need for efficient waste management policies that account for both environmental and public health aspects (Ferronato et al., 2019). In addition, some pollutants, such as particulate matter from industrial emissions and car exhaust, have severe effects on respiratory health. Medical evidence has found a direct association between elevated levels of air pollution and cases of conditions such as asthma, cardiovascular diseases, and lung cancer. Controlling these health impacts involves firm policy action and cutting-edge pollution-control techniques that aim to protect public health. Strict emissions regulations for industries and the use of cleaner energy sources can help reduce the adverse effects of pollution to a large extent. Additionally, education and community outreach are crucial for raising public awareness and inspiring collective action to curb pollution levels. These measures could serve as holistic frameworks to protect community health and support sustainable urban development (Mazzucato, 2018). Finally, the intersection of pollution and public health highlights the need for solutions that are interdisciplinary in scope but extend beyond traditional regulation. Adopting mission-oriented policies that create sustainable environments can yield sustainable public health dividends. These policies must include market co-creation and shaping, bringing multiple stakeholders together to catalyze whole and inclusive approaches to pollution management. Balanced collaboration among governments, the private sector, and community organizations can spearhead initiatives that promote pollution reduction while attaining health equity. With ongoing research to establish the extensive impact of pollution, there should be an emphasis in the future on implementing comprehensive solid waste management strategies that ensure environmental sustainability keeps pace with public health goals (Ferronato et al., 2019).

12.2.3. Sustainable Practices and Innovations

In response to today's environmental challenges, green innovations and practices have become critical components in addressing the world's major issues. With the engagement of multiple stakeholders, including universities and communities, collaborative partnerships can foster innovative education practices on the basis of sustainability. For instance, a four-step procedure for launching Science Education for Sustainable Living (SESL) has served as an effective springboard for preservice teachers to think about their practice within this paradigm.

The procedure not only intensifies teachers' knowledge about sustainable living but also writes environmental issues into the learning curriculum. Lastly, the focus on community involvement in teacher training provides a much-needed foundation for sustainability across generations by emphasizing the importance of shared effort in developing a more aware and ecologically responsible society (Hudson et al., 2006). The call for revolutionary innovation is increasingly recognized as imperative for achieving sustainability goals amid intensifying crises in climate, food security, and biodiversity. As recent research shows, policies and technologies should, more than ever, adopt innovative approaches tailored to unique contexts. The approaches should prioritize the concepts and views of grassroots actors involved in innovation, who understand the unique challenges that their communities face. For example, successful interventions in East African dryland agriculture and Latin American rural energy initiatives demonstrate the effectiveness of inclusivity in innovation design. By recognizing and enhancing the contributions of various stakeholders, sustainable measures can evolve into even more effective solutions for both local and global environmental problems in an integrated way (Arond et al., 2012). Sustainability's future directions involve researchers, policymakers, and practitioners work together to foster an ecosystem of innovation grounded in direction, diversity, and distribution.

Emphasizing collaboration on multiple scales enables a broader range of ideas and solutions to emerge and redirects community engagement models. Additionally, new sustainability brokering approaches can enable connections to provide the linkages needed to scale up grassroots innovations to larger populations, ensuring that solutions are context-relevant and mutually beneficial. Cooperative frameworks like these can provide inputs to decision-making mechanisms and analyses required to protect the planet for generations to come. As we proceed along this path, innovation and promotion of sustainable practice must be at the forefront of all initiatives towards global development (Arond et al., 2012).

Test Your Knowledge

1. How do environmental factors affect the preservation and analysis of skeletal remains in osteology?
2. What environmental challenges can impact fieldwork and laboratory research in osteological studies?

12.3. Technological Advancements

Learning Outcome

1. The digital divide and access to technology
2. Cybersecurity threats and responses
3. The role of artificial intelligence in society

The pace of technological advances is so rapid that it's making drastic impacts across numerous fields and leading the way to future innovation. New technologies such as robots and artificial intelligence (AI) are increasingly being incorporated into everyday life, which facilitates the development of solutions for the cyborgian age that enhance human potential. The merging of humans and technology creates new service modalities in which conventional roles are remolded, enabling unprecedented levels of efficiency and productivity in serving complex needs.

By integrating cyborg technologies into service environments, such as neural implants and interfaces, firms stand to redefine the scope of service interactions, creating opportunities for frontline service employees (FLEs) to enhance empathy and intuitive troubleshooting like never before (Garry et al., 2019). But with them come concerns about ethics and the need for new rules of engagement for the responsible use of such technologies. The conscious planning and implementation of strategic innovation becomes crucial to dealing with the challenges of rapid technological shifts. While developing a winning logic for innovation, the intersection of strategic management and innovation management becomes essential. The imperative to stay competitive necessitates a sharp understanding of emerging themes for strategic innovation (SI) in different contexts. The establishment of a thematic framework that categorizes the key elements of SI is important in aligning the industry practices with the scholarly results, hence establishing an environment conducive to innovative practices and outcomes (Paroutis et al., 2013). The framework, apart from outlining the various components of SI, such as environmental scanning and collective networks, serves as a checklist for the practitioners willing to implement effective innovation approaches. In the future, the trajectory of technological innovation will inevitably dictate sustained shifts in industry and academia. The interplay of such complexities to introduce cyborg technologies into the framework of workforce interactions, along with the strategic efforts required to assess such transitions, illustrates the necessity of sustaining study and discourse. Furthermore, as institutions attempt to capitalize on cyborg innovation, they will be required to balance development with ethical analysis, projecting the potential consequences of such integration. This futuristic strategy calls for active reimagining of existing frameworks and the formulation of new strategies to ensure that technological advancements serve societal ends. By establishing a participatory dialogue between strategic innovation researchers and practitioners, stakeholders are best placed to address the challenges and opportunities of the multifaceted landscape ahead (Figure 12.9).

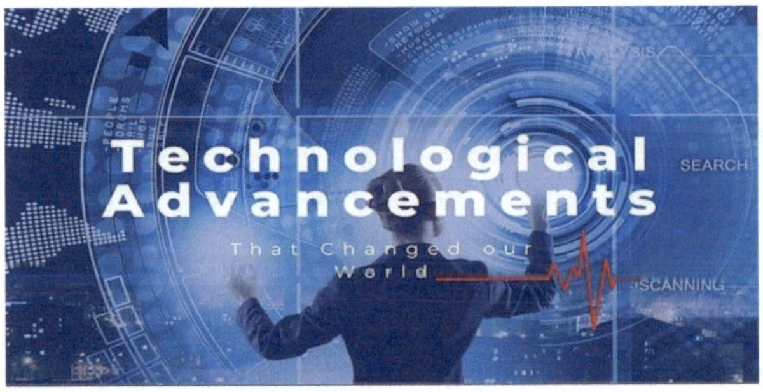

Figure 12.9. The landscape of technological advancements.

Source: https://external-content.duckduckgo.com/iu/?u=https%3A%2F%2Fwww.hindustanbusiness.in%2Fwp-content%2Fuploads%2F2024%2F07%2Ftechnological-advance_11zon-1.jpg&f=1&nofb=1&ipt=e95869c17b89b1edb0d84a017a2b1dbbe8e50cbb656386e5b93e0c2533ac4949.

12.3.1. Digital Divide and Access to Technology

In the current era, the digital divide is a major barrier to equal access to technology and its benefits. The digital divide is not merely a lack of devices and internet connections but also broader socio-economic disparities that influence people's ability to engage with digital spaces effectively. Citizens of underprivileged communities also have access to the necessary resources limited, and this further exacerbates the issues with education, healthcare, and employment opportunities. Telecommunication technologies have been developing rapidly, and they might be able to improve urban management systems, resulting in better living standards, but without bridging the digital divide, many remain excluded from such development. To bridge this gap, it is a collective effort to construct infrastructure that is inclusive and empowering for marginalized sections of society, enhancing their 21st-century quality of life (Yigitcanlar et al., 2009). In addition, technology-based interventions have become progressively significant tools in promoting equity, particularly in addressing vulnerable sections. For instance, technologies like mobile apps and networked sensors can enable access and communication for individuals who are consistently excluded by existing systems. However, for those whose challenges exist, they need attention to ethical conventions, to privacy concerns, and to inclusive design. Merging advanced data analytics, robots, and other emerging technologies could effectively address equity and access issues. Implemented correctly, they can empower individuals and households, shifting their experience, enhancing community resilience, and ultimately leading to a more inclusive online space (Apesoa-Varano et al., 2020). As we navigate today's digital divide, our future directions should focus on developing systems that not only address access but also the competencies for effective technology use. The focus needs to be on human-centered design, where solutions are made accessible and applicable to all socio-economic groups of people. Theoretical models need to highlight the convergence of technology, policy, and community engagement to build systems that give everyone access to the digital world. As society goes ahead, researchers and policymakers need to keep focus on activities that enhance the availability of meaningful technology, thereby developing a digital space that serves everyone equally. By identifying and conquering the barriers that continue to expand the digital divide, we can build a better future in a more integrated world (Apesoa-Varano et al., 2020).

12.3.2. Cybersecurity Threats and Responses

The rapid evolution of technology has led to a tremendous increase in the frequency and complexity of cybersecurity threats. Cybercriminals are exploiting advanced methods, such as artificial intelligence and machine learning, to execute advanced attacks ranging from ransomware to phishing. As highlighted in recent studies, integrating AI into cybersecurity tools can significantly enhance threat detection, enabling businesses to respond to breaches in real time (Oduri et al., 2022). However, this technological upgrade is accompanied by new challenges. For instance, the same technology used to combat cyber-attacks can be used by malicious actors to craft even more sophisticated attacks. Consequently, companies must remain vigilant and nimble, regularly updating their cybersecurity measures to stay ahead of evolving threats and vulnerabilities in their operations. This is a dynamic environment that demands continuous monitoring across research, funding, and learning in cybersecurity as part of a comprehensive strategy. The behavior of individual users has also become a crucial factor in the effectiveness of security measures, underscoring that technology alone is insufficient to protect against threats. Despite advances in defensive technologies, the human user remains the weakest link in cybersecurity due to behavioral factors such as complacency and ignorance. Studies have shown that active cybersecurity behavior (CSB) is associated with greater cybersecurity awareness, and individuals with high self-efficacy tend to adopt safer online behaviors (Conetta et al., 2019). Therefore, organizations must not only defend against technology threats but also establish a cybersecurity awareness culture among users. Proper implementation of targeted training programs that build users' knowledge and cybersecurity behaviors can significantly reduce risks. By tapping the human element of cybersecurity, companies can strengthen their security position and create a stronger defense against future attacks. To meet these emerging challenges, the future of cybersecurity needs to be multi-threaded with a synergy of technological advancement and human-influenced methods. With the ongoing development of artificial intelligence, organizations must invest in developing sophisticated algorithms that can anticipate and respond to cyberattacks before they occur (Oduri et al., 2022). Concurrently, education and training must also be improved to enable employees to detect and respond to cyber threats effectively. A harmony between technological progress and human empathy is needed to create a robust cybersecurity infrastructure. Additionally, ongoing research into the psychological aspect of cybersecurity behavior can help improve user engagement and compliance. With increasingly sophisticated cyber threats, an engaged and participatory mode that combines both cutting-edge technology and behavioral understanding will be crucial to address existing challenges as well as deciding future directions in the field of cybersecurity (Figure 12.10).

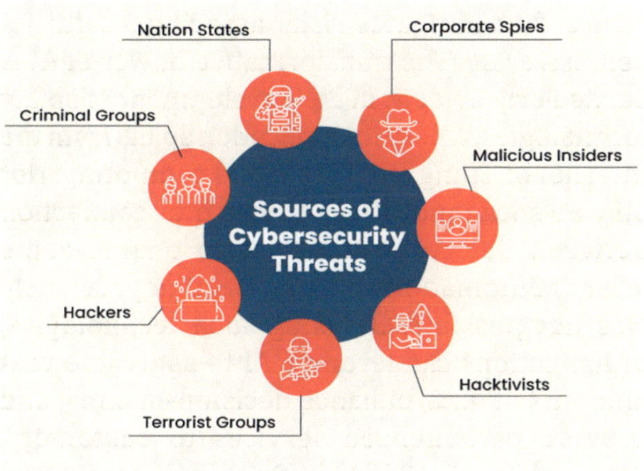

Figure 12.10. Cybersecurity threats and responses in health.

Source: https://external-content.duckduckgo.com/iu/?u=https%3A%2F%2Fwww.stealthlabs.com%2Fwp-content%2Fuploads%2F2020%2F12%2Fsources-of-cybersecurity-threats.jpg&f=1&nofb=1&ipt=f2c30e31d2aacaa45d7da949b6485c11ae406f874c8581b065f21da178c30d0d.

12.3.3. The Role of Artificial Intelligence (AI) in Society

The implementation of AI in various sectors of society is revolutionizing the manner in which we approach complex problems and enhancing the efficiency of our operations. In an effort to remain competitive in a more digitalized market economy, businesses have discovered that AI is an essential tool for data-driven decision-making. It enables firms to automate redundant tasks and handle massive amounts of data, thereby increasing efficiency and productivity. But while the potential benefits are enormous, so too are the potential pitfalls, such as data privacy, algorithmic bias, and ethical considerations in AI deployment. A thorough understanding of these concerns will be vital to developing accountable AI technologies that align with social norms and expectations. Organizations must navigate these complexities to harness AI's potential while ensuring trust and reliability in its implementation, shaping a future that mitigates risks associated with its pervasive use. The transformative power of AI is particularly evident in the development of smart technologies, where its application spans from the Internet of Things (IoT) to cloud computing. Not only do such innovations enable interconnection between devices, but they also enable some level of automation and analysis that previously was not possible. By using such technologies, organizations can leverage AI to aggregate vast amounts of data, enhance decision-making, and provide personalized services to customers. Alansari et al. (2021) affirm that combining AI with emerging technologies promises greater scalability and reliability, which is crucial in addressing the social challenges of the day. However, such developments do come with limitations, as scalability and reliability remain primary concerns. Hence, there is a need for endless research and innovation to overcome these issues and actualize AI's true potential in enhancing the well-being of society. With ongoing advancements in AI, industries are becoming increasingly aware of its potential, albeit with intimidating issues. The landscape of the digital economy is changing, and businesses will have to adapt to how AI influences market forces and consumer demand. Being aware of and taking advantage of these changes will be crucial to maintaining a competitive edge in the future. As explained by Badr et al. (2024), AI is not merely an automation technology but a paradigm shift that requires a rethink of current business models and strategies. The implications for society are not confined to firms alone, as AI-driven change impacts labor markets and broader economic systems. It compels stakeholders to confront ethics frameworks and governance approaches that make AI technologies available on fair terms, thereby developing a participatory society that maximizes the benefits of AI and minimizes the risk of social disruption (Figure 12.11).

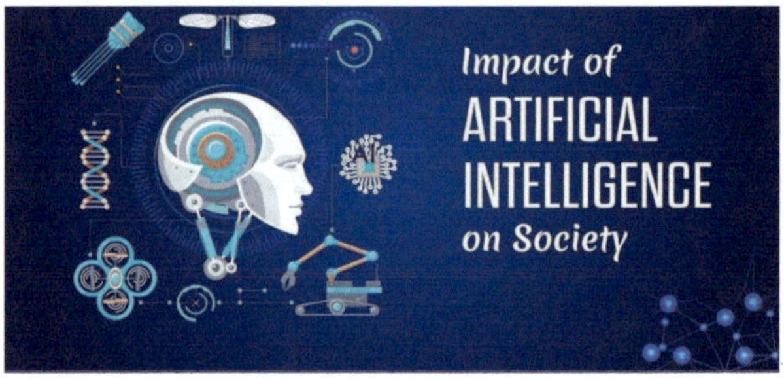

Figure 12.11. The role of artificial intelligence in society.

Source: https://external-content.duckduckgo.com/iu/?u=https%3A%2F%2Fdigitalzoneblog.com%2Fwp-content%2Fuploads%2F2024%2F04%2F0_vmPwP8-l5xTokf3S-1024x482.jpg&f=1&nofb=1&ipt=0da415d98674dbd2ada7cde72a4cf19d3c2d8e4c65ba973d8909b2e809f8df3f.

Test Your Knowledge

1. What recent technological advancements have improved the study and analysis of skeletal remains in osteology?
2. How have tools like 3D imaging, CT scans, and data analysis software enhanced osteological research?

12.4. Social and Cultural Challenges

Learning Outcome

1. Racial and ethnic tensions
2. Gender equality and women's rights
3. Mental health awareness and stigma

With a globalized world, social and cultural problems are enormous barriers to public health and well-being. Social problems such as discrimination, social inequality, and cultural dissonance adversely affect collective health outcomes by exacerbating variations in resources and service use. For instance, marginalized groups receive less access to proper healthcare, which in turn influences their ability to provide preventive care and manage chronic disease. The Shanghai Declaration on Promoting Health in the 2030 Agenda for Sustainable Development calls for addressing these social determinants to promote greater health equity and thereby underscores the need for targeted public health interventions. Resolution of these problems requires an all-encompassing approach that not only acknowledges the socio-economic and political factors at play but also engages populations affected by them in developing health-promoting interventions that operate within their specific cultural environments (Kilibarda, 2024). Cultural beliefs and norms play a pivotal role in shaping health attitudes and actions, thereby adding another layer of complexity to the intricacy of tackling social problems. In most societies, modern health advice may differ from traditional practices, and resistance to public health interventions follows. An example is the stigma for mental illness, which prevents individuals from accessing available care, and it creates a cycle of neglect and deteriorating health outcomes. Effective health promotion interventions should, as such, incorporate culturally competent approaches that respect and are sensitive to local beliefs, so that available interventions become relevant and acceptable. Behavioral science methods can be highly valuable for addressing these cultural context challenges, enabling the use of contextualized interventions that are effective at promoting community and individual health and are informed by culture (Kilibarda, 2024). In addition, as countries grapple with ongoing global issues such as climate change and economic disparities, efforts to address these social and cultural challenges are more crucial than ever. The rise of environmental justice social movements reflects greater awareness of the connections among health, social justice, and cultural values. In such a scenario, enhanced intersectoral cooperation is warranted, with Health in All Policies facilitating comprehensive public health strategies that integrate social determinants of health across all sectors. While there are still obstacles, such as the currently weak intersectoral policy structures, there is strong pressure towards equitable, sustainable innovations and people's participation in decision-making. Social mobilization can promote health promotion programs that not only meet the short-term needs of communities but also create resources for sustainable futures.

12.4.1. Racial and Ethnic Tensions

Racial and ethnic tensions are still the major issue facing society today, affecting all aspects, such as education and health. In schools, conflict on the grounds of race has been documented extensively, with data indicating an appalling climate that affects both the academic and social atmosphere for students. Incidents such as the Jena 6 and school-wide uprisings demonstrate the harsh reality of these tensions, which affect not only the parties directly involved, but also the larger school community, including administrators and staff. How school administrators choose to act in these conflicts is crucial to learn about. Still lacking is comprehensive research that delves into this decision-making process, emphasizing the need for school practitioners to be equipped with strategies for managing and resolving racial tensions in schools, as underscored in model studies (Martinez et al., 2010).

Beyond the problems in schools, racial and ethnic tensions at healthcare are an expression of greater societal issues of access and inequality. The intersection of race, culture, and socio-economic status strongly shapes individuals' perceptions and interactions with health resources. It has been demonstrated through qualitative research that marginal communities, particularly poorer African American women, encounter significant difficulties when they seek healthcare information. These difficulties often stem from historical distrust of the healthcare system and from issues with access to technology, such as the internet. Participants in studies have established that, despite these barriers, the internet is a viable solution for accessing valuable health information, thereby enabling patients to make more effective healthcare choices (Ahluwalia et al., 2012).

Removing such barriers and identifying them are significant steps toward making equity in health outcomes a reality. To move toward an answer to these lingering racial and ethnic tensions in the future, it is crucial to develop spaces that cherish inclusion and dialogue. Schools must provide structures that promote students' discussion of race, conflict resolution, and community building. Concomitantly, healthcare professionals need to prioritize cultural competence in practice, having all patients feel revered and understood. By implementing education interventions and training that address diverse population needs, barriers can be reduced and trust can be restored in the long run. The hour is there to collaborate to create a common strategy that bridges the gaps encountered in educational and healthcare settings towards a more equitable society where racial and ethnic tensions are recognized and explicitly treated (Figure 12.12).

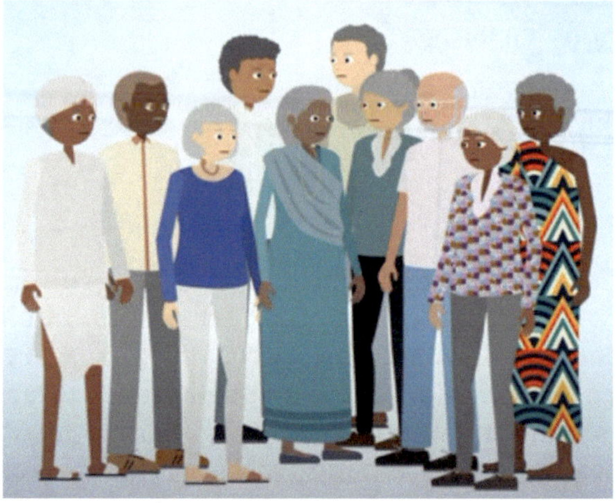

Figure 12.12. Racial and ethnic tensions continue to pose significant challenges in contemporary society.

Source: https://raceequalityfoundation.org.uk/wp-content/uploads/2023/02/recism-in-health-inequality.png.

12.4.2. Gender Equality and Women's Rights

The achievement of gender equality and women's rights has been met with numerous challenges across the world, many of which have been heightened by socio-economic factors as well as societal culture. Conventional gender roles remain major impediments to women's complete integration into the public as well as private domains, resulting in ongoing gaps in employment, education, and political participation. Activism around these issues has evolved, particularly with the advent of terminologies such as menstrual equity that illustrate more abstract concepts of gender justice. As the collaborative effort in menstrual equity activism has outlined, recognition of the webs of complications woven into gender rights that need an intersectional approach embracing the multidimensional experiences of women across contexts is growing. These analyses underscore the need for sustained legal reforms that not only enhance women's rights but also address the structural inequalities fueling gender discrimination (Crawford et al., 2020). The economic landscape under which women's rights organizations operate has also become increasingly precarious, underscoring a pressing dilemma in sustaining effective advocacy. According to the Association for Women's Rights in Development (AWID), funding for work on women's rights has experienced extreme dips and rises, making it increasingly difficult for organizations to sustain their trajectories. A recent survey of over 1,100 organizations reveals an acute need for a feminist collective resource mobilization strategy to address these changing times. Resources need to be strategically directed to ensure the programmes designed to counteract gender disparity and women's rights are sustainable. It becomes clear that there is a need for targeted funding, as it not only reflects the significance of the efforts but also the broader implications for social development toward gender justice (Arutyunova et al., 2013). In the future, the path to gender equality and women's rights will rely on cooperation, innovative advocacy, and comprehensive policy reform. Policymakers, activists, and scholars must join forces to create a broad-based movement that promotes grassroots mobilization and global agendas. The discourse around menstrual equity is a pertinent example of how intersectional perspectives can deepen gender justice scholarship. By broadening the discourse to include diverse voices, the movement can address the issues at hand for different groups of women. Lastly, witnessing a world where gender justice is realized is not only recognizing the accomplishments and failures of previous attempts but creating actionable pathways that will lead to tangible alterations in the future ahead, ensuring the progress achieved becomes lasting and inclusive (Crawford et al., 2020).

12.4.3. Mental Health Awareness and Stigma

The mental health knowledge environment is double-edged: increasing public understanding paired with combat against stigma simultaneously. Despite education and outreach advances regarding mental health illness, population misconceptions continue to exist, thereby generating hesitance in individuals to seek treatment. Mental health stigma may deter afflicted individuals from seeking necessary assistance and, accordingly, exacerbate their conditions. Efforts such as the research conducted by The Centre for Men's Health highlight the need for a social marketing approach to tackle these myths. With their focus on destigmatizing narratives and providing information about available resources, efforts such as these aim to reshape public opinion and encourage individuals—particularly young men aged 16-35 years—to seek help without stigma (Braybrook et al., 2012).

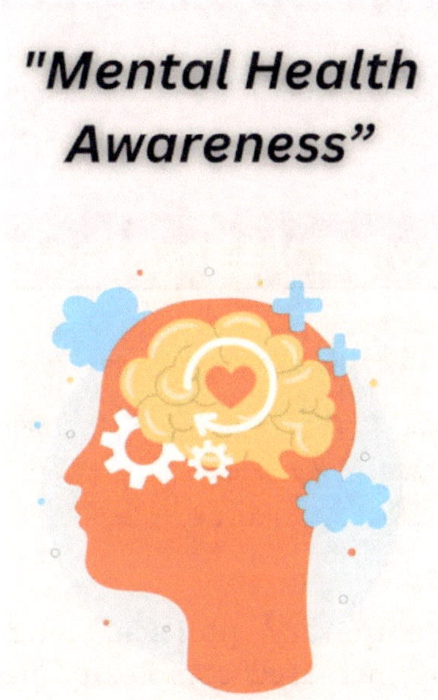

Figure 12.13. The landscape of mental health awareness illustrates a dual challenge.

Source: https://m.media-amazon.com/images/I/61JnmL2uaUL._UF1000,1000_QL80_.jpg.

Furthermore, the gender dynamics of mental illness complicate the dialogue about stigma. It has been found that boys and men have their specific barriers to accessing mental health problems, including societal norms of masculinity that exclude them from being vulnerable. This is more pronounced in the context of sexual abuse and exploitation, when boys can be further stigmatized by shame and confusion regarding their experiences (Barker et al., 2012). This in-built stigma not only deters them from institutional help-seeking behavior but also generates the silence around male mental illness. To address future plans for mental health awareness, the complex dynamics must be tackled to incorporate them in a manner that is inclusive and sensitive to the unique issues of various groups. As plans for awareness programs shift, the focus should shift towards solutions that promote inclusiveness and social sensitization. Community participation in community mental health initiatives helps make them more effective and community relevant. For instance, allowing local communities to express their concerns and needs ensures that strategies are created that effectively suit their needs. Closing the gap between services and service users makes activities create an enabling climate that reduces stigma. It is through comprehensive and adaptable strategies that mental health education can be disseminated, cultivating knowledge and dissolving barriers to care. Successful implementation of these steps could pave the way for future directions, positioning mental health as an integral part of overall wellness, making it possible for individuals to thrive without fear of stigma (Braybrook et al., 2012) (Figure 12.13).

Test Your Knowledge

1. What social and cultural challenges can researchers face when studying human skeletal remains?
2. How do cultural beliefs and community perspectives influence osteological research and its ethical practices?

12.5. Political Landscape

Learning Outcome

1. Polarization and its effects on governance
2. Globalization and national sovereignty
3. The rise of populism and its implications

The contemporary political landscape is marked by increased complexity, particularly as it overlaps with prominent environmental and social issues. It has been noted that the evolution of political ecology has significantly helped us understand power dynamics in resource management, particularly in the American West. The area has long grappled with socio-environmental conflicts arising from contests over land use, identity, and control. The revitalized attention to political ecology in recent decades has expanded its scope, with fresh visions and ideas joining the battle. Energy development and climate change challenges now face entrenched governance structures, calling for an overarching strategy that can effectively respond to these interconnected issues. Such a question is important in that it seeks collaborative constructs that move past stark environment-society dualisms, instead uncovering interdependent consequences for resource stewardship and community engagement (Bergmann et al., 2019). As stakeholder communities encounter the complexity of a governance regime characterized by competing interests, landscape stewardship becomes an appealing vector for cooperative engagement. The development of social-ecological approaches emphasizes the need for multistakeholder partnerships to address the complexity of multifunctional landscapes. These environments typically feature diverse social priorities, economic constraints, and ecological considerations, making it challenging to combine them into effective governance. Indications are that successful collaboration is contingent on a variety of variables—contextual, institutional, social-relational, individual, and political-historical. This complex approach prioritizes the value of acknowledgment of historical legacies and existing power dynamics in a bid to establish strong governance systems that are long-term, equitable, and sustainable (Cokburn et al., 2019). The political issues intensify when the trajectory of future collaboration and governance is considered. An imperative is necessary to analyze innovative methods that foster social cohesion and collective potential, particularly in environments with many interests and significant contestation. A bottom-up approach grounded in pluralism and relational enablers presents a valuable path to achieving effective stewardship. By developing interpersonal connections and facilitating small-scale collective action, constituents can work together on common objectives, representing an array of perspectives. Ultimately, the way forward to a more equitable political setting relies on the concerted efforts of diverse actors willing to defy conventional governance patterns and endure the obstacles of changing environmental and social realities. Such an ongoing debate is necessary in a bid to counter obstacles that may lie ahead and advance toward more sustainable futures (Cokburn et al., 2019).

12.5.1. Polarization and Its Effects on Governance

Polarization also significantly impacts governance, as it tints political discourse toward extremes rather than open dialogue. Political extremism is likely to override attempts to build consensus in the current political environment, making it harder for policymakers to effectively address complex problems. Polarization discourages cooperation because representatives are more interested in partisan wins than in addressing their constituents' material interests. The resulting legislative gridlock hinders action on critical matters like climate change, health care, and economic equity, generating an atmosphere of disillusionment among the electorate. The effects are endemic, eroding popular faith in the government and feeding cycles of dissatisfaction, requiring an understanding of the processes driving polarization in contemporary governance. The effects of polarization extend beyond legislative gridlock, as they directly shape public perceptions of governance institutions. The more deeply citizens are entrenched in their partisanship, the more likely they are to view government agencies and policies with suspicion. This sets up an endless cycle in which citizens withdraw from civic activities, intensifying polarization even further. Furthermore, as expounded in the articulation of environmental governance challenges, agents responsible for governing public resources are likely to be working in the turbulent waters of political scandal and widespread frustration. This introduces blindness or illegibility to the actualities they face, limiting their capacity to engage with stakeholders and eroding the overall performance of governance systems (Martin et al., 2020). Since the scandal around policies like trade agreements makes clear, political division constrains policymakers' abilities to collaborate in an increasingly polarized environment. The latest reports on the Transatlantic Trade and Investment Partnership (TTIP) reveal that trade negotiations have become extremely politicized, microcosms of the broader polarization debate. The issues with TTIP reveal how the politicization of trade not only complicates negotiations but also puts in sharp relief the necessity of governance in handling public opinion and in exercising accountability within policymaking (Gheyle et al., 2016). Understanding of these dynamics will be of utmost significance to scholars and practitioners in today's world as they operate at the intersection of societal contestation and policy-based governance over the coming years (Figure 12.14).

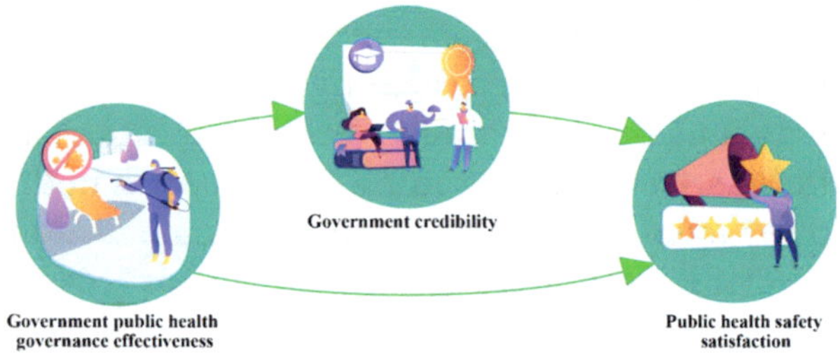

Figure 12.14. Polarization and its effects on governance in health.

Source: https://pub.mdpi-res.com/ijerph/ijerph-20-03286/article_deploy/html/images/ijerph-20-03286-g001.png?1676293790.

12.5.2. Globalization and National Sovereignty

As globalization persistently reshapes the configuration of global interaction, national sovereignty remains a controversial topic at the heart of policy debates. The meaning of sovereignty—the monopoly of power—remains central to how states engage with international norms, laws, and institutions. Yet, leaders will typically invoke sovereignty as a rhetorical device in order to shield against such discussions of changing global governance dynamics. Not only does this mask the complexities involved with globalization, but it can also prevent effective policymaking. To overcome these challenges, there is an imperative for a sophisticated conceptualization of sovereignty beyond conventional interpretations that affirms the complex dynamics between local authority and global interdependence. Critical analysis of the dominant paradigms thus becomes essential, as it can illuminate other avenues for policymakers to pursue amid the impact of globalization on national governments (Jackson et al., 2003). Formation of transnational networks and associations has also complicated the concept of national sovereignty. As nations increasingly cooperate across various global levels, such as through commercial agreements and multinational configurations, the constraints on unipolar decision-making intensify. This has created a new day in which sovereignty is possible only through awareness of the supranational forces that overshadow national interests. The core feature here is the legitimacy that such transnational networks, such as the European Union, impose on member states. The concept of decentration arises, challenging the notion that centralization necessarily leads to greater legitimacy and effectiveness in governance. Instead, the contradiction between democratic participation and legal-social proper access must be rethought as countries move into an international system that requires coordinated action in tackling universal challenges (Aliu et al., 2013). Essentially, dealing with the intersection of globalization and sovereignty is one of the most significant challenges policymakers today confront. States must recognize that, in a more interdependent world, maintaining sovereignty does not equate to isolationism. Instead, it calls for innovative approaches that prioritize cooperation without sacrificing core national interests. As international realities shift, countries can no longer dogmatically cling to old expressions of sovereignty. Entering into multilateral discussions and reshaping policy goals is essential to benefiting from the dividends of globalization without betraying the values of sovereignty. The following steps involve a commitment to constructing solid policy frameworks that address not only the short-run effects of globalization but also consider its long-run effects on national regulation, producing a viable path forward that balances these two often conflicting trends (Jackson et al., 2003; Aliu et al., 2013).

12.5.3. The Rise of Populism and Its Implications

The trend of populism in recent years has been at the forefront of reshuffling political landscapes globally. Populism is characterized by a populist discourse that defends the people's cause against corrupt elites. Populism has found traction based on a combination of socio-economic factors, ranging from economic inequality, loss of confidence in traditional political powers, to the decline of media monopolies. Though populist leaders employ discontent to rally their supporters, they reduce complex issues into a simple choice between two extremes, often stereotyping opponents as the public's adversaries. The simplification approach might diminish democratic discourse and mask policy complexities, leading to political debate that becomes sensationalized. Besides, the shift towards populism signals more profound social cleavages and suggests the inadequacy of prevailing political systems in meeting the diverse needs of modern electorates. The impact of populism extends beyond the short-run electoral consequences; it has significant implications for socioeconomic policy and the institutions of governance. Populist movements tend to disturb welfare state models, calling for the re-prioritization of governmental competencies and resources. As welfare states struggle to catch up with the times of rising populism, they are faced with the challenge of reframing the private and public spaces of welfare provision. The shift in welfare policies is apt to reflect a renewed focus on national security and identity, evoking concerns of inclusivity and equity in social services. This shift will lead to a paradox in which populist policies vow to protect the vulnerable and simultaneously disenfranchise minorities. Examination of these trends will assist researchers in better understanding the impact of populism on domestic and global welfare systems, necessitating further studies on this new terrain (Clarke et al., 2008). Moreover, the populist wave consequences also intersect with practice research to reveal a need for enhanced practitioner-policymaker communication. As the Fourth International Conference on Practice Research controversies have argued, there is an imperative need for a more sufficient vocabulary to outline the practitioners' dilemma when engaged in research (Begum et al., 2017). This need points to the broader field in which populism is unfolding—one that requires not only a rethinking of practice within welfare regimes but also a richer investigation of how knowledge production and dissemination occur in an era of populism. As practitioners navigate this complex terrain, it falls on scholars and policymakers to encourage collaboration that brings empirical evidence into practice, thereby creating frameworks that are not just responsive to populist moods but also guided by robust research and inclusivity. The resolution of these issues will ultimately matter in preventing populism from deteriorating the fabric of democracy and social justice in the future.

Test Your Knowledge

1. How can political factors influence the study, access, and repatriation of human skeletal remains?
2. In what ways do government policies and international relations impact osteological research practices?

12.6. Education System

Learning Outcome

1. Access to quality education
2. The impact of online learning
3. Curriculum relevance in a changing world

The contemporary education system has been faced with an array of imperative issues that undermine its ability to prepare students for the complexities of an emerging world. The greatest challenge is the unequal access to education resources and opportunities between communities and regions. This inequity has implications for both students' performance as well as the development of communities at large. Closing these gaps requires a multi-faceted approach that includes financial reforms, increased access to technology, and the equitable distribution of talented teachers. These systemic inequalities fuel cycles of poverty and limit individuals' potential for advancement, necessitating swift action from policymakers, schools, and community partners to ensure every child has an equal opportunity for success. A collective approach with a focus on equitable resource distribution is critical for responding to the current context and creating an inclusive education system that is responsive to the heterogeneous needs of all learners. While education systems aim to innovate and evolve, they must also address the effects of integrating technology into learning spaces. The success of online and blended learning strategies has attracted attention, particularly amid the shifts introduced by the COVID-19 pandemic. Technology has the potential to increase educational access and participation, but also brings challenges of digital equity and learner support. According to results from discussions with California's stakeholders, policymakers, and the public, there is a large desire to reform K-12 education to enable districts to exercise more control and receive more funding to develop tailored solutions according to state standards. However, to make this shift successful, education leaders must concentrate not only on implementing technology but also on training teachers and establishing comprehensive support systems that cater to different learning styles. Looking ahead, the education system needs to embrace flexibility and resilience to effectively respond to current challenges and evolving societal needs. This means reassessing ancient curricula and teaching methods to ensure they remain relevant and engaging for students. Insights from observing Jewish education institutions underscore the imperative to value particular community settings and to build connections between programs and educational foundations. With the focus placed on the successes and failures of various schools, the stakeholders may refer to one another when establishing the best practices and strategic options that facilitate comprehensive learning experiences. The use of such community perspectives is critical to creating an education system that not only addresses current issues but also looks to the future, ensuring that students are adequately prepared for global dynamics in a transforming world.

12.6.1. Access to Quality Education

Access to adequate education is a widespread concern in society today, compounded by socioeconomic disparities and institutional barriers to access. While community colleges have become pivotal institutions in higher education, many students never reach their full potential due to inadequate support systems. With over 7-million-degree candidates at community colleges, there is an urgent need to address the high attrition rates and incomplete degrees for these groups. The American Association of Community Colleges (N/A, 2013) presented issues regarding unacceptably low student success and inadequate employment preparation, both tied directly to labor market demand. These statistics reveal the need for integrated reforms, not just enhancing institutional support but also developing a success-friendly culture accessible to all, particularly marginalized communities of students. Additionally, integrating community participation into education systems can significantly enhance and tailor quality education to effectiveness and relevance. By connecting classroom learning to real-world applications, institutions foster a more participatory and socially responsive student population. University-community partnership models have also held promise in bridging the gap between practice and theory, allowing students to find relevant connections applicable to their own communities. Such programs allow students to develop essential skills in teamwork, social interaction, and self-responsibility, thereby equipping them for academic and professional success (Rudd et al., 2006).

As institutions accept service-learning approaches and develop public-private partnerships, not only do they enrich their curriculum but also proactively respond to the needs of society, thereby making the relevance of education robust in an evolving world. Looking ahead, addressing the issue of access to high-quality education requires a multifaceted approach that encompasses innovative practices and collaborative leadership. School leaders must embrace potent, metamorphic practices that will be able to enhance student performance for students across all demographics effectively. By prioritizing inclusive policies and equal access to resources, institutions can overcome longstanding barriers that have cemented the position of underrepresented groups. Facilitating strong community relationships, along with ongoing assessment of the education strategy, can lead to sustained improvement in student learning and achievement. Lastly, through creating inclusive environments that promote responsiveness and equity, education leaders and policymakers can lay the groundwork for a more equitable and accessible education environment, vital to the advancement of society and individuals (Figure 12.15).

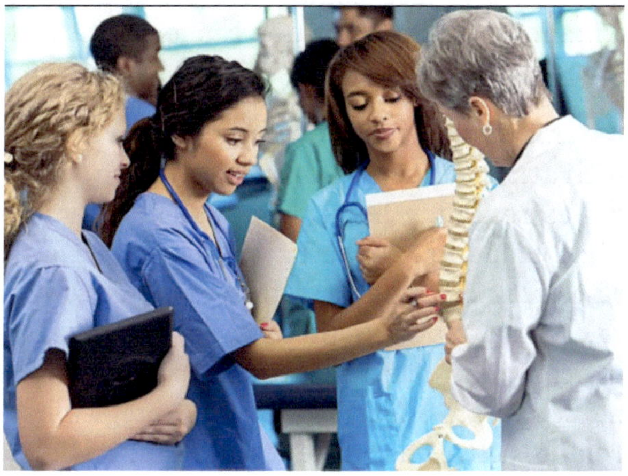

Figure 12.15. Access to quality education in health.

Source: https://etimg.etb2bimg.com/photo/107843846.cms.

12.6.2. The Impact of Online Learning

The mass adoption of online learning has revolutionized the landscape of education, offering never-before-seen levels of access to learning materials and possibilities. Encouraged by technological advancement, such as cloud computing, the online learning platform has evolved, enabling educational institutions to deliver content more effectively than ever. This transition has provided opportunities for students who would otherwise have been disadvantaged by geographical location or the absence of finances. The use of online learning, though, has not been without challenges. As institutions embrace online platforms, they must grapple with the inequality in technology access, which exacerbates existing disadvantages among students. Teachers and policymakers must be aware of these difficulties so that online learning can realize its promise of inclusiveness and fair access to education in the future. In addition to access issues, the rise of online learning poses particular challenges for learner engagement and retention. Unlike conventional classrooms, where face-to-face contact fosters a sense of community, online education can leave students feeling isolated.

This sort of isolation can dampen student motivation and performance, with some studies revealing higher dropout rates among online students compared to their on-campus counterparts. To address this issue, educators are turning to new methods to enhance student participation, including interactive technologies and cooperative learning. Such strategies both promote active engagement and foster an online learning community that is supportive in its construction. Through an understanding of the interactivity of online engagement, teachers are better able to tailor their approaches to meet the diverse demands of their learners, thus optimizing performance in the online learning environment. Moreover, the expansion of e-learning has ushered in a new information age of unprecedented proportions, underscoring the importance of digital literacy in a technology-driven world. Students today have access to a plethora of information sources and can be empowered and overwhelmed in the process. Misinformation poses particular problems since students may find it difficult to distinguish between credible and untrustworthy sources. As quoted in literature, disinformation erodes people's ability to make informed decisions and influences decision-making in various fields like politics and health (Alani et al., 2018). It is thus imperative that teachers not only teach the curriculum but also equip students with critical thinking abilities necessary for survival in the digital era. By cultivating these skills, schools can prepare students to thrive in a more complex global world and reap the full benefits of e-learning.

12.6.3. Curriculum Relevance in a Changing World

In the contemporary learning environment, the dynamic interplay between the relevance of curriculum and the evolving demands of an ever-changing environment has become the prevailing topic of discussion. With emerging changes in industries due to technology and globalization forces, schools and other educational institutions must adapt the curriculum to equip students to deal with challenges they will face in the job market. Such a change is especially evident in logistics and supply chain management, where a clear need exists for programs aligned with emerging trends and practices. This change can be promoted by close collaboration between academia and industry, allowing instructors to align educational content to fit employer requirements and skills of the labor market, as highlighted by the review of literature on teaching in logistics (Farris et al., 2008).

Moreover, curricula must also keep pace with broader social and cultural transformations, such as the need for diversity and inclusivity within learning spaces. Institutions need to design curricula that equip students with technical know-how, critical thinking, ethical judgment, and intercultural competence. Such a convergent approach to learning is all the more pertinent as globalization promotes maximum interaction among various segments of the population. Hence, the curriculum needs to address the needs of a globalized economy. By fostering a curriculum that embraces these values, educational institutions play a crucial role in shaping responsible citizens prepared to contribute meaningfully to society (President\u27s Office, 2007). Lastly, maintaining curriculum relevance in a changing world requires ongoing assessment and a willingness to adapt. Educational institutions should prioritize continuous evaluation and improvement frameworks, ensuring that content remains impactful and relevant in light of new developments. The integration of technology in teaching styles, for instance, has revolutionized access to information as well as learning processes. As a result, teachers must use data-driven insights and feedback loops to efficiently optimize teaching strategies and curricular content. Such foresight adjustments will not only render students more interactive and productive, but also position institutions as responsive to the evolving landscape of higher education and labor markets (Farris et al., 2008).

Test Your Knowledge

1. How does the education system contribute to training professionals in osteology and related fields?
2. What are the key challenges and opportunities in osteology education for students and researchers?

SUMMARY

Reflecting on the challenges currently being experienced across industries, it is clear that a thorough understanding of these challenges is vital for shaping future directions. The mismatch between increasing demand for organic produce and local capacity to produce elucidates the intricacy of farming practices in the current age. Notably, UK farmers are still navigating how to meet demand for adequate organic cereals, with the majority of their supplies coming from imports to sustain consumers' expectations. Overcoming this deficit requires careful examination of the implications of switching to organic production systems on pest and disease trends, as indicated in the publication of Anon (2001). Switching is not only a challenge but also presents a chance to establish new agricultural practice methods that are capable of leading to sustainability and resilience in food systems. Moreover, the challenges encountered in applying metabolomics to clinical research highlight the intricate nature of developing scientific strategies. The reliance on various resources for metabolic phenotyping has created logistical barriers that undermine the internal validity of the research results. As defined in Kang et al. (2020), end-to-end systems integrating quality assurance protocols and machine learning features are critical for overcoming such constraints. By developing robust protocols and workflows, researchers can improve the reliability and transferability of outcomes, thereby enabling the translation of metabolomics into practical healthcare interventions. These innovations are pivotal in redesigning the clinical research landscape and making scientific innovation accountable to the pressing needs of today's health challenges. Last but not least, where converging challenges meet future directions is the calling for cross-disciplinary solutions to address complex problems across sectors. The farming and medical sectors are at a turning point, with the potential to spearhead innovations that enhance productivity and health outcomes. By encouraging collective work among stakeholders, embracing technological innovations, and raising the level of research aimed at addressing current gaps, a revolutionary path can be achieved. Organic agriculture practices and metabolomic analyses indicate the spectacular impact of strategic planning and adaptability in addressing uncertainty. Therefore, synthesizing lessons from Anon (2001) and Kang et al. (2020) for future work will be crucial to developing adaptive systems that can address society's changing demands.

One of the most critical issues in addressing global food security is the need for a collective effort to move beyond traditional silos. Food scientists need to collaborate with agricultural specialists, nutritionists, and policymakers to develop integrated solutions that build sustainable capacity to feed an increasingly large population. Contemporary food sustainability discourses are primarily focused on agricultural production, with critical areas such as food processing neglected as an important connecting link between raw material farming and the processing of these materials into edible products. Augustin et al. (2020) posit that, in the absence of greater attention to food processing, aspirations to deliver sustainable diets are unlikely to be achieved. This highlights the requirement for a cross-disciplinary solution that encompasses varied indicators of sustainability and impact analysis, culminating in well-informed strategies for future food supply challenges. Federated Edge deployment management and networking are another key challenge that will have to be tackled in the future. With advances in technology, the concept of an Edge-based fabric spanning multiple geographic locations presents opportunities and challenges for decentralizing computation from data centers. The process is currently hindered by a myriad of technical challenges, intertwined with socio-legal and geopolitical hurdles. As highlighted by Baktir et al. (2018), effective management and communication principles are key to addressing the gaps. An accurate understanding of modeling and resource allocation will be essential to creating a good template for implementing Edge technology in many different situations. Addressing these challenges will not only result in enhanced operations but it will also enable a more flexible means of addressing and processing data at a global scale. Examining the food system's sustainability reveals the cumulative issues that must be addressed to improve the world's nutrition and food security. Perhaps the most challenging is the lack of synergy in food production, processing, and consumption behaviors, which most frequently manifests inefficiency and wastage. Furthermore, the sustainability definition is usually uncoupled from economic realities, so stakeholders remain unwilling to invest in sustainability. The reliance on traditional farming practices, coupled with the absence of proper innovation in the field of food technology, exacerbates such issues. In light of the data reported by Augustin et al. (2020), the development of actionable steps to establish economic incentives for sustainable practices is significant. Fostering an environment that facilitates interdisciplinary collaboration will ultimately create improved solutions, making sure that food systems are resilient when faced with emerging challenges.

KEY TERMS FROM THIS CHAPTER

- Additive manufacturing (AM)
- Brain-computer interfaces (BCIs)
- Collaboration
- Communication
- complexities
- Dementia
- Environmental consciousness
- Financial challenges
- Geopolitical
- Healthcare
- Human societal
- Insufficient
- Non-pharmacological treatments (NPTs)
- Proactive management
- Public education
- Rehabilitation
- Scholarship of Teaching and Learning (SOTL)
- Social sciences

CRITICAL THINKING QUESTIONS

1. **Which of the following is a major ethical concern in osteological research today?**
   a. Accurate measurements
   b. Repatriation of human remains
   c. Use of new technologies
   d. Preservation of artifacts
2. **A significant challenge in forensic osteology is:**
   a. DNA extraction from fresh tissue
   b. Bone aging in children
   c. Accurate identification from fragmentary remains
   d. Preserving ancient manuscripts
3. **Which technology is increasingly used to analyze bone microstructure in non-destructive ways?**
   a. MRI
   b. CT Scanning
   c. Sonography
   d. UV Spectroscopy
4. **What is one future direction in osteology to increase accessibility and collaboration?**
   a. Isotope analysis
   b. Bone boiling
   c. 3D scanning and digital databases
   d. Taxonomic classification
5. **Which of the following is a current challenge in global osteological collections?**
   a. Overuse of imaging tools
   b. Lack of educational interest
   c. Limited access and decolonization issues
   d. Excess funding

Short Answer Questions

1. What are some ethical concerns associated with the study of human skeletal remains in contemporary osteology?
2. How has digital imaging technology transformed modern osteological analysis?
3. Explain the importance of repatriation in osteological research.
4. How can artificial intelligence (AI) and machine learning contribute to future osteological studies?
5. What does the term "decolonizing osteology" mean, and why is it significant today?
6. Why is interdisciplinary collaboration important in modern osteological research?
7. Describe one example of how 3D scanning is used in skeletal analysis.
8. Discuss the challenge of standardizing methodologies in global osteological research.
9. Explain how forensic osteology is adapting to mass disaster and conflict scenarios.
10. What future directions could improve ethical practices in osteological fieldwork and research?

Answers to Critical Thinking Questions

1. (b); 2. (c); 3. (b); 4. (c); 5. (c)

REFERENCES

1. Addison, T., Arndt, C., & Tarp, F. (2025). The triple crisis and the global aid architecture. https://core.ac.uk/download/pdf/6348662.pdf (accessed on 21st July 2025).
2. Adelman, H. S., & Taylor, L. (2018). Improving school improvement. https://core.ac.uk/download/286362371.pdf (accessed on 21st July 2025).
3. Adelman, H. S., & Taylor, L. L. (2018). Addressing barriers to learning: In the classroom and schoolwide. https://core.ac.uk/download/286362370.pdf (accessed on 21st July 2025).
4. Ahluwalia, J. S., Burgess, D., Hecht, M. L., Kvasny, L., et al. (2012). Barriers, control and identity in health information seeking among African American women. https://digitalscholarship.unlv.edu/cgi/viewcontent.cgi?article=1044&context=jhdrp (accessed on 21st July 2025).
5. Phillipson, J., Gorton, M., Turner, R., Shucksmith, M., Aitken-McDermott, K., Areal, F., Cowie, P., Hubbard, C., Maioli, S., McAreavey, R., Souza-Monteiro, D., Newbery, R., Panzone, L., Rowe, F., & Shortall, S. (2020). The COVID-19 pandemic and its implications for rural economies. *Sustainability*, *12*(10), 3973. https://doi.org/10.3390/su12103973Alani, H., & Fernandez, M. (2018). Online misinformation: Challenges and future directions. https://core.ac.uk/download/151394134.pdf (accessed on 21st July 2025).
6. Alansari, Z., Belgaum, M. R., Mansoor Alam, M., Mazliham, M. S., et al. (2021). Role of artificial intelligence in cloud computing, IoT and SDN: Reliability and scalability issues. https://core.ac.uk/download/389319023.pdf (accessed on 21st July 2025).
7. Aliu, A., & Aliu, D. (2013). Power of global transnational networks: Civilizing of world order. https://core.ac.uk/download/16213826.pdf (accessed on 21st July 2025).
8. Allison, B. Z., Dunne, S., Leeb, R., Nijholt, A., et al. (2012). Recent and upcoming BCI progress: Overview, analysis, and recommendations. https://core.ac.uk/download/pdf/11484486.pdf (accessed on 21st July 2025).
9. Anon. (2001). *Review on the Possible Interactions of Pests, Diseases & Weeds in Cereals Grown in Organic and Conventional Agriculture.* https://core.ac.uk/download/10923156.pdf (accessed on 21st July 2025).
10. Apesoa-Varano, E. C., Gladstone, C., Kim, K. K., Lindeman, D., et al. (2020). Technology and caregiving: Emerging interventions and directions for research. https://core.ac.uk/download/323070528.pdf (accessed on 21st July 2025).
11. Arond, E., Ely, A., Folke, C., Leach, M., et al. (2012). Transforming innovation for sustainability. https://core.ac.uk/download/9051809.pdf (accessed on 21st July 2025).
12. Arutyunova, A., & Clark, C. (2013). *Watering the Leaves, Starving the Roots.* https://core.ac.uk/download/75784937.pdf (accessed on 21st July 2025).
13. Augustin, M. A., Knorr, D., & Tiwari, B. (2020). Advancing the role of food processing for improved integration in sustainable food chains. https://core.ac.uk/download/322792504.pdf (accessed on 21st July 2025).
14. Badr, Y., Balungu, D. M., & Kumar, A. (2024). Transforming the digital economy through artificial intelligence: A review of current trends and future directions. https://elar.urfu.ru/bitstream/10995/137665/1/978-5-91256-667-7_2024_002.pdf (accessed on 21st July 2025).

15. Bahar-Fuchs, A., Brodaty, H., Cassidy-Eagle, E., Chételat, G., et al. (2020). Toward a theory-based specification of non-pharmacological treatments in aging and dementia: Focused reviews and methodological recommendations. https://core.ac.uk/download/360955448.pdf (accessed on 21st July 2025).

16. Baktir, C., Ersoy, C., Ozgovde, A., Sonmez, M., et al. (2018). Addressing the challenges in federating edge resources. http://arxiv.org/abs/1803.05255 (accessed on 21st July 2025).

17. Barišić, M., Brinkmann, H., Dierks, B., Ponattu, A., et al. (2017). *Inclusive Growth–An Agenda for Germany: Five Action Areas for a New Growth Strategy*. https://core.ac.uk/download/287647944.pdf (accessed on 21st July 2025).

18. Barker, G., & Pawlak, P. (2012). Hidden violence: Preventing and responding to sexual exploitation and sexual abuse of adolescent boys. https://core.ac.uk/download/71362142.pdf (accessed on 21st July 2025).

19. Bechara, G. H., Chagas, A. C. de S., Chorilli, M., Constantini, V., et al. (2025). Current tick control strategies and prospects for using nanotechnology as an efficient alternative. https://core.ac.uk/download/643634195.pdf (accessed on 21st July 2025).

20. Begum, R., Chin, C. S., Ciro, D., Fisher, C., et al. (2017). *ICPR2017–The Fourth International Conference on Practice Research: Overview*. https://core.ac.uk/download/132608371.pdf (accessed on 21st July 2025).

21. Bergmann, N., Epstein, K., Gosnell, H., Kroepsch, A., et al. (2019). Revisiting and revitalizing political ecology in the American West. https://core.ac.uk/download/305124848.pdf (accessed on 21st July 2025).

22. Braybrook, D., Robertson, S., & Robinson, M. (2012). Evaluation of the Choose Life North Lanarkshire Awareness Programmed: Final Report. https://core.ac.uk/download/29018946.pdf (accessed on 21st July 2025).

23. Buyya, R., & Varghese, B. (2017). Next generation cloud computing: New trends and research directions. https://core.ac.uk/download/96664300.pdf (accessed on 21st July 2025).

24. Chen, Y., & Ely, A. (2011). Health biotechnology innovation for social sustainability: A perspective from China. https://core.ac.uk/download/2731317.pdf (accessed on 21st July 2025).

25. Clarke, J. (2008). *Reconstructing Nation, State and Welfare: The Transformation of Welfare States*. https://core.ac.uk/download/2731318.pdf (accessed on 21st July 2025).

26. Cokburn, J., Cornelius, S. F. (Ancia), Cundill, G., Metcalfe, J., et al. (2019). Collaborative stewardship in multifunctional landscapes: Toward relational, pluralistic approaches. https://core.ac.uk/download/288641960.pdf (accessed on 21st July 2025).

27. Conetta, C. (2019). Individual differences in cyber security. https://core.ac.uk/download/215423371.pdf (accessed on 21st July 2025).

28. Crawford, B. J., Johnson, M. E., Karin, M. L., Strausfeld, C., et al. (2020). The ground on which we all stand: A conversation about menstrual equity law and activism. https://core.ac.uk/download/322808787.pdf (accessed on 21st July 2025).

29. Dehghanghadikolaei, A., Emamian, S. S., Fotovvati, B., Gisario, A., et al. (2019). The potential of additive manufacturing in the smart factory industrial 4.0: A review. https://core.ac.uk/download/231748826.pdf (accessed on 21st July 2025).

30. Ely, A., Stirling, A., & Van Zwanenberg, P. (2011). New models of technology assessment for development. https://core.ac.uk/download/2731319.pdf (accessed on 21st July 2025).

31. Farris, M. T., & Gravier, M. (2008). An analysis of logistics pedagogical literature: Past and future trends in curriculum, content, and pedagogy. https://core.ac.uk/download/56737709.pdf (accessed on 21st July 2025).

32. Gantwerk, H., Furth, I., & Rosell, S. A. (2008). Moving along the learning curve: From values to public judgment: Citizen dialogues on K-12 education reform. https://core.ac.uk/download/71353319.pdf (accessed on 21st July 2025).

33. Garry, T., & Harwood, T. (2019). Cyborgs as frontline service employees: A research agenda. https://core.ac.uk/download/228181962.pdf (accessed on 21st July 2025).

34. Gheyle, N. (2016). Trade policy with the lights on: Linking trade and politicization. https://core.ac.uk/download/55824356.pdf (accessed on 21st July 2025).

35. Hudson, P., & Hudson, S. (2006). Initiating community engagement for enhancing preservice teacher education. https://core.ac.uk/download/10876425.pdf (accessed on 21st July 2025).

36. International Labor Office. (2005). *Global Employment Trends: Brief, February 2005*. https://core.ac.uk/download/5129404.pdf (accessed on 21st July 2025).

37. Jackson, J. H. (2003). Sovereignty–modern: A new approach to an outdated concept. https://core.ac.uk/download/70373715.pdf (accessed on 21st July 2025).

38. Kamyab, H., Razmfarsa, A., & Talaie, A. (2024). Advancing environmental engineering: The role of artificial intelligence in sustainable solutions–A short review. https://core.ac.uk/download/639366135.pdf (accessed on 21st July 2025).

39. Kang, Y. P., Kim, H. M., Kwon, S. W., Nghi, T., et al. (2020). Toward a standardized strategy of clinical metabolomics for the advancement of precision medicine. https://core.ac.uk/download/288117835.pdf (accessed on 21st July 2025).

40. Kilibarda, B. (2024). Global challenges and opportunities in health promotion. *Proceedings of the International Congress Public Health–Achievements and Challenges–zbornik radova*. https://www.semanticscholar.org/paper/bce0d1aea33eb6a60140ae55c6a164aab5840c49 (accessed on 21st July 2025).

41. Mackenzie, J., & Meyers, A. (2012). International collaboration in SoTL: Current status and future direction. https://core.ac.uk/download/229071351.pdf (accessed on 21st July 2025).

42. Martin, J. V. (2020). Between Scylla and Charybdis: Environmental governance and illegibility in the American West. https://core.ac.uk/download/305124793.pdf (accessed on 21st July 2025).

43. Martinez, M. J. (2010). Racial conflicts in schools. https://core.ac.uk/download/67748405.pdf (accessed on 21st July 2025).

44. Mazzucato, M. (2018). Mission-oriented innovation policies: Challenges and opportunities. *Industrial and Corporate Change, 27*, 803–815. https://doi.org/10.1093/icc/dty034 (accessed on 21st July 2025).

45. N/A. (2013). Crisis and opportunity: Aligning the community college presidency with student success. https://core.ac.uk/download/71362234.pdf (accessed on 21st July 2025).

46. Naumova, M. A. (2019). The impact of global challenges on the functioning of labor market.

https://core.ac.uk/download/201099370.pdf (accessed on 21st July 2025).

47. Navarro Ferronato, V., & Torretta, V. (2019). Waste mismanagement in developing countries: A review of global issues. *International Journal of Environmental Research and Public Health, 16*, 1060–1060. https://doi.org/10.3390/ijerph16061060 (accessed on 21st July 2025).
48. Oduri, S. (2022). The convergence of AI and cloud engineering for robust cybersecurity. https://core.ac.uk/download/654637285.pdf (accessed on 21st July 2025).
49. Orton, M., & Rowlingson, K. (2006). A problem of riches: Towards a new social policy research agenda on the distribution of economic resources. https://core.ac.uk/download/48843.pdf (accessed on 21st July 2025).
50. Paroutis, S., & Sammut-Bonnici, T. (2013). Developing a dominant logic of strategic innovation. https://core.ac.uk/download/17031009.pdf (accessed on 21st July 2025).
51. President's Office. (2007). *Strategic Directions for Gettysburg College, June 2007*. https://cupola.gettysburg.edu/cgi/viewcontent.cgi?article=1000&context=presoffice (accessed on 21st July 2025).
52. Rudd, C. J. (2006). Forging partnerships in health care: Process and measuring benefits. https://core.ac.uk/download/41533991.pdf (accessed on 21st July 2025).
53. Sales, A. L., Koren, A., Terry, J., Reimer, J., Saxe, L., Gribetz, M., & Samuel, N. (2006). *Mapping Jewish Education: The National Picture*. https://core.ac.uk/download/71352942.pdf (accessed on 21st July 2025).
54. Van Horn, C. E., King, C. T., & Smith, T. (2011). Identifying gaps and setting priorities for employment and training research. https://core.ac.uk/download/71345987.pdf (accessed on 21st July 2025).
55. Wu, A. S., & Hollander, C. D. (2025). The current state of normative agent-based systems. https://core.ac.uk/download/pdf/6560523.pdf (accessed on 21st July 2025).
56. Yigitcanlar, T. (2009). Managing ubiquitous eco cities: The role of urban telecommunication infrastructure networks and convergence technologies. https://core.ac.uk/download/10895362.pdf (accessed on 21st July 2025).

INDEX

C

D

E

M

N

O

P